Public Health Consequences of **E-Cigarettes**

Committee on the Review of the Health Effects of
Electronic Nicotine Delivery Systems

Kathleen Stratton, Leslie Y. Kwan, and David L. Eaton, *Editors*

Board on Population Health and Public Health Practice

Health and Medicine Division

A Consensus Study Report of

The National Academies of
SCIENCES · ENGINEERING · MEDICINE

THE NATIONAL ACADEMIES PRESS
Washington, DC
www.nap.edu

THE NATIONAL ACADEMIES PRESS **500 Fifth Street, NW** **Washington, DC 20001**

This activity was supported by Contract No. HHSF223201610054C between the National Academy of Sciences and the U.S. Department of Health and Human Services: Food and Drug Administration. Any opinions, findings, conclusions, or recommendations expressed in this publication do not necessarily reflect the views of any organization or agency that provided support for the project.

International Standard Book Number-13: 978-0-309-46834-3
International Standard Book Number-10: 0-309-46834-5
Digital Object Identifier: https://doi.org/10.17226/24952
Library of Congress Control Number: 2018932760

Additional copies of this publication are available for sale from the National Academies Press, 500 Fifth Street, NW, Keck 360, Washington, DC 20001; (800) 624-6242 or (202) 334-3313; http://www.nap.edu.

Printed in the United States of America

Suggested citation: National Academies of Sciences, Engineering, and Medicine. 2018. *Public health consequences of e-cigarettes*. Washington, DC: The National Academies Press. doi: https://doi.org/10.17226/24952.

The National Academies of

SCIENCES • ENGINEERING • MEDICINE

The **National Academy of Sciences** was established in 1863 by an Act of Congress, signed by President Lincoln, as a private, nongovernmental institution to advise the nation on issues related to science and technology. Members are elected by their peers for outstanding contributions to research. Dr. Marcia McNutt is president.

The **National Academy of Engineering** was established in 1964 under the charter of the National Academy of Sciences to bring the practices of engineering to advising the nation. Members are elected by their peers for extraordinary contributions to engineering. Dr. C. D. Mote, Jr., is president.

The **National Academy of Medicine** (formerly the Institute of Medicine) was established in 1970 under the charter of the National Academy of Sciences to advise the nation on medical and health issues. Members are elected by their peers for distinguished contributions to medicine and health. Dr. Victor J. Dzau is president.

The three Academies work together as the **National Academies of Sciences, Engineering, and Medicine** to provide independent, objective analysis and advice to the nation and conduct other activities to solve complex problems and inform public policy decisions. The National Academies also encourage education and research, recognize outstanding contributions to knowledge, and increase public understanding in matters of science, engineering, and medicine.

Learn more about the National Academies of Sciences, Engineering, and Medicine at **www.nationalacademies.org**.

The National Academies of

SCIENCES · ENGINEERING · MEDICINE

COMMITTEE ON THE REVIEW OF THE HEALTH EFFECTS OF ELECTRONIC NICOTINE DELIVERY SYSTEMS

DAVID L. EATON (*Chair*), Dean and Vice Provost, Graduate School, University of Washington

ANTHONY J. ALBERG, Professor and Chair, Department of Epidemiology and Biostatistics, Arnold School of Public Health, University of South Carolina

MACIEJ GONIEWICZ, Associate Professor of Oncology, Roswell Park Comprehensive Cancer Center

ADAM LEVENTHAL, Director, USC Health, Emotion, & Addiction Laboratory, Professor of Preventive Medicine and Psychology, USC Norris Comprehensive Cancer Center, Keck School of Medicine, University of Southern California

JOSÉ E. MANAUTOU, Professor of Pharmacology & Toxicology, Interim Head, Department of Pharmaceutical Sciences, University of Connecticut

SHARON McGRATH-MORROW, Professor, Department of Pediatrics, Eudowood Division of Pediatric Respiratory Sciences, Johns Hopkins University School of Medicine

DAVID MENDEZ, Associate Professor, Health Management and Policy, University of Michigan

RICHARD MIECH, Research Professor, Department of Youth and Social Issues, University of Michigan

ANA NAVAS-ACIEN, Professor, Department of Environmental Health Sciences, Mailman School of Public Health, Columbia University

KENT E. PINKERTON, Professor and Director, Center for Health and the Environment, Department of Anatomy, Physiology, and Cell Biology, University of California, Davis

NANCY A. RIGOTTI, Professor of Medicine, Harvard Medical School; Director, Tobacco Research and Treatment Center; Associate Chief, Division of General Internal Medicine, Massachusetts General Hospital

DAVID A. SAVITZ, Professor of Epidemiology, School of Public Health, Professor of Obstetrics and Gynecology and Pediatrics, Warren Alpert Medical School, Brown University

GIDEON St.HELEN, Assistant Professor of Medicine, Division of Clinical Pharmacology, Department of Medicine, University of California, San Francisco

Study Staff

KATHLEEN STRATTON, Study Director
LESLIE Y. KWAN, Associate Program Officer
AIMEE MEAD, Research Associate (*from July 2017*)
ALEXIS WOJTOWICZ, Senior Program Assistant
JORGE MENDOZA-TORRES, Senior Research Librarian
REBECCA MORGAN, Senior Research Librarian
DORIS ROMERO, Financial Associate (*until March 2017*)
MISRAK DABI, Financial Associate (*from April 2017*)
HOPE HARE, Administrative Assistant
ROSE MARIE MARTINEZ, Senior Director, Board on Population Health and Public Health Practice

Christine Mirzayan Science and Technology Policy Graduate Fellow

ANDREW MERLUZZI, Ph.D. Candidate at the University of Wisconsin–Madison (*until April 2017*)

Reviewers

This Consensus Study Report was reviewed in draft form by individuals chosen for their diverse perspectives and technical expertise. The purpose of this independent review is to provide candid and critical comments that will assist the National Academies of Sciences, Engineering, and Medicine in making each published report as sound as possible and to ensure that it meets the institutional standards for quality, objectivity, evidence, and responsiveness to the study charge. The review comments and draft manuscript remain confidential to protect the integrity of the deliberative process.

We thank the following individuals for their review of this report:

R. GRAHAM BARR, Columbia University Medical Center
NEAL L. BENOWITZ, University of California, San Francisco
JOHN BRITTON, University of Nottingham
CRISTINE D. DELNEVO, Rutgers, The State University of New Jersey
JOANNA S. FOWLER, Brookhaven National Laboratory and National Institutes of Health
MARIANNA D. GAÇA, British American Tobacco Research and Development Centre
STEPHEN S. HECHT, University of Minnesota
HARLAN R. JUSTER, New York State Department of Health
PAULA M. LANTZ, University of Michigan

RAFAEL MEZA, University of Michigan
MEIR STAMPFER, Harvard Medical School and Harvard T.H. Chan School of Public Health
THOMAS A. WILLS, University of Hawaii Cancer Center
JUDITH T. ZELIKOFF, New York University School of Medicine
SHU-HONG ZHU, University of California, San Diego

Although the reviewers listed above provided many constructive comments and suggestions, they were not asked to endorse the conclusions or recommendations of this report nor did they see the final draft before its release. The review of this report was overseen by **ERIC B. LARSON,** Kaiser Permanente Washington Health Research Institute, and **HUDA AKIL,** University of Michigan. They were responsible for making certain that an independent examination of this report was carried out in accordance with the standards of the National Academies and that all review comments were carefully considered. Responsibility for the final content rests entirely with the authoring committee and the National Academies.

Preface

On May 10, 2016, the Food and Drug Administration (FDA) issued a rule to extend regulatory authority to all tobacco products, including e-cigarettes, that meet the statutory definition of a tobacco product. This so-called "Deeming Regulation" allows FDA to regulate the manufacturing, distribution, and marketing of tobacco products such as e-cigarettes and includes automatic provisions such as youth access restrictions on sales. Although various forms of battery-powered "electronic nicotine delivery systems" (ENDS) devices have existed for more than a decade, their popularity, especially among youth, has increased in the past 5 years, although most recent data show a slight decline. In contrast to combustible tobacco cigarettes, e-cigarettes do not "burn," and do not contain most of the estimated 7,000 chemical constituents present in tobacco smoke. Thus, it is generally believed that e-cigarettes are "safer" than combustible tobacco cigarettes, yet exposures to nicotine and a variety of other potentially harmful constituents do occur. Harm might also occur if youth who begin their "tobacco" use with e-cigarettes then transition to combustible tobacco cigarettes or if adult cigarette smokers use e-cigarettes to supplement their smoking, rather than quitting combustible tobacco cigarettes completely.

In order to inform the public about the consequences of e-cigarettes and in support of future FDA and congressional action, a thorough and objective analysis of the state of scientific evidence relating to e-cigarettes and public health is needed. To that end, the ENDS Committee was established in December 2016 under the National Academies of Sciences, Engineering, and Medicine, with an ambitious timeline to complete a review of the science that can inform the understanding of public health risks and benefits of e-cigarettes. What are the short- and long-term health risks of regular use of e-cigarettes? What variables of the numerous types of devices and use patterns are important determinants of risk? Are e-cigarettes an effective means to quit smoking combustible tobacco cigarettes? Are e-cigarettes an "initiation pathway" of youth to smoking combustible tobacco cigarettes? These are just some of the important questions addressed by the committee in this report. Where feasible, the committee applied the most important attributes of systematic review methodology to the scientific literature to establish the strength of evidence surrounding the health risks (e.g., direct harmful effects, initiation of smoking) and benefits (e.g., smoking cessation) associated with e-cigarette use. Although the use of these products is relatively new, the committee identified more than 800 peer-reviewed scientific studies in this report. Based on this review, the committee has provided a summary of the current state of knowledge about the health risks and benefits of e-cigarette use, and has provided a series of research recommendations.

I am deeply gratified by the remarkable hard work and insights provided by my fellow committee members and indebted to the tireless and thoughtful work of the National Academies staff that so ably kept us on task throughout the duration of this study.

David L. Eaton, *Chair*
Committee on the Review of the Health Effects of
Electronic Nicotine Delivery Systems

Contents

SECTION I: E-CIGARETTE DEVICES, CONSTITUENTS, AND EXPOSURES

SECTION II: EFFECTS OF E-CIGARETTES ON HEALTH

SECTION III: PUBLIC HEALTH IMPLICATIONS OF E-CIGARETTES

Boxes, Figures, and Tables

BOXES

FIGURES

TABLES

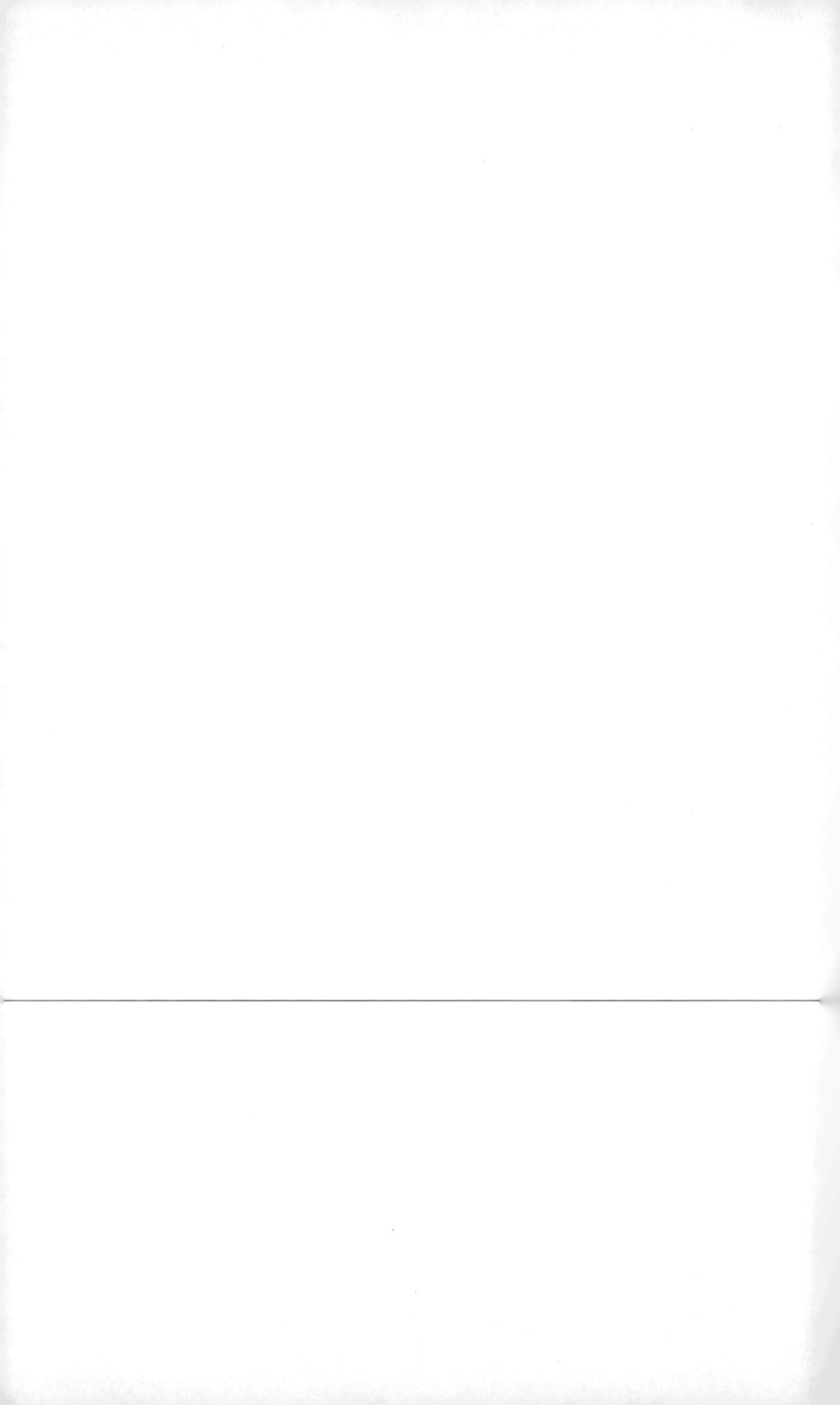

Summary

E-cigarette aerosol contains fewer numbers and lower levels of most toxicants than does smoke from combustible tobacco cigarettes. Exposure to nicotine and to toxicants from the aerosolization of e-cigarette ingredients is dependent on user and device characteristics. Laboratory tests of e-cigarette ingredients, in vitro toxicological tests, and short-term human studies suggest that e-cigarettes are likely to be far less harmful than combustible tobacco cigarettes. However, the absolute risks of the products cannot be unambiguously determined at this time. Long-term health effects, of particular concern for youth who become dependent on such products, are not yet clear.

Although e-cigarette use might cause youth to transition to combustible tobacco products, it might also increase adult cessation of combustible tobacco cigarettes. The net public health effect, harm or benefit, of e-cigarettes depends on three factors: their effect on youth initiation of combustible tobacco products, their effect on adult cessation of combustible tobacco products, and their intrinsic toxicity. If e-cigarette use by adult smokers leads to long-term abstinence from combustible tobacco cigarettes, the benefit to public health could be considerable. Without that health benefit for adult smokers, e-cigarette use could cause considerable harm to public health in the short and long term due both to the inherent harms of exposure to e-cigarette toxicants and to the harms related to subsequent combustible tobacco use by those who begin using e-cigarettes in their youth.

Population modeling is a useful strategy to help estimate the balance of potential benefits and harms from e-cigarettes in the short term before more definite scientific data are available. Factors that would promote the potential health benefits associated with these products include determining with more precision under which conditions e-cigarettes could serve as an effective smoking cessation aid, discouraging their use among youth through tobacco control strategies such as education and restrictions on products particularly appealing to youth, and increasing their safety through data-driven product engineering and design.

Millions of Americans use electronic cigarettes (e-cigarettes), even as rates of smoking[1] combustible tobacco cigarettes continue to decline among youth and adults. In 2016, youth e-cigarette use was substantially higher than cigarette smoking or use of any other tobacco product. A common picture emerges from national surveys. Prevalence of use increases with age in children and youth. E-cigarette use also varies by gender, with typically greater use among boys than girls. E-cigarette use also varies by race and ethnicity, with higher rates of use among youth who identify as Hispanic and non-Hispanic white compared with black, Asian, and other races. Early results suggest that use stabilized or decreased in youth between 2015 and 2016, despite increases between 2011 and 2015 across a range of measures and surveys. Substantial proportions of youth report using non-nicotine electronic cigarettes. Rates of e-cigarette use among adults are relatively low when compared with youth e-cigarette use and to adult combustible tobacco cigarette smoking. Most adult e-cigarette users report currently using other tobacco products. Among adults, as among youth, patterns of use vary by demographic subgroups—age, gender, and race and ethnicity. E-cigarette use is generally greatest among young adults and decreases with age in adults. Few adults begin using e-cigarettes who are not already using combustible tobacco cigarettes.

Despite their popularity, little is known about their health effects, and perceptions of potential risks and benefits of e-cigarette use vary widely among the public, users of e-cigarettes, health care providers, and the public health community. For example, whether e-cigarette use confers lower risk of addiction compared with combustible tobacco cigarettes is one point of controversy. Electronic cigarettes contain constituents that are not inert and are likely to have some negative health effects on their own. However, because the known risks of combustible tobacco are so great, understanding the net public health effect of e-cigarettes requires understanding not only the inherent risks of e-cigarettes, but also the relationship between e-cigarette use and combustible tobacco cigarette use.

Furthermore, concerns have been raised that e-cigarettes will induce youth to begin using combustible tobacco cigarettes. E-cigarette use among youth and young adults is especially worrying if e-cigarettes cause

[1] The committee uses the verb "smoke" to refer to use of combustible tobacco cigarettes and "vape" to refer to use of e-cigarettes. Similarly "smoker" refers to someone who uses combustible tobacco cigarettes.

dependence or the normalization of smoking behavior, and subsequently lead youth and young adults to start smoking combustible tobacco cigarettes. This is of particular concern for youth who otherwise would never have smoked. Among adult populations, to the extent that e-cigarette use promotes either reduction or complete abstinence from combustible tobacco smoking, e-cigarettes may help to reduce health risks.

E-cigarettes are regulated as tobacco products[2] by the Center for Tobacco Products of the Food and Drug Administration (FDA), which requested that the National Academies of Sciences, Engineering, and Medicine convene a committee of experts to conduct a review of the emerging evidence about e-cigarettes and health, make recommendations for the improvement of this research, and highlight gaps that are a priority for future research. The Statement of Task can be found in Box S-1.

The committee undertook a comprehensive review of the scientific literature regarding key constituents in e-cigarettes, human health effects, initiation and cessation of combustible tobacco cigarette use, and harm reduction. The committee considered the quality of individual studies, as well as the totality of the evidence to provide structured and consistent conclusions on the strength of the evidence. See Box S-2 for a summary of the framework the committee used for those conclusions. The committee notes that the framework is a guide, but that a great deal of expert judgment—in the evaluation of individual studies and in bodies of evidence—is always involved. The Annex to this Summary includes a compilation of the conclusions grouped by level of evidence, whereas they are listed by type of outcome in the sections that follow.

CONSTITUENTS

E-cigarettes contain liquids (referred to as e-liquids) that are aerosolized upon operation of the device. E-liquids typically contain nicotine (although some users prefer zero-nicotine solutions), flavorings, and humectants. Nicotine is a well-understood compound with known central and peripheral nervous system effects. It causes dependence and addiction, and exposure to nicotine from e-cigarettes likely elevates the cardiovascular disease risk in people with pre-existing cardiovascular disease(s), but the cardiovascular risk in people without cardiovascular disease(s) is uncertain. Based on studies of long-term users of nicotine replacement

---

[2] If an e-cigarette manufacturer made a claim in packaging or advertising that the products were useful for smoking cessation, the product would be regulated as a drug-delivery device under different statutory authorities and not by the Center for Tobacco Products. E-cigarettes are regulated as tobacco products because the nicotine in the e-liquids derives from tobacco plants. The Food and Drug Administration recently exerted authority over e-cigarettes; those that do not contain nicotine may be reviewed on a case-by-case basis.

BOX S-1
Statement of Task

The Health and Medicine Division of the National Academies of Sciences, Engineering, and Medicine shall convene a committee to evaluate the available evidence of the health effects related to the use of electronic nicotine delivery systems (ENDS) and identify future federally funded research needs. As part of its work, the committee will conduct a comprehensive and systematic assessment and review of the literature. The literature review shall include analysis of data on both short- and long-term health effects in:

- Users of ENDS, including health effects associated with the use of the full range of these devices (e.g., "cig-a-likes," tank systems, mods).
- Vulnerable populations of users (e.g., youth, pregnant women, individuals with underlying medical conditions [e.g., heart disease, pulmonary disease]).
- Non-users of ENDS exposed to secondhand and thirdhand aerosol generated by use of these devices.

A committee report will document the findings and provide a list of recommendations for future research. The list of research needs to inform the Food and Drug Administration and ENDS regulation will be prioritized with respect to:

- Research to gather information of most importance for the regulation of ENDS to protect the population health.
- Research that should be a priority for federal funding.

therapy or smokeless tobacco, nicotine exposure from e-cigarette use will likely pose minimal cancer risk to users. Most flavorings in e-liquids are designated as generally recognized as safe (also known as GRAS) by FDA, but those designations are for oral consumption in food and do not apply to flavorings used in e-cigarettes; most of these were never studied for toxicity via the inhalation route. The primary humectants are propylene glycol and glycerol, compounds also in widespread use for other purposes and about which significant scientific literature exists.

In reviewing the literature about the constituents in and exposures from e-cigarettes, the committee made nine conclusions:

> *Conclusion 3-1. There is **conclusive evidence** that e-cigarette use increases airborne concentrations of particulate matter and nicotine in indoor environments compared with background levels.*

BOX S-2
Levels of Evidence Framework for Conclusions

Conclusive evidence: There are many supportive findings from good-quality controlled studies (including randomized and non-randomized controlled trials) with no credible opposing findings. A firm conclusion can be made, and the limitations to the evidence, including chance, bias, and confounding factors, can be ruled out with reasonable confidence.

Substantial evidence: There are several supportive findings from good-quality observational studies or controlled trials with few or no credible opposing findings. A firm conclusion can be made, but minor limitations, including chance, bias, and confounding factors, cannot be ruled out with reasonable confidence.

Moderate evidence: There are several supportive findings from fair-quality studies with few or no credible opposing findings. A general conclusion can be made, but limitations, including chance, bias, and confounding factors, cannot be ruled out with reasonable confidence.

Limited evidence: There are supportive findings from fair-quality studies or mixed findings with most favoring one conclusion. A conclusion can be made, but there is significant uncertainty due to chance, bias, and confounding factors.

Insufficient evidence: There are mixed findings or a single poor study. No conclusion can be made because of substantial uncertainty due to chance, bias, and confounding factors.

No available evidence: There are no available studies; health endpoint has not been studied at all. No conclusion can be made.

*Conclusion 3-2. There is **limited evidence** that e-cigarette use increases levels of nicotine and other e-cigarette constituents on a variety of indoor surfaces compared with background levels.*

*Conclusion 4-1. There is **conclusive evidence** that exposure to nicotine from e-cigarettes is highly variable and depends on product characteristics (including device and e-liquid characteristics) and how the device is operated.*

*Conclusion 4-2. There is **substantial evidence** that nicotine intake from e-cigarette devices among experienced adult e-cigarette users can be comparable to that from combustible tobacco cigarettes.*

Conclusion 5-1. There is ***conclusive evidence*** *that in addition to nicotine, most e-cigarette products contain and emit numerous potentially toxic substances.*

Conclusion 5-2. There is ***conclusive evidence*** *that, other than nicotine, the number, quantity, and characteristics of potentially toxic substances emitted from e-cigarettes are highly variable and depend on product characteristics (including device and e-liquid characteristics) and how the device is operated.*

Conclusion 5-3. There is ***substantial evidence*** *that except for nicotine, under typical conditions of use, exposure to potentially toxic substances from e-cigarettes is significantly lower compared with combustible tobacco cigarettes.*

Conclusion 5-4. There is ***substantial evidence*** *that e-cigarette aerosol contains metals. The origin of the metals could be the metallic coil used to heat the e-liquid, other parts of the e-cigarette device, or e-liquids. Product characteristics and use patterns may contribute to differences in the actual metals and metal concentrations measured in e-cigarette aerosol.*

Conclusion 5-5. There is ***limited evidence*** *that the number of metals in e-cigarette aerosol could be greater than the number of metals in combustible tobacco cigarettes, except for cadmium, which is markedly lower in e-cigarettes compared with combustible tobacco cigarettes.*

Taken together, the evidence in support of these conclusions suggests that e-cigarette aerosol contains fewer numbers and lower levels of toxicants than smoke from combustible tobacco cigarettes. Nicotine exposure can mimic that found with use of combustible tobacco cigarettes, but is highly variable. However, the exposure to nicotine and toxicants from the aerosolization of flavorings and humectants is dependent on user and device characteristics.

HUMAN HEALTH EFFECTS

Combustible tobacco cigarettes pose serious risks to human health; these risks are well documented and well understood. Many of those health effects emerge only after decades of cigarette smoking. E-cigarettes have only been on the market in the United States since 2006, making scientific comparisons between e-cigarettes and combustible tobacco cigarettes about most health effects difficult. However, research on short-term exposures to e-cigarettes and effects on disease symptoms and intermediate outcomes exist. An important distinction when considering these data is whether the effects are seen in an e-cigarette user who had never used combustible tobacco cigarettes (usually children or youth) or in a combustible tobacco cigarette user, with and without preexisting tobacco-related disease, usually adults. The committee reviewed evidence on the effects of e-cigarettes in several health domains: dependence, cardiovascular disease, cancer, respiratory diseases, oral diseases, maternal and fetal outcomes, and injuries and poisonings. Although the amount of literature is relatively scant and complicated by the multiple types of e-cigarettes in use even within a given study, the committee made 26 conclusions about the effects of e-cigarettes on health.

Conclusion 7-1. There is ***substantial evidence*** *that e-cigarette aerosols can induce acute endothelial cell dysfunction, although the long-term consequences and outcomes on these parameters with long-term exposure to e-cigarette aerosol are uncertain.*

Conclusion 7-2. There is ***substantial evidence*** *that components of e-cigarette aerosols can promote formation of reactive oxygen species/oxidative stress. Although this supports the biological plausibility of tissue injury and disease from long-term exposure to e-cigarette aerosols, generation of reactive oxygen species and oxidative stress induction is generally lower from e-cigarettes than from combustible tobacco cigarette smoke.*

Conclusion 8-1. There is ***substantial evidence*** *that e-cigarette use results in symptoms of dependence on e-cigarettes.*

Conclusion 8-2. There is ***moderate evidence*** *that risk and severity of dependence are lower for e-cigarettes than combustible tobacco cigarettes.*

Conclusion 8-3. There is ***moderate evidence*** *that variability in e-cigarette product characteristics (nicotine concentration, flavoring, device type, and brand) is an important determinant of risk and severity of e-cigarette dependence.*

Conclusion 9-1. There is ***no available evidence*** *whether or not e-cigarette use is associated with clinical cardiovascular outcomes (coronary heart disease, stroke, and peripheral artery disease) and subclinical atherosclerosis (carotid intima-media thickness and coronary artery calcification).*

Conclusion 9-2. There is ***substantial evidence*** *that heart rate increases shortly after nicotine intake from e-cigarettes.*

Conclusion 9-3. There is ***moderate evidence*** *that diastolic blood pressure increases shortly after nicotine intake from e-cigarettes.*

Conclusion 9-4. There is ***limited evidence*** *that e-cigarette use is associated with a short-term increase in systolic blood pressure, changes in biomarkers of oxidative stress, increased endothelial dysfunction and arterial stiffness, and autonomic control.*

Conclusion 9-5. There is ***insufficient evidence*** *that e-cigarette use is associated with long-term changes in heart rate, blood pressure, and cardiac geometry and function.*

Conclusion 10-1. There is ***no available evidence*** *whether or not e-cigarette use is associated with intermediate cancer endpoints in humans. This holds true for e-cigarette use compared with use of combustible tobacco cigarettes and e-cigarette use compared with no use of tobacco products.*

Conclusion 10-2. There is ***limited evidence*** *from in vivo animal studies using intermediate biomarkers of cancer to support the hypothesis that long-term e-cigarette use could increase the risk of cancer; there is* ***no available evidence*** *from adequate long-term animal bioassays of e-cigarette aerosol exposures to inform cancer risk.*

Conclusion 10-3. There is ***limited evidence*** *that e-cigarette aerosol can be mutagenic or cause DNA damage in humans, animal models, and human cells in culture.*

Conclusion 10-4. There is ***substantial evidence*** *that some chemicals present in e-cigarette aerosols (e.g., formaldehyde, acrolein) are capable of causing DNA damage and mutagenesis. This supports the biological plausibility that long-term exposure to e-cigarette aerosols could increase risk of cancer and adverse reproductive outcomes. Whether or not the levels of exposure are high enough to contribute to human carcinogenesis remains to be determined.*

Conclusion 11-1. There is ***no available evidence*** *whether or not e-cigarettes cause respiratory diseases in humans.*

Conclusion 11-2. There is ***limited evidence*** *for improvement in lung function and respiratory symptoms among adult smokers with asthma who switch to e-cigarettes completely or in part (dual use).*

Conclusion 11-3. There is ***limited evidence*** *for reduction of chronic obstructive pulmonary disease (COPD) exacerbations among adult smokers with COPD who switch to e-cigarettes completely or in part (dual use).*

Conclusion 11-4. There is ***moderate evidence*** *for increased cough and wheeze in adolescents who use e-cigarettes and an association with e-cigarette use and an increase in asthma exacerbations.*

Conclusion 11-5. There is ***limited evidence*** *of adverse effects of e-cigarette exposure on the respiratory system from animal and in vitro studies.*

Conclusion 12-1. There is ***limited evidence*** *suggesting that switching to e-cigarettes will improve periodontal disease in smokers.*

Conclusion 12-2. There is ***limited evidence*** *suggesting that nicotine- and non-nicotine–containing e-cigarette aerosol can adversely affect cell viability and cause cell damage of oral tissue in non-smokers.*

Conclusion 13-1. There is ***no available evidence*** *whether or not e-cigarettes affect pregnancy outcomes.*

Conclusion 13-2. There is ***insufficient evidence*** *whether or not maternal e-cigarette use affects fetal development.*

Conclusion 14-1. There is ***conclusive evidence*** *that e-cigarette devices can explode and cause burns and projectile injuries. Such risk is significantly increased when batteries are of poor quality, stored improperly, or modified by users.*

Conclusion 14-2. There is ***conclusive evidence*** *that intentional or accidental exposure to e-liquids (from drinking, eye contact, or dermal contact) can result in adverse health effects including but not limited to seizures, anoxic brain injury, vomiting, and lactic acidosis.*

Conclusion 14-3. There is ***conclusive evidence*** *that intentionally or unintentionally drinking or injecting e-liquids can be fatal.*

Taken together, the evidence reviewed by the committee suggests that e-cigarettes are not without physiological activity in humans, but the implications for long-term effects on morbidity and mortality are not yet clear. Use of e-cigarettes instead of combustible tobacco cigarettes by those with existing respiratory disease might be less harmful.

INITIATION AND CESSATION

The Family Smoking Prevention and Tobacco Control Act of 2009, which is the basis for FDA's regulatory authority over tobacco products, including e-cigarettes, defined a unique regulatory standard, the public health standard. This requires that tobacco products introduced on the market after February 15, 2007, be shown to have a net population health benefit to users and non-users of the product. Operationally, if a product caused more people to begin harmful tobacco use and fewer people to quit tobacco use, even if the product itself poses less risk to the user than other products, it could be determined that the product poses a public health burden and would be kept off the market. Thus, the tobacco control field must pay close attention to the effects of e-cigarette use on initiation and cessation of combustible tobacco use, regardless of the effects of e-cigarettes on health outcomes. Although the studies reviewed had limitations, the committee was able to make seven conclusions:

> *Conclusion 16-1. There is* ***substantial evidence*** *that e-cigarette use increases risk of ever using combustible tobacco cigarettes among youth and young adults.*

> *Conclusion 16-2. Among youth and young adult e-cigarette users who ever use combustible tobacco cigarettes, there is* ***moderate evidence*** *that e-cigarette use increases the frequency and intensity of subsequent combustible tobacco cigarette smoking.*

> *Conclusion 16-3. Among youth and young adult e-cigarette users who ever use combustible tobacco cigarettes, there is* ***limited evidence*** *that e-cigarette use increases, in the near term, the duration of subsequent combustible tobacco cigarette smoking.*

> *Conclusion 17-1. Overall, there is* ***limited evidence*** *that e-cigarettes may be effective aids to promote smoking cessation.*

> *Conclusion 17-2. There is* ***moderate evidence*** *from randomized controlled trials that e-cigarettes with nicotine are more effective than e-cigarettes without nicotine for smoking cessation.*

> *Conclusion 17-3. There is* ***insufficient evidence*** *from randomized controlled trials about the effectiveness of e-cigarettes as cessation aids compared with no treatment or to Food and Drug Administration–approved smoking cessation treatments.*

> *Conclusion 17-4. While the overall evidence from observational trials is mixed, there is* ***moderate evidence*** *from observational studies that more frequent use of e-cigarettes is associated with an increased likelihood of cessation.*

Taken together the evidence suggests that while e-cigarettes might cause youth who use them to transition to use of combustible tobacco products, they might increase adult cessation of combustible tobacco cigarettes.

HARM REDUCTION

The committee reviewed evidence from the sections discussed above to specifically look at what is known about e-cigarette exposures and health effects when compared with combustible tobacco cigarettes. The committee reached five conclusions.

Conclusion 18-1. There is ***conclusive evidence*** *that completely substituting e-cigarettes for combustible tobacco cigarettes reduces users' exposure to numerous toxicants and carcinogens present in combustible tobacco cigarettes.*

Conclusion 18-2. There is ***substantial evidence*** *that completely switching from regular use of combustible tobacco cigarettes to e-cigarettes results in reduced short-term adverse health outcomes in several organ systems.*

Conclusion 18-3. There is ***no available evidence*** *whether or not long-term e-cigarette use among smokers (dual use) changes morbidity or mortality compared with those who only smoke combustible tobacco cigarettes.*

Conclusion 18-4. There is ***insufficient evidence*** *that e-cigarette use changes short-term adverse health outcomes in several organ systems in smokers who continue to smoke combustible tobacco cigarettes (dual users).*

Conclusion 18-5. There is ***moderate evidence*** *that secondhand exposure to nicotine and particulates is lower from e-cigarettes compared with combustible tobacco cigarettes.*

The evidence about harm reduction suggests that across a range of studies and outcomes, e-cigarettes pose less risk to an individual than combustible tobacco cigarettes.

MODELING

The committee used population dynamic modeling to examine the possible effects of e-cigarette use at the population level. The specific time frame and magnitude of population health effects of e-cigarettes will depend on their impact on the rates of initiation and cessation of combustible tobacco cigarettes and on their intrinsic harm. Any population health effect includes the possibility of some groups incurring harm (e.g., youth who initiate smoking combustible tobacco cigarettes), while others benefit (e.g., adult combustible tobacco cigarette users who completely quit or reduce smoking). As with other models of population health effects of tobacco use, the effects of changing cessation rates are seen earlier than effects of changing initiation rates, due to the lag time for serious chronic health effects of combustible tobacco cigarettes to manifest.

Under the assumption that the use of e-cigarettes increases the net cessation rate of combustible tobacco cigarette use among adults (i.e., the increase in permanent quitting offsets the potential relapse of former smokers because of e-cigarettes), the modeling projects that use of these products will generate a net public health benefit, at least in the short run. The harms from increased initiation by youth will take time to manifest, occurring decades after the benefits of increased cessation are seen. However, for long-range projections (e.g., 50 years out), the net public health benefit is substantially less and is negative under some scenarios. With the range of assumptions used, the model projects that there would be net public health harm in the short and long terms if the products do not increase combustible tobacco cessation in adults.

Factors that would maximize potential health benefits associated with these products include determining with more precision whether and under which conditions e-cigarettes could serve as an effective smoking cessation aid, discouraging their use among youth through standard tobacco control strategies such as education and access restrictions, and increasing their safety through data-driven product engineering and design.

RESEARCH RECOMMENDATIONS

Given the relatively short time that e-cigarettes have been used, it is understandable that the evidence base regarding their effects is limited. There is a great need for more evidence. Manufacturers will need to produce this research in a short amount of time if current statutory deadlines remain in place. Researchers from academia will also be involved directly (in contracts with manufacturers and in grants from government and others) in the generation of these data. Some types of research involve a long-term horizon; other important and informative research requires much less time to conduct. One type of research does not substitute for the other; a complete portfolio of research is needed. The committee understands that, in any new field, researchers struggle to conduct optimal research due to limitations of knowledge. Also, researchers feel the urgency to study an important new question and adapt what they know,

BOX S-3
Research Needs:
E-Cigarette Devices, Constituents, and Exposures

The following specific suggestions illustrate the range of priority research areas provided in the body of the report:

Recommendation 6-1: The committee recommends that the Food and Drug Administration and other federal research sponsors and/or device manufacturers prioritize e-cigarette research that addresses key gaps regarding knowledge about e-cigarette devices, constituents, and exposures. This might include rapid response funding opportunities.

- Study the stability of e-liquid ingredients when heated, identify potential byproducts of thermal degradation and of compounds that were not initially present in the e-liquid, and ascertain determinants of change in aerosol composition.
- Study the impact of e-cigarette use on indoor air quality and biomarkers of secondhand e-cigarette exposure in scenarios and exposure surveys that are relevant for the populations exposed, including workers in vape shops and vaping convention attendees, children, pregnant women, and patients with cardiorespiratory disease who live with adults who use e-cigarettes.

Recommendation 6-2: The committee recommends that the Food and Drug Administration and other federal research sponsors and/or device manufacturers prioritize research that improves the quality of e-cigarette research to better understand the devices, constituents, and exposures. This includes protocol and methods validation and development and use of appropriate study design, including the use of the appropriate control groups.

- Develop and validate methods to produce aerosols and to analyze target constituents in e-cigarettes; the standardized method should reflect not only the average puffing conditions observed among the users in real-life settings, but also intensive puffing behaviors.
- Use exposure conditions and animal models that are relevant to real-life inhalation exposure in humans.

without complete adjustments in research design or methods sufficient to address the nuances of the problem. Finally, the rapidly changing nature of the devices has made comparisons among studies difficult.

The committee identified gaps in the literature in every aspect in its work and provides overarching categories of research needs and specific research suggestions within the final chapters of each of the three major sections of the report. These overarching categories include (1) address-

BOX S-4
Research Needs: Effects of E-Cigarettes on Human Health

The following specific suggestions illustrate the range of priority research areas provided in the body of the report:

Recommendation 15-1: The committee recommends that the Food and Drug Administration and other federal research sponsors and/or device manufacturers prioritize e-cigarette research that addresses key gaps regarding health effects in individuals. This might include rapid response funding opportunities.

- Particle deposition in the human airways should be evaluated to assess where e-cigarette–derived particles impact the upper versus lower airways and alveoli and how area of impaction in the lung may influence health effects caused by e-cigarettes. Such studies should also include evaluation of airway epithelium repair.
- Studies are needed on the association of secondhand and thirdhand exposures with health outcomes in vulnerable populations, such as pregnant women, infants, young children, the elderly, and patients with cardiovascular and respiratory disease compared with secondhand tobacco smoke and the absence of secondhand exposure to both combustible tobacco smoke or to e-cigarettes.
- Longitudinal cohort studies are needed of youth and young adults to understand the trajectory of dependence over time in users with little or no combustible tobacco product exposure.

Recommendation 15-2: The committee recommends that the Food and Drug Administration and other federal research sponsors and/or device manufacturers prioritize research that improves the quality of e-cigarette research on health outcomes. This includes protocol and methods validation and development and use of appropriate study design, including the use of the appropriate control groups and relevant biomarkers.

- In clinical and epidemiological studies, use as comparison groups individuals who continue to smoke, those who try to quit with other evidence-based tobacco cessation treatments, and those who are not users of tobacco products, including e-cigarettes.
- Use methods development research to create or adapt existing abuse liability testing for e-cigarettes to better understand the development of dependence on e-cigarettes.

ing gaps in substantive knowledge and (2) improving research methods and quality through protocol and methods validation and development, including the use of appropriate study design. The six specific research recommendations and select suggestions can be found in Boxes S-3, S-4,

BOX S-5
Research Recommendations:
Public Health Implications of E-Cigarettes

The following specific suggestions illustrate the range of priority research areas provided in the body of the report:

Recommendation 20-1: The committee recommends that the Food and Drug Administration and other federal research sponsors and/or device manufacturers prioritize e-cigarette research that addresses key gaps regarding harm reduction and the public health implications of e-cigarettes. This might include rapid response funding opportunities.

- Research on the mechanisms through which e-cigarette use affects combustible tobacco cigarette smoking (both ever use among youth and quitting among current combustible tobacco cigarette smokers).
- Research on potential harm reduction to bystanders exposed involuntarily to tobacco smoke after secondhand or thirdhand exposure to combustible tobacco smoke is replaced by secondhand or thirdhand exposure to emissions of e-cigarettes.

Recommendation 20-2: The committee recommends that the Food and Drug Administration and other federal research sponsors and/or device manufacturers prioritize research on the public health implications of e-cigarettes that improves the quality of e-cigarette research. This includes protocol and methods validation and development and use of appropriate study design, including the use of appropriate control groups.

- Studies that build on existing nationally representative population surveys of adults to monitor patterns of e-cigarette use in detail on an ongoing basis to include characterization of patterns of e-cigarette use such as the frequency and duration of use, type of device used, and reason for use.

and S-5. The specific suggestions illustrate the range of priority research areas provided in the body of the report.

FINAL OBSERVATIONS

Much of the research on e-cigarettes suffers from methodological flaws, and many important areas have not yet been researched. Nonetheless, the committee found sufficient literature to suggest that, while there are risks associated with e-cigarettes, compared with combustible tobacco cigarettes, e-cigarettes contain fewer toxicants; can deliver nicotine in a manner similar to combustible tobacco cigarettes; show significantly less biological activity in a number of in vitro, animal, and human systems; and might be useful as a cessation aid to smokers who use e-cigarettes exclusively. However, youth who begin with e-cigarettes are more likely to transition to combustible tobacco cigarette use and become smokers who may be at risk to suffer the known health burdens of combustible tobacco cigarettes. Moreover, although infrequent, e-cigarettes can explode, leading to burns and other injuries, and consumption of or dermal exposure to e-liquids is dangerous, even fatal.

More and better research on short- and long-term health effects of e-cigarettes, as well as their effects on initiation and cessation of combustible tobacco product use, will bring clarity to the question of whether e-cigarettes will prove to reduce harm or induce harm at the individual and the population levels. Given how rapidly the e-cigarette product marketplace and user population are changing, there will undoubtedly be many new issues, which are currently unknown and will require careful surveillance and scientific scrutiny. The approach taken by the committee to evaluate the health effects of e-cigarettes in this report is anticipated to provide a generalizable template for future evaluations of the evidence.

Summary Annex

Report Conclusions by Level of Evidence

CONCLUSIVE EVIDENCE

- Conclusion 3-1. There is **conclusive evidence** that e-cigarette use increases airborne concentrations of particulate matter and nicotine in indoor environments compared with background levels.
- Conclusion 4-1. There is **conclusive evidence** that exposure to nicotine from e-cigarettes is highly variable and depends on product characteristics (including device and e-liquid characteristics) and how the device is operated.
- Conclusion 5-1. There is **conclusive evidence** that in addition to nicotine, most e-cigarette products contain and emit numerous potentially toxic substances.
- Conclusion 5-2. There is **conclusive evidence** that, other than nicotine, the number, quantity, and characteristics of potentially toxic substances emitted from e-cigarettes are highly variable and depend on product characteristics (including device and e-liquid characteristics) and how the device is operated.
- Conclusion 14-1. There is **conclusive evidence** that e-cigarette devices can explode and cause burns and projectile injuries. Such risk is significantly increased when batteries are of poor quality, stored improperly, or modified by users.
- Conclusion 14-2. There is **conclusive evidence** that intentional or accidental exposure to e-liquids (from drinking, eye contact, or dermal contact) can result in adverse health effects including but

not limited to seizures, anoxic brain injury, vomiting, and lactic acidosis.

- Conclusion 14-3. There is **conclusive evidence** that intentionally or unintentionally drinking or injecting e-liquids can be fatal.
- Conclusion 18-1. There is **conclusive evidence** that completely substituting e-cigarettes for combustible tobacco cigarettes reduces users' exposure to numerous toxicants and carcinogens present in combustible tobacco cigarettes.

SUBSTANTIAL EVIDENCE

- Conclusion 4-2. There is **substantial evidence** that nicotine intake from e-cigarette devices among experienced adult e-cigarette users can be comparable to that from combustible tobacco cigarettes.
- Conclusion 5-3. There is **substantial evidence** that except for nicotine, under typical conditions of use, exposure to potentially toxic substances from e-cigarettes is significantly lower compared with combustible tobacco cigarettes.
- Conclusion 5-4. There is **substantial evidence** that e-cigarette aerosol contains metals. The origin of the metals could be the metallic coil used to heat the e-liquid, other parts of the e-cigarette device, or e-liquids. Product characteristics and use patterns may contribute to differences in the actual metals and metal concentrations measured in e-cigarette aerosol.
- Conclusion 7-1. There is **substantial evidence** that e-cigarette aerosols can induce acute endothelial cell dysfunction, although the long-term consequences and outcomes on these parameters with long-term exposure to e-cigarette aerosol are uncertain.
- Conclusion 7-2. There is **substantial evidence** that components of e-cigarette aerosols can promote formation of reactive oxygen species/oxidative stress. Although this supports the biological plausibility of tissue injury and disease from long-term exposure to e-cigarette aerosols, generation of reactive oxygen species and oxidative stress induction is generally lower from e-cigarettes than from combustible tobacco cigarette smoke.
- Conclusion 8-1. There is **substantial evidence** that e-cigarette use results in symptoms of dependence on e-cigarettes.
- Conclusion 9-2. There is **substantial evidence** that heart rate increases shortly after nicotine intake from e-cigarettes.
- Conclusion 10-4. There is **substantial evidence** that some chemicals present in e-cigarette aerosols (e.g., formaldehyde, acrolein) are capable of causing DNA damage and mutagenesis. This supports the biological plausibility that long-term exposure to

e-cigarette aerosols could increase risk of cancer and adverse reproductive outcomes. Whether or not the levels of exposure are high enough to contribute to human carcinogenesis remains to be determined.

- Conclusion 16-1. There is **substantial evidence** that e-cigarette use increases risk of ever using combustible tobacco cigarettes among youth and young adults.
- Conclusion 18-2. There is **substantial evidence** that completely switching from regular use of combustible tobacco cigarettes to e-cigarettes results in reduced short-term adverse health outcomes in several organ systems.

MODERATE EVIDENCE

- Conclusion 8-2. There is **moderate evidence** that risk and severity of dependence are lower for e-cigarettes than combustible tobacco cigarettes.
- Conclusion 8-3. There is **moderate evidence** that variability in e-cigarette product characteristics (nicotine concentration, flavoring, device type, and brand) is an important determinant of risk and severity of e-cigarette dependence.
- Conclusion 9-3. There is **moderate evidence** that diastolic blood pressure increases shortly after nicotine intake from e-cigarettes.
- Conclusion 11-4. There is **moderate evidence** for increased cough and wheeze in adolescents who use e-cigarettes and an association with e-cigarette use and an increase in asthma exacerbations.
- Conclusion 16-2. Among youth and young adult e-cigarette users who ever use combustible tobacco cigarettes, there is **moderate evidence** that e-cigarette use increases the frequency and intensity of subsequent combustible tobacco cigarette smoking.
- Conclusion 17-2. There is **moderate evidence** from randomized controlled trials that e-cigarettes with nicotine are more effective than e-cigarettes without nicotine for smoking cessation.
- Conclusion 17-4. While the overall evidence from observational trials is mixed, there is **moderate evidence** from observational studies that more frequent use of e-cigarettes is associated with an increased likelihood of cessation.
- Conclusion 18-5. There is **moderate evidence** that secondhand exposure to nicotine and particulates is lower from e-cigarettes compared with combustible tobacco cigarettes.

LIMITED EVIDENCE

- Conclusion 3-2. There is **limited evidence** that e-cigarette use increases levels of nicotine and other e-cigarette constituents on a variety of indoor surfaces compared with background levels.
- Conclusion 5-5. There is **limited evidence** that the number of metals in e-cigarette aerosol could be greater than the number of metals in combustible tobacco cigarettes, except for cadmium, which is markedly lower in e-cigarettes compared with combustible tobacco cigarettes.
- Conclusion 9-4. There is **limited evidence** that e-cigarette use is associated with a short-term increase in systolic blood pressure, changes in biomarkers of oxidative stress, increased endothelial dysfunction and arterial stiffness, and autonomic control.
- Conclusion 10-2. There is **limited evidence** from in vivo animal studies using intermediate biomarkers of cancer to support the hypothesis that long-term e-cigarette use could increase the risk of cancer; there is **no available evidence** from adequate long-term animal bioassays of e-cigarette aerosol exposures to inform cancer risk.
- Conclusion 10-3. There is **limited evidence** that e-cigarette aerosol can be mutagenic or cause DNA damage in humans, animal models, and human cells in culture.
- Conclusion 11-2. There is **limited evidence** for improvement in lung function and respiratory symptoms among adult smokers with asthma who switch to e-cigarettes completely or in part (dual use).
- Conclusion 11-3. There is **limited evidence** for reduction of chronic obstructive pulmonary disease (COPD) exacerbations among adult smokers with COPD who switch to e-cigarettes completely or in part (dual use).
- Conclusion 11-5. There is **limited evidence** of adverse effects of e-cigarette exposure on the respiratory system from animal and in vitro studies.
- Conclusion 12-1. There is **limited evidence** suggesting that switching to e-cigarettes will improve periodontal disease in smokers.
- Conclusion 12-2. There is **limited evidence** suggesting that nicotine- and non-nicotine–containing e-cigarette aerosol can adversely affect cell viability and cause cell damage of oral tissue in non-smokers.
- Conclusion 16-3. Among youth and young adult e-cigarette users who ever use combustible tobacco cigarettes, there is **limited evidence** that e-cigarette use increases, in the near term, the duration of subsequent combustible tobacco cigarette smoking.

- Conclusion 17-1. Overall, there is **limited evidence** that e-cigarettes may be effective aids to promote smoking cessation.

INSUFFICIENT EVIDENCE

- Conclusion 9-5. There is **insufficient evidence** that e-cigarette use is associated with long-term changes in heart rate, blood pressure, and cardiac geometry and function.
- Conclusion 13-2. There is **insufficient evidence** whether or not maternal e-cigarette use affects fetal development.
- Conclusion 17-3. There is **insufficient evidence** from randomized controlled trials about the effectiveness of e-cigarettes as cessation aids compared with no treatment or to Food and Drug Administration–approved smoking cessation treatments.
- Conclusion 18-4. There is **insufficient evidence** that e-cigarette use changes short-term adverse health outcomes in several organ systems in smokers who continue to smoke combustible tobacco cigarettes (dual users).

NO AVAILABLE EVIDENCE

- Conclusion 9-1. There is **no available evidence** whether or not e-cigarette use is associated with clinical cardiovascular outcomes (coronary heart disease, stroke, and peripheral artery disease) and subclinical atherosclerosis (carotid intima-media thickness and coronary artery calcification).
- Conclusion 10-1. There is **no available evidence** whether or not e-cigarette use is associated with intermediate cancer endpoints in humans. This holds true for e-cigarette use compared with use of combustible tobacco cigarettes and e-cigarette use compared with no use of tobacco products.
- Conclusion 11-1. There is **no available evidence** whether or not e-cigarettes cause respiratory diseases in humans.
- Conclusion 13-1. There is **no available evidence** whether or not e-cigarettes affect pregnancy outcomes.
- Conclusion 18-3. There is **no available evidence** whether or not long-term e-cigarette use among smokers (dual use) changes morbidity or mortality compared with those who only smoke combustible tobacco cigarettes.

1

Introduction

Millions of Americans use e-cigarettes. Despite their popularity, little is known about their health effects, and perceptions of potential risks and benefits of e-cigarette use vary widely among the public, users of e-cigarettes, health care providers, and the public health community. For example, whether e-cigarette use confers lower risk of addiction compared with combustible tobacco cigarettes is one point of controversy. Likewise, there are uncertainties about the harm of e-cigarettes themselves, because of the exposure to potentially toxic substances contained in e-cigarette emissions, especially in individuals, such as youth and young adults, who have never used tobacco products. Furthermore, concerns have been raised that e-cigarettes will induce youth to begin using combustible tobacco cigarettes. Given their relatively recent introduction, there has been little time for a scientific body of evidence to develop on the health effects of e-cigarettes. The purpose of this report is to (1) conduct a critical, objective, and evidence-based review of the scientific evidence that addresses the various competing views on the public health consequences of e-cigarettes; (2) make recommendations for the improvement of this research; and (3) highlight gaps that are a priority for future research.

STATEMENT OF TASK

The Consolidated Appropriations Act of 2016 includes language directing the Center for Tobacco Products (CTP) of the Food and Drug

BOX 1-1
Statement of Task

The Health and Medicine Division of the National Academies of Sciences, Engineering, and Medicine shall convene a committee to evaluate the available evidence of the health effects related to the use of electronic nicotine delivery systems (ENDS) and identify future federally funded research needs. As part of its work, the committee will conduct a comprehensive and systematic assessment and review of the literature. The literature review shall include analysis of data on both short- and long-term health effects in:

- Users of ENDS, including health effects associated with the use of the full range of these devices (e.g., "cig-a-likes," tank systems, mods).
- Vulnerable populations of users (e.g., youth, pregnant women, individuals with underlying medical conditions [e.g., heart disease, pulmonary disease]).
- Non-users of ENDS exposed to secondhand and thirdhand aerosol generated by use of these devices.

A committee report will document the findings and provide a list of recommendations for future research. The list of research needs to inform the Food and Drug Administration and ENDS regulation will be prioritized with respect to:

- Research to gather information of most importance for the regulation of ENDS to protect the population health.
- Research that should be a priority for federal funding.

Administration (FDA) to "contract with the Institute of Medicine[1] to conduct an in-depth evaluation of available evidence of health effects from e-cigarettes and recommendations for future federally funded research" (U.S. Congress, 2016, p. 31). In accordance with this directive, CTP contracted with the National Academies of Sciences, Engineering, and Medicine to convene an ad hoc committee to conduct such an evaluation. (See Box 1-1 for the complete Statement of Task and Appendix A for a list of questions CTP provided for the committee to consider in addition to the Statement of Task.) The Committee on the Review of the Health Effects of Electronic Nicotine Delivery Systems includes experts in toxicology, nicotine pharmacology, adolescent and adult tobacco use patterns, epidemiology, public health, inhalation toxicology/pulmonology, cardiology,

[1] As of March 2016, the Health and Medicine Division continues the consensus studies and convening activities previously undertaken by the Institute of Medicine (IOM).

pediatrics, obstetrics, and oncology (see Appendix F for the committee biosketches). The committee held five meetings, including a public workshop (see Appendix E for the public workshop agenda).

A NOTE ON TERMINOLOGY: WHAT ARE E-CIGARETTES?

E-cigarette products, their components, and their use lack standard nomenclature, and thus even manufacturers and users refer to them using different terms (Alexander et al., 2016). Throughout this report the committee uses the terms "electronic cigarettes" and "e-cigarettes" interchangeably to refer to any device with a heating element that produces an aerosol from a liquid that users can inhale. Characteristics of e-cigarette devices and products are described in more detail in Chapter 3. During a discussion at the first meeting, Mitchell Zeller, director of CTP, clarified that the use of the term "ENDS" in the Statement of Task does not refer exclusively to nicotine-containing e-cigarettes. Rather, CTP used the term to capture a heterogeneous group of products that are referred to using widely variable terminology. Thus, Zeller urged the committee to interpret the term broadly and not to limit the committee's scope to nicotine-containing products, as e-liquids that do not contain nicotine or other substances made or derived from tobacco may still be subject to FDA's tobacco control authorities. At the same time, a representative from CTP also noted that because CTP does not have regulatory authority over controlled substances such as marijuana, the committee should not focus on the effects of other controlled substances that could be consumed via an e-cigarette. Finally, Zeller also clarified that this class of products excludes electronic devices that do not contain liquids and instead heat tobacco, such as those referred to as "heat-not-burn" products. The committee's use of the term e-cigarettes encompasses all products envisioned by CTP in the Statement of Task.

THE RAPID RISE OF E-CIGARETTE USE IN THE UNITED STATES

Several nationally representative surveys reported patterns of electronic cigarette use in the United States. These include three cross-sectional surveys with data on youth use, the National Youth Tobacco Survey (NYTS), Monitoring the Future (MTF), and Youth Risk Behavioral Surveillance (YRBS), and two cross-sectional surveys of adult use, the National Adult Tobacco Survey (NATS) and the National Health Interview Survey (NHIS). In addition, the Population Assessment of Tobacco and Health (PATH) study of youth and adults and the Tobacco Use Supplement to the Current Population Survey (TUS-CPS) also provide longitudinal surveillance data. These surveys usually capture several measures of e-cigarette use. Typical measures include ever use, current use, and frequent use. Ever or lifetime use captures whether an individual has used an electronic cigarette, even once or twice. Current use or use within the past 30 days typically captures whether someone has used an electronic cigarette on at least 1 day in the past 30 days. Frequent use generally describes e-cigarette use on 20 or more days of the past 30 days. Ever use is the most sensitive, but least specific, measure of use. Ever use collapses across low levels of use, such as experimentation (a temporary period of use that does not progress to regular or established use) and higher levels of use, including current, past 30-day, and frequent use. Cross-sectional data using such measures do not monitor patterns of use progression over time (trajectories), which leaves unclear whether people classified in one of these use patterns are on increasing, decreasing, or stable trajectories of use.

This section summarizes rates of electronic cigarette use as reported in these sources, including rates among subpopulations. Of note, although e-cigarettes entered the U.S. market in the middle of the first decade of the 2000s, little data on their use at a national level are available before 2011. Thus, little trend data are available even among surveys that collect data on e-cigarettes across multiple years. The lack of standard terminology also contributes to this problem because different surveys use different terms and definitions, and the terminology and definitions used to describe e-cigarettes across multiple years of the same survey change over time.

Youth Electronic Cigarette Use

Youth (age 17 and younger) have rapidly taken up e-cigarette use. The 2015 NYTS reported that 27.1 percent of middle and high school students ever used e-cigarettes (HHS, 2016b). Rates of ever use were similar in the 2016 MTF survey, ranging from 17.5 percent among 8th grade students to 29.0 percent among 10th graders, and 33.8 percent among high school seniors (Schulenberg et al., 2017). The most recent youth rates reported from the PATH survey (Wave 1 in 2013–2014) indicate much lower rates of ever use, with only 10.7 percent of youth ages 12 to 17 reporting ever using an e-cigarette even once or twice (Backinger, 2017). Conversely, rates in the 2015 YRBS are substantially higher, with 44.9 percent of high school students reporting ever using "electronic vapor products" (Kann et al., 2016). As can be seen, the proportion of youth who reported ever using e-cigarettes varies substantially across surveys. With respect to use in the past 30 days, the 2016 NYTS reported that 4.3 percent of middle school students and 11.3 percent of high school students reported any e-cigarette use in the past 30 days (Jamal et al., 2017). Table 1-1 shows

TABLE 1-1 Percentage of High School and Middle School Students Who Have Ever Used E-Cigarettes; National Youth Tobacco Survey (NYTS) 2011–2016

	2011	2012	2013	2014	2015	2016
	% (95% CI)	% (95% CI)	% (95% CI)	% (95% CI)	% (95% CI)	% (95% CI)
High School	1.5 (1.2–2.0)	2.8 (2.3–3.5)	4.5 (3.8–5.3)	13.4 (11.2–16.1)	16.0 (14.1–18.0)	11.3 (9.9–12.9)
Middle School	0.6 (0.4–0.9)	1.1 (0.9–1.5)	1.1 (0.8–1.5)	3.9 (3.0–5.0)	5.3 (4.6–6.2)	4.3 (3.7–4.9)

SOURCES: HHS, 2016b; Jamal et al., 2017.

the percentage of high school and middle school students who have ever used e-cigarettes, 2011 to 2016, in NYTS. MTF rates for 2016 are similar, with 6.2 percent of 8th graders, 11.0 percent of 10th graders, and 12.5 percent of 12th grade students reporting e-cigarette use in the past 30 days (Schulenberg et al., 2017). Again, youth use rates reported in the PATH Wave 1 survey in 2013–2014 are the lowest, with only 3.1 percent of youth age 12 to 17 reporting current use (Backinger, 2017), while rates among high school students in the 2015 YRBS are again the highest, at 24.1 percent (Kann et al., 2016).

Rates of frequent e-cigarette use among youth are quite low overall. The 2015 NYTS reported that 0.6 percent of all middle school students (comprising 11.7 percent of current middle school users) and 2.5 percent of all high school students (comprising 15.5 percent of current high school users) use e-cigarettes frequently (HHS, 2016b). Rates in PATH Wave 1 (2013–2014) among all youth age 12 to 17 are similarly low overall, at just 0.1 percent (Backinger, 2017).

As described above, little trend data are available. NYTS reports an increase in current use among middle schoolers from 0.6 percent in 2011 to a high of 5.3 percent in 2015, and among high schoolers from 1.5 percent in 2011 to 16.0 percent in 2015 (HHS, 2016b). Current use declined in 2016 to 4.3 percent among middle schoolers and 11.3 percent among high schoolers (Jamal et al., 2017). Due to changing terminology and definitions in MTF, it was only able to report trends from 2015 to 2016, but similar to NYTS, MTF reported a statistically significant decline in current use between these 2 years (Johnston et al., 2017). Trend data are not available for the YRBS or PATH.

Electronic cigarette use varies substantially across demographic subgroups, including age, gender, and race and ethnicity. In terms of age, e-cigarette use tends to increase with age among youth across all measures of use. For example, rates of ever, past 30-day, and frequent e-cigarette use are lower for middle school students compared with high school students in NYTS (HHS, 2016b; Jamal et al., 2017). Similarly, both ever and past 30-day use are lower in 8th compared with 10th and 12th and 10th compared with 12th grade students in MTF (Schulenberg et al., 2017). E-cigarette use also varies by gender, with typically greater use among boys than girls (Jamal et al., 2017). E-cigarette use also varies by race and ethnicity and generally is highest among youth who identify as Hispanic and non-Hispanic white (HHS, 2016b; Jamal et al., 2017).

In 2016, among youth who reported using tobacco, e-cigarettes were the most common form used. The 2016 MTF shows that 6.2 percent of 8th graders, 11.0 percent of 10th graders, and 12.5 percent of 12th graders reported e-cigarette use in the past 30 days (Schulenberg et al., 2017). This compares with 2.6 percent of 8th graders, 4.9 percent of 10th graders, and

10.5 percent of 12th graders reporting past 30-day combustible tobacco cigarette smoking (Schulenberg et al., 2017). Similarly, according to the 2016 NYTS, nearly double the number of middle school students (4.3 percent) reported currently using e-cigarettes compared with the next three products—combustible tobacco cigarettes, cigars, and smokeless tobacco (each at 2.2 percent), which were followed by hookah (2.0 percent), pipe tobacco (0.7 percent), and trailed by bidis (0.3 percent) (Jamal et al., 2017). Among high school students, 11.3 percent reported using e-cigarettes in the past 30 days, compared with only 8.0 percent combustible tobacco cigarette use, 7.7 percent cigar use, 5.8 percent smokeless tobacco use, 4.8 percent hookah use, 1.4 percent pipe tobacco use, and 0.5 percent bidi use. This pattern holds for all subgroups by race and ethnicity except among black middle and high school males who reported highest rates of cigar smoking followed by e-cigarette use (4.5 percent compared with 4.0 percent among middle schoolers and 9.5 percent compared with 6.2 percent among high schoolers) (Jamal et al., 2017).

Among those who reported having ever used an e-cigarette, youth most commonly reported using rechargeable/refillable tank-style devices, with more than half (53.4 percent) of middle and high school students reporting using only this kind of device (Singh et al., 2016). A total of 14.5 percent reported using only disposable models, and nearly one-third (32.1 percent) reported using both (Singh et al., 2016).

Even given the patterns of use described above, it remains unclear what precisely youth are vaping. Substantial proportions of youth report using non-nicotine electronic cigarettes. Among middle and high school students in the 2015 NYTS, nearly one-third (32.5 percent) of ever users of electronic cigarettes reported ever using an electronic cigarette device for any other substance other than for nicotine (Singh et al., 2016). Rates were similar among middle school students (33.7 percent) and high school students (32.2 percent). By contrast, analysis of the 2015 MTF found that nearly two-thirds of e-cigarette–ever users reported vaping "just flavoring" at last use. Again, rates were similar among 8th (66.0 percent), 10th (65.2 percent), and 12th (64.7 percent) grade students (CTP, 2017c). After "just flavoring," e-cigarette–ever users of all ages next most commonly reported last vaping nicotine (22.2 percent among 12th grade students, 19.9 percent among 10th grade students, and 13.3 percent among 8th graders). Among ever users of all ages, roughly 6 percent reported vaping marijuana, and 13.7 percent of 8th graders, 7.7 percent of 10th graders, and 6.3 percent of 12th graders reported not knowing what they last vaped. Rates of last vaping just flavoring among past 30-day users are slightly lower compared with ever users, but still most common, except among 12th grade students who reported vaping six or more times in the past 30 days who most commonly vaped nicotine; 62.7 percent of 8th,

59.5 percent of 10th, and 59.2 percent of 12th graders reported last vaping just flavoring. After "just flavoring," past 30-day vapers most commonly reported vaping nicotine (16.2 percent in 8th grade, 27.4 percent in 10th grade, 30.7 percent in 12th grade), followed by marijuana (10.6 percent in 8th grade, 8.75 percent in 10th grade, 5.2 percent in 12th grade), and don't know (7.9 percent in 8th grade, 3.7 percent in 10th grade, 4.0 percent in 12th grade) (Miech et al., 2017).

Adults

Rates of e-cigarette use among adults (age 18 and older) are relatively low when compared with youth e-cigarette use and to adult combustible tobacco cigarette smoking. The 2014 NHIS survey reported that 12.6 percent of adults ever used e-cigarettes (Schoenborn and Gindi, 2015). The 2014–2015 TUS-CPS reported a substantially lower rate of ever use among adults, at 8.5 percent (Zhu et al., 2017). In terms of current (past 30-day) use, the PATH Wave 1 survey in 2013–2014 reported the highest rates of current use of e-cigarettes, at 5.5 percent (Coleman et al., 2017). NHIS data from 2014 show that 3.7 percent of adults reported currently using e-cigarettes (Schoenborn and Gindi, 2015). The rate of current use was lowest in the 2014–2015 TUS-CPS, at 2.4 percent (Zhu et al., 2017). According to PATH Wave 1 data, among current users, 21.3 percent reported daily use, 36.5 percent reported moderate use (more than 2 of the past 30 days), and 42.2 percent reported infrequent use (0 to 2 of the past 30 days) (Coleman et al., 2017).

Most adult e-cigarette users report currently using other tobacco products. According to data from Wave 1 of the PATH survey, among current users of e-cigarettes, 69.7 percent were current smokers, 8.6 percent quit smoking combustible tobacco cigarettes within the past year, and 5.7 percent were former smokers (abstained from smoking for more than 1 year) (Coleman et al., 2017). Interestingly, 16 percent of adult current users of e-cigarettes reported having never smoked combustible tobacco cigarettes. Additionally, 39.2 percent of current e-cigarette users reported current use of other combustible tobacco products (filtered cigars, cigarillos, traditional cigars, hookahs, and pipes) and 8.9 percent reported current use of non-combustible tobacco products (smokeless tobacco [snus pouches, loose snus, moist snuff, dip, spit, or chewing tobacco] and dissolvable tobacco) (Coleman et al., 2017).

As with data on youth use, limited trend data are available on e-cigarette use among adults. MTF reported no significant change in ever use among college students from 2015 to 2016 (26.0 percent to 26.8 percent), a non-significant decrease in ever use among all young adults ages 19 to 30 (30.3 percent to 26.9 percent), a non-significant decrease in past

30-day use among college students from 8.8 percent to 6.9 percent, and a significant decrease in past 30-day use among all young adults (9.2 percent to 6.0 percent) (Schulenberg et al., 2017). These MTF data for young adults echo the decreases in youth use.

Among adults as among youth, patterns of use vary by demographic subgroups—age, gender, and race and ethnicity. With respect to age, e-cigarette use is generally greatest among young adults, and decreases with increasing age. According to 2016 MTF data, 26 percent of college students and young adults reported ever using electronic cigarettes, and 5.8 percent reported past 30-day use (Schulenberg et al., 2017). Past 30-day use is highest among those age 19 to 22 (8 percent) and declines steadily by age groups through those age 25 to 30 (Schulenberg et al., 2017). Similarly, the rate of ever use is highest among adults age 18 to 24 (21.6 percent), declining steadily with increased age in the 2014 NHIS (Schoenborn and Gindi, 2015). According to the 2013–2014 NATS, 35.8 percent of young adults age 18 to 24 reported ever using an electronic cigarette and 13.6 percent reported current use (HHS, 2016b). This compares with 16.4 percent of adults age 25 and older who reported ever using an e-cigarette and 5.7 percent who reported current use (HHS, 2016b). The PATH Wave 1 data on e-cigarette use also differ significantly by age for all use groups (daily, moderate, and frequent users) (Coleman et al., 2017). However, the PATH data show a slightly different pattern, with the highest use rates among adults age 25 to 34 (26.4 percent), followed by young adults age 18 to 24 (20.9 percent), and then decreasing with age among those 35 years and older.

Similar to youth use, differences in e-cigarette use among adults by gender typically show greater use among men compared with women. Significantly more men (14.2 percent) reported ever using electronic cigarettes compared with women (11.2 percent) in the 2014 NHIS data (Schoenborn and Gindi, 2015). In the PATH Wave 1 survey, current e-cigarette use was higher for men compared with women overall (53.5 percent compared with 46.5 percent, respectively). Among current users, use was also higher for men compared with women when stratified by intensity of use (daily, moderate, and infrequent use), but differences were not significant (Coleman et al., 2017). Similarly, according to the 2013–2014 NATS, among adults age 25 years and older, more men reported ever (18.3 percent), currently (6.6 percent), and frequently (23.0 percent among current users, 1.5 percent among all adults) using e-cigarettes than women (14.7 percent ever use, 5.0 percent current use, 20.6 percent frequent use among current users, and 1.0 percent current use among all adults) (HHS, 2016b).

Adult e-cigarette use also varies by racial and ethnic group. Data from the 2014 NHIS show that a significantly greater percentage of non-Hispanic whites (14.8 percent) reported ever using electronic cigarettes, followed by

Hispanic (8.6 percent), black (7.1 percent), and Asian (6.2 percent) adults. American Indian or Alaska Native (AI/AN) adults reported the highest rates of ever use, with greater than one in five reporting ever using e-cigarettes (Schoenborn and Gindi, 2015). Ever use of e-cigarettes was significantly higher among AIs/ANs compared with Hispanic, black, and Asian subgroups. PATH Wave 1 data (2013–2014) on current e-cigarette users show similar patterns by race and ethnicity. Among adult current users, significantly higher proportions of non-Hispanic whites (71.0 percent) currently use e-cigarettes, followed by Hispanics (12.7 percent), blacks (9.3 percent), those identifying as other race or multiracial (3.8 percent), and Asians (2.7 percent) (Coleman et al., 2017). Interestingly, in contrast to the highest rates of ever use among AIs/ANs in the NHIS data, rates of AI/AN current use from the PATH data are the lowest among all racial and ethnic subgroups, at only 0.6 percent (Coleman et al., 2017).

Among adults, device characteristics vary significantly by frequency of use. Among daily users, 73.6 percent used a refillable device and 91.6 percent used a rechargeable device (Coleman et al., 2017). Among those daily users who reported using a rechargeable device, only 42.3 percent reported use of cartridges. Among moderate e-cigarette users, 51.4 percent reported using a refillable device, 78.0 percent reported using a rechargeable device, and 61.5 percent of those using rechargeable devices reported using cartridges. By contrast, fewer than one-third (32.4 percent) of infrequent e-cigarette users reported using a refillable device and 58.6 percent reported using a rechargeable device; among those using rechargeable devices, 71.0 percent reported using cartridges. With respect to what substance adults are vaping, most adults reported vaping e-cigarettes that contain nicotine—91.2 percent of daily users, 88.2 percent of non-daily users, and 89.5 percent of both daily and non-daily users overall (Coleman et al., 2017). Approximately two-thirds of current users also reported using a non-tobacco flavored brand; these flavors include menthol, mint, clove, spice, candy, fruit, chocolate, alcohol (e.g., wine or cognac), or other sweet flavors (Coleman et al., 2017).

POTENTIAL PUBLIC HEALTH RISKS AND BENEFITS OF E-CIGARETTES

Electronic cigarettes contain constituents that are not inert and are likely to have some negative health effects on their own. Although toxic combustion products associated with cancers are less likely to be present, e-cigarettes emit potentially toxic substances including fine particulate matter, metals, and nicotine. These substances are known to cause adverse health consequences such as cardiovascular and respiratory illnesses. However, understanding the public health consequences of electronic cigarettes requires an understanding of the context of tobacco control in the United States. Because e-cigarette use is understood not as a unitary and isolated phenomenon and because the known risks of combustible tobacco are so great, the net public health impact of e-cigarettes is expected to result from the effects of e-cigarette use on combustible tobacco cigarette smoking. Therefore, understanding the net public health effect of e-cigarettes requires understanding not only the inherent risks of e-cigarettes, but also the relationship between e-cigarette use and combustible tobacco cigarette use.

A central issue addressed in this report is the use of e-cigarettes as a harm-reduction tool, with a thorough evaluation of the evidence base for the hypothesis that electronic cigarettes are substantially less harmful and are a less toxic alternative to combustible tobacco cigarettes, because combustion, which produces substantial toxic substances, does not occur. Thus, among adult populations, to the extent that e-cigarette use promotes either reduction or complete abstinence from combustible tobacco smoking, e-cigarettes may help to reduce health risks. E-cigarettes could similarly reduce risks to youth who take up e-cigarettes instead of combustible tobacco cigarettes. This may be especially beneficial for certain vulnerable populations, such as pregnant women or smokers with physical (e.g., chronic respiratory or cardiovascular illness) or mental health comorbidities. Pregnancy is a vulnerable life stage because deleterious exposures to women during pregnancy may negatively impact child development (Bruin et al., 2010). Some evidence suggests that pregnant women increasingly switch from smoking combustible tobacco cigarettes to e-cigarettes because of their perceived lower harm (Bruin et al., 2010). This may bear out, but e-cigarettes also typically contain nicotine, which is known to harm child development (Bruin et al., 2010). Thus, the possible health effects of maternal e-cigarette exposure on the developing fetus remain unclear. Similarly, smokers with illnesses that could be caused or worsened by smoking, such as asthma, chronic obstructive pulmonary disease, cardiovascular disease, and cancer already experience heightened health risks of continued cigarette use. If e-cigarettes are effective for reducing or abstaining from combustible tobacco cigarette smoking, those with medical comorbidities may experience the greatest benefits from reducing their overall tobacco-related risks (Kruse et al., 2017). In these scenarios, the concern is the health effects of e-cigarettes compared with combustible tobacco cigarette use.

To the extent that laboratory tests of e-cigarette ingredients, in vitro toxicological tests, and short-term human studies suggest that e-cigarettes are likely less harmful than combustible tobacco cigarettes, due to lack of long-term epidemiological studies and large clinical trials, the implications for long-term effects on morbidity and mortality are not yet clear and the absolute safety of the products cannot be unambiguously assessed at this time and concerns about the uptake of e-cigarettes among youth and young adults remain. Youth are a particularly vulnerable group, as they may be more likely to engage in risky behavior and experiment with illicit drugs and alcohol, and are differentially affected by nicotine or other toxicants throughout development (IOM, 2015). Thus, e-cigarette use among youth and young adults is especially worrying if e-cigarettes cause dependence or the normalization of smoking behavior, and subsequently lead youth and young adults to start smoking combustible tobacco cigarettes. This is of particular concern for youth who otherwise would never have smoked. Furthermore, concerns have been raised that e-cigarettes may deter current combustible tobacco cigarette smokers from quitting smoking or cause them to relapse. In these scenarios, the concern is the health effect of e-cigarettes (including transition to combustible tobacco cigarette use) compared with no use of either product.

In short, understanding the potential health risks and benefits of e-cigarettes requires an understanding of the risks of e-cigarettes relative to both cigarette smoke as well as never using any tobacco. Future regulatory strategies will determine whether the risks associated with electronic cigarettes (i.e., their potential to cause harm on their own, or through initiation of combustible tobacco cigarette smoking among individuals and populations) are sufficiently balanced with benefits (e.g., positive harm-reduction potential among individuals and populations).

REGULATORY BACKGROUND

The Family Smoking Prevention and Tobacco Control Act of 2009 (the Tobacco Control Act) granted FDA authority to regulate tobacco products manufactured, marketed, and distributed in the United States. While this included cigarettes, cigars, loose tobacco, and smokeless tobacco products, it did not include provisions specifically for electronic cigarettes. Rather, the law stated that any other tobacco products that the Secretary of Health and Human Services deems as relevant to the law may be included under FDA's regulatory jurisdiction. Importantly, the Tobacco Control Act considers any product a "tobacco product" if it includes any constituent "made or derived from tobacco," but is not otherwise regulated as a "drug," "device," or "combination product."[2] To regulate electronic cigarettes as tobacco products, FDA was required to undertake the rulemaking process. In May 2016, FDA published the final "deeming rule" (HHS, 2016a). Major provisions of the rule are listed in Box 1-2.

Given the possibility of pending product standards, marketing restrictions, and other regulations, the deeming rule has received both praise

[2] Family Smoking Prevention and Tobacco Control Act of 2009, Public Law 111-31 § 906, 111th Cong. (June 22, 2009).

BOX 1-2
Major Provisions of the Food and Drug Administration Deeming Tobacco Products to Be Subject to the Federal Food, Drug, and Cosmetic Act, as Amended by the Family Smoking Prevention and Tobacco Control Act

- Restricts adulterated and misbranded products
- Requires disclosure of ingredient lists and documented health effects
- Requires registration of manufacturers
- Requires disclosure of a list of all tobacco products, including information related to labeling and advertising
- Requires premarket review of new tobacco products, or those not on the market as of February 15, 2007
- Restricts products marketed with claims about harm reduction
- Prohibits sales to minors
- Prohibits products without a nicotine warning
- Prohibits vending machine sales of electronic cigarette products, except in facilities that never admit youth
- Grants the Food and Drug Administration the authority to:
  - Institute product standards, including on device specifications, flavoring, other constituents, package sizes, child-resistant packaging, health warnings, and nicotine levels.
  - Restrict marketing and advertising, including the promotion of products on self-service displays and sponsorship of events by electronic cigarette manufacturers.

and criticism. Some scientific researchers believe the deeming rule can set in motion more rigorous and thoughtful research practices on e-cigarettes, thereby providing a strong evidence base for regulation and eventually reducing mortality from combustible tobacco product use (Backinger et al., 2016). Yet various stakeholders, including manufacturers, retailers, and consumers, are likely to hold different opinions about provisions in the deeming rule. For instance, under the deeming rule, anyone who "makes, modifies, mixes, manufactures, fabricates, assembles, processes, labels, repacks, relabels, or imports" any electronic cigarette product qualifies as a tobacco product "manufacturer," and is therefore subject to the existing rules governing tobacco products (CTP, 2017c). Manufacturers will need to bear the burden of proof for their products to remain on the market after August 8, 2022, undergoing the premarket application submission process to obtain FDA authorization.

Given the regulatory hurdle, many independent manufacturers may not have the capital to remain in the market, whereas larger companies will more easily overcome these financial barriers (Russell, 2016). Similarly, retailers may also feel encumbered by regulation, including restrictions on selling from vending machines, providing free samples, or selling any e-cigarette products or posting advertisements without visible and clear health warnings (CTP, 2017d). These regulatory changes may affect consumer behaviors. It has been suggested, for instance, that consumers may buy their current product of choice in bulk before it is removed from the market. Some may continue to buy products from an unlicensed vendor. Others still may begin mixing their own e-liquids at home, or begin smoking combustible tobacco cigarettes (Russell, 2016). Determining how manufacturers, retailers, and consumers will react to government policies is an important element in designing regulation and in predicting subsequent public health impacts.

The U.S. regulatory approach toward e-cigarettes is grounded in and shaped by its past regulation of tobacco, and other countries have followed different paths and arrived at very different approaches. Table 1-2 summarizes key events in the history of e-cigarette regulation in the United States. At least 68 different countries currently regulate e-cigarettes

TABLE 1-2 Summary of the Key Events in the History of E-Cigarette Regulation

Year	Event
1964	Luther L. Terry, Surgeon General, releases first report of the Surgeon General's Advisory Committee on Smoking and Health.[a]
1965	Herbert A. Gilbert's patent request for an early approximation of an e-cigarette is approved on August 17.[b]
1992	Passage of the Synar Amendment to Alcohol, Drug Abuse, and Mental Health Administration Reorganization Act on July 10 requires states to restrict sale and distribution of tobacco products to minors.[c] Prescription nicotine patches are introduced to the U.S. market as smoking cessation aids.[d]
1995	FDA declares cigarettes "drug delivery devices" and proposes marketing and sales restrictions to reduce youth initiation.[e]
2000	On March 21, the Supreme Court affirms the 1998 court case ruling that FDA lacks the jurisdiction under the Federal Food, Drug, and Cosmetic Act to regulate tobacco. FDA subsequently revokes the final rule issued in 1995 as it is invalid.[f]
2003	Chinese pharmacist Hon Lik develops modern e-cigarette as it is currently known. It is entered into the market under the company Ruyan.[g]

TABLE 1-2 Continued

Year	Event
2006	On August 22, the first import ruling in the U.S. Customs database appears. Electronic cigarettes have been officially introduced to the United States.[h]
2009	In April, FDA denies import of e-cigarettes and accessories, as products appear to be unapproved drug-delivery devices.[i]
	In June, President Barack Obama signs the Family Smoking Prevention and Tobacco Control Act into law, giving FDA the authority to regulate tobacco products to protect public health. CTP is established; FDA announces a ban on combustible tobacco cigarettes with fruit, candy, or clove flavorings.[j]
2010	U.S. District Court for the District of Columbia enters judgment in favor of Smoking Everywhere and NJOY, ruling that e-cigarettes are not drug-delivery devices, as the intended use of e-cigarettes is to encourage nicotine use, not discourage, prevent, or mitigate.[k]
2011	On April 25, CTP issues a press release announcing its intention to regulate e-cigarettes as tobacco products.[l]
2016	On May 10, FDA issues final deeming rule: all products that meet definition of tobacco product (including e-cigarettes) are subject to CTP regulation.[m]
	HHS releases the report *E-Cigarette Use Among Youth and Young Adults: A Report of the Surgeon General*.[n]
2017	On July 28, FDA announces intentions to regulate nicotine levels in tobacco products.[o]

NOTE: CTP = Center for Tobacco Products; FDA = Food and Drug Administration; HHS = Department of Health and Human Services.
SOURCES:
[a] CDC, 2009.
[b] Gilbert, 1965.
[c] Alcohol, Drug Abuse, and Mental Health Administration Reorganization Act of 1992, Public Law 102-321, 102nd Cong. (July 10, 1992).
[d] Pastore et al., 2015.
[e] FDA, 2014.
[f] CDC, 2015.
[g] HHS, 2016b.
[h] CBP, 2006.
[i] *Smoking Everywhere, Inc., Sottera, Inc. and d/b/a NJOY v. U.S. Food and Drug Administration et al.*, 680 F. Supp. 2d 62 (D.C. Cir. 2010).
[j] FDA, 2014.
[k] *Smoking Everywhere, Inc., Sottera, Inc. and d/b/a NJOY v. U.S. Food and Drug Administration et al.*, 680 F. Supp. 2d 62 (D.C. Cir. 2010).
[l] CTP, 2011.
[m] CTP, 2017a.
[n] HHS, 2016b.
[o] CTP, 2017b.

in some fashion (Kennedy et al., 2017). Some policies are more permissive, such as in the United Kingdom, while others are more restrictive, such as in Australia. Implicit in many of the policies is an underlying assumption about the health effects of e-cigarette use, with the more permissive policies often based on the goal of maximizing the assumed health benefits of e-cigarette use and the more restrictive policies based on the goal of minimizing their assumed harm. An evaluation of the evidence on the health effects of e-cigarettes offers the opportunity to identify which harms and benefits are scientifically proven, which in turn would ultimately be the key outcomes to consider in evaluation of different e-cigarette policies and their population impact.

An important provision of the Tobacco Control Act is what is known as the public health standard. Unlike FDA regulation of pharmaceuticals under the standard of "safe and effective," FDA regulates tobacco products based on a public health standard that considers the risks and benefits of the tobacco product on the population as a whole.[3] Functionally, this means that FDA considers the effect of a tobacco product not only on those who use the product (e.g., smokers), but also on those who do not (e.g., people who have quit smoking combustible tobacco cigarettes but might relapse due to the presence on the market of a newly introduced product, or people who might begin to use tobacco who would not have otherwise). Products introduced onto the market after February 15, 2007 (such as most e-cigarettes) and products with a modified-risk claim must be shown to have a net population health benefit, for users and non-users of the product.

OUTLINE OF THE REPORT

Chapter 2 outlines the committee's approach to identifying, reviewing, and assessing evidence on the effects of e-cigarettes on individual and population health. The report is then organized into three sections. The same standards of evidence assessment were applied to any outcome assessed, in all three sections of the report, so as not to give preference to harms or benefits. Section I includes three chapters reviewing the evidence on e-cigarette devices, constituents, and exposures. Section I ends with research recommendations related to those chapters. Section II begins with a chapter on modes of action of e-cigarette constituents and their relevance to human health. Seven chapters follow describing the evidence regarding the effects of e-cigarettes on human health, ranging from dependence to cardiovascular disease to burns from exploding

[3] Family Smoking Prevention and Tobacco Control Act of 2009, Public Law 111-31 § 906, 111th Cong. (June 22, 2009).

device batteries. As shown in Appendix B, the committee did not limit its literature search to health outcomes that were "negative" or "harmful." These chapters are not limited to comparisons with the effects of combustible tobacco cigarettes, and much of the literature assesses the effects of e-cigarette exposure independent of combustible tobacco exposure. Section II concludes with research recommendations. Section III addresses the public health implications of e-cigarettes, including chapters reviewing the evidence on the effects of e-cigarettes on youth initiation of combustible tobacco cigarettes, on adult cessation of combustible tobacco cigarettes, and on harm reduction, that is, a comparison between the effects of e-cigarettes and combustible tobacco cigarettes. A chapter using population dynamic modeling presents the results of a range of scenarios of the possible effects of e-cigarettes on a population measure of mortality (years of life lost) and reflects the range of conclusions relevant to the public health standard FDA is statutorily obligated to use in its regulatory decision making about tobacco products. Section III concludes with a chapter on research needs. The report ends with a chapter of brief concluding observations.

REFERENCES

Alexander, J. P., B. N. Coleman, S. E. Johnson, G. K. Tessman, C. Tworek, and D. M. Dickinson. 2016. Smoke and vapor: Exploring the terminology landscape among electronic cigarette users. *Tobacco Regulatory Science* 2(3):204–213.

Backinger, C. L. 2017. *Youth use of electronic cigarettes.* http://c.ymcdn.com/sites/www.srnt.org/resource/resmgr/conferences/2017_annual_meeting/FDA_PreCon_Slides/Backinger_youth_e-cig_SRNT20.pdf (accessed September 18, 2017).

Backinger, C. L., H. Meissner, and D. L. Ashley. 2016. The FDA "deeming rule" and tobacco regulatory research. *Tobacco Regulatory Science* 2(3):290–293.

Bruin, J. E., H. C. Gerstein, and A. C. Holloway. 2010. Long-term consequences of fetal and neonatal nicotine exposure: A critical review. *Toxicological Sciences* 116(2):364–374.

CBP (U.S. Customs and Border Protection). 2006. *NY M85579: The tariff classification of a nicotine inhaler and parts from China.* https://rulings.cbp.gov/index.asp?ru=m85579&qu=NY+M85579&vw=detail (accessed September 18, 2017).

CDC (Centers for Disease Control and Prevention). 2009. *History of the Surgeon General's reports on smoking and health.* https://www.cdc.gov/tobacco/data_statistics/sgr/history/index.htm (accessed September 18, 2017).

CDC. 2015. *Highlights: Tobacco timeline.* https://www.cdc.gov/tobacco/data_statistics/sgr/2000/highlights/historical/index.htm (accessed September 14, 2017).

Coleman, B. N., B. Rostron, S. E. Johnson, B. K. Ambrose, J. Pearson, C. A. Stanton, B. Wang, C. Delnevo, M. Bansal-Travers, H. L. Kimmel, M. L. Goniewicz, R. Niaura, D. Abrams, K. P. Conway, N. Borek, W. M. Compton, and A. Hyland. 2017. Electronic cigarette use among U.S. adults in the Population Assessment of Tobacco and Health (PATH) study, 2013–2014. *Tobacco Control* 26:e117–e126.

CTP (Center for Tobacco Products). 2011. *Stakeholder letter: Regulation of e-cigarettes and other tobacco products.* https://www.fda.gov/newsevents/publichealthfocus/ucm252360.htm (accessed September 18, 2017).

CTP. 2017a. *Extension of certain tobacco product compliance deadlines related to the final deeming rule: Guidance for industry (revised).* https://www.fda.gov/downloads/TobaccoProducts/Labeling/RulesRegulationsGuidance/UCM557716.pdf (accessed September 18, 2017).

CTP. 2017b. *FDA announces comprehensive regulatory plan to shift trajectory of tobacco-related disease, death.* https://www.fda.gov/NewsEvents/Newsroom/PressAnnouncements/ucm568923.htm (accessed September 18, 2017).

CTP. 2017c. *Manufacturing.* https://www.fda.gov/TobaccoProducts/GuidanceComplianceRegulatoryInformation/Manufacturing/default.htm (accessed September 19, 2017).

CTP. 2017d. *Summary of federal rules for tobacco retailers.* https://www.fda.gov/TobaccoProducts/GuidanceComplianceRegulatoryInformation/Retail/ucm205021.htm (accessed September 19, 2017).

FDA (Food and Drug Administration). 2014. *Significant dates in U.S. food and drug law history.* https://www.fda.gov/aboutfda/whatwedo/history/milestones/ucm128305.htm (accessed September 14, 2017).

Gilbert, H. A., inventor. 1965. Smokeless non-tobacco cigarette. U.S. Patent 3,200,819. http://patft.uspto.gov/netacgi/nph-Parser?Sect1=PTO1&Sect2=HITOFF&d=PALL&p=1&u=%2Fnetahtml%2FPTO%2Fsrchnum.htm&r=1&f=G&l=50&s1=3200819.PN.&OS=PN/3200819&RS=PN/3200819 (accessed October 18, 2017).

HHS (U.S. Department of Health and Human Services). 2016a. Deeming tobacco products to be subject to the federal Food, Drug, and Cosmetic Act, as amended by the Family Smoking Prevention and Tobacco Control Act; restrictions on the sale and distribution of tobacco products and required warning statements for tobacco products. *Federal Register* 81(90):28973–29106.

HHS. 2016b. *E-cigarette use among youth and young adults: A report of the Surgeon General.* Atlanta, GA: U.S. Department of Health and Human Services, Centers for Disease Control and Prevention, National Center for Chronic Disease Prevention and Health Promotion, Office on Smoking and Health.

IOM (Institute of Medicine). 2015. *Public health implications of raising the minimum age of legal access to tobacco products.* Washington, DC: The National Academies Press.

Jamal, A., A. Gentzke, S. Hu, K. A. Cullen, B. J. Apelberg, D. M. Homa, and B. A. King. 2017. Tobacco use among middle and high school students—United States, 2011–2016. *Morbidity and Mortality Weekly Report* 66(23):597–603.

Johnston, L. D., P. M. O'Malley, R. Miech, J. G. Bachman, and J. E. Schulenberg. 2017. *Monitoring the Future national survey results on drug use, 1975–2016: Overview, key findings on adolescent drug use.* Ann Arbor: Institute for Social Research, University of Michigan.

Kann, L., T. McManus, W. A. Harris, S. L. Shanklin, K. H. Flint, J. Hawkins, B. Queen, R. Lowry, E. O. Olsen, D. Chyen, L. Whittle, J. Thornton, C. Lim, Y. Yamakawa, N. Brener, and S. Zaza. 2016. Youth risk behavior surveillance—United States, 2015. *Morbidity and Mortality Weekly Report* 65(6):1–174.

Kennedy, R. D., A. Awopegba, E. De León, and J. E. Cohen. 2017. Global approaches to regulating electronic cigarettes. *Tobacco Control* 26(4):440–445.

Kruse, G. R., S. Kalkhoran, and N. A. Rigotti. 2017. Use of electronic cigarettes among U.S. adults with medical comorbidities. *American Journal of Preventive Medicine* 52(6):798–804.

Miech, R., M. E. Patrick, P. M. O'Malley, and L. D. Johnston. 2017. What are kids vaping? Results from a national survey of U.S. adolescents. *Tobacco Control* 26(4):386–391.

Pastore, M. N., Y. N. Kalia, M. Horstmann, and M. S. Roberts. 2015. Transdermal patches: History, development and pharmacology. *British Journal of Pharmacology* 172(9):2179–2209.

Russell, C. 2016. Unintended consequences of the FDA's e-cigarette regulations. In *The Hill*: Capitol Hill Publishing Corp.

Schoenborn, C. A., and R. M. Gindi. 2015. Electronic cigarette use among adults: United States, 2014. *NCHS Data Brief* (217):1–8.

Schulenberg, J. E., L. D. Johnston, P. M. O'Malley, J. G. Bachman, R. Miech, and M. E. Patrick. 2017. *2016 Volume II: College students & adults ages 19–55*. http://www.monitoringthefuture.org/pubs/monographs/mtf-vol2_2016.pdf (accessed September 18, 2017).

Singh, T., S. Kennedy, K. Marynak, A. Persoskie, P. Melstrom, and B. A. King. 2016. Characteristics of electronic cigarette use among middle and high school students—United States, 2015. *Morbidity and Mortality Weekly Report* 65(5051):1425–1429.

U.S. Congress. 2016. *Division A-Agriculture, Rural Development, Food and Drug Administration, and Related Agencies Appropriations Act, 2016*. http://docs.house.gov/meetings/RU/RU00/20151216/104298/HMTG-114-RU00-20151216-SD002.pdf (accessed October 16, 2017).

Zhu, S. H., Y. L. Zhuang, S. Wong, S. E. Cummins, and G. J. Tedeschi. 2017. E-cigarette use and associated changes in population smoking cessation: Evidence from U.S. current population surveys. *BMJ* 358:j3262. https://doi.org/10.1136/bmj.j3262 (accessed February 6, 2018).

2

Committee Approach

The Statement of Task charges the committee with conducting a "comprehensive and systematic assessment and review of the literature" on the health effects of electronic cigarettes. The committee's approach to this task was informed by published guidelines for conducting systematic reviews, as well as the approaches taken by prior National Academies committees (CRD, 2009; Higgins and Green, 2011; IOM, 2011a, pp. 10–24, 2011b, 2016, pp. 8–10; NASEM, 2017; NRC, 2014; OHAT, 2015; Sena et al., 2014; Whiting et al., 2016). Notably, the committee's approach incorporated major attributes of systematic reviews. The committee systematically located, screened, and selected studies for review (including use of multiple databases to identify studies, predefined criteria to select studies for inclusion and exclusion, and systematically collecting data); evaluated individual studies for strengths and limitations; and synthesized findings into an assessment of the overall body of literature. The committee aims to be transparent about its process and thus describes its methods in this chapter and Appendix B with an eye to this goal.

The committee did not treat all bodies of evidence equally, and prioritized human studies (including studies on health effects as well as effects on combustible tobacco cigarette smoking initiation and cessation), which most relevantly bear on the committee's charge for its most structured assessments. The chapter begins with brief overviews of the committee's methods for identifying, reviewing, and assessing literature (more discussion of these methods is found in Appendix B). The chapter next describes the committee's approach to assessing causality and integrating data from human, animal, and in vitro studies. The chapter closes by presenting the standardized language the committee used to describe the weight of evidence assigned to its conclusions.

LITERATURE SEARCH

Working with a professional research librarian, the committee conducted a series of searches in six databases—PubMed, Scopus, World of Science, PsycINFO (ProQuest), MEDLINE (Ovid), and Embase (Ovid)—between February 1, 2017, and August 31, 2017,[1] to identify all literature on e-cigarettes. In all databases, the committee used the following key terms: e-cigarette, e-cigarettes, electronic cigarette, electronic cigarettes, electronic nicotine delivery, electronic nicotine device, vape, vaping, and e-liquid.[2] Searches in PubMed and MEDLINE also used the Medical Subject Headings (MeSH) term "electronic cigarettes." Special searches further restricting the results from the original searches were conducted to more precisely identify literature on e-cigarettes and dependence outcomes as well as combustible tobacco smoking initiation and cessation outcomes. The committee's literature search strategy is described comprehensively in Appendix B. After identifying literature, titles and abstracts of the search results were reviewed to identify studies for inclusion in the review. Inclusion criteria are listed in Appendix B. Studies that met the inclusion criteria were sorted by population (human, in vivo, animal, and in vitro) and outcomes for committee review and quality assessment.

LITERATURE REVIEW AND QUALITY ASSESSMENT

Health Effects Literature

For the assessment of studies on disease endpoints, in general, one committee member conducted an initial review of all literature identified pertaining to a set of outcomes. In its assessment of study strengths and limitations, the committee considered study design, elements of the design (e.g., sample size, setting, study population, exposure variables and methods of assessment, relevant controls or comparison groups, statistical methods, outcome measures assessed), other potential sources of

[1] Due to e-pub ahead of print and online first articles, 2018 citations were captured. In addition, a few 2016 and 2017 studies may not have been captured due to lags and discrepancies in database indexing.

[2] The committee excluded the term "e-liquid" from searches in Scopus and Web of Science, which are multidisciplinary databases, where the term produced results related to geothermal energy.

conflict of interest or bias,[3] and study results. After the initial review, a full committee discussion evaluated the first assessment, with particular attention to the strengths and weaknesses of individual studies. More information on the committee's qualitative assessment procedures can be found in Appendix B; special considerations for specific disease outcomes are discussed in Section II in the chapters on the relevant disease outcomes.

The committee used a modified approach to assess evidence from case studies, which are typically considered a weaker form of evidence. The committee looked for data on the patient (and patient characteristics where available), the exposure (including dose and other characteristics), and the conditions of the injury, accident, or other adverse outcome.

The committee also used a modified approach to assess in vivo animal and in vitro studies. The committee considered research design, conduct, analysis, and other sources of bias when assessing study strengths and weaknesses as it did for human studies.

Smoking Transitions Literature

The largest body of evidence was available on questions of e-cigarette use in relation to combustible tobacco cigarette smoking transitions (initiation and cessation). Not only are epidemiological studies available, but high-quality systematic reviews and meta-analyses also exist. Rather than replicating the efforts of these existing reviews, the committee began by assessing the quality of the existing reviews and then examined additional literature not included in the reviews. This supplemental literature was published after the search dates of the reviews or the committee judged that they contributed in some other way to the committee's ability to draw causal inferences about the relationship between e-cigarette use and subsequent smoking behavior. The committee's approach to causality is detailed in the next section. Methods to assess reviews were adapted from published guidelines and prior National Academies committees (NASEM, 2017; Whiting et al., 2016). Assessment of primary literature followed methods described above for assessment of literature on the

[3] The committee recognizes a range of non-scientific influences on research, including but not limited to the research sponsorship and source of employment. The committee also acknowledges particular concerns in literature on the health effects of tobacco products due to the tobacco industry's past involvement in manipulating evidence to support their interests. For completeness, the committee documented the source of research sponsorship (including the provision of e-cigarette products for use in trials), noting whether each study was funded by industry, a federal research agency, or other (e.g., university or foundation), or was not stated, as well as other industry participation in a table available as an online supplement at https://www.nap.edu/catalog/24952.

effects of e-cigarettes on health outcomes. Additional details and special considerations regarding the committee's approach to assessing causality for these combustible tobacco cigarette smoking outcomes are provided in Chapters 16 and 17.

The committee did not systematically or comprehensively review the health effects of known constituents and contaminants of e-cigarette devices or their refill solutions (e.g., nicotine, humectants, and certain metals). Because many of these constituents have been widely studied in other settings, the committee draws on existing bodies of evidence to describe the known health risks of these constituent parts.

APPROACH TO ASSESSING CAUSALITY

The committee faced some unique issues given the very recent introduction of e-cigarettes and limited empirical evidence for assessing their health effects. While there is a general consensus that high-quality epidemiological studies backed by solid toxicology and other mechanistic biological evidence provide the strongest basis for making firm inferences regarding causality, that simply does not exist for these devices. With only a few exceptions, the epidemiological literature is quite limited, and even where it is strongest (assessing short-term cardiovascular and respiratory effects), it does not address the etiology of chronic diseases. In other cases, such as cancer and reproductive health, there is simply no credible epidemiological research to consider.

Given this challenge, the committee drew upon indirect evidence based on knowledge of the health effects of some of the constituents of e-cigarette products, notably nicotine and humectants. While the nature of the devices makes the inferences based on analogy speculative, it does provide one line of evidence relevant to assessment of health effects of e-cigarettes. Another important source of evidence is from toxicology and other evidence with implications for biological mechanisms of e-cigarettes. The certainty, magnitude, and health relevance of these pathways bear on the value of such information for making causal inferences. For example, in vivo animal evidence may be more pertinent to inferences regarding human health effects than in vitro findings. Nevertheless, this toxicological and mechanistic literature provides evidence supporting the plausibility of various mechanisms by which e-cigarette exposure could influence health.

Tying these diverse threads of indirectly relevant evidence together to draw a summary conclusion is necessarily somewhat subjective, bringing together the knowledge and judgment of the committee as a whole to reach a consensus. To provide comparable inferences across the full array of health concerns, the committee modified approaches used in other National Academies reports and published guidelines on evidence synthesis (e.g., IOM, 2011a; NRC, 2007, 2014) to reach conclusions based on human evidence, animal evidence, and their integration.

Conceptual Framework

The committee developed a conceptual framework illustrating potential causal pathways by which e-cigarettes could affect health to help integrate and present evidence on known and likely e-cigarette exposures, potential mechanisms, intermediate outcomes, and disease endpoints. Figure 2-1 presents a simplified schematic of a generic plausible pathway between e-cigarettes and a health outcome. The committee presents modified frameworks applied to specific exposures, mechanisms, and

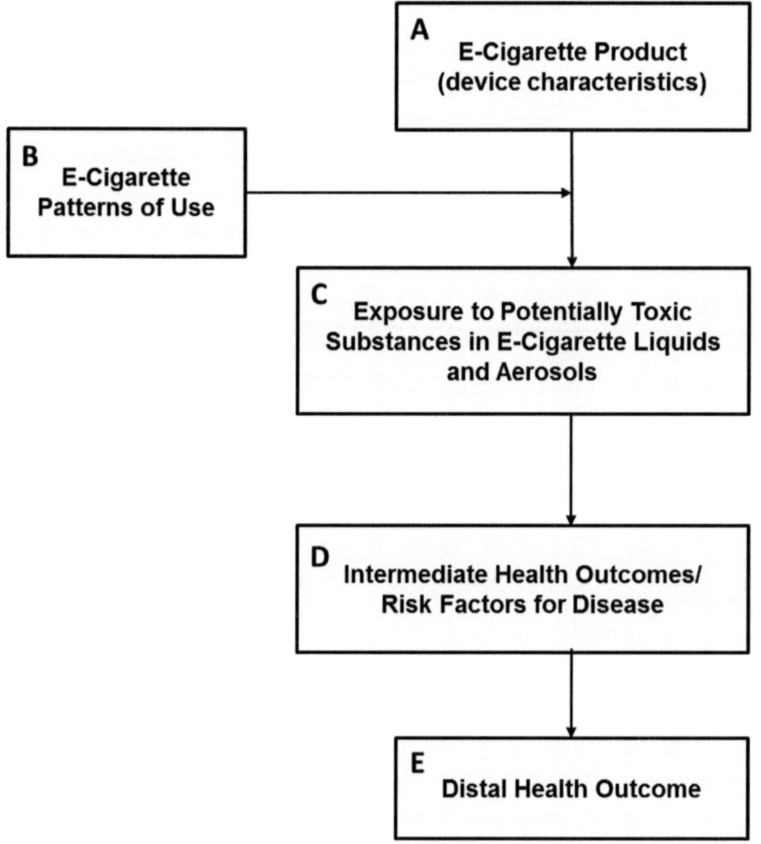

FIGURE 2-1 General and simplified conceptual framework of potential causal pathways by which e-cigarettes could affect health.

outcomes that represent plausible disease pathways for specific disease outcomes in Section II.

In Figure 2-1, the e-cigarette products used are shown at the top of the causal chain (Box A). Although e-cigarette devices and their components are not exposures per se, characteristics of e-cigarette products (e.g., nicotine concentration, power, etc.) influence the quantity and level of potential toxic substances emitted from the device. This emission, moderated by how the device is used (Box B), in turn influences users' exposure to potentially toxic substances in e-cigarette aerosols (i.e., what is inhaled, Box C). These exposures influence intermediate health outcomes (Box D) proximally before affecting disease endpoints more distally (Box E). Intermediate outcomes include biomarkers of exposure, mechanisms, and biomarkers or risk factors of disease; they also capture short-term effects of e-cigarettes on organ systems, such as short-term increases in blood pressure. Distal disease consequences relevant to e-cigarette exposure examined in this report include cardiovascular, respiratory, oral, cancer, developmental and reproductive, and dependence outcomes.

Because the committee is primarily concerned about distal health outcomes, evidence on the effects of e-cigarette exposure on these outcomes is most relevant for the committee's assessment of the health effects of e-cigarettes. In the absence of high-quality epidemiological evidence on these outcomes, the committee drew upon data further up the causal chain as additional evidence supportive of hypothesized disease pathways. Thus, to assess a given health risk, after examining evidence on long-term health outcomes, the committee looked to literature on intermediate or short-term outcomes, mechanisms, modes of action, and exposures from which it could draw inferences about potential health risk.

The committee considered data from humans to be most relevant for assessing human health risks of e-cigarettes, whereas additional animal data provide supporting evidence. For example, evidence of short-term effects of e-cigarette aerosol exposure from animal studies was considered weaker evidence compared with evidence of similar effects in humans. Although useful for hypothesis generation and critical for understanding mechanisms of health outcomes, because of important differences such as those pertaining to dose, duration of exposure, and changes in particles and constituents with aging, the relevance of in vitro data for establishing human health risk is uncertain.

Evidence Synthesis

The committee's assessment of data aimed to establish causation between e-cigarettes and a given health endpoint, not merely a statistical association. In the absence of high-quality epidemiological studies, the committee took into account several considerations to draw causal inferences from the evidence available. These considerations draw from criteria typically used to interpret and establish causation based on epidemiological data, and which are adapted from the approach taken in the 2014 Surgeon General's report on smoking and health (HHS, 2014; Hill, 1965). First, the committee sought to identify the *strength of an association* between e-cigarettes and any given outcome. The committee began by identifying a statistical association or a point estimate of an effect. Relevant studies to determine such an association include experimental and observational studies examining an e-cigarette exposure and a health outcome. In general, randomized controlled trials (RCTs) provide the strongest evidence, but in some cases are infeasible for ethical reasons—for example, assessing risks of e-cigarette use among never smokers. Where randomized studies were not possible, prospective longitudinal studies provided the next strongest evidence. Well-documented case reports and case series provide evidence for the committee's conclusion on injuries and poisonings. After establishing an association, the committee then considered the magnitude (strength) of the association, whereby effects of greater magnitude were considered stronger evidence than evidence of smaller effects. Relatedly, the committee looked for evidence of a *dose–response* relationship, meaning that increases in health risk correspond with increases in exposure. Across multiple studies, the committee considered the *consistency* of an observed association—for example, the replication of findings across multiple studies, especially those with different designs or populations, or those conducted by different investigators. Evidence from multiple epidemiological studies would provide the strongest evidence of a consistent effect.

The committee took into account several considerations of particular importance to assessing observational studies, including temporality and specificity. Establishing a *temporal relationship*, or that e-cigarette exposure occurred before the outcome was particularly relevant for effects on combustible tobacco cigarette smoking initiation, where reverse causation is plausible; temporality is less relevant for health effects because the likelihood that a disease endpoint or even an intermediate outcome would cause an individual to use cigarettes is unlikely. Establishing temporality is especially important in assessing observational data; longitudinal studies with multiple follow-up periods provide the strongest evidence of temporal precedence, whereas cross-sectional studies are considered weaker because they cannot exclude the possibility of reverse causation. *Specificity* of observed relationships describes whether the association was unique to e-cigarette exposure. For observational studies, statistically controlling for potential confounders could increase confidence in a

BOX 2-1
Levels of Evidence Framework for Conclusions

Conclusive evidence: There are many supportive findings from good-quality controlled studies (including randomized and non-randomized controlled trials) with no credible opposing findings. A firm conclusion can be made, and the limitations to the evidence, including chance, bias, and confounding factors, can be ruled out with reasonable confidence.

Substantial evidence: There are several supportive findings from good-quality observational studies or controlled trials with few or no credible opposing findings. A firm conclusion can be made, but minor limitations, including chance, bias, and confounding factors, cannot be ruled out with reasonable confidence.

Moderate evidence: There are several supportive findings from fair-quality studies with few or no credible opposing findings. A general conclusion can be made, but limitations, including chance, bias, and confounding factors, cannot be ruled out with reasonable confidence.

Limited evidence: There are supportive findings from fair-quality studies or mixed findings with most favoring one conclusion. A conclusion can be made, but there is significant uncertainty due to chance, bias, and confounding factors.

Insufficient evidence: There are mixed findings or a single poor study. No conclusion can be made because of substantial uncertainty due to chance, bias, and confounding factors.

No available evidence: There are no available studies; health endpoint has not been studied at all. No conclusion can be made.

specific effect. For RCTs, because both known and unknown confounders are randomized, they would affect all trial arms equally.

Finally, the committee looked for *coherence* across the body of evidence. For example, the committee draws *analogies* from exposure to e-liquid constituents as well as other tobacco products. The committee also uses animal and in vitro data as well as evidence on intermediate outcomes to establish the *biological plausibility* of a hypothesized disease pathway. Evidence of effects from animal and in vitro populations that were similar to and in the same direction as observed effects in human populations would be coherent with human studies. Therefore, if such research provided evidence of potential mechanisms or otherwise supporting biological plausibility, the committee considered it to bolster in vivo animal or epidemiological studies. However, animal or in vitro evidence was not necessary to draw causal conclusions. Additionally, the committee did not consider null, mixed, or negative in vitro findings to downgrade findings from robust, high-quality animal or human studies.

Additional considerations regarding these factors specific to organ systems or smoking transitions are discussed in the relevant chapters of Sections II and III.

CONCLUSIONS

Informed by reports of previous Institute of Medicine and National Academies committees (IOM, 2011a, 2016; NASEM, 2017), the committee developed standardized language to categorize the weight of evidence as described in the committee's conclusions. Box 2-1 presents the conclusion categories and describes the types of evidence that correspond to each conclusion category. Stronger evidence implies that observed associations between e-cigarette use and a given outcome are more likely to be causal, whereas weaker evidence is less supportive of causality. Of note, conclusions of moderate, substantial, conclusive, or limited evidence describe a direction of effect (i.e., increased risk of a health outcome), whereas conclusions of no available or insufficient evidence do not imply a direction. The level of evidence does not indicate the size, magnitude, or importance of the effect. The committee notes that the framework is a guide, but that a great deal of expert judgment—in the evaluation of individual studies and in bodies of evidence—is always involved.

REFERENCES

CRD (Centre for Reviews and Dissemination). 2009. *Systematic reviews: CRD's guidance for undertaking reviews in health care*. https://www.york.ac.uk/crd/SysRev/!SSL!/WebHelp/SysRev3.htm (accessed November 27, 2017).

HHS (U.S. Department of Health and Human Services). 2014. *The health consequences of smoking—50 years of progress: A report of the Surgeon General*. Atlanta, GA: U.S. Department of Health and Human Services, Centers for Disease Control and Prevention, National Center for Chronic Disease Prevention and Health Promotion, Office on Smoking and Health.

Higgins, J. P. T., and S. Green, eds. 2011. *Cochrane handbook for systematic reviews of interventions version 5.1.0*. The Cochrane Collaboration. http://www.handbook.-5-1-cochrane.org (accessed November 27, 2017).

Hill, A. B. 1965. The environment and disease: Association or causation? *Proceedings of the Royal Society of Medicine* 58:295–300.

IOM (Institute of Medicine). 2011a. *Adverse effects of vaccines: Evidence and causality*. Washington, DC: The National Academies Press.

IOM. 2011b. *Finding what works in health care: Standards for systematic reviews*. Washington, DC: The National Academies Press.

IOM. 2016. *Veterans and Agent Orange: Update 2014*. Washington, DC: The National Academies Press.

NASEM (National Academies of Sciences, Engineering, and Medicine). 2017. *The health effects of cannabis and cannabinoids: The current state of evidence and recommendations for research.* Washington, DC: The National Academies Press.

NRC (National Research Council). 2007. *Toxicity testing in the 21st century: A vision and a strategy.* Washington, DC: The National Academies Press.

NRC. 2014. *Review of EPA's Integrated Risk Information System (IRIS) process.* Washington, DC: The National Academies Press.

OHAT (National Toxicology Program Office of Health Assessment and Translation). 2015. *Handbook for conducting a literature-based health assessment using OHAT approach for systematic review and evidence integration.* https://ntp.niehs.nih.gov/ntp/ohat/pubs/handbookjan2015_508.pdf (accessed November 27, 2017).

Sena, E. S., G. L. Currie, S. K. McCann, M. R. Macleod, and D. W. Howells. 2014. Systematic reviews and meta-analysis of preclinical studies: Why perform them and how to appraise them critically. *Journal of Cerebral Blood Flow and Metabolism* 34(5):737–742.

Whiting, P., J. Savovic, J. P. Higgins, D. M. Caldwell, B. C. Reeves, B. Shea, P. Davies, J. Kleijnen, R. Churchill, and R. Group. 2016. ROBIS: A new tool to assess risk of bias in systematic reviews was developed. *Journal of Clinical Epidemiology* 69:225–234.

Section I

E-Cigarette Devices, Constituents, and Exposures

E-cigarette aerosol contains fewer numbers and lower levels of toxicants than smoke from combustible tobacco cigarettes. Nicotine exposure can mimic that found with use of combustible tobacco cigarettes, but is highly variable. However, exposure to nicotine and toxicants from the aerosolization of flavorings and humectants is dependent on user and device characteristics.

3

E-Cigarette Devices, Uses, and Exposures

CHARACTERISTICS OF E-CIGARETTE DEVICES

Electronic cigarettes are a diverse group of products that produce a heated aerosol, typically containing nicotine, which users inhale via a mouthpiece. E-cigarettes range widely in design, appearance, and complexity, but generally contain similar components and operate in a similar manner (Brown and Cheng, 2014). Common components of e-cigarettes include a battery, heating coil, atomizer that transforms the e-liquid to an aerosol, cartridge that contains the e-liquid, and mouthpiece. Each component has the potential to affect health outcomes independently. They may also interact to create an influence different from the sum of their individual parts, posing a challenge for research in this field. The basic operation of e-cigarettes generally follows several steps and includes drawing on the e-cigarette, activation of a heating element, which aerosolizes the contained liquid, and inhalation of the liquid aerosol.

Currently, a diverse and non-standardized terminology is used to refer to e-cigarette devices, their components, and their use. Terms used differ in non-systematic ways, often simply due to user preference. This non-standard nomenclature presents a key challenge for e-cigarette product surveillance and examining patterns of use (Alexander et al., 2016). Appendix C lists some commonly used terms related to e-cigarette devices and their use, along with their definitions.

The e-liquids typically contain nicotine, flavorings, and a humectant. The health effects of nicotine are well documented, although much remains unknown about the specific health effects of nicotine when delivered as an aerosol as compared with a constituent in combusted smoke. Many of the flavoring constituents have been thoroughly evaluated for safety when included in food, but their effects when they enter the bloodstream through the lungs are less well known. Similarly, much remains unknown about the effects of inhaling aerosolized humectants such as propylene glycol (PG) and glycerol. Chapter 5 presents a comprehensive discussion on the toxicology of e-liquid constituents and other contaminants found in e-cigarette aerosols.

The battery design and type may put the device at risk for a fire or in rare cases for an explosion, and in combination with the heating coils, the battery also influences the aerosol properties (discussed in more detail in the following paragraph). The majority of e-cigarette devices are powered by a rechargeable battery (a manufacturer-supplied unit), a non-rechargeable battery, or a user-replaceable battery (rechargeable or non-rechargeable). Portable chargeable carrying cases are available for remote e-cigarette charging for some brands. Nickel-cadmium (NiCad), nickel metal-hydride (NiMh), lithium ion (Li-ion), alkaline and lithium polymer (Li-poly), and lithium manganese (LiMn) batteries may be used to power e-cigarettes (Brown and Cheng, 2014). Many e-cigarettes use lithium batteries because they can store a large amount of energy in a compact space. However, the inherent characteristics of lithium batteries can pose a risk of fire and explosion. Poor design, use of low-quality materials, manufacturing flaws and defects, and improper use and handling can all contribute to a condition known as "thermal runaway," whereby the internal battery temperature can increase to the point of causing a battery fire or even an explosion. The use of overcharging protection circuits, thermal power cutoffs, and internal overpressure relief mechanisms can help prevent and mitigate thermal runaway.

The heating coils and atomizer influence the aerosol properties, and therefore potential health effects. When aerosolization settings are not optimal (e.g., when the heating power is too high), it creates a negative sensation called a "dry hit" in users. This unpleasant sensation may be related to the formation of thermal decomposition by-products of PG and glycerol, including toxic carbonyl compounds (Farsalinos et al., 2015b; Geiss et al., 2016). Of note, nicotine undergoes pyrolytic degradation at temperatures above 600°C (Schmeltz et al., 1979), which no studies on e-cigarettes have reported reaching, so the potential pyrolytic degradation of nicotine is very unlikely in e-cigarettes. The amount of power applied to the atomizer also affects the mass of aerosol produced from the e-cigarette device, with more power typically creating denser aerosol per puff (Gillman et al., 2016).

The characteristics of the heating coils and atomizer can be customized by users. They may add more coils and/or lower the standard resistance of the heating coils to generate more heat and create denser aerosols. In some devices it is possible for e-liquids to come into direct contact with the heating coils in a process known as "dripping," which may introduce metals and other constituents into the aerosol that users inhale.

Classification of E-Cigarettes

For the purpose of this report, e-cigarette devices are classified as first, second, and third generation based on their product characteristics and operational features. Figure 3-1 shows typical first-, second-, and third-generation e-cigarette devices.

First-generation devices refer to e-cigarettes devices designed to mimic the smoking experience as close as possible. These products served as stand-ins for cigarettes among users who wished to quit smoking or sought out an alternative product to a cigarette. First-generation e-cigarettes are often designed to look like a combustible tobacco cigarette, but some are designed to simulate a cigar or pipe. They are also called cigalikes (cig-a-likes) or "vape sticks." Other cigalikes are slightly longer or narrower than a combustible tobacco cigarette (so called "pen style").

Second-generation e-cigarettes are characterized by a clearomizer—a transparent cartridge that holds e-liquid and an atomizer—and a thin battery. Second-generation devices include products that are shaped like pens, are comparatively larger and cylindrical, and are often referred to as "tank systems" in reference to the transparent reservoir that holds larger amounts of e-liquid than previous cartridge-containing models.

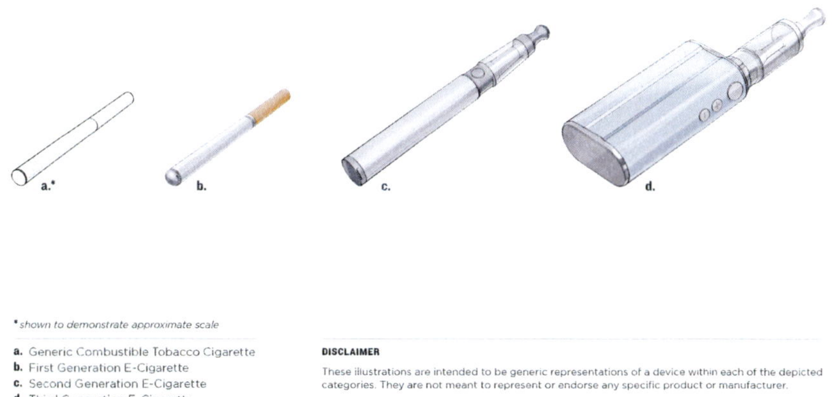

FIGURE 3-1 First-, second-, and third-generation e-cigarette devices.

Third-generation devices represent a diverse set of products and represent the greatest departure from combustible tobacco cigarettes. Often these devices are advertised as "vaping" products and the associated marketing makes no reference to cigarettes (Zhu et al., 2014). Aesthetically they bear little resemblance to cigarettes, as many are square or rectangular and feature customizable and rebuildable atomizers and batteries. In addition, since the beginning of the availability of e-cigarettes and their component parts, users have been modifying the devices or building their own devices, which are often referred to as "mods." The differences in design and engineering of the products are key factors in the size, distribution, and amount of aerosol particles. The variability in levels of chemicals and nicotine present in the e-liquid/aerosol determines the composition of the aerosol delivered to the user (Brown and Cheng, 2014).

E-CIGARETTE USE

The basic operation of e-cigarettes generally follows several steps. First, the user draws upon the e-cigarette. Then, a user either manually presses a switch button to activate a heating element, or draws upon the e-cigarette and an airflow sensor automatically activates it. In automatically activated devices, the airflow sensor detects pressure changes and prompts the flow of power to a heating element and (optionally) an LED. The e-liquid contained in the device saturates a wick via capillary action, which the heating element then aerosolizes. This process is commonly called "vaporization." Aerosolized droplets of liquid subsequently flow into the user's mouth and are inhaled into the lungs. Although e-cigarette use is commonly referred to as vaping, technically the device emits and the user inhales an aerosol, composed of a suspension of a mixture of gases, vapors, and aqueous particles, and not a vapor, which is a substance in gas phase. The exposure of a user to potentially hazardous chemicals depends on how the user inhales the aerosol, the physical characteristics of that aerosol, where the aerosol ends up in the respiratory tract, and the concentration of toxicants in the aerosol at different locations in the respiratory tract. The following sections review information about how to assess those exposures and illustrative results from the literature. The pharmacology and toxicology of those exposures is discussed in Chapters 4 and 5.

Puff Topography

For combustible tobacco cigarettes, smoking is understood to be a complex process that allows smokers to titrate their desired dose of nicotine and nicotine brain level on a puff-by-puff basis. The intake of nicotine during smoking depends on what are referred to as topography variables, such as puff volume, the depth of inhalation, the rate of puffing, and the intensity of puffing, as well as the extent of smoke dilution with room air (Hukkanen et al., 2005). Puffing patterns influence nicotine intake and exposure to hazardous substances in tobacco smoke. Similarly, puffing behavior or topography may also be an important determinant of nicotine intake and exposure to potentially toxic substances in e-cigarette aerosol, with implications for disease risks. (An examination of the relationship between puff topography and nicotine exposure in e-cigarette users is presented in Chapter 4.). Furthermore, understanding user puff topography is also useful to inform animal, in vitro, and machine-based studies of e-cigarette aerosol exposures that are relevant to human exposures.

Fourteen studies were identified that described e-cigarette puffing topography. A summary of the studies is presented in Table 3-1, including the e-cigarette(s) used, nicotine concentration of the e-liquids consumed, study population (whether experienced e-cigarette users or e-cigarette–naïve smokers), the study conditions and vaping protocol, and averages of vaping topography variables.

The methods or instruments used to measure e-cigarette puffing topography varied across studies. Four of the studies used a modified Clinical Research Support System (CReSS Pocket, Borgwaldt Ltd., Germany) (Behar et al., 2015; Goniewicz et al., 2013; Lee et al., 2015; Norton et al., 2014). Three studies from one research group used a device developed and manufactured by collaborators at the American University of Beirut (Lopez et al., 2016; Spindle et al., 2015, 2017). Two other studies, led by the same author, used a wireless personal use monitor (wPUM) designed by researchers at Rochester Institute of Technology (Robinson et al., 2015, 2016). Other studies used video recordings (St.Helen et al., 2016a), an e-cigarette that tracks puff number and puff duration (eVic) (Dawkins et al., 2016; Farsalinos et al., 2015a), or a modified SA7 (British American Tobacco [Investments]) (Cunningham et al., 2016). Differences in instruments/methods of measurement likely introduce variability among study findings.

One question of interest is whether e-cigarette puffing topography is comparable to that of combustible tobacco cigarette use. Three studies examined this question. Norton and colleagues (2014) conducted a pilot study to examine initial reactions to e-cigarette use and puffing behaviors among combustible tobacco cigarette smokers. Puffing topography was measured on day 1 while participants smoked a combustible tobacco cigarette and about 24 hours later during ad libitum (ad lib) use of a first-generation e-cigarette. Participants had been asked to use the e-cigarette exclusively over the previous 24 hours. The study found that e-cigarette–naïve smokers (n = 18) took more puffs when smoking a combustible

TABLE 3-1 Summary of E-Cigarette Puffing Topography Studies

Reference	Study Product	Nicotine Content	Sample Size	Study Conditions	Method
Norton et al., 2014	Smoke 51 TRIO (1st generation)	11 mg/ml	18	Lab; ad libitum (ad lib)	CReSS
	Usual combustible tobacco cigarette	n/a		Lab; 1 cigarette	
Farsalinos et al., 2015a	eVic by Joyetech (2nd generation)	18 mg/ml	E-cigarette–naïve, combustible tobacco smokers: 23 Experienced e-cigarette users: 24	Lab; 10 puffs in 5 minutes followed by ad lib use in 60 minutes	eVic
Lee et al., 2015	M201 (1st generation)	18 mg (11.0 ± 1.5 mg measured)	20	Lab; baseline, ad lib Lab; week 2, ad lib	CReSS
Lopez et al., 2016	eGO 3.3-V battery with 1.5-Ω Smoktech cartomizer	0 mg/ml 8 mg/ml 18 mg/ml 36 mg/ml	16	Lab; two 10-puff standardized sessions, 30-second interval, sessions were 1 hour apart	in-house device

Puff Count Mean (SD or SE)	Puff Duration Mean (SD or SE), seconds	Interpuff Interval Mean (SD or SE), seconds	Flow Rate Mean (SD or SE), ml/second	Puff Volume Mean (SD or SE), ml
8.7 (SE = 1.6)	3.0 (SE = 0.8)	29.6 (SE = 11.7)	52.0 (SE = 4.7)	118.2 (SE = 13.3)
13.2 (SE = 1.1)	3.0 (SE = 1.0)	21.3 (SE = 6.2)	36.1 (SE = 1.8)	67.5 (SE = 6.3)
n/a	E-cigarette–naïve, combustible tobacco smokers: 2.3 (SE = 0.2) Experienced e-cigarette users: 3.5 (SE = 0.2)	n/a	n/a	n/a
19.3 (SE = 2.5)	2.2 (SE = 0.1)	19.2 (SE = 2.7)	30.6 (SE= 2.3)	64.0 (SE = 4.8)
21.3 (SE = 2.4)	2.9 (SE = 0.2)	22.1 (SE = 4.9)	24.8 (SE = 1.9)	63.3 (SE = 5.2)
n/a	3.00 (SD = 1.38)	n/a	30.0 (SD = 25.7)	83.2 (SD = 62.6)
n/a	2.80 (SD = 1.41)	n/a	30.9 (SD = 20.1)	80.3 (SD = 53.8)
n/a	2.85 (SD = 1.49)	n/a	27.1 (SD = 13.1)	70.2 (SD = 28.8)
n/a	2.27 (SD = 0.99)	n/a	31.8 (SD = 33.1)	66.7 (SD = 55.9)

continued

TABLE 3-1 Continued

Reference	Study Product	Nicotine Content	Sample Size	Study Conditions	Method
Strasser et al., 2016	Five brands: NJOY, V2, Green Smoke, blu, White Cloud	NJOY: 18 mg; V2: 18 mg; Green Smoke: 18.9–20.7 mg; blu: 20–24 mg; White Cloud: 23–24 mg	28	Lab; ad lib over 10 minutes (day 5) Lab; ad lib over 10 minutes (day 10)	videotape
	Usual combustible tobacco cigarette	n/a		Lab; 1 cigarette (day 1)	
Goniewicz et al., 2013	Usual e-cigarette brands	n/a	10	Lab; ad lib	CReSS
Behar et al., 2015	blu and V2 (1st generation)	blu: 16 mg/ml; V2: 18 mg/ml	20	Lab; ad lib use for 10 minutes	CReSS
Robinson et al., 2015	blu (1st generation)	16 mg	22	Naturalistic environment, ad lib, 1 day	wPUM
Spindle et al., 2015	Usual battery with 1.5-Ω SmokTech cartomizer	Usual e-liquid: mean = 21.7 (SD = 3.9; range = 12–24) mg/ml	13	Lab; 10-puff standardized session, 30 seconds between puffs	in-house device

Puff Count Mean (SD or SE)	Puff Duration Mean (SD or SE), seconds	Interpuff Interval Mean (SD or SE), seconds	Flow Rate Mean (SD or SE), ml/second	Puff Volume Mean (SD or SE), ml
16.1 (SD = 11.9)	1.99 (SE = 0.7)	11.2 (SD = 5.2)	n/a	n/a
13.2 (SD = 9.4)	2.06 (SE = 0.7)	11.2 (SD = 5.2)		
13.6 (SD = 4.0)	1.64 (SD = 0.3)	25.3 (SD = 13.3)		
15 (SD = 6)	1.8 (SD = 0.9)	10 (SD = 13)	n/a	70 (SD = 68)
32 (SD = 8)	2.65 (SD = 0.98)	17.9 (SD = 7.5)	20 (SD = 6)	51 (SD = 21)
24-hours: 225 (SD = 272); per session: 15 (SD = 25)	3.5 (SD = 1.8)	n/a	37 (SD = 16)	133 (SD = 90)
n/a	4.16 (SE = 1.06)	n/a	24.17 (SE = 10.66)	101.37 (SE = 50.01)

continued

TABLE 3-1 Continued

Reference	Study Product	Nicotine Content	Sample Size	Study Conditions	Method
Cunningham et al., 2016	Vype Reload (1st generation)	4.5% nicotine (45 mg/ml)	32	Lab; ad lib over self-determined length; mean = 6:54 (SD = 3:43) minutes	modifed SA7
	Vype ePen (2nd generation)	3.0% nicotine (30 mg/ml)	28	Lab; ad lib over self-determined length; mean = 7:41 (SD = 6:17) minutes	
Dawkins et al., 2016	eVic by Joyetech (2nd generation)	6 mg/ml 24 mg/ml	11	Lab; ad lib over 60 min	eVic
Robinson et al., 2016	Usual device (1st generation)	Usual nicotine level	20	Naturalistic environment, ad lib, 1 day	wPUM
St.Helen et al., 2016a	Usual brands	Usual e-liquid: mean = 9.4 (SD = 4.1; range = 5.0–15.3) mg/ml	13	Lab; ad lib over 90 minutes	videotape
Spindle et al., 2017	Usual battery with 1.5-Ω SmokTech cartomizer	Usual e-liquid: mean = 18.9 (SD = 5.9) mg/ml	29	Lab; 10-puff session (30-second interpuff interval)	in-house device
				Lab; ad lib over 90 minutes	

NOTE: SD = standard deviation; SE = standard error.

Puff Count Mean (SD or SE)	Puff Duration Mean (SD or SE), seconds	Interpuff Interval Mean (SD or SE), seconds	Flow Rate Mean (SD or SE), ml/second	Puff Volume Mean (SD or SE), ml
21.1 (SD = 14.9)	2.0 (SD = 0.7)	23.2 (SD = 10.6)	Peak: 39.0 (SD = 10.3)	52.2 (SD = 21.6)
16.1 (SD = 8.0)	2.2 (SD = 0.9)	29.3 (SD = 19.2)	Peak: 60.6 (SD = 19.8)	83.0 (SD = 44.3)
70.73 (SD = 34.45) 48.36 (SD = 22.86)	5.20 (SD = 1.39) 3.84 (SD = 1.02)	n/a	n/a	n/a
78 (SD = 81)	2.0 (0.6)	n/a	30.4 (SD = 9.2)	65.4 (SD = 24.8)
64 (SD = 38)	3.5 (SD = 1.4)	118 (SD = 141)	n/a	n/a
9.97 (SD = 0.12)	4.51 (SD = 1.55)	25.19 (SD = 1.55)	27.78 (SD = 19.48)	124.56 (SD = 89.13)
62.55 (SD = 32.34)	5.29 (SD = 2.08)	102.77 (SD = 63.07)	27.47 (SD = 22.63)	148.52 (SD = 119.6)

tobacco cigarette, but per-puff volume, flow rate, and peak flow rate were significantly higher with e-cigarettes; puff duration was not significantly different. The relatively short period of e-cigarette use (~24 hours) before the lab session was likely inadequate to stabilize e-cigarette puffing behavior; the findings may not be generalizable to experienced e-cigarette users. Spindle and colleagues (2015) measured puffing topography of 13 experienced second-generation e-cigarette users during a 10-puff session in which puffing characteristics such as duration were not standardized. The authors compared the findings with a previously published study on combustible tobacco cigarette smokers (Kleykamp et al., 2008). By comparison, experienced e-cigarette users took larger volumes per puff and longer puffs, but flow rate with e-cigarettes was lower. Given that these comparisons are not within subject, the findings should be treated cautiously. In another study, Strasser and colleagues (2016) measured puff topography of combustible tobacco cigarette smokers who switch to first-generation e-cigarettes. Puff topography when smoking one combustible tobacco cigarette was measured on the first day and e-cigarette puff topography was measured on days 5 and 10 during a 10-minute ad lib session. The number of puffs taken did not differ when smoking the combustible tobacco cigarette compared with using the e-cigarettes. However, puff duration increased with e-cigarette use while interpuff interval decreased. Because the study used video analysis, other variables such as puff volume and flow rate were not reported. Based on these three studies, it appears that puff duration is longer and puff volume larger with e-cigarette use compared with combustible tobacco cigarette use. The findings on flow rate were less consistent.

Another question is whether e-cigarette puffing topography of experienced users differs from that of e-cigarette–naïve users. In other words, does puffing topography change as e-cigarette–naïve users gain experience with e-cigarettes? Four of the studies enrolled e-cigarette–naïve combustible tobacco cigarette smokers, nine studies enrolled experienced e-cigarette users, and one enrolled both groups. Farsalinos and colleagues (2015a) compared the number of puffs taken and puff duration between 24 experienced e-cigarette users and 23 e-cigarette–naïve users. Participants were given a second-generation e-cigarette (eVic by Joyetech) and were asked to take 10 puffs in 5 minutes followed by 60 minutes of ad lib use. The number of puffs and puff duration were recorded by the e-cigarette (eVic by Joyetech). The study found that while the number of puffs taken during the 65-minute period did not differ between the two groups, experienced e-cigarette users took significantly longer puffs than the e-cigarette–naïve users. Two studies examined changes in puffing topography in e-cigarette–naïve combustible tobacco smokers over time. Lee and colleagues (2015) found that puff duration increased and puff flow rate decreased significantly after e-cigarette–naïve smokers (n = 20) used a first-generation e-cigarette for one week compared with baseline (first use of the e-cigarette); these differences were sustained after 2 weeks of e-cigarette use. Strasser and colleagues (2016) reported similar average number of puffs, puff duration, and interpuff interval during a 10-minute ad lib session 5 and 10 days after switching from combustible tobacco cigarettes to e-cigarettes. Based on Table 3-1, in general, puff duration appears to be longer among experienced e-cigarette users (range of means = 1.8 to 5.29 seconds) compared with e-cigarette–naïve users (range of means = 1.64 to 3.0 seconds). Puff volume also appears to be larger with experienced e-cigarette users (range of means = 51.0 to 148.5 ml) compared with e-cigarette–naïve users (range of means = 63.0 to 118.2 ml).

A third question is whether e-cigarette device characteristics influence puffing topography. Device characteristics include the type of e-cigarette (first generation versus advanced models), voltage or power, and nicotine strength of e-liquids. In one study, Cunningham and colleagues (2016) assigned experienced e-cigarette users to either a first-generation device (Vype Reload, classic flavor bold containing 4.5 percent nicotine by volume) (n = 32) or to a button-activated, variable-voltage e-cigarette that uses prefilled cartridges containing e-liquid (Vype ePen with 3.0 percent nicotine by volume) (n = 28). Vaping topography was measured during ad lib sessions of self-determined durations during two lab visits. Participants used the same devices during each visit, but those with the variable-voltage Vype ePen alternated between a low or high voltage during each visit. No significant differences in puff topography were reported between different days of use of the first-generation e-cigarette or voltage of the advanced-model e-cigarette. However, compared with the first-generation e-cigarette (Vype Reload), average number of puffs taken was fewer, average puff volume was larger, mean interpuff interval was longer, and mean peak flow rate was higher with the advanced-model e-cigarette. These findings suggest that e-cigarette puffing topography is different among types of e-cigarettes. One likely explanation is the difference in power between types of devices, as more advanced e-cigarettes are operated at higher power (voltage) than first-generation e-cigarettes. However, this study found no differences in topography variables when the same participants switched between low and high voltage (the exact voltages were not stated), implying that, while plausible, power did not influence vaping topography in this study. Another plausible explanation for differences in puffing topography among types of devices is the nicotine concentration of the e-liquid. The first-generation had higher nicotine concentration compared with the second-generation e-cigarette.

Lopez and colleagues (2016) examined the effect of e-liquid nicotine concentration on puffing topography. Sixteen e-cigarette–naïve smokers crossed over among second-generation e-cigarettes with 0, 8, 18, and 36 mg/ml nicotine over 4 days. Participants engaged in two 10-puff sessions in which puff parameters were not standardized. Puff volume and puff duration tended to decrease with increasing nicotine concentration, while there was no clear trend with flow rate. In a similar study, Dawkins et al. (2016) found that experienced e-cigarette users took fewer and shorter puffs at high nicotine concentration (24 mg/ml) compared with low nicotine concentration (6 mg/ml) over a 60-minute period of ad lib access to a second-generation e-cigarette. Based on these studies, it appears that nicotine concentration of the e-liquid used is a major determinant of e-cigarette puffing topography (Cunningham et al., 2016; Dawkins et al., 2016; Lopez et al., 2016).

Most of the studies (12 of 14) measured puffing topography in controlled environments, where puffing behavior may or may not represent e-cigarette use behavior in the "real world." Two observational studies characterized puffing topography of experienced e-cigarette users of first-generation devices in their naturalistic environments. In the first study, Robinson and colleagues (2015) described puffing topography of e-cigarette users over a 24-hour period. Participants (n = 21) were given a day's supply of blu rechargeable e-cigarettes (a first-generation device), which was used in conjunction with a wPUM (Robinson et al., 2015). Average puff duration, flow rate, and puff volume were within the range of reported values from studies of experienced e-cigarette users in controlled environments (see Table 3-1). In addition, the researchers identified what they characterized as three representative puff topographies: "many short" puffs (1.4-second puff duration); "typical" puffs (3.7-second puff duration); and "fewer long" puffs (6.9-second puff duration). The average number of puffs taken was 225 (SD = 272). Given that the study enrolled only users of first-generation e-cigarettes, the findings may not be generalizable to users of more advanced models.

Robinson and colleagues (2016) conducted a second observational study of experienced first-generation e-cigarette users in their naturalistic environment, but over a 7-day period. Participants (n = 20) used their usual e-cigarettes in conjunction with the topography device (wPUM). Average puff duration was at the lower end of the range of values observed among experienced e-cigarette users in controlled settings and also lower than the first study by Robinson and colleagues (2015). Three groups of puffs based on duration were identified: "short" puff duration (1.8 seconds), "moderate" puff duration (2 seconds), and "long" puff duration (2.5 seconds). These groups were different from the three representative topographies identified in the first study. In addition, the study found that participants engaged in an average of 6 distinct vaping sessions (activation of a wireless personal use monitor, taking puffs, and turning the device off) per day, and took an average of 78 puffs per day. The average number of puffs taken per day was drastically lower than the average number of puffs taken per day in the first study. The lower number of puffs per day in the 7-day study compared with the 1-day study likely reflects variability in use patterns among days within subjects. In addition, it was uncertain to what extent participants complied with the study protocol by using the wPUM for every puff taken. Although studies of e-cigarette users in their naturalistic environments may offer realistic information on user behaviors, compliance with study protocol cannot be guaranteed, thus limiting the reliability of study findings.

In summary, puffing topography seems to differ between users of e-cigarettes and combustible tobacco cigarettes. E-cigarette users tend to take puffs of longer duration and larger volume. Furthermore, puffing topography changes as e-cigarette–naïve users become more experienced. Puff duration and puff volume increase with experience. Also, device characteristics such as type of device (first generation versus advanced models) and nicotine strength of e-liquids influence puffing topography. Number of puffs taken and puff duration tend to decrease as nicotine strength of the e-liquid increases. Finally, puffing topography of experienced e-cigarette users measured in their naturalistic environment was in the range of values measured in experienced users in controlled settings.

EXPOSURE TO AEROSOLS AND PARTICULATES

E-cigarette aerosol is best described as a mist, which is an aerosol formed by the condensation of spherical liquid droplets in the submicrometer to 200-µm size range. Methods for particle measurement have included spectral transmission using an electrical mobility analyzer. Pratte and colleagues (2016) used a light scattering methodology for droplet sizing of e-cigarette aerosols. Yet others have used the cascade impactors to determine the mass of various particle sizes.

Ingebrethsen and colleagues (2012) demonstrated particle size distribution of aerosols produced by electronic cigarettes in an undiluted state using a spectral transmission procedure after high dilution with an electrical mobility analyzer. They found particle diameters of average mass in the 250- to 450-nm size range with particle number concentrations of 10^9 particles/cm^3. These measurements are comparable to those observed for combustible tobacco cigarette smoke in prior studies and also measured in the current study with the spectral transmission method and with the electrical mobility procedure. Total particulate mass for the e-cigarettes calculated from the size distribution parameters measured by spectral transmission were in good agreement with replicate determinations of total particulate mass by gravimetric filter collection. By contrast, average particle diameters determined for e-cigarettes by the electrical mobility method were in the 50-nm range, and total particulate masses calculated based on the suggested diameters are orders of magnitude smaller than those determined gravimetrically. These small particle diameters observed are thought to arise from e-cigarette aerosol particle evaporation at the dilution levels and conditions of the electrical mobility analysis. By contrast, a smaller degree, approximately 20 percent by mass, of particle evaporation has been observed for combustible tobacco cigarette smoke.

Alderman and colleagues (2014) did follow-up studies using a cascade impactor to determine particle size distribution by collecting eight puffs total (four per e-cigarette) with a 30-second interpuff interval. Three e-cigarette brands were evaluated. E-cigarette 1 and e-cigarette 2 were both rechargeable models, with cartomizer-type cartridges, while the e-cigarette 3 was a disposable model. All components were connected by conductive silicone rubber tubing to minimize particle loss during sampling. Figure 3-2 presents the representative impactor-collected data,

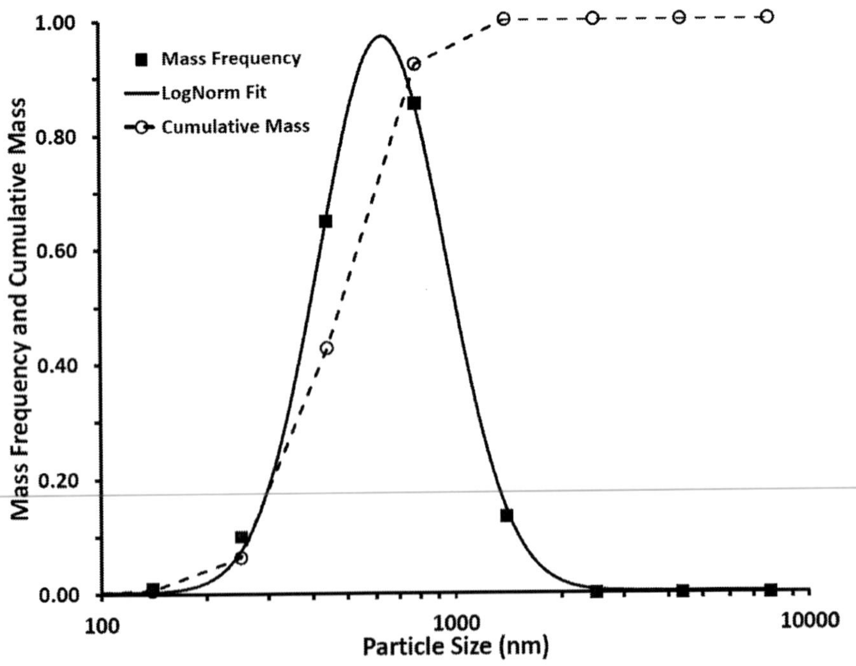

FIGURE 3-2 Mass frequency and cumulative mass distributions derived from impactor particle size distribution measurement of e-cigarette 1.
NOTE: The data shown here are representative of each e-cigarette brand evaluated.
SOURCE: Alderman et al., 2014.

TABLE 3-2 Particle Size Distribution Parameters Determined from Cascade Impactor Analysis

E-Cigarette	MMAD (nm)	CMD (nm)	GSD	Puff Mass (mg/puff)
1	631	319	1.50	2.16
2	487	262	1.52	3.07
3	534	261	1.52	1.95

NOTE: CMD = count mean diameter; GSD = geometric standard deviation; MMAD = mass mean aerodynamic diameter.
SOURCE: Alderman et al., 2014.

namely a mass frequency distribution curve and corresponding lognormal fit to the data, as well as the corresponding cumulative mass distribution. The data provided in Figure 3-2 are for e-cigarette 1 and are generally representative of each e-cigarette brand sampled. Figure 3-2 indicates that essentially all (95 percent) aerosol mass is confined to the particle size range of 280–1,420 nm. Further analysis of the particle size distribution from the cascade impactor analysis is shown in Table 3-2. Further analysis demonstrated that although the distribution of particle sizes represented by the mass median aerodynamic diameter and count mean diameter is heterogeneous, all particles are highly respirable throughout the respiratory tract.

Table 3-2 is a particle size summary for all products evaluated in the Alderman and colleagues (2014) study. The particle size distribution parameters in Table 3-2 are derived by fitting the mass frequency data to a lognormal function. In addition, the puff mass in Table 3-2 is based on the cumulative mass of particulate matter collected on the various impactor stages. Both curves from Figure 3-2 indicate that essentially all (95 percent) aerosol mass is confined to the particle size range of 280–1,420 nm, or in other words, highly respirable within the respiratory tract.

Fuoco and colleagues (2014) observed similar findings with different types of e-cigarettes, while also showing the total particle number concentration peak (using a 2-second puff), averaged across the different electronic cigarette types and liquids, at $4.4 \pm 0.4 \times 10^9$ particles/cm^3, compared with the combustible tobacco cigarette at $3.1 \pm 0.6 \times 10^9$ particles/cm^3. Puffing times and nicotine contents were found to influence the particle concentration, whereas no significant differences were recognized in terms of flavors and types of combustible tobacco cigarettes used. Particle number distribution modes of the e-cigarette–generated aerosol were in the 120- to 165-nm range. Marini and colleagues (2014) further confirmed similar particle concentrations. This striking contrast in particle size between Alderman and Fuoco might suggest the generation of different particle sizes due to the wattage and temperature used to generate the e-cigarette aerosol, as well as possible differences in e-cigarette composition.

Ji and colleagues (2016) generated and characterized e-cigarette aerosols using advanced technologies. In the gas phase, the particle number concentration (PNC) of e-cigarette aerosols was found to be positively correlated with puff duration, whereas the PNC and size distribution may vary with different flavors and nicotine concentration. In the liquid phase (water or cell culture media), the size of e-cigarette aerosol particles appeared to be significantly larger than those in the gas phase, which might be due to aggregation of aerosol particles in the liquid phase.

While the particle count in e-cigarette aerosols may not be substantially different than mainstream combustible tobacco smoke, the nature of the particles is substantially different. E-cigarette aerosol particulates consist largely of aqueous droplets and vapors of humectants, either PG or glycerol, whereas particulates in combustible tobacco smoke are complex, largely organic constituents that contain polycyclic aromatic hydrocarbons and a variety of other known or suspected carcinogens. Thus, it would be incorrect to assume that the long-term health risks of the two aerosols were similar just because particle count was similar.

Particle Deposition

Deposition by e-cigarette vaping within the human respiratory tract is essential to better understand the biological dosing of gases, aerosols, and aqueous particles generated during e-cigarette use. To address particle dosing, Pichelstorfer and colleagues (2016) implemented the aerosol dynamics in containments (ADiC) model to describe the dynamic changes of both inhaled combustible tobacco cigarette smoke as well as aerosols generated by e-cigarette vaping. The model involved particles present during puffing, mouth-hold, inspiration, and expiration. The authors included consideration of coagulation, phase transition, conductive heat and diffusive/convective vapor transport, as well as dilution/mixing into a single-path representation of the stochastic lung dosimetry model IDEAL (inhalation, deposition, and exhalation of aerosols in the lungs) to compute particulate-phase deposition as well as vapor-phase deposition in the airway generations of the human lung.

The ADiC model applied to the inhalation of combustible and electronic cigarette aerosols is a means to understand those aerosol dynamics processes that influence the physical properties of the particle and vapor phases in the human respiratory tract with the following observations:

(1) reduced inhaled aerosol particle number is caused primarily by coagulation and less by deposition for both types of aerosols; (2) hygroscopic growth rates are higher for e-cigarettes than for combustible tobacco cigarettes; (3) the effect of particle growth on deposition leads to a lower total deposition in the case of combustible tobacco cigarette smoke particles and a higher total deposition in the case of e-cigarette droplets relative to their initial size distributions; and (4) most of the nicotine is deposited by the vapor phase for both aerosols (Pichelstorfer et al., 2016).

Because of the complexity of the model and the resulting extensive computational time, Pichelstorfer and colleagues used a single-path version of the IDEAL airway geometry. Average airway dimensions for each airway generation were derived for the particle and vapor transport in the lungs, while average deposition fractions for each airway generation were based on the full stochastic deposition model.

Figure 3-3 illustrates the number/size distribution of inhaled particles of combustible tobacco cigarette smoke (panel A) and e-cigarette droplets (panel B) across time. These time points include after-puffing, mouth-hold, inhalation, and exhalation phases. The figure shows most particles in both aerosols are removed after the puffing and mouth-hold stages, eliminating initial size distribution disparities between the two aerosols (Pichelstorfer et al., 2016). This can largely be attributed to coagulation, which decreases particle concentration and increases particle diameter. For example, nicotine is almost eliminated in the alveolar region (as seen in that peak's split in panel B). Evaporation of water and glycerol in smaller e-cigarette particles also occurs in the mouth during the puffing and mouth-hold periods (as shown in the peak of particles near 40 nm in panel B).

Size-selective deposition by Brownian motion in the lungs and hygroscopic growth, which becomes greater as particle size increases (Winkler-Heil et al., 2014), remove additional particles in the respiratory tract. These three processes (coagulation, size-selective deposition, and hygroscopic growth) result in particles with larger diameters by the expiration phase. Indeed, e-cigarette droplets' higher hygroscopic growth rates make this change to larger diameters by the end stage more distinct than alterations to combustible tobacco cigarette smoke particle diameters. Furthermore, unlike combustible tobacco cigarettes, e-cigarette particles will not reach equilibrium with their surroundings because they have more volatile substances; combustible tobacco cigarettes' tar content helps stabilize the particles. Therefore, smaller particles are removed by processes such as coagulation, resulting in a larger median particle diameter. E-cigarette aerosols' higher growth rates increase total deposition in the lung. This deposition is powered mainly by inertia in bronchial airways and via gravity in alveolar spaces.

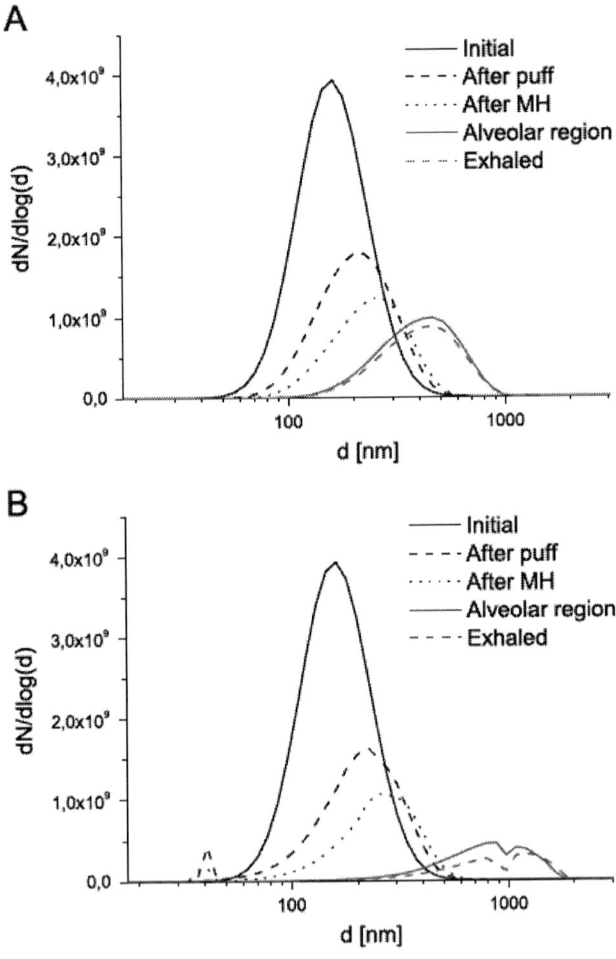

FIGURE 3-3 Temporal evolution of the number/size distribution of inhaled combustible tobacco cigarette smoke particles (panel A) and e-cigarette droplets (panel B) during puffing, mouth-hold (MH), inhalation, and exhalation, based on the same initial size distribution.
SOURCE: Pichelstorfer et al., 2016.

Finally, puff topography (Evans and Hoffman, 2014; Norton et al., 2014), on average, will not alter these results; the effects of longer puff duration with e-cigarettes on deposition fractions will be offset in general by their higher puff volume (Evans and Hoffman, 2014; Fuoco et al., 2014; Norton et al., 2014; Winkler-Heil et al., 2014).

Measurements of Constituents Found in E-Cigarettes

E-liquids generally contain four main components: nicotine, flavors, water, and carrier liquids (humectants). The carrier liquid dissolves flavors and nicotine and aerosolizes at a certain temperature on the atomizer of the e-cigarette. PG and glycerol, the principal carriers used in e-liquids, undergo partial decomposition in contact with the atomizer heating coil, forming volatile carbonyls. Some of these, such as formaldehyde, acetaldehyde, and acrolein, are of concern due to their adverse impact on human health when inhaled at sufficient concentrations. Physical, chemical, and toxicological characteristics of e-cigarette liquids and aerosols are discussed in Chapter 5.

Analytical methodology for qualitative and/or quantitative determination of a constituent in e-cigarette aerosol generally encompasses two areas of effort: sample preparation and instrumental analysis. Sample preparation involves aerosol generation, sample extraction, and sample collection. Instrumental analysis involves analyzing the sample to identify and quantify analytes of interest. The instrument is commonly selected based on the chemical characteristics of the target analyte, the applicable features of the instrument, and the instrument accessibility (Cheng, 2014).

Currently, there is no standardized method for generating and collecting aerosol from e-cigarettes for analytical purposes and laboratory studies. Factors influencing e-cigarette aerosol generation include the e-cigarette device and setup, puffing topography, machine aerosol generation parameters, and aerosol generation techniques. As described in the beginning of this chapter, the design and composition of e-cigarette devices (including e-liquid composition, device battery power, activation voltage, and coil resistance) vary considerably, and these variations influence the e-cigarette aerosol produced. Thus, it is crucial to understand each unique setup and test article prior to chemical analysis and in vitro biological exposure. Human puffing topography, described in detail above, is important in determining true levels of human exposure to constituents in e-cigarettes. Smoking machine parameters for laboratory studies are important in understanding the way that constituent yields delivered by a product can change over a range of different smoking conditions. With respect to aerosol generation techniques, current machine-based aerosol generation techniques pose several challenges for assessing different product aerosols because many smoking machines and exposure systems were originally designed for use with combustible tobacco cigarettes and do not easily translate to the standard production of e-cigarette aerosols. For example, e-cigarettes require a higher airflow rate and longer puff durations to produce aerosols than combustible tobacco cigarettes require to produce smoke. Furthermore, pressure drop (mmH_2O across e-cigarettes during each puff) varies greatly, including across cartridges used in the same models, across brands, and even within brands (Goniewicz et al., 2013, 2014; Trehy et al., 2011; Trtchounian et al., 2010; Williams and Talbot, 2011). Other important differences between e-cigarette aerosols and combustible tobacco cigarette smoke in such systems include aerosols condensing in transit tubing (possibly restricting aerosol flow and impeding syringe function) and some concerns with device button activation synchrony (either manually, or automated with a separate robot) with the syringe puffing to ensure the entire puff is activated and delivered (Goniewicz et al., 2014; Havel et al., 2016). These important methodological issues with generating e-cigarette aerosol for analytical and toxicological testing have important implications for analyzed dose and biological effects. A standardized protocol for evaluating emissions (particulate and gas phase) of e-cigarettes would facilitate interpretation of study results reported in literature.

Novel devices may help overcome the challenges of using smoking machines. For example, Herrington and Myers (2015) developed a simple sampling device to draw e-cigarette aerosol into a multisorbent thermal desorption tube, which was then thermally extracted and analyzed via gas chromatography (GC)–mass spectrometry (MS) methodology. The investigators found that this novel device was effective at providing detectable levels of numerous compounds from e-cigarette aerosol, including many not listed by the manufacturers and those not present in the e-liquid.

After producing aerosols, most studies conduct a multistep chemical analysis of emissions in e-cigarette aerosols. High performance liquid chromatography and GC-MS are analytical techniques commonly used for separation, identification, and measurement of chemicals in e-liquids. Aerosols also commonly require sample pretreatment such as extraction and/or derivatization (Geiss et al., 2015; Goniewicz et al., 2014; Ohta et al., 2011; Papousek et al., 2014; Schripp et al., 2013; Uchiyama et al., 2010). The instrument is typically selected based on the chemical characteristics of the target analyte, the applicable features of the instrument, and the instrument accessibility. For the identification of the major ingredients (PG and glycerol) and their relative concentrations, GC with flame ionization detector or with MS is usually used. For the identification and quantitative analysis of nicotine, GC with nitrogen-selective detector or with MS are typically used. Flavorings are commonly identified using GC with headspace sample delivery interface and tandem MS (GC-MS/MS) or time-of-flight mass spectrometer. Chromatography methods provide adequate sensitivity, but a main challenge includes a significant matrix effect, which results in peak suppression of analytes (Geiss et al., 2016; Herrington and Myers, 2015).

SECONDHAND EXPOSURE TO E-CIGARETTE AEROSOL

In 2006, the report of the Surgeon General on the health consequences of involuntary exposure to tobacco smoke concluded there is no risk-free level of exposure to secondhand tobacco smoke (Moritsugu, 2007). Consistently, the guidelines for the implementation of Article 8 of the World Health Organization (WHO) Framework Convention on Tobacco Control (FCTC) indicated there is no safe level of exposure to secondhand smoke, and the only effective measure to prevent exposure is the total elimination of smoking in indoor environments (WHO, 2003). Following those evidence-based conclusions, many cities and states in the United States and countries around the world have enacted comprehensive legislation banning smoking in all indoor public places. Many of those laws also include outside areas near the entrances to indoor areas. The spreading of the smoke-free movement and the banning of smoking indoors is probably one of the biggest achievements in public health in the first decade of the 21st century, protecting hundreds of millions of people from involuntary exposure to secondhand smoke around the world. Many people remain exposed, in venues that have been excluded from legislations (e.g., casinos), in states and countries that have not enacted legislation, and especially in private settings. While interventions rely mostly on educational and voluntary measures to eliminate secondhand tobacco smoke exposure in private spaces, legislation banning smoking in private places, such as in motor vehicles when children are present and in public housing, is increasing. For example, in 2016, the Department of Housing and Urban Development issued a mandate requiring housing authorities to adopt smoke-free policies, affecting 1.2 million households nationwide (PIH, 2016).

E-cigarettes were initially advertised as a form of tobacco that could circumvent existing smoke-free legislation (Paradise, 2014). Their increasing popularity brought initial confusion as to whether existing smoke-free legislation also applies to e-cigarettes (Stillman et al., 2015). Increasingly, legislation banning combustible tobacco cigarette smoking in indoor public places has been amended to expand coverage to e-cigarettes (Paradise, 2014). Many exceptions exist. For instance, vaping is allowed in e-cigarette shops and also in venues that hold vaping conventions (even if the use of e-cigarettes is banned in those venues during other events) (Jarmul et al., 2017) (see Figure 3-4). Overall, relatively few studies have investigated the characteristics and health effects of secondhand exposure to e-cigarette aerosol.

In this section, the committee reviews the evidence available on secondhand e-cigarette aerosol, its characteristics, and its possible health effects, compared with ambient air. Comparisons between secondhand

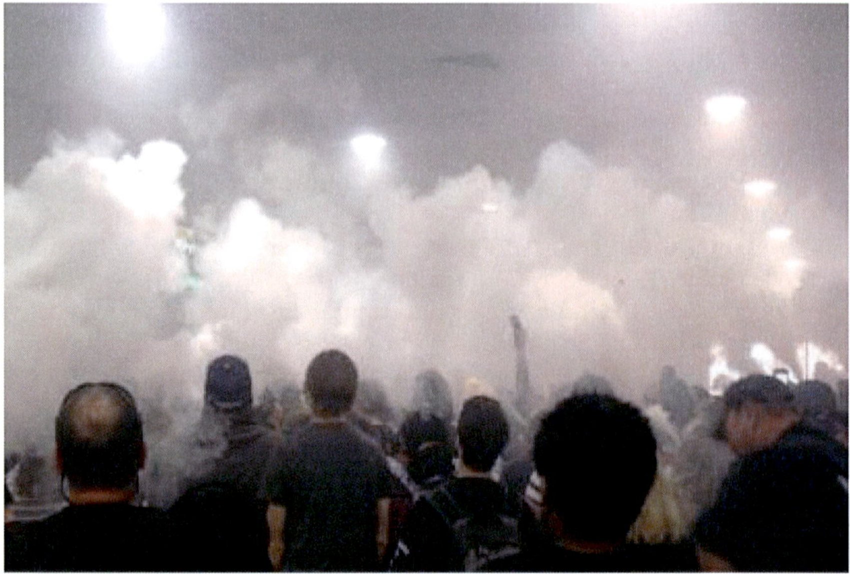

FIGURE 3-4 Photograph taken during a cloud competition at about 2 pm at a vaping convention, April 2016, Maryland.
SOURCE: Chen et al., 2017.

exposure from e-cigarettes and combustible tobacco cigarettes are discussed in Chapter 18 on harm reduction.

Characteristics and Chemical Composition of Secondhand E-Cigarette Aerosol

For combustible tobacco cigarettes, secondhand smoke is defined as the combination of mainstream (exhaled by the smoker) and sidestream (emitted from the burning cigarette) smoke, with sidestream smoke representing more than 80 percent of the total amount of secondhand tobacco smoke. Secondhand aerosol from e-cigarettes is very different from secondhand combustible tobacco smoke. First, e-cigarette aerosol is composed in large part by small liquid droplets while tobacco smoke contains mostly solid and semi-solid materials, resulting in different half-lives and deposition behavior in the environment. Second, the e-cigarette aerosol is directly inhaled by the user from the battery-powered device without generation of sidestream smoke. The secondhand aerosol from the e-cigarette thus originates from the aerosol that is exhaled by the vaper and is almost 100 percent mainstream. Multiple studies have characterized the inhaled secondhand smoke using smoking machines or other systems to generate the e-cigarette aerosol, and described it as an aerosol formed by the condensation or atomization of spherical liquid droplets in the submicrometer to 200-μm range. Those studies are not directly relevant for understanding the characteristics and health risks of secondhand aerosol from e-cigarettes as it has not been exhaled by a vaper. In this part of the report the committee only reviews studies in which the aerosol under study has been originated by a person vaping an e-cigarette, and thus reflects the exposure to bystanders. The number of such studies is relatively small, despite its potential impact on indoor air quality and the involuntary nature of exposure. Those studies have been conducted in exposure chambers or rooms that tried to recreate a room where vaping is occurring (Czogała et al., 2014; Liu et al., 2017; Melstrom et al., 2017; Protano et al., 2017; Schober et al., 2014), in a real-life setting in the homes of e-cigarette users (Ballbè et al., 2014; Fernández et al., 2015), and during vaping conventions (Chen et al., 2017; Soule et al., 2016).

In a study conducted in an exposure chamber with five dual users who used their personal e-cigarette devices (no details provided regarding type of device) ad lib twice for 5 minutes with a 30-minute interval, mean (standard deviation [SD]) 1-hour air nicotine concentration measured using active sampling was 3.32 (2.49) μg/m^3 compared with undetectable for 1-hour measure collected at baseline ($p < 0.05$) (Czogała et al., 2014). Real-time $PM_{2.5}$ concentrations increased shortly after the beginning of vaping. The mean (SD) $PM_{2.5}$ concentration was also higher following vaping (152 [86.8] μg/m^3) compared with baseline (32.4 μg/m^3) ($p < 0.05$). No differences were observed for CO (1.40 [0.55] versus 1.40 [0.55]). For volatile organic compounds (VOCs), toluene was the only one detected in the exposure chamber and the levels remained similar after vaping (3.79 [2.16] versus 4.09 [2.21]; $p = 0.85$) (Czogała et al., 2014). Another chamber study with four volunteers vaping e-cigarettes for 12 puffs with Smooke E-SMART device confirmed that particles increased in real time, although the concentrations were lower compared with secondhand tobacco smoke (Protano et al., 2017). In a chamber study with 37 volunteers using cigalikes and tank-style devices under controlled conditions and 4-hour ad lib use, nicotine, PG, and glycerol increased, but were several-fold below the time-weighted average limits used in workplace settings (Liu et al., 2017). The tank device produced the highest difference from baseline in the level of PG and glycerol. For nicotine, the air levels ranged from 0.38 to 2.83 μg/m^3. Of the 15 carbonyls measured, only hexaldehyde and acetaldehyde were significantly higher with either cigalikes or tank-style devices, respectively. Of the 12 VOCs measured, benzene, isoprene, and toluene increased with the use of cigalikes or tank-style devices. This study did not measure particulate matter.

In a study of nine volunteers using e-cigarettes (with a refillable tank) for 2 hours in groups of three trying to recreate a real-life scenario (café-like setting) and using different e-liquids with and without nicotine, the mean airborne concentration of $PM_{2.5}$ during the vaping sessions was 197 μg/m^3 versus 6 μg/m^3 for the control periods (Schober et al., 2014). PM_{10} (mean 229 versus 47 μg/m^3), particle number concentrations (61,682 versus 4,466 particles/cm^3), nicotine (2.2 versus less than 0.04 μg/m^3), total polycyclic aromatic hydrocarbons (PAHs) (515 versus 350 ng/m^3), and aluminum (483 versus 203 ng/m^3) also increased during the vaping sessions.

In real-life settings, studies in homes found small real-time increases in $PM_{2.5}$ concentrations in the home of an e-cigarette user that coincided with vaping use during a 60-minute sampling, although the median concentration (9.88 μg/m^3) was similar (8.32 μg/m^3) to the levels found in the home of the non-vaper (Fernández et al., 2015). In another study in homes by the same research team, median air nicotine (0.11 versus 0.01 μg/m^3; $p = 0.007$), salivary cotinine (0.24 versus 0.05 ng/ml; $p = 0.003$), and urinary cotinine (2.64 versus 0.72 ng/ml; $p = 0.008$) concentrations were higher in homes of participants who lived with somebody who vaped more than 2 hours/day versus control homes (Ballbè et al., 2014).

Two studies measured indoor air quality in e-cigarette convention events (Chen et al., 2017; Soule et al., 2016). Those events are often attended by tens to hundreds of e-cigarette users who often vape at the same time. In both studies levels of particulate matter (PM_{10} in one study, $PM_{2.5}$ in the other study) were markedly elevated, reaching levels that are typical of bars and hookah venues. One of the studies measured $PM_{2.5}$ the day before, during, and the day after the event (see Figure 3-5), showing that even on the day after, $PM_{2.5}$ concentrations were still markedly higher compared with the day before the event (Soule et al., 2016).

In the other study in a vaping convention, in addition to real-time PM_{10}, real-time CO_2 (a marker of how many people were in the room) and total volatile organic compounds (TVOCs) were measured, as well as a 7-hour nicotine concentration (Chen et al., 2017). The estimated 24-hour time-weighted average PM_{10} was 1,800 μg/m^3, 12 times higher than the Environmental Protection Agency 24-hour standard (150 μg/m^3). Median indoor TVOC concentration was 0.13 (range = 0.04–0.3) ppm. TVOC and PM_{10} were highly correlated with CO_2, indicating the high number of people using e-cigarettes and exposed to poor air quality. The concentrations of TVOC also increased markedly during a cloud competition (for PM_{10} the monitor stopped shortly after the beginning of the competition and the comparison is limited) (see Figure 3-6). The picture in Figure 3-6 shows a high moment during the cloud competition. Air nicotine concen-

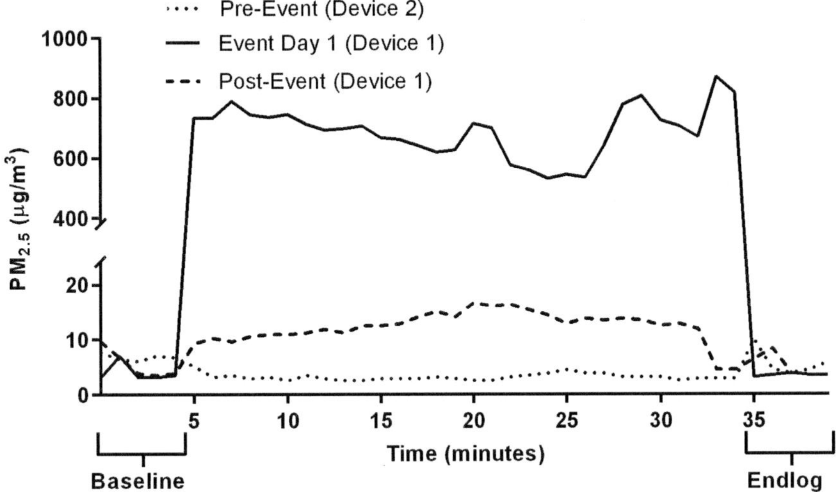

FIGURE 3-5 Event room $PM_{2.5}$ concentrations before, during, and after an e-cigarette convention.
NOTE: $PM_{2.5}$ = particulate matter 2.5 micrometers or less in diameter.
SOURCE: Soule et al., 2016.

tration was 125 µg/m^3, similar to concentrations measured in bars and nightclubs.

The findings from these two studies indicate that e-cigarette aerosol in vaping conventions where many e-cigarette users congregate is a major source of particulate matter, air nicotine, and VOCs, impairing air quality. These exposures can also be a concern for e-cigarette vendors and other venue workers who spend many hours in those places (Chen et al., 2017).

In addition to these studies based primarily on exposure assessment and environmental sampling, two studies have developed models to evaluate the secondhand aerosol generated by e-cigarettes under different conditions (Logue et al., 2017; Rostami et al., 2016). For instance, one model assessed real-life settings, such as a residential setting where a non-user lives with a user and a bar that allows vaping indoors (Logue et al., 2017). The contribution of secondhand e-cigarette aerosols to air pollutant concentrations in the home did not exceed the California Office of Environmental Health Hazard Assessment 8-hour reference exposure levels (RELs), except when a high-emitting device was used (4.8 V). In that extreme scenario, the contributions from vaping amounted to as much as 12 µg m^{-3} formaldehyde and 2.6 µg m^{-3} acrolein. In the bar scenario, the contributions from vaping to indoor air levels were markedly higher than those in the home scenario. Formaldehyde (mean 135

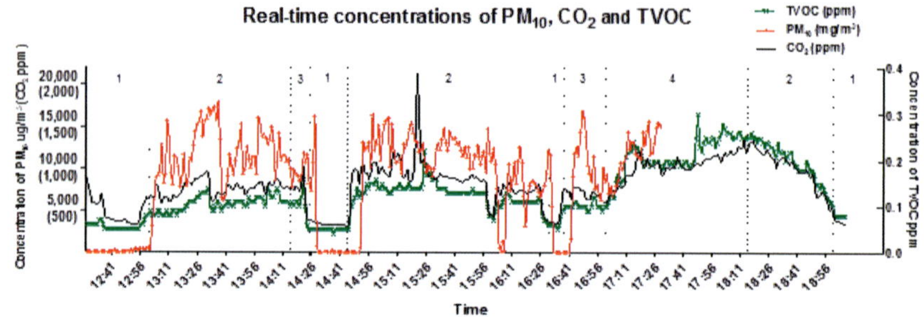

FIGURE 3-6 Real-time changes of PM_{10}, CO_2, and TVOC concentrations during a vaping convention in Maryland.
NOTES: 1 = outside the venue; 2 = inside the venue; 3 = trick competition; 4 = vaping competition. PM_{10} = particulate matter 10 micrometers or less in diameter; TVOC = total volatile organic compound.
SOURCE: Chen et al., 2017.

μg m^{-3}) and acrolein (28 μg m^{-3}) exceeded the acute 1-hour exposure REL for the highest emitting vaporizer/voltage combination. Predictions for these compounds also exceeded the 8-hour REL in several bars when less intense vaping conditions were considered. Benzene concentrations in a few bars approached the 8-hour REL, and diacetyl levels were near the lower limit for occupational exposures. These findings support the evidence that e-cigarettes can contribute to substantial air pollution, especially in places with a large number of e-cigarette users. The committee did not identify any studies evaluating health effects or early biomarkers of disease resulting from secondhand exposure to e-cigarette aerosols per se. One study conducted a health impact assessment based on computing disability-adjusted life-years (DALYs) lost due to exposure to secondhand e-cigarette aerosol (Logue et al., 2017). DALYs were estimated for residential and hospitality industry scenarios based on the recent incorporation of DALYs into health impact assessments of exposures to indoor pollutants, including tobacco smoke and particles, and estimating, on a compound-by-compound basis, the population-averaged health damage per year of exposure. The toxicants included were formaldehyde, acetaldehyde, benzene, acrolein, and glycidol. Formaldehyde, acetaldehyde, and benzene are established carcinogens and glycidol is a probable carcinogen according to the International Agency for Research on Cancer. Acrolein is not yet classified as a carcinogen but it was the dominant contributor to the aggregate harm (see Figure 3-7). DALYs for different combinations of device/voltage characteristics were lower, but in some instances comparable to those estimated for exposure to secondhand tobacco smoke.

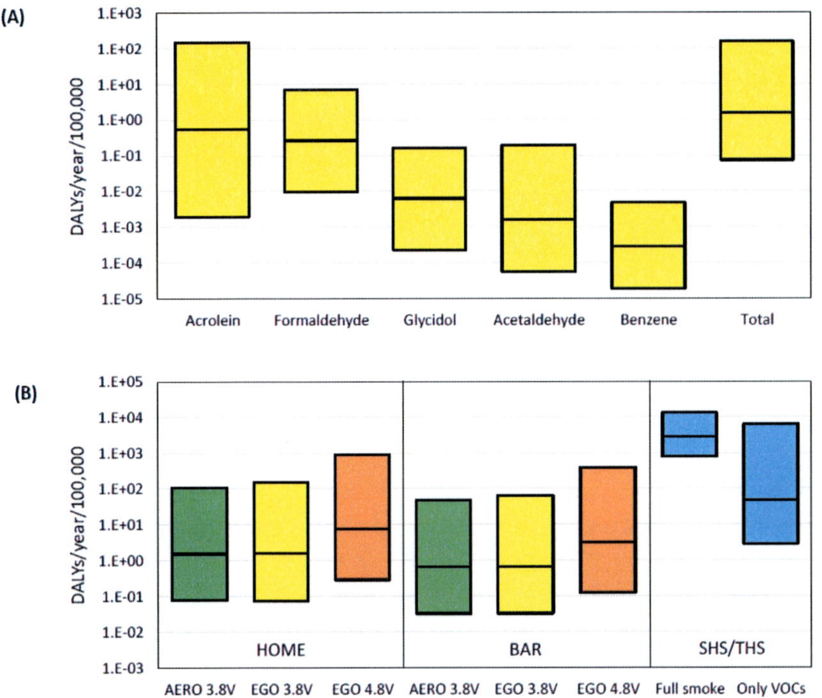

FIGURE 3-7 Estimated disability-adjusted life-years (DALYs) lost due to exposure to secondhand e-cigarette aerosol.
NOTES: The boxes show the median and 95th percentile range of predicted health damage. Panel A shows toxicant-specific impact estimated for the residential scenario in which the vaper consumes CT e-liquid using the EGO device at 3.8 V. Panel B shows aggregated damage for six scenarios of home and bar exposures using three device/voltage combinations. In all cases, emission rates correspond to typical vaping sessions of 25 puffs each. The figure includes the estimated damage due to second- and thirdhand smoke from combustible tobacco cigarettes as calculated in a previous study from St.Helen et al. (2016b). The DALYs are presented for full smoke and for the VOCs alone (excluding $PM_{2.5}$). DALY = disability-adjusted life-year; SHS/THS = secondhand smoke/thirdhand smoke; VOC = volatile organic compound.
SOURCE: Logue et al., 2017.

Synthesis

Several studies have measured airborne concentrations of particulate matter, nicotine, and other constituents in indoor environments, either in exposure chambers, rooms trying to recreate real-life settings, or real-life settings such as homes and conventions where vaping takes place. All studies measuring particulate matter and nicotine (for experiments with nicotine e-liquids) found statistically significant increases of those chemicals as compared with background. The levels of both particulate matter and nicotine were higher in experiments with more than one vaper, and they were extremely high in studies of vaping conventions, where levels of particulate matter and nicotine concentrations were comparable to those founds in bars and nightclubs. Among the other constituents, two studies detected airborne toluene and other VOCs in the air following vaping experiments. Total VOCs were markedly high and increased with increasing levels of vaping, during a vaping cloud competition, supporting the hypothesis that VOCs are released from the e-cigarettes into the environment during the exhalation of the e-cigarette aerosol. Overall, these exposure studies indicate that e-cigarette vaping contributes to some level of indoor air pollution, which, although lower than what has been observed from secondhand combustible tobacco cigarettes, is above the smoke-free level recommended by the Surgeon General and the WHO FCTC. As with secondhand smoke, children, pregnant women, the elderly, and patients with cardiorespiratory diseases may be at special risk. The e-cigarette convention studies also suggest that e-cigarette aerosol exposure could be substantial for workers in these venues, especially those who are exposed during multiple events. No available studies have evaluated health effects (either clinical effects or early biomarkers of disease) of secondhand e-cigarette exposure.

Conclusion 3-1. There is ***conclusive evidence*** *that e-cigarette use increases airborne concentrations of particulate matter and nicotine in indoor environments compared with background levels.*

This conclusion is supported by chamber experiments, real-setting experiments, and observational studies in homes and convention centers. In experiments with one single e-cigarette user, levels are markedly lower than for secondhand tobacco smoke. Levels increase markedly with the increase in the number of vapers, in particular at vaping conventions.

Conclusion 3-2. There is ***limited evidence*** *that e-cigarette use increases levels of nicotine and other e-cigarette constituents on a variety of indoor surfaces compared with background levels.*

REFERENCES

Alderman, S. L., C. Song, S. C. Moldoveanu, and S. K. Cole. 2014. Particle size distribution of e-cigarette aerosols and the relationship to Cambridge filter pad collection efficiency. *Beitrage zur Tabakforschung International/Contributions to Tobacco Research* 26(4):183–190.

Alexander, J. P., B. N. Coleman, S. E. Johnson, G. K. Tessman, C. Tworek, and D. M. Dickinson. 2016. Smoke and vapor: Exploring the terminology landscape among electronic cigarette users. *Tobacco Regulatory Science* 2(3):204–213.

Ballbè, M., J. M. Martínez-Sánchez, X. Sureda, M. Fu, R. Pérez-Ortuño, J. A. Pascual, E. Saltó, and E. Fernández. 2014. Cigarettes vs. e-cigarettes: Passive exposure at home measured by means of airborne marker and biomarkers. *Environmental Research* 135:76–80.

Behar, R. Z., M. Hua, and P. Talbot. 2015. Puffing topography and nicotine intake of electronic cigarette users. *PLoS ONE* 10(2):e0117222. https://doi.org/10.1371/journal.pone.0117222 (accessed February 6, 2018).

Brown, C. J., and J. M. Cheng. 2014. Electronic cigarettes: Product characterisation and design considerations. *Tobacco Control* 23(Supplement 2):ii4–ii10. http://tobaccocontrol.bmj.com/content/23/suppl_2/ii4 (accessed February 6, 2018).

Chen, R., A. Aherrera, C. Isicheye, P. Olmedo, S. Jarmul, J. E. Cohen, A. Navas-Acien, and A. M. Rule. 2017. Assessment of indoor air quality at an electronic cigarette (vaping) convention. *Journal of Exposure Science and Environmental Epidemiology* https://www.nature.com/articles/s41370-017-0005-x (accessed December 29, 2017).

Cheng, T. R. 2014. Chemical evaluation of electronic cigarettes. *Tobacco Control* 23:11–17.

Cunningham, A., S. Slayford, C. Vas, J. Gee, S. Costigan, and K. Prasad. 2016. Development, validation and application of a device to measure e-cigarette users' puffing topography. *Scientific Reports* 6:35071. https://www.nature.com/articles/srep35071 (accessed February 6, 2018).

Czogała, J., M. L. Goniewicz, B. Fidelus, W. Zielinska-Danch, M. J. Travers, and A. Sobczak. 2014. Secondhand exposure to vapors from electronic cigarettes. *Nicotine & Tobacco Research* 16(6):655–662.

Dawkins, L. E., C. F. Kimber, M. Doig, C. Feyerabend, and O. Corcoran. 2016. Self-titration by experienced e-cigarette users: Blood nicotine delivery and subjective effects. *Psychopharmacology (Berl)* 233(15–16):2933–2941.

Evans, S. E., and A. C. Hoffman. 2014. Electronic cigarettes: Abuse liability, topography and subjective effects. *Tobacco Control* 23(Supplement 2):ii23–ii29. http://dx.doi.org/10.1136/tobaccocontrol-2013-051489 (accessed February 6, 2018).

Farsalinos, K. E., A. Spyrou, C. Stefopoulos, K. Tsimopoulou, P. Kourkoveli, D. Tsiapras, S. Kyrzopoulos, K. Poulas, and V. Voudris. 2015a. Nicotine absorption from electronic cigarette use: Comparison between experienced consumers (vapers) and naïve users (smokers). *Scientific Reports* 5:11269. https://www.nature.com/articles/srep11269 (accessed February 6, 2018).

Farsalinos, K. E., V. Voudris, and K. Poulas. 2015b. E-cigarettes generate high levels of aldehydes only in "dry puff" conditions. *Addiction* 110(8):1352–1356.

Fernández, E., M. Ballbè, X. Sureda, M. Fu, E. Saltó, and J. M. Martínez-Sánchez. 2015. Particulate matter from electronic cigarettes and conventional cigarettes: A systematic review and observational study. *Current Environmental Health Reports* 2(4):423–429.

Fuoco, F. C., G. Buonanno, L. Stabile, and P. Vigo. 2014. Influential parameters on particle concentration and size distribution in the mainstream of e-cigarettes. *Environmental Pollution* 184:523–529.

Geiss, O., I. Bianchi, F. Barahona, and J. Barrero-Moreno. 2015. Characterisation of mainstream and passive vapours emitted by selected electronic cigarettes. *International Journal of Hygiene and Environmental Health* 218(1):169–180.

Geiss, O., I. Bianchi, and J. Barrero-Moreno. 2016. Correlation of volatile carbonyl yields emitted by e-cigarettes with the temperature of the heating coil and the perceived sensorial quality of the generated vapours. *International Journal of Hygiene and Environmental Health* 219(3):268–277.

Gillman, I. G., K. A. Kistler, E. W. Stewart, and A. R. Paolantonio. 2016. Effect of variable power levels on the yield of total aerosol mass and formation of aldehydes in e-cigarette aerosols. *Regulatory Toxicology and Pharmacology* 75:58–65.

Goniewicz, M. L., T. Kuma, M. Gawron, J. Knysak, and L. Kosmider. 2013. Nicotine levels in electronic cigarettes. *Nicotine & Tobacco Research* 15(1):158–166.

Goniewicz, M. L., J. Knysak, M. Gawron, L. Kosmider, A. Sobczak, J. Kurek, A. Prokopowicz, M. Jablonska-Czapla, C. Rosik-Dulewska, C. Havel, I. P. Jacob, and N. Benowitz. 2014. Levels of selected carcinogens and toxicants in vapour from electronic cigarettes. *Tobacco Control* 23(2):133–139.

Havel, C. M., N. L. Benowitz, P. Jacob, 3rd, and G. St.Helen. 2016. An electronic cigarette vaping machine for the characterization of aerosol delivery and composition. *Nicotine & Tobacco Research* 19(10):1224–1231.

Herrington, J. S., and C. Myers. 2015. Electronic cigarette solutions and resultant aerosol profiles. *Journal of Chromatography A* 1418:192–199.

Hukkanen, J., P. Jacob, 3rd, and N. L. Benowitz. 2005. Metabolism and disposition kinetics of nicotine. *Pharmacological Reviews* 57(1):79–115.

Ingebrethsen, B. J., S. K. Cole, and S. L. Alderman. 2012. Electronic cigarette aerosol particle size distribution measurements. *Inhalation Toxicology* 24(14):976–984.

Jarmul, S., A. Aherrera, A. M. Rule, P. Olmedo, R. Chen, and A. Navas-Acien. 2017. Lost in e-cigarette clouds: A culture on the rise. *American Journal of Public Health* 107(2):265–266.

Ji, E. H., B. B. Sun, T. K. Zhao, S. Shu, C. H. Chang, D. Messadi, T. Xia, Y. F. Zhu, and S. Hu. 2016. Characterization of electronic cigarette aerosol and its induction of oxidative stress response in oral keratinocytes. *PLoS ONE* 11(5):e0154447. https://doi.org/10.1371/journal.pone.0154447 (accessed February 6, 2018).

Kleykamp, B. A., J. M. Jennings, C. Sams, M. F. Weaver, and T. Eissenberg. 2008. The influence of transdermal nicotine on tobacco/nicotine abstinence and the effects of a concurrently administered cigarette in women and men. *Experimental and Clinical Psychopharmacology* 16(2):99–112.

Lee, Y. H., M. Gawron, and M. L. Goniewicz. 2015. Changes in puffing behavior among smokers who switched from tobacco to electronic cigarettes. *Addictive Behaviors* 48:1–4.

Liu, J., Q. Liang, M. J. Oldham, A. A. Rostami, K. A. Wagner, I. G. Gillman, P. Patel, R. Savioz, and M. Sarkar. 2017. Determination of selected chemical levels in room air and on surfaces after the use of cartridge- and tank-based e-vapor products or conventional cigarettes. *International Journal of Environmental Research & Public Health* 14(9):E969.

Logue, J. M., M. Sleiman, V. N. Montesinos, M. L. Russell, M. I. Litter, N. L. Benowitz, L. A. Gundel, and H. Destaillats. 2017. Emissions from electronic cigarettes: Assessing vapers' intake of toxic compounds, secondhand exposures, and the associated health impacts. *Environmental Science & Technology* 51(16):9271–9279.

Lopez, A. A., M. M. Hiler, E. K. Soule, C. P. Ramoa, N. V. Karaoghlanian, T. Lipato, A. B. Breland, A. L. Shihadeh, and T. Eissenberg. 2016. Effects of electronic cigarette liquid nicotine concentration on plasma nicotine and puff topography in tobacco cigarette smokers: A preliminary report. *Nicotine & Tobacco Research* 18(5):720–723.

Marini, S., G. Buonanno, L. Stabile, and G. Ficco. 2014. Short-term effects of electronic and tobacco cigarettes on exhaled nitric oxide. *Toxicology and Applied Pharmacology* 278(1):9–15.

Melstrom, P., B. Koszowski, M. H. Thanner, E. Hoh, B. King, R. Bunnell, and T. McAfee. 2017. Measuring $PM_{2.5}$, ultrafine particles, air nicotine and wipe samples following the use of electronic cigarettes. *Nicotine & Tobacco Research* 19(9):1055–1061.

Moritsugu, K. P. 2007. The 2006 report of the Surgeon General: The health consequences of involuntary exposure to tobacco smoke. *American Journal of Preventive Medicine* 32(6):542–543.

Norton, K. J., K. M. June, and R. J. O'Connor. 2014. Initial puffing behaviors and subjective responses differ between an electronic nicotine delivery system and traditional cigarettes. *Tobacco Induced Diseases* 12(1):17.

Ohta, K., S. Uchiyama, Y. Inaba, H. Nakagome, and N. Kunugita. 2011. Determination of carbonyl compounds generated from the electronic cigarette using coupled silica cartridges impregnated with hydroquinone and 2,4-dinitrophenylhydrazine. *Bunseki Kagaku* 60(10):791–797.

Papousek, R., Z. Pataj, P. Novakova, K. Lemr, and P. Bartak. 2014. Determination of acrylamide and acrolein in smoke from tobacco and e-cigarettes. *Chromatographia* 77(17–18): 1145–1151.

Paradise, J. 2014. Electronic cigarettes: Smoke-free laws, sale restrictions, and the public health. *American Journal of Public Health* 104(6):e17–e18.

Pichelstorfer, L., W. Hofmann, R. Winkler-Heil, C. U. Yurteri, and J. McAughey. 2016. Simulation of aerosol dynamics and deposition of combustible and electronic cigarette aerosols in the human respiratory tract. *Journal of Aerosol Science* 99:125–132.

PIH (Office of the Assistant Secretary for Public and Indian Housing). 2016. Instituting smoke-free public housing. *Federal Register* 81(233):87430–87444.

Pratte, P., S. Cosandey, and C. Goujon-Ginglinger. 2016. A scattering methodology for droplet sizing of e-cigarette aerosols. *Inhalation Toxicology* 28(12):537–545.

Protano, C., M. Manigrasso, P. Avino, and M. Vitali. 2017. Second-hand smoke generated by combustion and electronic smoking devices used in real scenarios: Ultrafine particle pollution and age-related dose assessment. *Environment International* 107:190–195.

Robinson, R. J., E. C. Hensel, P. N. Morabito, and K. A. Roundtree. 2015. Electronic cigarette topography in the natural environment. *PLoS ONE* 10(6):e0129296. https://doi.org/10.1371/journal.pone.0129296 (accessed February 6, 2018).

Robinson, R. J., E. C. Hensel, K. A. Roundtree, A. G. Difrancesco, J. M. Nonnemaker, and Y. O. Lee. 2016. Week long topography study of young adults using electronic cigarettes in their natural environment. *PLoS ONE* 11(10):e0164038. https://doi.org/10.1371/journal.pone.0164038 (accessed February 6, 2018).

Rostami, A. A., Y. B. Pithawalla, J. M. Liu, M. J. Oldham, K. A. Wagner, K. Frost-Pineda, and M. A. Sarkar. 2016. A well-mixed computational model for estimating room air levels of selected constituents from e-vapor product use. *International Journal of Environmental Research and Public Health* 13(8):E828.

Schmeltz, I., A. Wenger, D. Hoffmann, and T. C. Tso. 1979. Chemical studies on tobacco smoke. 63. On the fate of nicotine during pyrolysis and in a burning cigarette. *Journal of Agricultural and Food Chemistry* 27(3):602–608.

Schober, W., K. Szendrei, W. Matzen, H. Osiander-Fuchs, D. Heitmann, T. Schettgen, R. A. Jorres, and H. Fromme. 2014. Use of electronic cigarettes (e-cigarettes) impairs indoor air quality and increases FeNO levels of e-cigarette consumers. *International Journal of Hygiene and Environmental Health* 217(6):628–637.

Schripp, T., D. Markewitz, E. Uhde, and T. Salthammer. 2013. Does e-cigarette consumption cause passive vaping? *Indoor Air* 23(1):25–31.

Soule, E. K., S. F. Maloney, T. R. Spindle, A. K. Rudy, M. M. Hiler, and C. O. Cobb. 2016. Electronic cigarette use and indoor air quality in a natural setting. *Tobacco Control* 26(1):109.

Spindle, T. R., A. B. Breland, N. V. Karaoghlanian, A. L. Shihadeh, and T. Eissenberg. 2015. Preliminary results of an examination of electronic cigarette user puff topography: The effect of a mouthpiece-based topography measurement device on plasma nicotine and subjective effects. *Nicotine & Tobacco Research* 17(2):142–149.

Spindle, T. R., M. M. Hiler, A. B. Breland, N. V. Karaoghlanian, A. L. Shihadeh, and T. Eissenberg. 2017. The influence of a mouthpiece-based topography measurement device on electronic cigarette user's plasma nicotine concentration, heart rate, and subjective effects under directed and ad libitum use conditions. *Nicotine & Tobacco Research* 19(4):469–476.

St.Helen, G., K. C. Ross, D. A. Dempsey, C. M. Havel, P. Jacob, 3rd, and N. L. Benowitz. 2016a. Nicotine delivery and vaping behavior during ad libitum e-cigarette access. *Tobacco Regulatory Science* 2(4):363–376.

St.Helen, G., C. Havel, D. Dempsey, P. Jacob, 3rd, and N. L. Benowitz. 2016b. Nicotine delivery, retention and pharmacokinetics from various electronic cigarettes. *Addiction* (111)3:535–544.

Stillman, F. A., A. Soong, L. Y. Zheng, and A. Navas-Acien. 2015. E-cigarette use in air transit: Self-reported data from US flight attendants. *Tobacco Control* 24(4):417–418.

Strasser, A. A., V. Souprountchouk, A. Kaufmann, S. Blazekovic, F. Leone, N. L. Benowitz, and R. A. Schnoll. 2016. Nicotine replacement, topography, and smoking phenotypes of e-cigarettes. *Tobacco Regulatory Science* 2(4):352–362.

Trehy, M. L., W. Ye, M. E. Hadwiger, T. W. Moore, J. F. Allgire, J. T. Woodruff, S. S. Ahadi, J. C. Black, and B. J. Westenberger. 2011. Analysis of electronic cigarette cartridges, refill solutions, and smoke for nicotine and nicotine related impurities. *Journal of Liquid Chromatography and Related Technologies* 34(14):1442–1458.

Trtchounian, A., M. Williams, and P. Talbot. 2010. Conventional and electronic cigarettes (e-cigarettes) have different smoking characteristics. *Nicotine & Tobacco Research* 12(9): 905–912.

Uchiyama, S., Y. Inaba, and N. Kunugita. 2010. Determination of acrolein and other carbonyls in cigarette smoke using coupled silica cartridges impregnated with hydroquinone and 2,4-dinitrophenylhydrazine. *Journal of Chromatography A* 1217(26):4383–4388.

WHO (World Health Organization). 2003. *WHO framework convention on tobacco control.* Geneva, Switzerland: World Health Organization. http://www.who.int/fctc/text_download/en (accessed February 6, 2018).

Williams, M., and P. Talbot. 2011. Variability among electronic cigarettes in the pressure drop, airflow rate, and aerosol production. *Nicotine & Tobacco Research* 13(12):1276–1283.

Winkler-Heil, R., G. Ferron, and W. Hofmann. 2014. Calculation of hygroscopic particle deposition in the human lung. *Inhalation Toxicology* 26(3):193–206.

Zhu, S. H., J. Y. Sun, E. Bonnevie, S. E. Cummins, A. Gamst, L. Yin, and M. Lee. 2014. Four hundred and sixty brands of e-cigarettes and counting: Implications for product regulation. *Tobacco Control* 23(Supplement 3):iii3–iii9. http://tobaccocontrol.bmj.com/content/23/suppl_3/iii3 (accessed February 6, 2018).

4

Nicotine

Electronic cigarettes are designed to deliver a nicotine-containing aerosol to the user. According to the 1988 Surgeon General's report *The Health Consequences of Smoking: Nicotine Addiction*, "Nicotine is the drug in tobacco that causes addiction" (HHS, 1988, p. 9). Because dependence on tobacco is produced primarily through the pharmacological effects of nicotine (Benowitz, 2009), an understanding of the pharmacology (i.e., disposition kinetics, metabolism, and pharmacodynamics) of nicotine, concentration of nicotine in commercial e-cigarette liquids and aerosols, systemic nicotine exposure among users, and factors that may affect nicotine exposure are essential to understanding the potential addictiveness of e-cigarettes. In addition, although most of the harm caused by tobacco smoking is attributed to combustion products, nicotine contributes to health outcomes such as cardiovascular disease in smokers (HHS, 2014). Therefore it is important to understand mechanisms of action of nicotine to understand its role in the overall health effects of e-cigarettes.

CONCENTRATION OF NICOTINE IN COMMERCIAL E-CIGARETTES

Although some e-cigarettes/e-liquids do not contain nicotine, most do, and the nicotine contents of e-cigarettes are variable. Based on vaping machine studies, higher nicotine concentration of e-liquids results in higher nicotine yield of any given e-cigarette (Talih et al., 2015). As with combustible tobacco cigarettes, machine-derived nicotine yield of e-cigarettes is not necessarily predictive of users' systemic exposures to nicotine. Other factors such as power of the e-cigarette and user behavior and use patterns are also critical. Nevertheless, e-liquid nicotine concentration may be a determinant of systemic nicotine exposure. Here, the committee reviews current evidence related to the range of nicotine concentrations in commercially available e-cigarettes, whether cartridges of first-generation and closed-tank e-cigarettes or refill liquids used in other open-system e-cigarettes. The committee also discusses labeling accuracy of nicotine content.

There is no consensus in the way nicotine strength is reported on labels of products or in studies. The nicotine strength on the label of some products is qualitative (e.g., zero, low, medium, high, super high) or quantitative on others. The unit of quantitative measure of nicotine strength is often reported on labels or in studies as amount per cartridge (mg), percentage per volume (e.g., 2.4 percent nicotine), concentration (mg/ml), or amount of nicotine per amount of e-liquid (µg/mg or mg/g).

A previous systematic review of the evidence evaluating chemicals in refill solutions and cartridges included studies published between January 2007 and September 2013 (Cheng, 2014). Based on 10 of the 29 studies included in this review, which reported on nicotine concentration of e-liquids, the review found that nicotine levels in e-liquids varied considerably, with a range of 0–87.2 mg/ml. For example, one study assessed the level of nicotine in popular brands of refill liquids from the United States and Western Europe (Etter et al., 2013). Among the 20 samples from 10 different brands, the range of nicotine on the labels was 6–30 mg. The range of measured nicotine concentration was 6–29.0 mg/ml; the measured concentration ranged from 85 to 107 percent of the labeled nicotine content. Another study assessed the nicotine content of 16 e-cigarette brands (20 cartridges and 15 refill liquids) based on high popularity in markets in Poland, the United Kingdom, and the United States (Goniewicz et al., 2013). Measured nicotine in cartridges ranged from 0.3 to 19 mg (per cartridge) and 0 to 25 mg in refill liquids. In another study, nicotine concentration was measured in a convenience sample of seven e-cigarette refill liquids (Cameron et al., 2014). Measured mean nicotine concentration across the seven brands ranged from 8.5 to 22.2 mg/ml, and were equivalent to or lower than labeled concentrations.

A number of studies have assessed nicotine concentration in e-liquids since the 2014 review by Cheng. Goniewicz and colleagues (2015) measured nicotine in 32, 29, and 30 popular brands of e-liquids purchased between 2013 and 2014 in the United States, South Korea, and Poland, respectively. In samples from the United States, nicotine in the e-liquid ranged from below limit of quantitation (BLQ) to 36.6 mg/ml. Of 32 samples, 9 (28 percent) had measured nicotine levels that deviated from the labeled nicotine strength by more than 20 percent. In South Korea, two-thirds of the products tested did not have detectable levels of nicotine while the higher concentration was 150 mg/ml (this product was labeled "Pure Nicotine"). The range of nicotine strength in Polish samples was BLQ to 24.7 mg/ml. Ten percent of the Polish products tested showed deviations from the label of greater than 20 percent, while none of the products labeled nicotine-free contained detectable amounts of nicotine. Lisko and colleagues (2015) measured nicotine concentration in 36 cartridge and refill e-liquids in the U.S. market that had favorable online reviews. Nicotine content ranged from undetected to 20.5 mg/g. The measured nicotine concentrations were 5.8–41.7 percent lower than the labeled nicotine content. Tierney and colleagues (2016) reported a range of 6 to 24 mg/ml in a sample of 30 cartridge and refill e-liquids.

Etter and Bugey (2017) assessed the agreement between labeled and measured nicotine content across brands and across batches within the same brand. Eighteen e-liquids from 11 frequently used brands in the United States, the United Kingdom, France, and Switzerland were purchased in 2013. Nicotine on the labels ranged from 16 to 48 mg/ml. The measured nicotine concentrations ranged from 15.5 to 52.0 mg/ml. A majority of the sample, 82 percent, had measured nicotine concentration within 10 percent of the labeled content. Differences across batches within the same brands were small (0.5 percent). By contrast, Goniewicz and colleagues (2014), in a study that measured nicotine content of e-liquids from six popular products in the United Kingdom that were purchased 4 weeks apart, found the mean difference between batches of the same brand ranged from 1 to 31 percent.

Some clinical studies have reported the nicotine content of their participants' usual brands of e-cigarettes. St.Helen and colleagues (2016a,b) characterized nicotine delivery and e-cigarette nicotine pharmacokinetic profiles among experienced e-cigarette users. Among the 13 enrolled participants, the labeled nicotine content of their usual e-liquids ranged from 6 to 24 mg/ml. The measured nicotine content ranged from 5.0 to 15.3 mg/g (note the difference in units). In another study of experienced e-cigarette users by St.Helen and colleagues (2017), the average nicotine on the label of the participants' usual e-liquids was 7.9 mg/ml (range = 3–18 mg/ml). The measured nicotine concentration averaged 7.4 mg/ml (range = 1.6–19.9 mg/ml).

The preferred nicotine strength may differ across types of e-cigarettes used, particularly based on the power of the e-cigarettes. Users of high-powered e-cigarettes tend to use e-liquids with lower nicotine concentrations. Wagener and colleagues (2017) enrolled 9 second-generation and 11 third-generation e-cigarette users in a clinical study. The average power of the second-generation e-cigarettes was 8.6 W compared with 71.6 W of the third-generation e-cigarettes. The average nicotine concentration of users of second-generation e-cigarettes was 22.3 mg/ml (range = 11–36 mg/ml) compared with 4.1 mg/ml (range = 1.5–6 mg/ml).

In summary, these studies show that nicotine content varies widely among products. Some studies show agreement between the nicotine content on the label and what was chemically measured while other studies show greater deviation of measured nicotine content from labeled content. One study showed that nicotine content is similar across batches of the same brand while another showed wider variability. Finally, the choice of preferred nicotine strength may be influenced, in part, by the characteristics of the e-cigarette used, including the power of the device.

NICOTINE CONCENTRATION IN E-CIGARETTE EMISSIONS

Nicotine concentration in e-cigarette emissions is an important determinant of systemic exposure to nicotine, and likely directly affects the abuse liability of e-cigarettes. E-cigarettes are designed to deliver nicotine to the user. Device characteristics that alter nicotine concentration in the aerosol are expected to also affect the abuse liability of e-cigarettes.

The systematic review by Cheng (2014) also included a review of nicotine delivery. As discussed above, Cheng identified five studies between January 2007 and September 2013 that reported amounts of nicotine in e-cigarette aerosol (Cobb et al., 2010; Goniewicz et al., 2013; Pellegrino et al., 2012; Trehy et al., 2011; Westenberger, 2009). The unit of measurement of nicotine in e-cigarette aerosol varied among the studies and included amount in a certain number of puffs (e.g., 100 or 150 puffs) and amount per volume of air (e.g., μg/100 ml puff, mg/m^3). One major finding was that delivery of nicotine is not consistent across products.

For example, Goniewicz and colleagues (2013) assessed nicotine in aerosol in a study described previously. Sixteen popular e-cigarettes, including 20 cartridges, were obtained from Poland, the United Kingdom, and the United States based on popularity. Aerosol was generated from 300 puffs from each e-cigarette in 20 series of 15 puffs. Puffing conditions were based on average puff topography from 10 experienced e-cigarette users (70-ml puff volume, 1.8-second puff duration, and 10-second inter-puff interval). As mentioned before, nicotine in the cartridges ranged from 0.3 to 19 mg. Nicotine in the aerosol varied by brand and ranged from 0.5 to 15.4 mg per 300 puffs. Also, nicotine in the aerosol varied from 21 percent to 85 percent of the nicotine present in the cartridge.

Adamson and colleagues (2016) compared nicotine delivery from a commercially available e-cigarette (Vype ePen) with 3R4F reference cigarettes (University of Kentucky) using the Health Canada Intense smoking regime (2-second puff duration, 55-ml puff volume, 30-second interpuff interval). The e-cigarette was used at 4.0 V (5.7 W) and contained e-liquid with nicotine concentration of 18 mg/ml. Two different smoking machines were used, namely, Borgwaldt RM20S and Vitrocell VC10. Mean nicotine per puff from the 3R4F combustible tobacco cigarette was 0.171 (SD = 0.055) mg and 0.193 (SD = 0.055) mg on the RM20S and VC10, respectively. In comparison, mean amount of nicotine per puff from the e-cigarette was 0.049 (SD = 0.006) mg and 0.053 (SD = 0.012) mg. Interestingly, the nicotine concentration per puff increased from puff to puff when generating the combustible tobacco cigarette smoke. This is because tar and nicotine deposit down the cigarette rod on burning, enriching the distillable material in the rod for later puffs (Adamson et al., 2016). By contrast, the e-cigarette nicotine concentration was found to be highly consistent from puff to puff. The implications for variation or lack thereof in nicotine concentration per puff between combustible tobacco cigarette use versus e-cigarette use are not clear. However, this study shows that at a power of 5.7 W, e-cigarettes deliver less nicotine per puff than combustible tobacco cigarettes. Nicotine delivery per puff is expected to increase with power. The study mentioned that delivery at a power of 4.6 W was 0.032 mg of nicotine per puff. This was based on another study by the same research group, which compared nicotine delivery from Vype ePen at low voltage with 3R4F reference combustible tobacco cigarettes (Margham et al., 2016).

Talih and colleagues (2015) examined the influence of puff duration and puff velocity (or flow rate), as well as device power and nicotine concentration, on vaping machine-derived emissions from e-cigarettes. One type of e-cigarette cartridge, V4L CoolCart, was used in the study, and aerosols were generated by a machine designed and manufactured by the American University of Beirut. Five distinct puff profiles representing a combustible tobacco cigarette smoker and four types of e-cigarette user profiles (different puff duration and puff velocity) were examined. Power and e-liquid nicotine concentration were varied. The study found that nicotine yield ranged by more than 50-fold across conditions, from 0.11 mg to 4.70 mg in 15 puffs. Nicotine yield in 15 puffs was positively related to puff duration, power (voltage), and nicotine concentration of the e-liquid. Interestingly, puff velocity was not related to nicotine yields. This study showed that the concentration of nicotine in e-cigarette aerosols is determined both by e-cigarette characteristics and user behavior.

In summary, nicotine concentration in e-cigarette aerosol is variable among e-cigarettes. In the conditions tested, nicotine yield from an e-cigarette was lower than that of a reference combustible tobacco cigarette. However, the concentration of nicotine in e-cigarette aerosol is a product of device characteristics and user behavior. Nicotine yield increases with e-cigarette power and e-liquid nicotine concentration, and with increasing puff duration.

pH OF E-LIQUIDS

Nicotine is a weak base with a pKa of 8.5. The absorption and renal excretion of nicotine is highly pH dependent (IOM, 2001). In acidic environments, nicotine is in its protonated, charged state and does not cross membranes rapidly. For example, the smoke of flue-cured cigarettes (the most common form) has pH ranging from 5.5 to 6.0, resulting in nicotine existing primarily in the protonated form (Benowitz et al., 2009). Studies have shown little buccal absorption of nicotine from flue-cured cigarette smoke (Gori et al., 1986). On the other hand, smoke from air-cured tobacco, the dominant form used in pipes and cigars, has a pH of 6.5 or greater, results in a higher fraction of unprotonated (free-base) nicotine, and is absorbed in the mouth (Armitage et al., 1978).

The proportion of free-based (unprotonated) nicotine, which is the more volatile and readily absorbed form, increases with pH (Pankow, 2001; Pankow et al., 1997). Given its relatively high volatility, more free-base nicotine in combustible tobacco cigarette smoke is thought to lead to greater deposition of free-base nicotine in the mouth and throat (Henningfield et al., 2004). Although free-base nicotine is absorbed in the mouth and upper respiratory tract, the rate of such absorption into the blood is slower than in the lungs (Bergstrom et al., 1995). On the other hand, deposition of free-base nicotine in the mouth and throat leads to greater sensory effects due to possible activation of peripheral nerves (Henningfield et al., 2004).

The pH of e-liquids and its implications for nicotine absorption and pharmacological effects of e-cigarettes have not been extensively studied. By definition, pH is relevant to aqueous solutions (water as the solvent). To measure the apparent pH of e-liquids, which have propylene glycol (PG) and/or glycerol as the solvent, the e-liquid is first dissolved in a known amount of deionized water and pH measured over a time period (El-Hellani et al., 2015). Using this method, Lisko and colleagues (2015) found that the pH of a sample of 36 cartridges and refill liquids ranged from 5.1 to 9.1. The pH was positively correlated with the nicotine concentration of the e-liquid. Interestingly, this relationship was stronger in laboratory-prepared e-liquids than commercial e-liquids, indicating a potential effect of flavor additives on pH. El-Hellani and colleagues (2015) reported that cartridges from three brands with various nicotine concentrations and refill liquids had pH ranging from 7.4 to 9.7. This study found wide variability in nicotine partitioning between the unprotonated and protonated states of nicotine in the e-liquid and aerosols. Unprotonated nicotine was found to account for 18–95 percent of the total nicotine, depending on the product in question and the pH. Based on high agreement between measured and predicted amounts of protonated nicotine in laboratory-prepared e-liquids and poorer agreement in commercial e-liquids, the authors inferred, similar to Lisko and colleagues, that flavor additives in commercial e-liquids likely affect e-liquid pH (El-Hellani et al., 2015). Etter and Bugey (2017) reported pH of 18 e-liquids ranging from 8.1 to 9.9 (average = 9.1). The pH of 14 usual brand e-liquids of participants in a clinical study by St.Helen and colleagues (2017) ranged from 4.33 to 9.10 (average = 6.80).

Given that nicotine partitioning in the protonated and unprotonated forms in e-liquid and aerosol varies widely among products (El-Hellani et al., 2015), it is important to understand how such variation impacts nicotine deposition in the airways, rates of absorption, systemic exposure, and sensory effects. A pilot study by St.Helen and colleagues (2017) found elevated rates of nicotine absorption and maximum plasma nicotine concentration when participants used a strawberry e-liquid (18 mg/ml nicotine, 50/50 glycerol/PG, pH 8.29) compared with a tobacco e-liquid (18 mg/ml nicotine, 50/50 glycerol/PG, pH 9.10). After 15 puffs (30-second interpuff) with the same e-cigarette on separate days, 5-, 15-, and 30-minute areas under the plasma nicotine concentration-time curve (AUC) were 17–23 percent higher and maximum plasma nicotine concentration was 22 percent higher with the less basic strawberry e-liquid compared with the tobacco. This study was not a systematic study of the effect of pH, but suggests that a potential effect of flavorants is through pH. Systematic studies of the effect of e-liquid and aerosol pH on e-cigarette pharmacology are needed for more definitive answers. The pH of e-liquids is one e-liquid characteristic that the Food and Drug Administration may consider regulating, but more research is needed.

NICOTINE SALTS

Nearly all e-cigarettes use solvents such as PG and glycerol as the carrier compounds in the aerosol. However, novel e-cigarettes are being developed that do not contain glycerol or PG, but contain nicotine base and a weak organic acid that forms a nicotine salt. These devices are patterned after technology described by Rose and colleagues (2008). One example is JUUL™ by JUUL Labs. Chemical analysis of the liquid in JUUL™ pods, which are prefilled cartridges, found benzoic acid and nicotine in a 0.97–1 molar concentration ratio (44.8 ± 0.6 and 61.6 ± 1.5 mg/ml, respectively) (Pankow et al., 2017), indicating that benzoic acid is a major ingredient of this device. The nicotine salt, nicotine benzoate, likely forms when the device is activated, and is delivered to the user in an aerosol form. Furthermore, Philip Morris Products S.A. recently developed a novel e-cigarette called P3L (Teichert et al., 2017). The device consists of a cartridge containing nicotine base and lactic acid in separate cavities. On activation and controlled heating, the nicotine salt (nicotine lactate) is released as an aerosol. In a clinical study, maximum plasma nicotine concentrations from use of three formulations of P3L, namely, 50, 80, and 150 μg/puff P3L, were 9.7, 11.2, and 9.8 ng/ml, respectively (Teichert et al., 2017). JUUL™ and new products such as P3L show the potential use of nicotine salts to deliver nicotine in electronic nicotine delivery systems.

TOXICOLOGY AND MODES OF ACTION

In this section, the pharmacology of nicotine is summarized, but it is not intended to be a systematic review of the topic. Several authoritative reviews have been published on nicotine and were identified as the primary sources for this summary. They include the 1988 Surgeon General's report on smoking, *The Health Consequences of Smoking: Nicotine Addiction* (HHS, 1988); the 2001 Institute of Medicine report *Clearing the Smoke: Assessing the Science Base for Tobacco Harm Reduction* (IOM, 2001); the 2010 Surgeon General's report *How Tobacco Smoke Causes Disease* (HHS, 2010b); and reviews on nicotine chemistry, metabolism, disposition kinetics, and pharmacology (e.g., England et al., 2017). Individual adverse outcomes of nicotine are covered in greater detail in the specific health outcomes sections.

General Pharmacology of Nicotine

Nicotine, 3-(1-methyl-2-pyrrolidinyl) pyridine, consists of a pyridine and a pyrrolidine ring, is volatile, and has a molecular weight of 162.23 (Benowitz, 2009). It is the most abundant tobacco alkaloid, making up about 95 percent of the alkaloid content of combustible tobacco cigarettes and 1.5 percent by weight in cigarette tobacco (Benowitz et al., 2009). The nicotine content of commercially available e-liquids varies from low to high (commonly 0.3–5 percent by volume) (Cameron et al., 2014; Cheng, 2014; Etter and Bugey, 2017; Etter et al., 2013; Goniewicz et al., 2015). Most of the nicotine in tobacco is the levorotary (S)-isomer; (R)-nicotine is found in much smaller quantities (0.1–0.6 percent) (Benowitz et al., 2009).

On activation of the e-cigarette, nicotine is released from the e-liquid on aerosol particles or volatilized to gas-phase nicotine, which are then inhaled. Nicotine bound to particles can be deposited into the lungs, where it is expected to be rapidly absorbed into the pulmonary venous circulation, or to evaporate from particles on impact in the mouth and upper airways and absorbed into the circulation, but slower than in the lungs.

As with tobacco smoke, gas-phase nicotine is expected to be absorbed in the mouth and upper airways, which may contribute to the sensory effects of nicotine in the mouth and throat. Once nicotine enters the pulmonary venous circulation, it then enters the arterial circulation and rapidly moves across the blood–brain barrier into the brain (Benowitz, 2009). Nicotine then diffuses readily in brain tissue and (S)-nicotine, the predominant form, binds stereoselectively to nicotine cholinergic receptors (nAChRs) (Benowitz, 2009). nAChRs are ligand-gated ion channels, which open when a cholinergic agonist binds to the outside of the channel. When the channels open, they allow the entry of cations such as calcium and sodium, which activates signal transduction pathways, including activation of voltage-dependent calcium channels that allow further entry of calcium (Benowitz, 2009).

Nicotine-induced stimulation of central nervous system nAChRs results in the release of multiple neurotransmitters in the brain, dopamine being dominant, which have been related to nicotine's pharmacodynamic effects. The action of nicotine leads to the release of dopamine, which is associated with pleasure and appetite suppression, in the mesolimbic area, the frontal cortex, and the corpus striatum (Benowitz, 2009). Dopamine release in the shell of the nucleus accumbens and the dopaminergic neurons in the ventral tegmental area of the midbrain are especially important because this pathway is involved in drug-induced reward (HHS, 2014). The pleasurable experience from dopamine release plays a critical role in the reinforcing effects of nicotine. When dopamine neurons in rat brain are chemically or anatomically lesioned, self-administration of nicotine is prevented (Benowitz, 2009; IOM, 2001). Other nicotine-induced behaviors are mediated by a variety of neurotransmitters that are also released, including norepinephrine (arousal, appetite suppression), acetylcholine (arousal, cognitive enhancement), serotonin (mood modulation, appetite suppression), γ-aminobutyric acid (reduction of anxiety and tension), glutamate (learning, memory enhancement), and endorphins (reduction of anxiety and tension) (Benowitz, 2008).

Nicotine addiction develops as a neurobiological adaptation to chronic nicotine exposure (HHS, 2014). An important characteristic of nicotine dependence is the emergence of withdrawal symptoms on abrupt cessation of nicotine administration (compulsory nicotine administration is the other characteristic of nicotine dependence). Tolerance (neuroadaptation) to nicotine develops for some nicotinic effects on repeated exposure to nicotine. The number of nAChR binding sites in the brain increases, which is thought to represent upregulation in the response of nicotine-mediated desensitization of receptors (Benowitz, 2009). During periods of abstinence in chronic smokers, such as during nighttime sleep, previously desensitized $\alpha_4\beta_2$ nAChRs become unoccupied and recover to a responsive state. Abstinence symptoms are believed to develop when these nAChRs revert to this unoccupied and responsive state. Craving and withdrawal symptoms are alleviated through nicotine binding and desensitization of the receptors.

nAChRs are also located at the interganglionic junctions of the autonomic nervous system and on organs throughout the body as part of the parasympathetic autonomic nervous system (HHS, 2010b, 2014). Stimulation of these globally expressed nAChRs causes wide-ranging physiological effects such as nicotine intoxication syndrome. Symptoms of nicotine intoxication syndrome include nausea and vomiting. More severe poisoning can progress to diarrhea, increased salivation and respiratory secretions, bradycardia, seizures, and respiratory depression. The rapid development of tolerance to nicotine with repeated administration helps counter the development of acute nicotine toxicity (HHS, 2014).

Nicotine Receptor Pharmacology

The nAChR complex, a pentamer, includes combinations of α, β, γ, and δ subunits (IOM, 2001), and is found in the peripheral and central nervous systems (Benowitz, 2009; Gotti et al., 2006). nAChRs have been located in the brain, neuromuscular junctions, autonomic ganglia, and adrenal medulla (Gundisch, 2000; IOM, 2001). The varied effects of nicotine in both the peripheral and central nervous systems are mediated by the specific configurations of the subunits. While nicotine exerts diverse pharmacological effects in the peripheral nervous system (e.g., stimulation in the trachea that may enhance the reinforcing effect of self-administration), it is generally believed that the actions of nicotine in the central nervous system are pivotal to reinforcing tobacco use (HHS, 1988). Neuronal subunits that are thought to be attributed to the effects of nicotine contain $\alpha_{3,4,7}$ and $\beta_{2,4}$ subunits (IOM, 2001). The mammalian brain contains up to nine α subunits (α_2 to α_{10}) and three β subunits (β_2 to β_4). In the human brain, $\alpha_4\beta_2$, $\alpha_3\beta_4$, and α_7 (homomeric) are the most abundant receptor subtypes; $\alpha_4\beta_2$, with or without the presence of other subunits, is predominant and is thought to be the primary receptor mediating nicotine dependence in humans (Benowitz, 2009). The $\alpha_4\beta_2$ receptor may also include subunits such as α_5, α_6, and/or β_3. The additional subunits on the $\alpha_4\beta_2$ receptor can modulate the sensitivity and function of the receptor. Furthermore, it appears that the β_2 subunit is particularly important in reinforcing effects of nicotine. β_2 subunit gene knockout mice did not show the behavioral effects of nicotine (Benowitz, 2009; Picciotto, 1998). The behavioral effects of nicotine were restored on reinsertion of the β_2 subunit into the ventral tegmental area of the β_2 knockout mice (Benowitz, 2009; Maskos et al., 2005). The α_4 subunit seems to play a role in determining sensitivity to nicotine while the α_7 subunit appears to play an important role in withdrawal, learning, and sensory gating, and is involved in rapid synaptic transmission (Benowitz, 2009; IOM, 2001). In addition, the cardiovascular effects of nicotine are thought to be mediated by the $\alpha_3\beta_4$ nAChR.

Pharmacokinetics and Pharmacodynamics of Nicotine

The amount of nicotine delivered and the way in which it is delivered influences the addictiveness of a tobacco product (HHS, 2010b). The abuse liability of tobacco products increases with greater delivery, faster rate of absorption, and higher blood nicotine concentrations. Furthermore, the route of administration and dose of nicotine influence the time course of nicotine in the brain and the resulting pharmacological effects (Hukkanen et al., 2005). Nicotine in tobacco smoke, once it reaches the small airways and alveolar region of the lungs, is rapidly absorbed into the pulmonary venous circulation. From there, nicotine moves quickly to the left ventricle of the heart, then to the systemic arterial circulation, and then to the brain (Hukkanen et al., 2005). High levels of nicotine reach the brain in about 15 seconds after a puff on a combustible tobacco cigarette (Berridge et al., 2010). This rapid increase in nicotine levels in the brain, faster than with intravenous administration, leads to activation of the dopaminergic reward system, as discussed before, and produces rapid behavioral reinforcement (Hukkanen et al., 2005). Given the rapid rise of nicotine and associated psychoactive effects, smoking allows the smoker to titrate the level of nicotine and related effects during smoking. This makes smoking the most reinforcing and dependence-producing form of nicotine administration.

Nicotine is delivered from e-cigarettes through the pulmonary route in a manner that is very similar to that of combustible tobacco cigarettes. As discussed above and in detail later in this chapter under Exposure to Nicotine and Nicotine Derivatives from E-Cigarettes, e-cigarettes can deliver nicotine levels comparable to combustible tobacco cigarettes (St.Helen et al., 2016a), and the plasma nicotine profile can resemble that of combustible tobacco cigarette smokers (Dawkins et al., 2016; Ramoa et al., 2016; St.Helen et al., 2016a; Wagener et al., 2017). With the potential for high and rapid delivery of nicotine to the user, e-cigarettes are expected to produce nicotine-related psychoactive effects that can cause or maintain nicotine dependence. Whether or not e-cigarettes are as reinforcing and dependence producing as combustible tobacco cigarettes is an important question, with implications for both smoking cessation and transitioning from e-cigarettes to combustible tobacco cigarettes. The abuse liability of e-cigarettes relative to tobacco cigarettes is discussed in greater detail in Chapter 8.

Nicotine from chewing tobacco and snuff are rapidly absorbed because these products are buffered to alkaline pH. However, blood nicotine concentration rises gradually and plateaus at about 30 minutes, with levels remaining elevated and slowly decreasing over a nicotine half-life (2 hours) or more (Hukkanen et al., 2005). The rise in brain nicotine concentrations is slower than with smoking. Formulations of nicotine replacement therapy (NRT) are also buffered to alkaline pH to facilitate oral absorption. A considerable amount of nicotine administered orally is swallowed and undergoes first-pass metabolism. Because gastric fluid is acidic, nicotine is poorly absorbed in the stomach. On the other hand, nicotine is absorbed more efficiently in the small intestine due to the alkaline pH there and the large surface area. Given the slower rate of increase of nicotine levels in the blood and the brain from NRT administered orally, the abuse liability of NRT is considered to be low (Hukkanen et al., 2005). The gradual rise of nicotine levels in the brain allows for the development of tolerance to the pharmacological effects of nicotine, resulting in less intense central nervous system stimulation.

Nicotine base absorbs readily through the skin. This is the basis for nicotine transdermal systems, such as nicotine patches, and is also the reason for some nicotine toxicities in the occupational setting (green tobacco sickness). Nicotine-containing e-liquids can potentially make contact with the skin of users or non-users, such as children and infants. Therefore, dermal contact with nicotine-containing e-liquids can lead to systemic nicotine exposure.

Once absorbed into the circulation, nicotine is distributed extensively to body tissues with average steady-state volume of distribution ranging from 2.2 to 3.3 L/kg (see Table 4-1). Less than 5 percent of nicotine dose binds to plasma proteins (Hukkanen et al., 2005). Nicotine has low affinity for adipose tissue and high affinity for liver, kidney, spleen, lung tissues, and the brain. The receptor-binding capacity of nicotine in the brain is higher in smokers compared with non-smokers because of the upregulation of nicotinic cholinergic receptors in the brain of smokers (Hukkanen et al., 2005). Due to ion-trapping, nicotine accumulates in gastric juice and saliva. Nicotine also accumulates in breast milk as well as in fetal serum and amniotic fluids (once it crosses the placental barrier) in slightly higher concentrations than maternal serum.

Peak-to-trough blood nicotine levels oscillate considerably from cigarette to cigarette (Benowitz, 2009). During daily smoking, typical peak blood nicotine concentrations range from 19 to 50 ng/ml, while typical trough concentrations range from 10 to 37 ng/ml; depending on how the cigarette is smoked, each cigarette increases blood nicotine concentra-

TABLE 4-1 Pharmacokinetic Parameters of (*S*)-Nicotine and (3′R,5′S)-*Trans*-3′-Hydroxycotinine After Intravenous Administration

	Clearance (ml/minute)	Renal Clearance (ml/minute)	Non-Renal Clearance (ml/minute)	Volume of Distribution (Steady State) (L/kg)	Elimination Half-Life (minute)
Nicotine	1,110–1,500	35–90	1,050–1,460	2.2–3.3	100–150
Cotinine	42–55	3–9	36–52	0.69–0.93	770–1,130
Trans-3′-hydroxycotinine	82	50	32	0.66	396

SOURCE: Hukkanen et al., 2005.

tions by 5–30 ng/ml (Benowitz et al., 2009). Given the rapid delivery and absorption of nicotine from smoking, blood nicotine concentration rises while smoking and peaks at the end of smoking. Blood nicotine levels then decline rapidly over the next 20 minutes as nicotine distributes to tissue, with a distribution half-life of 8 minutes (Hukkanen et al., 2005). The elimination half-life of nicotine is about 2 hours. Consistent with this half-life, nicotine from regular smoking over 6–9 hours accumulates in the body. Smoking, therefore, results in exposure to nicotine in an intermittent and transient manner, but importantly, exposure to nicotine lasts 24 hours per day (Benowitz, 2009). The persistent systemic exposure to nicotine leads to persistent presence of nicotine in the brain throughout the day and night and results in structural and functional changes in nicotinic receptors and in intracellular processes of neuroadaptation (Benowitz, 2009). There is wide variability in patterns of e-cigarette use during the day. Nonetheless, as discussed later, e-cigarette users also administer nicotine throughout the day, likely leading to persistent systemic exposure to nicotine and associated neuroadaptation and tolerance to pharmacological effects of nicotine observed in combustible tobacco cigarette smokers.

Biotransformation of Nicotine

The metabolism of nicotine has been reviewed in depth elsewhere (Benowitz et al., 2009; Hukkanen et al., 2005) and is summarized in this section (see also Figure 4-1). The main site of nicotine metabolism is the liver, where it is extensively metabolized. Nicotine contains both aromatic and aliphatic carbon and nitrogen atoms, which can be sites for metabolic oxidation and subsequent conjugation reactions (IOM, 2001). Cotinine is

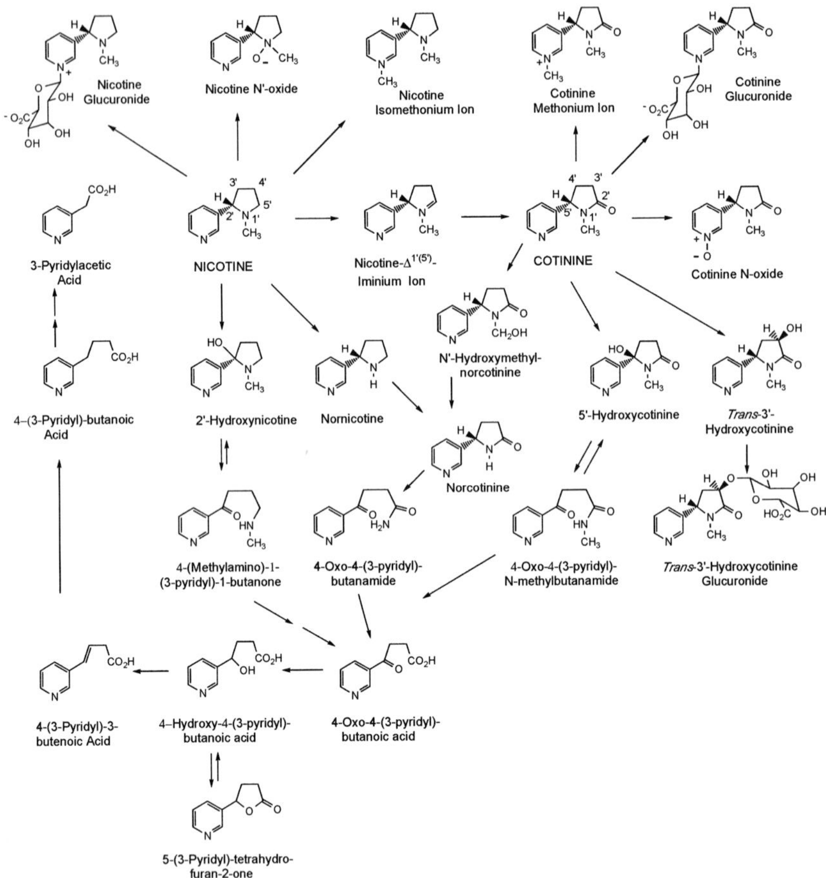

FIGURE 4-1 Nicotine metabolic pathways.
SOURCE: Hukkanen et al., 2005.

quantitatively the most important nicotine metabolite in mammals. About 70–80 percent of nicotine is metabolized through the cotinine pathway. Nicotine is converted to cotinine via a two-step metabolic process, consisting of a cytochrome P450–mediated reaction (CPY2A6) to produce nicotine-$\Delta^{1'(5')}$-iminium ion followed by a cytoplasmic aldehyde oxidase reaction (Hukkanen et al., 2005). Cotinine is further metabolized to a number of metabolites. About 4 to 7 percent of nicotine absorbed in smokers is converted to nicotine *N′*-oxide through the action of flavin-containing monooxygenase 3 (FMO3). Nicotine *N′*-oxide is not metabolized further and is excreted in this form or reduced back to nicotine. Cotinine and nicotine *N′*-oxide are formed through oxidation of the pyrrolidine ring.

Nonoxidative methylation of the pyridine nitrogen and glucuronidation of nicotine are two additional metabolic pathways. The methylation pathway is catalyzed by *N*-methyltransferase, forming the nicotine isomethonium ion in small amounts in smokers. Formation of (*S*)-nicotine-*N*-β-glucuronide, which constitutes about 3–5 percent of nicotine metabolites excreted in urine, is catalyzed by the uridine diphosphate-glucuronosyltransferase (UGT) enzyme (Hukkanen et al., 2005).

Nornicotine, which is also a constituent of tobacco leaves, is formed from absorbed nicotine through oxidative *N*-demethylation through the CYP450 system. About 0.41 and 0.65 percent of nicotine is excreted as nornicotine in users of transdermal nicotine and smokers, respectively (Hukkanen et al., 2005). Finally, nicotine undergoes 2´-hydroxylation through CYP450 activity to produce 2´-hydroxynicotine as an intermediate. 2-Hydroxynicotine yields 4-(methylamino)-1-(3-pyridyl)-1-butanone and nicotine-$\Delta^{1'(2')}$-iminium ion. 4-Oxo-4-(3-pyridyl)butanoic acid and 4-hydroxy-4-(3-pyridyl)-butanoic acid are derived from 4-(methylamino)-1-(3-pyridyl)-1-butanone and form about 10–15 percent of excreted nicotine and metabolites (Hukkanen et al., 2005).

Despite the cotinine pathway being the predominant metabolic route of nicotine, only 10–15 percent of nicotine absorbed by smokers is excreted as unchanged cotinine. Cotinine has six primary metabolites in humans: 3´-hydroxycotinine, 5´-hydroxycotinine, cotinine-*N*-oxide, cotinine methonium ion, cotinine glucuronide, and norcotinine (Benowitz et al., 2009). 3´-Hydroxycotinine, the most abundant nicotine metabolite in smokers' urine, and its *O*-glucuronide conjugate account for 40–60 percent of the nicotine dose in urine. Conversion of cotinine to cotinine *N*-oxide is formed by CYP450 enzymes, unlike formation of nicotine *N*-oxide, and accounts for 2–5 percent of the excreted nicotine and metabolites in urine. Norcotinine, making up about 1 percent of excreted nicotine and metabolites in urine, is formed either through demethylation of cotinine or oxidation of nornicotine (Hukkanen et al., 2005).

Nicotine and metabolites measured in urine, referred to as the total nicotine equivalents, account for approximately 90 percent of the systemic dose of nicotine (Benowitz et al., 2009). To summarize quantitatively the pattern of nicotine metabolism in humans, nicotine and metabolites are excreted in urine as nicotine *N*-oxide (4–7 percent), nicotine glucuronide (3–5 percent), cotinine (10–15 percent), *trans*-3´-hydroxycotinine (33–40 percent), cotinine glucuronide (12–17 percent), and *trans*-3´-hydroxycotinine glucuronide (7–9 percent).

Based on measurement of blood nicotine levels after administration of a known dose, average total clearance of nicotine is about 1,200 ml/minute. Given that nonrenal clearance makes up about 70 percent of liver blood flow, about 70 percent of the nicotine dose is removed from the blood in each pass through the liver (Benowitz et al., 2009). On the other hand, clearances of cotinine and *trans*-3´-hydroxycotinine are slower and average about 45 ml/minute and 82 ml/minute, respectively (Hukkanen et al., 2005). The ratio of plasma or saliva 3´-hydroxycotinine to cotinine (3HC/cotinine), which is highly correlated with oral clearances of nicotine and cotinine and half-life of cotinine, is a validated non-invasive proxy of CYP2A6 metabolism of nicotine (Dempsey et al., 2004). The ratio of 3HC/cotinine in urine is also used as a proxy of CYP2A6 nicotine metabolism, with forms including unconjugated, glucuronidated, or total (unconjugated + glucuronidated) 3´-hydroxycotinine and cotinine. The validity of the ratio of 3´-hydroxycotinine to cotinine in urine as a proxy of CYP2A6 nicotine metabolism when using glucuronidated 3´-hydroxycotinine and/or cotinine may be influenced by observed differences in rates of glucuronidation of nicotine and cotinine among individuals or groups (Berg et al., 2010a,b).

CYP2A6 is the major enzyme involved in oxidation of nicotine to cotinine and cotinine to 3´-hydroxycotinine. CYP2A6 is also involved in 2´-hydroxylation of nicotine and in the formation of 5´-hydroxycotinine and norcotinine from cotinine (Hukkanen et al., 2005). Other enzymes involved in nicotine oxidation include CYP2B6 (second most active), CYP2D6, CYP2E1, and CYP2A13. CYP2A13 is a close relative of CYP2A6, is highly expressed in the respiratory tract, and includes shared substrates with CYP2A6 such as 4-(methylnitrosamino)-1-(3-pyridyl)-1-butanone (NNK) (Hukkanen et al., 2005). Aldehyde oxidase is the enzyme involved in the conversion of nicotine-$\Delta^{1'(5')}$-iminium ion to cotinine. FMO3 catalyzes the formation of nicotine *N*´-oxide. Amine *N*-methyltransferase, whose expression is highest in human thyroid, adrenal gland, and lung, catalyzes *N*-methylation of nicotine. UDP-glucuronosyltransferase (UGT) catalyzes the phase II *N*-glucuronidation of nicotine and cotinine and *N*- and *O*-glucuronidation of 3´-hydroxycotinine. UGT2B10 and UGT1A4 are the main enzymes involved in *N*-glucuronidation of nicotine and cotinine, while UGT1A9 plays a minor role; UGT2B10 is thought to be a more efficient catalyst of *N*-glucuronidation (Benowitz et al., 2009; Berg et al., 2010a; Chen et al., 2007; Ehmer et al., 2004; Hukkanen et al., 2005; Kaivosaari et al., 2007). It is yet unknown which enzyme(s) catalyzes *O*-glucuronidation of 3´-hydroxycotinine but evidence suggests that UGT1A9 and UGT2B7 are involved given their action in NNAL *O*-glucuronidation and the high correlation between 3´-hydroxycotinine *O*-glucuronide and NNAL-*O*-glucuronide. Evidence suggests that UGT2B17 plays a major role in *O*-glucuronidation of 3´-hydroxycotinine while UGT2B10 and UGT1A4 are involved in its *N*-glucuronidation (Chen et al., 2012).

Gender and Racial Differences in Nicotine Metabolism and Genetic Polymorphisms

The rate of elimination of nicotine and cotinine varies considerably in humans and across species. A number of factors contribute to this observed interindividual variation, including physiological factors such as diet, age, gender, pathological conditions, medications, smoking, and racial and ethnic differences. These factors and known polymorphisms in genes encoding nicotine-metabolizing enzymes have been discussed in detail elsewhere (Benowitz et al., 2009).

Given that most nicotine is cleared through hepatic extraction, factors that change liver blood flow such as meals, exercise, and other physiological events can influence nicotine clearance. After eating a meal, hepatic blood flow increases by an estimated 30 percent and nicotine clearance increases by about 40 percent (Hukkanen et al., 2005). Some food constituents and additives are also known to mediate enzymes involved in nicotine metabolism. Menthol, a flavorant used in foods, toothpaste, combustible tobacco cigarettes, and e-cigarettes, moderately inhibits CYP2A6. Metabolism of nicotine to cotinine and glucuronidation of nicotine were inhibited after smoking mentholated cigarettes compared with after smoking non-mentholated cigarettes (Benowitz et al., 2004; Hukkanen et al., 2005). Although their effects on nicotine metabolism have not been studied, grapefruit and wheatgrass juice inhibit metabolism of coumarin, a CYP2A6 substrate, indicating that these foods likely inhibit nicotine metabolism.

Age is another physiological influence on the rate of nicotine metabolism. Clearance of nicotine decreases with age among adults. Compared with young adults, total clearance was 23 percent lower and renal clearance was 49 percent lower in the elderly (Hukkanen et al., 2005). Hepatic blood flow is lower in the elderly, leading to reduction in hepatic extraction of nicotine. At the other end, the half-life of nicotine in neonates has been shown to be three to four times longer than in adults, indicative of much slower rates of nicotine metabolism.

Hepatic clearance of nicotine slows during sleep as blood flow to the liver declines. The combination of this variation in hepatic blood flow and effect of meals on hepatic blood flow and nicotine clearance results in circadian variations in blood nicotine levels even during constant nicotine dosing (Hukkanen et al., 2005).

Gender-related differences in nicotine metabolism have been noted, with some studies reporting alternative conclusions. However, studies support that nicotine and cotinine clearances are higher in women compared with men; oral contraceptives further induce nicotine metabolism; and pregnancy markedly increases nicotine metabolism (Hukkanen et al., 2005). These gender and pregnancy differences are attributed to sex hormones, given that estrogens and progesterone are higher in women than men, higher in women using oral contraceptives compared those who are not, and even higher during pregnancy (Hukkanen et al., 2005). Compared with men, nicotine and cotinine clearances were 13 percent and 16 percent higher in women not using oral contraceptives. Nicotine and cotinine clearances were induced by 30 percent and 33 percent, respectively, in women using oral contraceptives compared with women not using oral contraceptives (Hukkanen et al., 2005). Differences in coumarin metabolism have also been reported between women and men, supporting the idea that these gender differences are associated with CYP2A6 activity (Hukkanen et al., 2005). Pregnancy increases clearance of nicotine and cotinine by 60 percent and 140 percent, respectively, through increased induction of CYP2A6. Gender differences in nicotine glucuronidation has not been found in human studies, but studies using human liver microsomes suggest slower glucuronidation in women (Ghosheh and Hawes, 2002; Pulvers et al., 2016).

Significant racial differences in nicotine and cotinine metabolism have been noted. These differences may be a result of genetic variations in nicotine-metabolizing enzymes as well as other external factors, such as predominant types of cigarettes smoked by a racial/ethnic group (e.g., menthol versus non-menthol). The fractional clearance of nicotine to cotinine, metabolic clearance of nicotine to cotinine, and total and non-renal clearance of cotinine were significantly lower in blacks compared with whites (Benowitz et al., 1999; Perez-Stable et al., 1998). Nicotine and cotinine glucuronidation, although polymorphic in blacks (i.e., presence of both people who formed *N*-glucuronide fast and those who formed it slowly), were lower compared with whites, who showed unimodal distribution of glucuronidation (Berg et al., 2010a; Hukkanen et al., 2005). In comparisons among Chinese Americans, Latinos, and whites, total and non-renal clearance of nicotine and cotinine, and metabolic clearance of nicotine via the cotinine pathway were lowest among Chinese Americans (Benowitz et al., 2002; Hukkanen et al., 2005). Chinese are known to have higher frequencies of reduced function or dysfunctional *CYP2A6* alleles compared with whites (Hukkanen et al., 2005; Pitarque et al., 2001; Wang et al., 2003). Japanese are also known to have higher frequencies of null and reduced activity *CYP2A6* alleles, resulting in slower nicotine metabolism.

Polymorphisms in genes encoding nicotine-metabolizing enzymes are important determinants of the rate of nicotine metabolism in individuals and across racial groups, and have been discussed in detail elsewhere (Hukkanen et al., 2005). The rate of nicotine metabolism is associated with the likelihood of being an adult smoker (Schoedel et al., 2004), number of cigarettes smoked per day (Benowitz et al., 2003; Schoedel et al., 2004), exposure to tobacco-related toxicants (Derby et al., 2008), and efficacy of smoking cessation with NRT (Lerman et al., 2006, 2010; Schnoll et al., 2009). Several polymorphisms have been noted in *CYP2A6*. The wild-type allele is denoted by *CYP2A6*1A*. Fully inactive *CYP2A6* alleles are associated with substantial reduction in *CYP2A6* activity. *CYP2A6* whole gene deletion alleles include *CYP2A6*4A*, *CYP2A6*4B*, and *CYP2A6*4D*. Reduced activity also comes from alleles containing a single nucleotide change such as *CYP2A6*2* and *CYP2A6*5*. Slow nicotine metabolizers include those with alleles such as *CYP2A6*6*, *CYP2A6*7*, *CYP2A6*8*, and *CYP2A6*9*, which produce functional enzymes with reduced metabolic capacities. Other alleles such as *CYP2A6*1XN* produce enzymes with increased metabolic activity. Polymorphisms have also been noted in other genes that encode enzymes involved in nicotine metabolism, such as in *CYP2B6*, *CYP2D6*, *CYP2E1*, and *CYP2A13*. Polymorphisms in the genes for aldehyde oxidase have not been reported while several polymorphisms have been detected in the human *FMO3* gene.

Other factors that lead to variation in nicotine metabolism include pathological conditions, medications, and tobacco smoke itself. Hepatic pathologies impact nicotine metabolism. Based on coumarin metabolism as a proxy for CYP2A6 activity, hepatitis A and alcoholic liver disease are expected to slow hepatic extraction of nicotine while liver fluke parasite infection induces nicotine metabolism. Kidney failure decreases both renal clearance of nicotine and also hepatic clearance due to inhibition of CYP2A6 activity or downregulation of hepatic CYP2A6 expression by accumulated uremic toxins (Benowitz et al., 2009). Drugs such as rifampicin, dexamethasone, phenobarbital, and other anticonvulsant drugs are known to induce CYP2A6. Other compounds such as pilocarpine, metyrapone, methoxsalen, naphthalene, rifampicin, and others that are known to reduce coumarin metabolism through inhibition of CYP2A6 are expected to inhibit nicotine metabolism (Hukkanen et al., 2005). Studies with smokers as well as those with coumarin support that tobacco smoke inhibits CYP2A6-mediated metabolism of nicotine. While the exact CYP2A6 inhibitor(s) in tobacco smoke have not been identified, β-nicotyrine, a minor tobacco alkaloid, inhibits CYP2A6 in vitro (Benowitz et al., 2009; Denton et al., 2004). Downregulation of CYP2A6 expression, but not CYP2A6 inhibition, is another explanation for smoking-induced reduction of nicotine clearance. While smoking reduces nicotine C-oxidation, it appears that it induces 3′-hydroxycotinine *O*-glucuronidation. Rates of *N*-glucuronidation of nicotine and cotinine have not been shown to be affected by smoking.

Species Differences in Nicotine Metabolism

The highest total metabolism of nicotine has been seen in guinea pig and hamster hepatocytes followed by those of mice and humans, indicating cross-species differences in nicotine metabolism. All mammal species produce cotinine and 3′-hydroxycotinine as the major metabolites of nicotine. However, guinea pigs and rats form as much nicotine *N*′-oxide as cotinine and 3′-hydroxycotinine. Other differences exist across species, including rates of nicotine metabolism, relative amounts of metabolites produced, as well as differences in the major CYP enzymes involved in nicotine metabolism. For example, CYP2A is inactive in nicotine metabolism in rats while CYP2B is the main active enzyme. In nonhuman primates, nicotine metabolism resembles that of humans. Nicotine *N*′-glucuronidation also differs across species, with highest activity in the human liver and no activity in rats, mice, dogs, and rabbits. Cotinine glucuronidation has only been detected in humans (Hukkanen et al., 2005).

Other Effects of Nicotine

Carcinogenesis

Concerns about the potential carcinogenic risk of nicotine is important due to the growing prevalence of use of alternative forms of nicotine delivery such as e-cigarettes and other non-combustible tobacco products, as well as smokers who attempt to quit through extended use of NRT. Carcinogenesis consists of initiation, promotion, and progression. A complete carcinogen is an agent (physical, chemical, or biological, e.g., viruses) that can, by itself, induce tumors, usually with initiating, promoting, and progressing properties (Haussmann and Fariss, 2016). Initiation, the first stage of the cancer process, consists of genetic alterations such as mutations and deletions made by the initiating agent. Promotion involves the selective clonal expansion of initiated cells to produce preneoplastic lesions; both endogenous and exogenous agents that stimulate cell growth can act as tumor promoters. Importantly, repeated applications of or continuous exposure to agents that promote tumors is required for continued growth of preneoplastic lesions (Klaassen and Watkins, 2015). Progression entails conversion of benign preneoplastic lesions into invasive cancer.

Current evidence does not support the idea that nicotine is a human carcinogen, let alone a complete carcinogen. Specifically with respect to initiation, the 2014 Surgeon General's report found mixed data for a genotoxic effect of nicotine; most studies were negative (HHS, 2014). The Lung Health Study, a 5-year randomized trial to assess the effects of smoking cessation on chronic lung disease and lung function, investigated the cancer risk from using NRT products (Murray et al., 2009). This has been the only study to provide information on long-term NRT users. It found no evidence for an effect of NRT use on overall cancer risk or specifically for lung or gastrointestinal tract cancers. One study reported no additional mutagenic potential from increasing nicotine yield in cigarette smoke (Chen et al., 2008). In fact, the only exception was an animal study which found sarcomas in the muscle and uterus of A/J mice exposed to nicotine; no other tumors were found (Galitovskiy et al., 2012). In this study, A/J mice were subcutaneously injected with a nicotine dose of 3 mg/kg five times per week for 24 months (equivalent to 2.1 mg/kg/day of nicotine) (Grando, 2014), a dose comparable to that from consuming regular Scandinavian snus (Wickholm et al., 2012). The Surgeon General's report (HHS, 2014, p. 114) found that the current body of evidence from animal and human studies on this topic failed to support the hypothesis that nicotine is a human carcinogen, concluding that "there is insufficient data to conclude that nicotine causes or contributes to cancer in humans."

The Surgeon General's report (HHS, 2014, p. 114) went on to conclude that "there is evidence showing possible oral, esophageal, or pancreatic cancer risks" (HHS, 2014, p. 114); the risks are indirect evidence based on some evidence of endogenous formation of the carcinogenic tobacco-specific nitrosamine (TSNA), *N'*-nitrosonornicotine (NNN), in users of NRT (Carmella et al., 1997; Knezevich et al., 2013; Stepanov et al., 2009a,b) and elevated risk of these cancers in users of smokeless tobacco products (IARC, 2012). NNN is a potent carcinogen that has been shown to induce tumors locally and systemically (Hecht, 1998), and is associated with increased risk of esophageal cancer in smokers (Yuan et al., 2011). Although the Surgeon General's report did not find evidence to conclude that nicotine causes cancer, the report also stated that "there is some biological basis for proposing that nicotine may promote cancer based on experimental studies that have limitations in replicating human exposure and on mechanistic studies, but human evidence is lacking" (HHS, 2014, p. 113). Of importance to the potential tumor-promoting properties of nicotine are nAChRs located in organs such as the lungs, which can be involved in triggering signaling pathways in lung cells. As discussed in the 2014 Surgeon General's report, nicotine's effects on carcinogenic pathways include (1) inhibition of apoptosis; (2) stimulation of the release of epidermal growth factor and activation of Ras-Raf-ERK cascade, which affects cell proliferation; (3) activation of ERK, PI3-K, and mTOR and the expression of PPAR-β/δ by stimulating fibroblast production; and (4) possible promotion of metastases because nicotine stimulates cell motility and migration, loss of cell adhesion, and induction of the transition of well-differentiated epithelial cells to highly invasive carcinoma via epithelial-mesenchymal transition (HHS, 2014). The potential for nicotine to promote and spread tumors through its effects on cancer cell survival and protection from apoptosis, nAChR mediation of nicotine-dependent upregulation of proliferative and survival genes, effects on metastasis, and nicotine-related induction of pathological angiogenesis that facilitates tumor survival and spreading have been discussed extensively in a review by Grando (2014).

In addition to the 2014 Surgeon General's report, other studies also found that there is insufficient evidence to determine whether nicotine is a human carcinogen. A systematic review was conducted to determine the potential carcinogenic effect of nicotine at levels found in users of nicotine delivery systems (Haussmann and Fariss, 2016). The only epidemiological study included was the study on long-term NRT use after smoking cessation, same as the 2014 Surgeon General's report. The review concluded that "for human studies (NRT use), there appears to be inadequate evidence for an association between nicotine exposure and the presence of or lack of a carcinogenic effect due to a limited number of studies" (Haussmann and Fariss, 2016, p. 709). Based on animal studies, the review concluded that "limited evidence suggests an association between long-term nicotine exposure and a *lack* of a complete carcinogenic effect" (Haussmann and Fariss, 2016, p. 715). The review of approximately 70 animal studies also concluded that there is inadequate evidence to conclude that nicotine exposure does or does not modulate (stimulate) carcinogenesis in humans.

An additional line of evidence to inform our understanding of whether nicotine can contribute to increased cancer risk is to assess the occurrence of cancer in smokeless tobacco users. Smokeless tobacco products used in Scandinavia have lower levels of TSNAs compared with traditional smokeless tobacco products and combustible tobacco products (HHS, 2014; Stepanov et al., 2006), but deliver as much nicotine as combustible tobacco cigarettes (Digard et al., 2013). In Sweden, the prevalence of smokeless tobacco use is 12.3 percent (20.7 percent in men, 3.5 percent in women) (Leon et al., 2016). In a longitudinal cohort of male Swedish construction workers, use of snus by never-smoking users was independently associated with increased risk of pancreatic cancer (higher risk compared with never users of any tobacco), but was unrelated to incidence of oral and lung cancers (Luo et al., 2007). Exposure to the TSNA NNK is the likely explanation for the observed increased in pancreatic cancer risk among snus users. NNK exposure is known to induce pancreatic cancer in rats when administered orally (Rivenson et al., 1988). Furthermore, a study of smokeless tobacco users enrolled in the National Longitudinal Mortality Study in the United States found that current smokeless tobacco users did not have elevated mortality from all cancers combined, and pancreatic, esophageal, and oral cavity cancers separately, compared with never users of tobacco (Timberlake et al., 2017). These studies provide additional evidence to suggest that nicotine per se is not contributing to human cancer risk.

When the evidence is viewed in total, while there is a biological rationale for how nicotine could potentially act as a carcinogen in humans, there is no human evidence to support the hypothesis that nicotine is a human carcinogen. While it is biologically plausible that nicotine can act as a tumor promoter, the existing body of evidence indicates this is unlikely to translate into increased risk of human cancer. Studies of NRT users, which show no increase in cancer risk (Murray et al., 2009), and studies of smokeless tobacco users, which show increase in risk of cancers related to TSNA exposure but not an increase in risk of other cancers (Luo et al., 2007; Timberlake et al., 2017), indicate that it is unlikely that nicotine exposure acts as a tumor promoter to increase the risk of cancer in humans. Based on the existing body of evidence, it is reasonable to infer there is likely no significant increase in risk of cancer from exposure to nicotine delivered by e-cigarettes.

Cardiovascular Effects

The cardiovascular effects of nicotine have been reviewed in the 2010 and 2014 Surgeon General's reports and elsewhere (Benowitz and Burbank, 2016; HHS, 2010b, 2014). Given that epidemiological studies cannot effectively disentangle smoking-related cardiovascular disease caused by nicotine and that caused by other toxic substances in tobacco smoke, analysis of epidemiological studies of long-term NRT or smokeless tobacco users facilitates evaluation of the cardiovascular risk of nicotine. The factors that mediate the effects of nicotine on the cardiovascular system are complex. Many of these effects are thought to be related to activation of nAChRs. As stated before, nAChRs are found in endothelial, immune, neuronal, and muscle cells (HHS, 2014).

Activation of the sympathetic nervous system produces hemodynamic effects manifested as increased heart rate, blood pressure, myocardial contractility, and cutaneous and coronary vasoconstriction (Benowitz and Fraiman, 2017; Bhatnagar, 2016). Stimulation of the sympathetic nervous system by nicotine is thought to be a result of activation of nAChRs in the peripheral nervous system, as well as those in the central nervous system (Benowitz and Burbank, 2016). Nicotine increases adrenal release of epinephrine and adrenergic neuron release of norepinephrine (HHS, 2010a). Heart rate and blood pressure increase regardless of the nicotine source or route of administration. Blood vessels constrict in response to nicotine, including coronary blood vessels and blood vessels in the skin, but those in skeletal muscle dilate (Benowitz and Burbank, 2016). Increased sympathetic activity from acute exposure to nicotine is also associated with a decrease in heart rate variability in both smokers and nicotine-naïve healthy human subjects (Bhatnagar, 2016).

Nicotine also impacts coronary blood flow, but the net effect is a balance of two actions with opposite effects (Benowitz and Burbank, 2016). Through its action on α_1-adrenergic receptors in vascular smooth muscle, nicotine can constrict coronary arteries and decrease blood flow. On the other hand, nicotine-induced accelerated heart rate increases cardiac output, which causes flow-mediated dilation (FMD). FMD directly stimulates β_2 receptors in the coronary artery for vasodilation. While the pathophysiological significance of the sympathomimetic-driven hemodynamic effects of nicotine are unclear, increases in heart rate, reduction in heart rate variability, and endothelial dysfunction can lead to reduced myocardial blood flow, coronary occlusion, and increased myocardial demand for oxygen and nutrients, all of which are known to be associated with increased risks of myocardial ischemia/infarction and sudden death (Bhatnagar, 2016).

Other effects of nicotine on the cardiovascular system are believed to include myocardial remodeling, arrhythmogenesis, thrombogenesis, endothelial dysfunction, inflammation, and angiogenesis (Benowitz and Burbank, 2016). Persistent sympathetic stimulation by nicotine, particularly through β-adrenergic activation, can enhance myocardial tissue remodeling. Tissue remodeling (hypertrophy and fibrosis) creates heart failure. The arrhythmogenic effect of nicotine is mediated through catecholamine release, which can contribute to ventricular tachycardia and fibrillation. The thrombogenic effect of nicotine varies. Some animal studies have reported increased platelet activation from acute exposure to nicotine, whereas long-term exposure in rodents leads to reduced platelet activation. Studies of NRT and smokeless tobacco do not show increased platelet activation following nicotine intake. Endothelial dysfunction, which consists of impaired FMD (the vasodilatory response to increased local blood flow), is mediated primarily by oxidative stress and chronic inflammation. It is not clear what additional effect nicotine has on endothelial dysfunction above that of the effects of powerful oxidants and pro-inflammatory agents. Nevertheless, impaired endothelial function has been observed in people following local infusion of nicotine and use of a nicotine inhaler (Bhatnagar, 2016; Neunteufl et al., 2002). Inflammation plays an important role in several mechanisms that lead to cardiovascular diseases, namely atherogenesis and acute ischemic events. However, nicotine appears to have both anti-inflammatory and pro-inflammatory effects. Nicotine can act on the immune system directly by activating nAChRs that modulate immune function or indirectly by activating the sympathetic nervous system. Nicotine can also act on the cholinergic immune system by activating non-neuronal α_7

nAChRs, which has an anti-inflammatory effect. On the other hand, by acting as a chemotactic agent, nicotine can contribute to inflammation by facilitating migration of neutrophils (HHS, 2010a). In other studies, nicotine enhanced leukocyte–endothelium interactions, resulting in greater leukocyte rolling and adhesion in mice; nicotine stimulated an inflammatory response by acting on human monocyte-derived dendritic cells; and nicotine increased secretion of pro-inflammatory cytokines in cultured dendritic cells (HHS, 2010a). Nevertheless, based on studies showing significant decline in inflammatory markers after switching from smoking to transdermal nicotine and similar levels of inflammatory markers between smokeless tobacco users and non-tobacco users, nicotine is not believed to be the main determinant of an inflammatory response in smokers (HHS, 2010a). Similarly, acute exposure to nicotine enhanced angiogenesis through its action on α_7 nAChRs, but chronic exposure to nicotine in rodents led to impairment of angiogenesis, which indicates that nicotine is not an important driver of tobacco smoke-related angiogenesis (Benowitz and Burbank, 2016).

Smoking is associated with a more atherogenic lipid profile, progression of chronic hypertension to accelerated or malignant hypertension, and type 2 diabetes, which raises questions about the role of nicotine. While nicotine is known to induce lipolysis via catecholamine action at β-adrenoreceptors, and increasing plasma-free fatty acid concentrations, which possibly results in enhanced synthesis of low-density lipoproteins (LDLs) and lowering of high-density lipoproteins (HDLs), cessation studies using NRT and nicotine nasal sprays report improvement in HDL/LDL ratios and reduced dyslipidemia (Benowitz and Burbank, 2016; HHS, 2010a; Murray et al., 1996). Smoking causes transient increases in blood pressure, but is not associated with high blood pressure. A majority of smokeless tobacco studies have also not reported an increased incidence or prevalence of hypertension in users. However, smoking is likely associated with progression of chronic hypertension to accelerated or malignant hypertension; nicotine-induced vasoconstriction can play a role in this escalation. Finally, smokers have increased insulin resistance compared with non-smokers and cigarette smoking is recognized as an important risk factor for type 2 diabetes. It appears that nicotine is the main constituent in tobacco smoke responsible for increased insulin resistance in people. This is based on studies showing a dose–response association between hyperinsulinemia and insulin resistance in people with long-term use of nicotine gum (HHS, 2010a). Nicotine-induced release of hormones such catecholamine, cortisol, and growth hormone, which are insulin antagonists, can enhance insulin resistance. In addition, nicotine produces insulin resistance by directly activating AMP-activated protein kinase via α7 nAChR effects in adipose tissue (Benowitz and Burbank, 2016).

Because e-cigarettes are designed to deliver nicotine to the user, the cardiovascular effects of nicotine must be considered when assessing the overall potential cardiovascular effects of e-cigarettes. The evidence related to the cardiovascular effects of e-cigarettes is reviewed in Chapter 9. However, based on known cardiovascular effects of nicotine (Benowitz and Burbank, 2016; HHS, 2010b), exposure to nicotine from e-cigarettes likely elevates the risk in people with preexisting cardiovascular disease(s), but the risk in people without cardiovascular disease(s) is uncertain.

EXPOSURE TO NICOTINE AND NICOTINE DERIVATIVES FROM E-CIGARETTES

The abuse liability of e-cigarettes and their potential to help combustible tobacco cigarette smokers quit smoking and/or sustain dual use of combustible tobacco cigarette and e-cigarettes depend to a great extent on the amount of nicotine delivered and how it is delivered. E-cigarettes, which deliver more nicotine and facilitate faster nicotine absorption and higher blood nicotine concentrations, are expected to be more satisfying and addictive.

This section primarily addresses the question: *What is the nicotine exposure profile of e-cigarettes?* In short, how fast is nicotine from e-cigarettes absorbed, and what is the systemic exposure to nicotine? These questions can be answered through clinical studies that measure biomarkers of nicotine exposure after e-cigarette use, including pharmacokinetic parameters such as the maximum blood nicotine concentration (C_{max}) and time to maximum concentration (T_{max}). Studies that assess nicotine exposure biomarkers in smokers who switch to e-cigarettes over a study period are also useful in describing nicotine exposure from e-cigarettes. Furthermore, other studies measure biomarkers of nicotine exposure longitudinally in long-term e-cigarette users, thus providing information on the stability or progression of nicotine intake in e-cigarette users.

The committee identified 27 clinical studies that investigated acute nicotine exposure from e-cigarette use. Details of each study, including product used, nicotine content of e-cigarettes, sample size, puffing protocol, and biomarker concentrations or pharmacokinetic parameters are presented in Table 4-2. The studies entailed nicotine administration during either a controlled session (bout of fixed number of puffs), during ad lib use over a period of time, or both. The studies enrolled either combustible tobacco cigarette smokers who had not used e-cigarettes before or were infrequent users (often referred to as inexperienced users or e-cigarette–naïve smokers) or current e-cigarette users (often referred to as experienced users). Two studies enrolled both experienced users and e-cigarette–naïve smokers (Farsalinos et al., 2015; Fearon et al., 2017).

Comparisons of nicotine exposure from e-cigarettes with other inhaled forms of nicotine such as combustible tobacco cigarettes or nicotine inhalers can inform questions of the relative addictiveness of e-cigarettes or their ability to serve as a substitute for combustible tobacco cigarettes among smokers who want to quit (Benowitz et al., 2009). Some studies included combustible tobacco cigarettes or inhalers as comparators. For general reference, combustible tobacco cigarette smokers absorb about 1 mg (range = 0.3–2 mg) of nicotine systemically from smoking, which represents about 80 to 90 percent of the amount of nicotine inhaled (Armitage et al., 1975). Average venous blood nicotine C_{max} ranges from 15 to 30 ng/ml and T_{max} ranges from 5 to 8 minutes from the first puff (Benowitz et al., 2009). Typical average venous plasma nicotine C_{max} from a 1-mg nicotine spray ranges from 5 to 8 ng/ml, and T_{max} ranges from 11 to 18 minutes from the start of administration.

Clinical Studies with E-Cigarette–Naïve Smokers (Inexperienced Users)

Seventeen studies, including the ones by Fearon and colleagues (2017) and Farsalinos and colleagues (2015), enrolled smokers with no or little experience with e-cigarettes. The study by Bullen and colleagues (2010) was the first such study. Study participants were randomized to use an e-cigarette (Ruyan V8) with or without nicotine (16-mg nicotine cartridge), nicotine inhaler (Nicorette) or their usual combustible tobacco cigarette over 4 study days. A subset (n = 8) gave venous blood samples for nicotine pharmacokinetic analysis. Participants used the e-cigarette and combustible tobacco cigarette ad lib over 5 minutes and the inhaler over 20 minutes. Use of the e-cigarette with nicotine (16 mg cartridge) resulted in only a small increase in plasma nicotine (C_{max} = 1.3 ng/ml). By comparison, average C_{max} for the combustible tobacco cigarette and inhaler were 13.4 ng/ml and 2.1 ng/ml, respectively. The fastest T_{max} was achieved with the combustible tobacco cigarette (14.3 minutes after first puff) followed by the nicotine e-cigarette (19.6 minutes after first puff) and the inhaler (32 minutes after first administration). While the authors concluded that the pharmacokinetic profile of the e-cigarette was similar to the inhaler, they also suggested that the shorter T_{max} with the e-cigarette compared with the inhaler may be due to absorption of nicotine from e-cigarette aerosol in the respiratory tract while nicotine from the inhaler is absorbed buccally.

Eissenberg (2010) presented preliminary findings of a within-sub-

TABLE 4-2 Summary of Clinical Studies Examining Nicotine Exposure from E-Cigarette Use

	Study Characteristics		
Reference	Study Product	Nicotine Content	Sample Size
Clinical Studies with E-Cigarette–Naïve Smokers			
Bullen et al., 2010	Ruyan V8	16-mg cartridge	8
Eissenberg, 2010	NPRO by NJOY or Hydro by Crown Seven	16-mg cartridge (both brands)	16
Vansickel et al., 2010	NPRO by NJOY or Hydro by Crown Seven	NPRO: 18-mg cartridge; Hydro, 16-mg cartridge	32
Vansickel et al., 2012	Vapor King	18-mg/ml cartridge	20
Flouris et al., 2013	Giant by Nobacco G.P.	11-mg/ml cartridge	15
Farsalinos et al., 2015	eVic by Joyetech (2nd generation)	18-mg/ml	23

	Results	
Puffing Protocol	Biomarker	Study Comparison
e-cigarette: 5 minutes ad lib; inhaler: 20 minutes ad lib; usual cigarette: 5 minutes ad lib	plasma nicotine: C_{max}: 1.3 (0–2.6) ng/ml (mean and 95% CI); T_{max}: 19.6 (4.9–34.2) minutes following initial puff	inhaler: C_{max}: 2.1 (1.0–3.1) ng/ml, T_{max}: 32 (18.7–45.3) minutes; usual cigarette: C_{max}: 13.4 (6.5–20.3) ng/ml, T_{max}: 14.3 (8.8–19.9) minutes
two 10-puff standardized sessions, 30-second interval, sessions were 1 hour apart	plasma nicotine: after first session: NPRO, 3.5 (0.5) ng/ml (mean, SEM); Hydro, 2.5 (0.2) ng/ml	usual brand cigarette: 16.8 (3.4) ng/ml
two 10-puff standardized sessions, 30-second interval, sessions were 1 hour apart	no significant change in plasma nicotine	usual brand cigarette: baseline: 2.1 (0.32) ng/ml (mean, SD); 5 minutes after session 18.8 (11.8) ng/ml
six 10-puff standardized sessions, 30 seconds between puffs; sessions were 30 minutes apart	plasma nicotine: baseline: 2.2 (0.78) ng/ml (mean, SD); 5 minutes after last session: 7.4 (5.1) ng/ml	N/A
median = 11 puffs; puffs varied between participants; took equivalent puffs to be equivalent to two usual brand cigarettes based on a ratio of 1.5 cigarettes to e-cigarette nicotine absorption ratio	plasma cotinine: increased significantly immediately after and 1 hour after e-cigarette use	usual brand cigarette: no significant difference in plasma cotinine between e-cigarette and cigarette use
10 puffs in 5 minutes followed by ad lib use in 60 minutes	plasma nicotine: baseline: 1.6 (0.3) ng/ml (mean, SEM); 5 minutes after first puff: 4.3 (0.7) ng/ml; after 65 minutes: 13.8 (1.6) ng/ml	N/A

continued

TABLE 4-2 Continued

	Study Characteristics		
Reference	Study Product	Nicotine Content	Sample Size
Nides et al., 2014	King Bold by NJOY	26-mg cartridge	25
Hajek et al., 2015	Green Smoke	2.4% cartridge (24 mg/ml)	6
Oncken et al., 2015	Joye eGo-C	18-mg/ml e-liquid with tobacco or tobacco and menthol	20
Yan and D'Ruiz, 2015	blu e-cigs	5 different formulations: 3 with 24 mg/ml and 2 with 16 mg/ml	23

	Results	
Puffing Protocol	Biomarker	Study Comparison
two 10-puff standardized sessions, 30-second interval, sessions were 1 hour apart	plasma nicotine: 30 seconds after first 10 puffs: 3.5 (0.69) ng/ml (mean, SEM); 10 minutes after 10 puffs of second session: 5.1 (1.1–7.1) ng/ml (mean, range)	N/A
two 5-minute ad lib sessions: the first was at baseline and the second 4 weeks later	plasma nicotine: baseline: C_{max}: 4.6 (3.0) ng/ml (mean, SD); T_{max}: 5.0 (0.0) minutes; week 4: C_{max}: 5.7 (3.3) ng/ml; T_{max}: 5.0 (0.0) minutes	N/A
two 5-minute ad lib sessions; each session was preceded by 7–10 days of e-cigarette use with a different e-liquid	plasma nicotine: session 1: baseline: 4.2 (1.1) ng/ml (mean, SE); 5 minutes after first puff: 8.2 (1.7) ng/ml; session 2: baseline: 4.2 (0.7) ng/ml; 5 minutes after first puff: 9.3 (0.73) ng/ml	N/A
50-puff standardized session, 5-second puff, 30-second interval,1-hour ad lib session	plasma nicotine: baseline: range of mean: 0.01 (0.05)–0.04 (0.13) ng/ml (mean, SD); 5 minutes after first puff: range of mean: 1.99 (1.47)–3.00 (1.38) ng/ml; 30 minutes after first puff: range of mean: 9.96 (3.59)–17.05 (6.64) ng/ml	one Marlboro Gold King Size: baseline: 0.03 (0.12) ng/ml (mean, SD); 5 minutes after first puff: 14.42 (9.42) ng/ml; 30 minutes after first puff: 7.86 (1.99)
	plasma nicotine: range of mean at end of ad lib session: 13.70 (5.95)–22.42 (7.66) ng/ml	end of ad lib: 29.23 (10.84) ng/ml

continued

TABLE 4-2 Continued

	Study Characteristics		
Reference	Study Product	Nicotine Content	Sample Size
D'Ruiz et al., 2015	Not specified (but same study as Yan and D'Ruiz, 2015)	5 different formulations: 3 with 24 mg/ml and 2 with 16 mg/ml	23
Antoniewicz et al., 2016	eGo XL 3.7-V battery with dual-coil CE5 atomizer	12 mg/ml e-liquid	16
Lopez et al., 2016	eGO 3.3-V battery with 1.5-Ω Smoktech cartomizer	4 different e-liquids: 0, 8, 18, or 36 mg/ml nicotine	16
Walele et al., 2016	e-cigarette prototype	2 mg/ml nicotine (flavored and unflavored)	12
		0%, 0.4%, 0.9%, 2.0% nicotine	12

	Results	
Puffing Protocol	Biomarker	Study Comparison
50-puff standardized session, 5-second puff, 30-second interval	plasma nicotine: C_{max} within first 30 minutes: 10.3 (3.7)–18.1 (6.47) (range of mean, SD)	tobacco cigarette: C_{max} within first 30 minutes: 15.8 (8.64) ng/ml (mean, SD)
1-hour ad lib session	plasma nicotine: range of mean at end of ad lib session: 13.7 (5.98)–22.4 (7.65) ng/ml	end of ad lib: 29.2 (10.86) ng/ml
10 puffs in 10 minutes	plasma cotinine: 4 hours after 10 puffs: 4.1 ng/ml (median); IQR: 3.5, 4.7 ng/ml	John Silver cigarette (1 mg): plasma cotinine using similar protocol: 7.8 ng/ml (median), IQR: 4.6, 14.2
two 10-puff standardized sessions, 30-second interval, sessions were 1 hour apart	plasma nicotine: 5 minutes after 1 puff: 3.8 (3.30) ng/ml for 0 mg/ml e-liquid (mean, SD); 8.8 (6.3) ng/ml for 8 mg/ml; 13.2 (13.2) ng/ml for 18 mg/ml: 17.0 (17.9) ng/ml for 36 mg/ml e-liquid	N/A
10-puff standardized session, 4-second puff, 30-second interval (e-cigarette and inhaler), 2-second puff for tobacco cigarette	plasma nicotine: unflavored: C_{max}: 3.6 (33.9) ng/ml (mean, CV%); T_{max}: 9 (range, 1–15) minutes; flavored: C_{max} 2.5 (41.6) ng/ml; T_{max}: 10 (3–45) minutes	JPS Silver King Size cigarette: C_{max}: 21.2 (43.1) ng/ml; T_{max}: 3.0 (1–6) minutes; inhaler: C_{max}: 2.5 (45.2); T_{max}: 13 (5–15) minutes
10-puff standardized session, 4-second puff, 30-second interval	plasma nicotine: 0%: C_{max}: 0.6 (346.4) ng/ml (mean, CV%); T_{max}: 60 minutes (median); 0.4%: C_{max} 1.0 (41) ng/ml; T_{max}: 5 (1–60) minutes; 0.9%: C_{max} 1.9 (33) ng/ml; T_{max}: 7 (1–15) minutes; 2.0% C_{max} 3.6 (20.9) ng/ml; T_{max}: 7 (3–30) minutes	N/A

continued

TABLE 4-2 Continued

	Study Characteristics		
Reference	Study Product	Nicotine Content	Sample Size
Fearon et al., 2017	Vype vPro ePen (Nicoventures, Ltd.)	1.86%	23
Papaseit et al., 2016	Nhoss (tank)	16 mg/ml	9
Stiles et al., 2017	Vuse Solo	14-, 29-, and 36-mg cartridge	45
Clinical Studies with Experienced E-Cigarette Users			
Vansickel and Eissenberg, 2013	usual brands	average of e-liquid: 17.6 mg/ml; range: 9–24 mg/ml	8
Dawkins and Corcoran, 2014	SKYCIG	18-mg cartridge	14

	Results	
Puffing Protocol	Biomarker	Study Comparison
10-puff standardized session, 30 seconds between puffs; followed by 15–60 minutes ad lib use	plasma nicotine: standardized: C_{max}: 2.5 (0.5–6.9) ng/ml (GM, range); T_{max}: 6.0 (median); ad lib: C_{max}: 5.9 (1.6–12.5) ng/ml; T_{max}: 75 minutes (median)	JPS Blue: plasma nicotine: standardized: C_{max}: 13.0 (5.3–35.5) ng/ml; T_{max}: 7 minutes (median); ad lib: C_{max}: 14.1 (6.9–40.6) ng/ml; T_{max}: 75 minutes
two 10-puff sessions (30-second interpuff interval); 1 hour apart	plasma nicotine: first bout: C_{max}: 5.8 (0.0–14.5) ng/ml (median, range); T_{max}: 15 (0–55) minutes; second bout: C_{max}: 5.9 (0.0–24.6) ng/ml; T_{max}: 75 (55–120) minutes	Marlboro: first bout: C_{max}: 7.3 (2.9–16.4) ng/ml (median, range); T_{max}: 5 (5–45) minutes; second bout: C_{max}: 9.0 (3.7–19.6) ng/ml; T_{max}: 90 (65–120) minutes
up to 10 minutes of ad lib use of e-cigarette or cigarette; 30 minutes chewing nicotine gum	plasma nicotine: C_{max}: 14 mg: 3.01 ng/ml; 29 mg: 4.67 ng/ml; 36 mg: 5.36 ng/ml; T_{max}: 14 mg: 27.35 minutes; 29 mg: 21.83 minutes; 36 mg: 24.17 minutes	usual brand cigarette: C_{max}: 17.98 ng/ml; T_{max}: 8.13 minutes; nicotine gum: C_{max}: 5.26; T_{max}: 50.88 min
10-puff standardized session, 30 seconds between puffs	plasma nicotine: baseline: 2 (0) ng/ml (mean, SEM); 5 minutes after first puff: 10.3 (2) ng/ml	N/A
1-hour ad lib session	16.3 (4.5) ng/ml	
10 puffs within 5 minutes; ad lib interval	plasma nicotine: baseline: 0.74 (0.12) ng/ml (mean, SEM); 10 minutes after start of 10 puffs: 6.77 (1.23) ng/ml	N/A
1-hour ad lib session	13.91 (2.12) ng/ml	

continued

TABLE 4-2 Continued

	Study Characteristics		
Reference	Study Product	Nicotine Content	Sample Size
Farsalinos et al., 2015	eVic by Joyetech (2nd generation)	18 mg/ml	24
Ramoa et al., 2016	eGO 3.3-V battery with 1.5-Ω cartomizer	4 different e-liquids: 0, 8, 18, or 36 mg/ml nicotine	16
Spindle et al., 2015	usual battery with 1.5-Ω SmokTech cartomizer	usual e-liquid: 21.7 (3.9) mg/ml (mean, SD); range: 12–24 mg/ml	13
Dawkins et al., 2016	eVic Supreme (3.9 V) with Nautilus Aspire tank (1.8 Ω)	6 and 24 mg/ml nicotine	11
St.Helen et al., 2016a	usual brands	usual e-liquid: 12.5 (7.1) mg/ml (mean, SD); range: 6–24 mg/ml	13
Wagener et al., 2017	usual brands	2nd generation: 22.3 (7.5) mg/ml (mean, SD) (range; 11–36 mg/ml); 3rd generation: 4.1 (2.9) mg/ml (range; 1.5–6 mg/ml)	20

	Results	
Puffing Protocol	Biomarker	Study Comparison
10 puffs in 5 minutes followed by ad lib use in 60 minutes	plasma nicotine: baseline: 2.1 (0.3) ng/ml (mean, SEM); 5 minutes after first puff: 7.9 (0.9) ng/ml; after 65 minutes: 24.1 (2.0) ng/ml	N/A
two 10-puff standardized sessions, 30-second interval, sessions were 1 hour apart	plasma nicotine: change from baseline: –4.4 (17.9) ng/ml for 0 mg/ml e-liquid (mean, SD); 11.1 (9.4) ng/ml for 8 mg/ml; 18.1 (15.5) ng/ml for 18 mg/ml; and 24.1 (18.2) ng/ml for 36 mg/ml	N/A
10-puff standardized session, 30 seconds between puffs, with or without topography device	plasma nicotine: baseline: 2.4 (0.2) ng/ml (mean, SEM); 5 minutes after first puff: 19.2 (2.3) ng/ml	N/A
60-minute ad lib session	plasma nicotine: 10 minutes after first puff: 8.59 (7.52) ng/ml (mean, SD) for 6 mg/ml e-liquid and 33.77 (34.88) ng/ml for 24 mg/ml; end of session: 22.03 (16.19) for 6 mg/ml and 43.57 (34.78) ng/ml for 24 mg/ml e-liquid	N/A
standardized session of 15 puffs, 30-second interval	plasma nicotine: C_{max}: 8.4 (5.1) ng/ml (mean, SD) (range: 2.3–19.8 ng/ml); T_{max}: 5.1 (7.6) minutes (range: 2–30 minutes)	N/A
10-puff standardized session, 30 seconds between puffs	5 minutes after first puff: 2nd generation: 7.3 (2.8) ng/ml (mean, SD); 3rd generation: 17.5 (12.9) ng/ml	N/A

continued

TABLE 4-2 Continued

	Study Characteristics		
Reference	Study Product	Nicotine Content	Sample Size
Fearon et al., 2017	Vype vPro ePen (Nicoventures, Ltd.) and Nicolites (Nicocigs Ltd.)	Vype (1.86%) and Nicolites (1.33%)	18
Hajek et al., 2017	usual brand and 8 other common brands	range: 16–48 mg/ml	11
Spindle et al., 2017	usual battery with 1.5-Ω SmokTech cartomizer	usual e-liquid: 18.9 (5.9) mg/ml (mean, SD)	29
St.Helen et al., 2017	KangerTech mini Protank 3	two test e-liquids (18 mg/ml); usual e-liquid: 7.9 (6.0) mg/ml (mean, SD) (range: 3–18 mg/ml)	14

	Results	
Puffing Protocol	Biomarker	Study Comparison
115-minute ad lib session	plasma nicotine: after last puff: 2nd generation: 23.5 (12.8) ng/ml; 3rd generation: 24.8 (11.6) ng/ml	
5-minute ad lib use session	plasma nicotine: Vype: standardized: C_{max}: 7.8 (0.0–40.2) ng/ml (GM, range); T_{max}: 6.0 (median); Nicolites: C_{max}: 4.7 (1.2–18.2) ng/ml; T_{max}: 9 minutes (median)	Marlboro Ultralights tobacco cigarette: plasma nicotine: C_{max}: 7.2 (0.7–37.6) ng/ml; T_{max}: 6 minutes (median)
5-minute ad lib session	plasma nicotine: C_{max}: 7.5 (5.0)–13.6 (9.7) ng/ml (range of means (SD)); T_{max}: 4–6 minutes after first puff (range of means)	usual tobacco cigarette: C_{max}: 17.9 (16.0) ng/ml; T_{max}: 4 minutes
10-puff standardized session, 30 seconds between puffs, with or without topography device	plasma nicotine: baseline: 4.0 (0.7) ng/ml (mean, SEM); immediately after 10 puffs: 20.6 (2.8) ng/ml	N/A
90-minute ad lib, with or without topography device	plasma nicotine: end of session: 35.0 (4.6) ng/ml	
standardized session of 15 puffs, 30-second interval	plasma nicotine: test e-liquids: C_{max}: 12.1 (2.0) ng/ml and 9.5 (1.2) ng/ml (mean, SEM); T_{max}: 5.4 (1.4) and 4.9 (1.2) minutes after last puff; usual e-liquids: C_{max}: 6.2 (1.0) ng/ml; T_{max}: 3.1 (0.4) minutes after last puff	N/A
90-minute ad lib	plasma nicotine: test e-liquids: after 90 minutes: 16.5 (3.1) ng/ml and 11.3 (2.3) ng/ml; usual e-liquids: 11.2 (1.7) ng/ml	

ject study that compared nicotine exposure from two e-cigarette brands (NPRO by NJOY and Hydro by Crown Seven), both 16 mg nicotine. Participants (n = 16) engaged in two 10-puff sessions, with 30-second interpuff intervals, and sessions were 1 hour apart. Other conditions include smoking their usual brand of combustible tobacco cigarettes and sham smoking (puffing an unlit cigarette). The committee presents the results from the first session, which reflected nicotine exposure after a period of abstinence (more than 12 hours). Only the combustible tobacco cigarette significantly increased plasma nicotine levels. Mean plasma nicotine levels immediately after the first session were: NPRO (3.5 ng/ml); Hydro (2.5 ng/ml); and usual brand of combustible tobacco cigarette (16.8 ng/ml).

Vansickel and colleagues (2010) present the results of the full study described above by Eissenberg. The NPRO cartridge used was 18 mg nicotine while the Hydro cartridge was 16 mg nicotine. Participants took 10 puffs at two separate times during each session, as described before. The participants' usual tobacco cigarette brand significantly increased plasma nicotine concentration 5 minutes after the first puff, while NPRO, Hydro, and sham smoking did not alter blood nicotine levels.

Vansickel and colleagues (2012) conducted another study, this time with the e-cigarette Vapor King (18-mg/ml nicotine cartridge). Participants (n = 20) vaped the e-cigarette in six sessions (or six bouts), each time taking 10 puffs, one puff every 30 seconds and 1 hour between sessions. Average plasma nicotine concentration at baseline was 2.2 ng/ml, was significantly different after the fourth session, and reached 7.4 ng/ml 5 minutes after the final bout. This study indicated that prolonged use was required with these e-cigarettes before significantly elevating plasma nicotine levels. Still, the plasma nicotine levels after six 10-puff sessions were still lower than that from one typical combustible tobacco cigarette.

Flouris and colleagues (2013) examined the impact of e-cigarette use on serum cotinine and lung function in smokers. Fifteen smokers with no history of e-cigarette use crossed over among three conditions: their usual brand of cigarettes, an e-cigarette (Giant, 11-mg/ml nicotine cartridge), and sham smoking. Participants smoked two of their usual cigarettes over a 30-minute period. The number of puffs on the e-cigarette that would lead to equivalent amounts of nicotine delivered from the e-cigarette compared with their usual e-cigarettes was estimated using data from a pilot survey of 141 e-cigarette users who were former smokers. Information on nicotine content of the participants' combustible tobacco cigarettes, nicotine concentration of e-liquids, and number of puffs required to consume 1 ml of e-liquid were used to obtain a tobacco/e-cigarette absorption ratio of 1.5. Based on this ratio, participants took a median of 11 puffs (mean ± SD = 10.4 ± 2.7 puffs) over a 30-minute period. Serum cotinine immediately after and 1 hour after active smoking or e-cigarette use was significantly higher than baseline but there was no significant difference in serum cotinine between e-cigarette use and combustible tobacco cigarette use. This study suggests that when e-cigarettes deliver levels of nicotine comparable with combustible tobacco cigarettes, the overall systemic exposure to nicotine from e-cigarettes is similar to that of combustible tobacco cigarettes.

Nides and colleagues (2014) conducted a study of nicotine exposure from NJOY e-cigarettes. Participants (n = 25) were given King Bold by NJOY (26-mg nicotine cartridge) and were involved in two 10-puff standardized sessions (30-second interpuff interval, 1 hour between sessions). Average plasma nicotine concentration 30 seconds after the first session was 3.5 ng/ml, a fraction of that from smoking a typical combustible tobacco cigarette.

In another study, Yan and D'Ruiz (2015) randomized 23 smokers to five different formulations of blu e-cigarettes (three with 24 mg/ml nicotine and two with 16 mg/ml nicotine). For each cigarette, participants took 50 puffs (5-second duration, 30-second interpuff interval) during a standardized session followed by a 1-hour ad lib session. Participants also smoked a Marlboro Gold King Size cigarette (usual puff duration, 30-second interpuff interval). The range of average baseline plasma nicotine concentrations across all e-cigarette formulations ranged from 0.01 to 0.04 ng/ml, which increased to 1.99–3.00 ng/ml after 10 puffs and 7.86–17.05 ng/ml after 50 puffs. By comparison, average baseline plasma nicotine concentration was 0.03 ng/ml and increased to 14.42 ng/ml after smoking one cigarette. At the end of the 1-hour ad lib session, average plasma nicotine concentration ranged from 13.70 to 22.42 ng/ml with the e-cigarettes compared with 29.23 ng/ml with the combustible tobacco cigarettes. This study again showed that prolonged use of this e-cigarette was required before reaching plasma nicotine levels typically obtained after smoking just one combustible tobacco cigarette.

Farsalinos and colleagues (2015) compared plasma nicotine from acute e-cigarette use in 23 e-cigarette–naïve smokers with 24 experienced e-cigarette users. All participants were asked to take 10 puffs from a second-generation e-cigarette with 18 mg/ml e-liquid over 5 minutes followed by 60 minutes of ad lib use. Plasma nicotine levels were significantly higher in the experienced e-cigarette users 5 minutes after initiating puffing and at the end of the ad lib session. This study demonstrates that experience contributes to the ability of e-cigarette users to self-dose with nicotine from e-cigarettes.

Hajek and colleagues (2015) described differences in nicotine exposure among e-cigarette–naïve users who learned how to use the e-cigarette over a 4-week period. Six smokers interested in quitting, who were taking part in a larger study assessing toxicant exposure and nicotine intake (McRobbie et al., 2015), provided pharmacokinetic data. Participants used a Green Smoke first-generation e-cigarette (2.4 percent nicotine on label or 24 mg/ml) over a 5-minute ad lib period on the targeted quit smoking date (baseline) and 4 weeks later. While average plasma nicotine C_{max} increased from baseline (week 1) to week 4 (4.6–5.7 ng/ml), that change was not significant; T_{max} stayed the same (5 minutes). However, AUC from 0 to infinity was significantly higher at week 4, indicating higher systemic nicotine exposure. This study suggests that nicotine intake and systemic exposure from e-cigarettes can increase with practice.

Oncken and colleagues (2015) examined nicotine exposure with e-cigarette use in smokers who were not seeking treatment. The e-cigarette used was Joye e-Go-C. Participants crossed over between two e-liquid flavors, tobacco with menthol and tobacco, both 18 mg/ml nicotine. During each arm, participants used the e-cigarette over the previous 7–10 days at home. On the last day of each arm, participants were involved in a 5-minute ad lib session at the laboratory. Twenty participants completed at least one session and 18 completed both. Average plasma nicotine concentration increased significantly from baseline to 5 minutes after the first puff during both laboratory sessions. Average plasma nicotine increased from 4.2–8.2 ng/ml at session one and 4.2–9.3 at session two. There was no effect of laboratory session, flavor, or sex on change in plasma nicotine levels. However, women who were given their preferred flavor of e-liquid had significantly higher increase in plasma nicotine levels. The same effect was not seen among men.

Antoniewicz and colleagues (2016) conducted a study on the effects of e-cigarette aerosol on vascular function, and also reported plasma cotinine levels. Sixteen healthy seldom smokers who were also naïve e-cigarette users crossed over between use of an e-cigarette and a control condition of no e-cigarette use. The e-cigarette used was a second-generation CE5 atomizer with eGo XL 3.7-V battery, and 12 mg/ml nicotine e-liquid. Participants took 10 puffs in 10 minutes and cotinine was measured in plasma collected before and 4 hours after use. Median plasma cotinine at 4 hours was 4.1 ng/ml (participants with baseline cotinine were omitted from the study). By comparison, median plasma cotinine in smokers of John Silver cigarettes (1 mg) following a similar protocol by the same authors was significantly higher (7.8 ng/ml) (Antoniewicz et al., 2016; Mobarrez et al., 2014), suggesting that exposure to nicotine was lower from e-cigarettes compared with combustible tobacco cigarettes among seldom smokers.

Lopez and colleagues (2016) presented preliminary results of a study that examined the influence of e-liquid nicotine concentration on plasma cotinine levels. Sixteen smokers were enrolled and crossed over among e-liquids with 0, 8, 18, and 36 mg/ml nicotine. Participants used a 3.3-V eGo battery with a 1.5-Ω dual-coil cartomizer (Smoktech) and were involved in two 10-puff standardized sessions (30-second interval, 1 hour between sessions). Five minutes after the first puff, plasma nicotine concentrations for the 0, 8, 18, and 36 mg/ml e-liquids were 3.8 ng/ml, 8.8 ng/ml, 13.2 ng/ml, and 17.0 ng/ml, respectively. This study indicated that for naïve users, plasma nicotine increased with e-liquid nicotine concentration.

Walele and colleagues (2016) described a study examining the nicotine pharmacokinetics of an e-cigarette prototype. The first part of the study entailed testing the effect of flavoring (menthol versus non-menthol) on nicotine exposure (2.0 percent nicotine for flavored and unflavored e-liquid). The second part examined nicotine exposure using e-liquids with 0 percent, 0.4 percent, 0.9 percent, and 2.0 percent nicotine (0, 4 mg/ml, 9 mg/ml, and 20 mg/ml, respectively). Twelve participants were enrolled in each part. In the first part, participants also smoked a JPS Silver King Size cigarette and a nicotine inhaler (15 mg). For the e-cigarette and inhaler, participants took 10 puffs (4-second duration, 30-second interpuff interval) and for the cigarette, 2-second puffs. Mean C_{max} was significantly higher for the unflavored compared with the flavored e-cigarette (3.6 versus 2.5 ng/ml). Mean C_{max} for the cigarette was 21.2 ng/ml and that of the inhaler was 2.5 ng/ml. Average T_{max} for the unflavored and flavored e-liquid was 9 and 10 minutes after the first puff, respectively. The average T_{max} for the cigarette and inhaler was 3 and 13 minutes after the first puff, respectively. The plasma nicotine profile was similar between the e-cigarette and the nicotine inhaler. In part two, the average C_{max} for the 0 percent, 0.4 percent, 0.9 percent, and 2.0 percent nicotine was 0.6 ng/ml, 1.0 ng/ml, 1.9 ng/ml, and 3.6 ng/ml, respectively, increasing with the nicotine concentration of the e-liquid. T_{max} did not vary across e-liquid nicotine concentration. This study was the first to examine the effect of flavors on nicotine pharmacokinetics of e-liquids and suggests that nicotine exposure was higher with the unflavored e-liquid compared with the flavored e-liquid (menthol). The role of e-liquid flavors on nicotine absorption and systemic exposure to nicotine is not well understood and needs further study.

Fearon and colleagues (2017) conducted a study to describe nicotine exposure from use of Vype vPro ePen e-cigarettes (Nicoventures, Ltd.). This study involved two parts; the first part is described here. E-cigarette–naïve smokers (n = 23) were enrolled in the first part and used a cartridge with 1.86 percent nicotine (18.6 mg/ml nicotine). Participants took part in a 10-puff standardized session (30-second interpuff interval) which was followed by 15–60 minutes of ad lib use starting at 15 minutes after the start of the initial standardized puffing session. Mean C_{max} after 10 puffs was significantly lower with the e-cigarette (geometric mean [GM] = 2.5 ng/ml) than with the conventional cigarette (GM = 13.4 ng/ml).

Papaseit and colleagues (2016) conducted a crossover study with nine e-cigarette–naïve users who were randomized to a second-generation e-cigarette (Nhoss) with 16 mg/ml e-liquid or Marlboro cigarette (0.8 mg nicotine per cigarette, USA) on each of 2 days. Participants took 10 puffs from each product (30-second interpuff interval) during two administrations, 1 hour apart. Plasma nicotine C_{max} and T_{max} did not differ significantly between products at either administration. Plasma AUC from 0 to 55 minutes was significantly higher with the combustible tobacco cigarette during the first administration, indicating higher systemic nicotine exposure from combustible tobacco cigarettes compared with e-cigarettes. It should be noted that plasma nicotine C_{max} of 7.3 and 9.0 ng/ml from smoking the Marlboro cigarette are lower than typical C_{max} from smoking combustible tobacco cigarettes.

Stiles and colleagues (2017) examined nicotine exposure from use of three different Vuse Solo e-cigarette formulations (14, 29, and 36 mg nicotine/cartridge) in e-cigarette–naïve smokers. Participants used the designated e-cigarette ad lib for up to 10 minutes. The comparators were their usual brand of combustible tobacco cigarettes, which was also smoked during a 10-minute ad lib period, and a nicotine gum (4 mg), which was chewed for 30 minutes. Average C_{max} was significantly higher with smoking compared with the e-cigarettes. There were no significant differences in C_{max} between the Vuse Solo 29 mg and Vuse Solo 36 mg e-cigarettes compared with the nicotine gum but C_{max} was significantly lower with the Vuse Solo 14 mg compared with the nicotine gum. T_{max} was shorter for the cigarette (8.1 minutes) compared with e-cigarettes (21.8–27.4 minutes) and nicotine gum (50.9 minutes). Based on the pharmacokinetic profiles of the products tested, the authors concluded that the abuse liability for the Vuse Solo e-cigarettes was lower than that of combustible tobacco cigarettes, but higher than that of nicotine gum.

These studies suggest that e-cigarettes deliver lower levels of nicotine when used by e-cigarette–naïve smokers compared with levels delivered from combustible tobacco cigarettes, which is about 1 mg (Djordjevic and Doran, 2009). Studies that include direct comparisons with combustible tobacco cigarettes show that, among these naïve users, plasma nicotine levels are much lower with e-cigarettes compared with their usual combustible tobacco cigarettes. All but three of the studies examined nicotine exposure from cigalikes (Antoniewicz et al., 2016; Farsalinos et al., 2015; Lopez et al., 2016).

Clinical Studies with Experienced E-Cigarette Users

Twelve studies reported nicotine exposure in experienced or current e-cigarette users. Vansickel and Eissenberg (2013) conducted a study that described systemic nicotine exposure among e-cigarette users who used their usual devices. Participants (n = 8) used their e-cigarettes during a 10-puff standardized session (30-second interpuff interval) followed by a 1-hour ad lib session. Nicotine concentration of the e-liquids ranged from 9 to 24 mg/ml (mean = 17.6 mg/ml). Plasma nicotine increased significantly from 2 ng/ml at baseline to 10.3 ng/ml 5 minutes after the first puff of 10, and increased to 16.3 ng/ml at the end of the 1-hour ad lib session. This study demonstrated significant nicotine delivery among experienced e-cigarette users who use their own e-cigarettes.

Dawkins and Corcoran (2014) enrolled 14 experienced e-cigarette users in a study to examine nicotine delivery from SKYCIG, a cigalike. Participants used the e-cigarette (18-mg cartridge) during a 10-puff session (puffs were taken within 5 minutes but puff interval was not controlled) and during a 1-hour ad lib session. Plasma nicotine increased from 0.74 ng/ml at baseline to 6.77 ng/ml 10 minutes after the start of the 10-puff session and increased to 13.91 ng/ml at the end of the ad lib session. Plasma nicotine concentration from use of this first-generation e-cigarette was consistent with levels measured in some e-cigarette–naïve users (Lopez et al., 2016; Stiles et al., 2017; Vansickel et al., 2012).

Ramoa and colleagues (2016) presented the preliminary results of a study that examined the relationship between e-liquid nicotine concentration and plasma nicotine concentration. Sixteen experienced e-cigarette users were involved in a within-subject comparison of e-liquids containing 0, 8, 18, and 36 mg/ml nicotine. All participants used a 1.5-Ω cartomizer that was powered by an eGO 3.3-V battery. Participants were involved in two 10-puff standardized sessions (30-second interpuff interval, sessions 1 hour apart). Plasma nicotine concentrations were related to the concentration of nicotine in the e-liquid. The change from baseline for the 0, 8, 18, and 36 mg/ml nicotine e-liquids was –4.4 ng/ml, 11.1 ng/ml, 18.1 ng/ml, and 24.1 ng/ml. This study also demonstrated that e-cigarettes can elevate blood nicotine levels in experienced users within the range of that of combustible tobacco cigarettes.

Spindle and colleagues (2015) examined the impact of using a topography device with e-cigarettes on plasma nicotine levels. Thirteen e-cigarette users were given their usual e-cigarette battery and a study cartomizer (1.5-Ω SmokTech) and their usual e-liquid (mean = 21.7 mg/ml nicotine, range = 12–24 mg/ml) and participated in a 10-puff standardized session (30-second interpuff interval) with or without the topography device, on different days. The topography device did not influence plasma nicotine concentration. Plasma nicotine increased from an average of 2.4

ng/ml at baseline to an average of 19.3 ng/ml immediately following e-cigarette use. This study again demonstrated that e-cigarettes can cause blood nicotine concentration to be elevated into the range of that of combustible tobacco cigarettes.

Dawkins and colleagues (2016) conducted another study in which they evaluated blood nicotine levels from using e-cigarettes with different e-liquid nicotine concentrations. In this study, 11 e-cigarette users used a Nautilus Aspire tank (1.8 Ω) with an eVic Supreme (3.9 V) and used e-liquids with 6 and 24 mg/ml. Participants used the e-cigarette over a 60-minute ad lib session. Ten minutes after the first puff, plasma nicotine concentrations for the 6 and 24 mg/ml e-liquids were 8.59 ng/ml and 33.77 ng/ml, respectively. At the end of the session, plasma nicotine concentrations for the 6 and 24 mg/ml e-liquids were 22.03 ng/ml and 43.57 ng/ml, respectively. These results are consistent with other studies which show that for a given e-cigarette, plasma nicotine concentration increases with the concentration of nicotine in the e-liquid, and that e-cigarettes can elevate plasma nicotine concentrations to combustible-tobacco-cigarette-like levels (Ramoa et al., 2016; Vansickel and Eissenberg, 2013).

St.Helen and colleagues (2016a) conducted a study of nicotine delivery, retention, and systemic exposure among experienced e-cigarette users. Participants (n = 13) used their usual e-cigarette during a standardized session of 15 puffs (30-second interpuff interval). Systemic nicotine retention was determined by measuring the amount of nicotine inhaled and the amount exhaled into gas traps. Nicotine concentration of the usual e-liquids used in this study ranged from 6 to 24 mg/ml (average = 12.5 mg/ml). An average of 1.3 mg (range = 0.42–2.64 mg) of nicotine was inhaled and an average of 1.22 mg (range = 0.42–2.34 mg) was systemically retained. This represents an average of 93.8 percent systemic retention of the inhaled dose, similar to combustible tobacco cigarettes (80–90 percent). Average C_{max}, having controlled for baseline plasma nicotine, was 8.4 ng/ml (range = 2.3–19.8 ng/ml), and average T_{max} was 5.1 minutes (all 2–5 minutes and one at 30 minutes) after the last of 15 puffs. This study demonstrated that the shape of the plasma nicotine concentration-time curve was, on average, similar to that of combustible tobacco cigarettes, albeit with a lower average C_{max} compared with combustible tobacco cigarettes. However, there was variation, including some profiles that resembled that of smokeless tobacco, that is, slow rise to peak and sustained plasma nicotine levels, which are indicative of buccal absorption. Nevertheless, consistent with several other studies, the short time to peak for most e-cigarette users indicates rapid absorption of nicotine in the lungs. The study also demonstrated that, on average, e-cigarettes deliver comparable levels of nicotine to combustible tobacco cigarettes among experienced users.

Wagener and colleagues (2017) compared nicotine exposure from use of second- and third-generation e-cigarettes. Twenty participants (9 second-generation and 11 third-generation users) took 10 puffs in a standardized session (30-second puff interval) with their own devices and usual e-liquid brands. The average e-liquid concentrations used were 22.3 (SD = 7.5) mg/ml for the second-generation devices and 4.1 (2.9) mg/ml for the third-generation devices. Average power for the second generation devices was 8.6 (1.9) W and 71.6 (50.0) W for the third-generation devices. Plasma nicotine concentration 5 minutes after the 10th puff was 7.3 ng/ml for the second-generation e-cigarettes and 17.5 ng/ml for the third-generation e-cigarettes. The study showed that third-generation devices are able to mimic the plasma nicotine concentration of combustible tobacco cigarettes, likely due to their high power levels. The study also showed that users of third-generation devices consume significantly higher amounts of e-liquid compared with users of second-generation e-cigarettes. This implies that users of third-generation devices can potentially be exposed to higher levels of toxic substances that may be present in the e-liquid or given off in the aerosol.

Eighteen experienced e-cigarette users were enrolled in the second part of the study by Fearon and colleagues (2017). Participants crossed over between a Vype vPro ePen (Nicoventures, Ltd.) with 1.86 percent nicotine (18.6 mg/ml) and Nicolites (Nicocigs, Ltd.) with 1.33 percent nicotine (13.3 mg/ml). Participants took part in a 5-minute ad lib use session. A comparator was the Marlboro Ultralights tobacco cigarette. Average plasma nicotine C_{max} was 7.8 ng/ml (geometric mean) and 4.7 ng/ml for Vype and Nicolites, respectively, compared with 7.2 ng/ml with the tobacco cigarette. Average plasma nicotine C_{max} with the Vype e-cigarette was higher among experienced users compared with that of e-cigarette–naïve participants discussed in part 1 of this study, above.

Hajek and colleagues (2017) described the pharmacokinetic profiles of eight common e-cigarette brands in the United Kingdom as well as the participants' usual brands. Eleven participants were enrolled. The test e-cigarettes had nicotine concentrations ranging from 16 to 48 mg/ml. Participants used each e-cigarette over a 5-minute ad lib session. Average C_{max} ranged between 7.5 and 13.6 ng/ml and average T_{max} ranged from 4 to 6 minutes from the first puff for the different e-cigarette brands. Average C_{max} and T_{max} for the cigalike (first-generation) e-cigarette were 8.5 ng/ml and 6 minutes compared with 11.7 ng/ml and 6 minutes for the refillable model e-cigarettes. Average C_{max} for the usual combustible tobacco cigarette was 17.9 ng/ml and T_{max} was 4 minutes. While the plasma nicotine C_{max} for e-cigarettes was lower than for combustible tobacco cigarettes, there was variability among e-cigarettes; plasma nicotine C_{max} was higher with use of the refillable e-cigarettes. This is likely related to higher power of refillable (second-generation e-cigarettes) compared with cigalikes (Wagener et al., 2017).

In a second study by Spindle and colleagues (2017), which presents the full results of the study, experienced e-cigarette users (n = 29) were given a SmokTech cartomizer (1.5 Ω) to use with their usual e-cigarette battery and usual e-liquid (mean = 18.9 mg/ml nicotine). Participants used the e-cigarette in a 10-puff standardized session (30-second interpuff interval) followed by a 90-minute ad lib session, with or without a topography device attached. Consistent with preliminary results, plasma nicotine was not influenced by the topography device. Average baseline plasma nicotine concentration across conditions was 4.0 ng/ml, which increased to 20.6 ng/ml immediately after the 10 puffs. At the end of the 90-minute ad lib session, mean plasma nicotine concentration was 35.0 ng/ml. This study showed that the e-cigarette can be effective nicotine delivery devices.

St.Helen and colleagues (2017) conducted one of the first studies to examine the effect of e-liquid flavors on e-cigarette nicotine pharmacokinetics. Fourteen experienced e-cigarette users participated in the study and crossed over between two test flavors, strawberry and tobacco (both 18 mg/ml nicotine), and the participants' usual e-liquid flavors (average = 7.9 mg/ml, range = 3–18 mg/ml nicotine). Each e-liquid was administered on a different day. Participants used the e-cigarette during a 15-puff standardized session (30-second interpuff interval) followed by a 90-minute ad lib session. Average amount of nicotine delivered ranged between 0.9 and 1.7 mg (depending on nicotine concentration of e-liquid) and average systemic retention of nicotine ranged from 98.6 percent to 99.2 percent (there was no flavor effect on nicotine delivery and systemic retention). Average plasma nicotine C_{max} for two test flavors was 12.1 ng/ml and 9.5 ng/ml, respectively (strawberry versus tobacco); T_{max} was 5.4 versus 4.9 minutes after the last of 15 puffs. Based on AUCs at various early time points, it appeared as if the rate of absorption of nicotine was faster with the strawberry compared with the tobacco e-liquid. The differences were not statistically significant, but AUCs from 0 minutes to 5, 15, and 30 minutes for the strawberry e-liquid were 23 percent, 20 percent, and 17 percent higher than that of the tobacco e-liquid, respectively. C_{max} and T_{max} for the usual flavors were 6.2 ng/ml and 3.1 minutes, respectively. Plasma nicotine concentrations after the 90-minute ad lib session were 16.5 ng/ml (strawberry), 11.3 ng/ml (tobacco), and 11.2 ng/ml (usual brand of e-liquids).

In summary, studies of nicotine delivery and systemic retention in experienced users suggest that e-cigarettes can deliver nicotine in the range of a typical combustible tobacco cigarette, and most of the nicotine is systemically retained under experimental conditions. While variability remains between products and users, clinical studies with experienced users also indicate that e-cigarettes deliver nicotine in a way that resembles the pharmacokinetic profile of combustible tobacco cigarettes. Several studies reported plasma nicotine concentrations after 10 to 15 puffs or ad lib use (60–90 minutes), which were in the range of that of combustible tobacco cigarettes, particularly after use of high-powered third-generation e-cigarettes or high nicotine concentration e-liquids. These studies support the idea that exposure to nicotine from e-cigarettes is dependent, in part, on user experience. The type of e-cigarette, which is associated with the power used, as well as nicotine concentration of the e-liquid, are also important determinants of systemic nicotine exposure. Studies are needed to understand the role of flavors on the rate of nicotine absorption and systemic exposure in e-cigarette users.

Switching Studies

Studies in which tobacco cigarette smokers are given e-cigarettes to use instead of combustible tobacco cigarettes can be used to compare daily nicotine intake from combustible tobacco cigarettes and e-cigarettes, and answer whether e-cigarettes can effectively replace combustible tobacco cigarettes as a source of nicotine. The committee identified eight publications in which biomarkers of nicotine exposure were reported. Of these, two appear to describe the same parent study and present the same nicotine exposure results (D'Ruiz et al., 2016; O'Connell et al., 2016). Thus, seven studies are described. The seven studies measure biomarkers of nicotine exposure (cotinine and/or total nicotine equivalents, which is the molar sum of nicotine and its metabolites in urine) before and after switching to e-cigarettes.

McRobbie and colleagues (2015) assessed exposure to nicotine (as well as other toxic substances) before and after 4 weeks of e-cigarette use in 40 smokers who wanted to quit smoking. The study used a Green Smoke e-cigarette (first generation) with 2.4 percent nicotine (24 mg/ml) on the label. Participants were initially supplied with two cartridges per day, which was adjusted based on use, and were told to use the e-cigarette ad lib. Thirty-three participants were using the e-cigarette 4 weeks after the quit date. Of these, 16 (8 women) did not smoke combustible tobacco cigarettes during the previous week and 17 (8 women) smoked combustible tobacco cigarettes as well as the e-cigarette (dual users). Overall, urinary cotinine decreased 36 percent, from 1,655 ng/mg creatinine at baseline to 1,063 ng/mg creatinine at 4 weeks. Among the abstinent group, urinary cotinine decreased 17 percent, from 1,073 ng/mg creatinine to 889 ng/mg creatinine. Among the dual users, urinary cotinine decreased 44 percent, from 2,203 ng/mg creatinine to 1,227 ng/mg creatinine. This study suggests a decrease in daily nicotine intake when smokers replace combustible tobacco cigarettes fully or partially with a first-generation e-cigarette.

Adriaens and colleagues (2014) investigated the efficacy of second-generation e-cigarettes to reduce craving and reduce combustible tobacco cigarette consumption in an 8-month randomized controlled trial. Forty-eight e-cigarette–naïve smokers (27 women) with no intention to quit combustible tobacco cigarettes were randomized into two e-cigarette groups and a control group. The two e-cigarette groups were assigned to use Joye eGo-C or Kanger T2-CC with 18 mg/ml nicotine e-liquid while the control group smoked their usual combustible tobacco cigarette. Cotinine was measured in saliva samples collected by participants immediately before their visit to the laboratory at week 1, week 4, and week 8. During each of these visits, participants used their e-cigarette or combustible tobacco cigarette over a 5-minute ad lib session based on assigned group. Between visits, participants in the e-cigarette groups could use the assigned e-cigarette or smoke ad lib, whereas those in the control group could only smoke. Nicotine biomarkers were measured before or after laboratory sessions. After 8 weeks, the control group was also given e-cigarettes. Saliva cotinine was measured in samples collected before the final follow-up visit in the eighth month. No differences in saliva cotinine concentrations were found between the e-cigarette groups and the control group. Furthermore, saliva cotinine decreased significantly in the e-cigarette groups as well as the control group over the first 8 weeks (the period in which the control group was not given e-cigarettes) but increased in the e-cigarette groups at the last follow-up visit (month 8) and did not increase in the control group. At the last follow-up visit, no differences in saliva cotinine concentrations were observed between the e-cigarette groups and the control group (the control group had been allowed to use e-cigarettes over the last 6 months of the study). The average cotinine levels across all participants decreased from 663.50 ng/ml (SD = 350.15) at baseline to 449.96 ng/ml (SD = 193.19) at the end of the study. Saliva cotinine concentrations were examined across levels of combustible tobacco cigarette reduction (i.e., no reduction; greater than or equal to 50 percent reduction; greater than or equal to 80 percent reduction; and 100 percent reduction or quitters). No significant differences in saliva cotinine levels were seen between these groups at the times measured. The results of this study indicate that there was no significant difference in daily nicotine intake among smokers who switched completely to e-cigarettes, those who used both e-cigarettes and combustible tobacco cigarettes, and those who only smoked combustible tobacco cigarettes. In addition, the study also showed that e-cigarette–naïve smokers can titrate their nicotine intake with practice.

Cravo and colleagues (2016) conducted a study to evaluate the safety profile of an e-cigarette prototype (2.0 percent nicotine) in smokers who switch to the e-cigarette. The nicotine pharmacokinetic profile of this e-cigarette was discussed previously (Walele et al., 2016). Participants were randomized to the e-cigarette or usual cigarette and followed for 12 weeks. Of 419 enrolled participants, 408 (182 women) used the product at least once (full analysis set), and 387 completed the study. A subset of the participants (cohort 2) (40 total, 12 women) was confined to a research facility until day 6. Urinary total nicotine equivalents (molar sum of nicotine, cotinine, nicotine-*N*-glucuronide, cotinine-*N*-glucuronide, *trans* 3′-hydroxycotinine, and *trans* 3′-hydroxycotinine glucuronide) were used to measure daily nicotine intake. Overall, 40.2 percent of participants were compliant during the unconfined phase of the study, that is, self-reported smoking no combustible tobacco cigarettes on 80 percent or more of the study days (e-cigarette compliant), while 59.8 percent were less e-cigarette compliant. Total nicotine equivalents decreased rapidly in the e-cigarette arm and were significantly lower than the combustible tobacco cigarette arm at weeks 4, 8, and 12. Reductions in total nicotine equivalent were observed from day 2 in the confined participants (fully compliant). Participants in the e-cigarette arm saw average reductions in urinary total nicotine equivalents of 33.3 percent, 29.3 percent, and 25.3 percent in weeks 4, 8, and 12, respectively, relative to baseline. Levels of total nicotine equivalents were even lower among compliant participants of the e-cigarette arm. Participants in the combustible tobacco cigarette arm had stable total nicotine equivalents throughout the study, with reductions of 1.0 percent and 5.9 percent in weeks 4 and 12, respectively, and an increase of 3.0 percent in week 8, relative to baseline. A decrease in urine nicotine equivalents coincided with an increase in nicotine withdrawal symptoms. The results of this study suggest that the e-cigarette product could not effectively deliver nicotine to smokers who switch and resulted in significant decrease in daily nicotine intake. This is consistent with the low blood nicotine levels reported from acute use of this product (Walele et al., 2016).

Two publications, one by D'Ruiz and colleagues (2016), and the other by O'Connell and colleagues (2016), seem to describe the same parent study and nicotine exposure results. The authors of both publications reported changes in nicotine exposure among different groups following a 5-day forced switch from usual brand of tobacco cigarette to exclusive use of commercial e-cigarettes; dual use of commercial e-cigarettes and participants' usual combustible tobacco cigarette; or discontinued use of all tobacco or nicotine products (O'Connell et al., 2016). Three commercially available blu e-cigarettes (all 24 mg/ml nicotine) were used. A total of 105 participants (37 women) were enrolled and clinically confined over the study duration. Total nicotine equivalents decreased significantly from baseline to day 5 in the e-cigarette group. Average total nicotine equivalents ranged from 14.5–17.6 mg/24 hours at baseline for the three formulations of e-cigarettes to 10.5–12.7 mg/24 hours at day 5. There was no significant change in total nicotine equivalents in the dual-use group: baseline, 15.7–16.6 mg/24 hours to 15.8–18.4 mg/24 hours. Smoking/nicotine cessation resulted in a significant decrease in total nicotine equivalents: 20.0 mg/24 hours at baseline to 0.5 mg/24 hours at day 5. There were significant reductions in blood nicotine and cotinine from baseline to day 5 in the e-cigarette group for all three e-cigarettes. In the dual-use group, plasma cotinine did not change significantly, but plasma nicotine decreased significantly for one e-cigarette. Nicotine cessation resulted in significant reductions in plasma nicotine and cotinine from baseline to day 5. The study showed that use of e-cigarettes alone (blu e-cigarettes) resulted in significant reductions in daily nicotine intake compared with baseline (before switching). Daily nicotine intake of participants in the dual-use group did not change significantly from baseline.

Pulvers and colleagues (2016) described a study of 40 cigarette smokers (73 percent male) enrolled in a 4-week observational study. The enrolled smokers were interested in e-cigarettes, but not necessarily interested in quitting. The study e-cigarette was an e-Go C (second generation, non-variable voltage) and participants had a choice of seven flavor categories, which included tobacco, mint, fruit, candy, sweets, chocolate, and drink/soda, in nicotine strength of 12 or 24 mg/ml. Biomarkers were measured at baseline and at 4 weeks. Thirty-seven of 40 participants provided follow-up and used the e-cigarette. Sixteen participants (40 percent) reported no cigarettes at week 2 and 6 (15 percent) reported no cigarette use at week 4. Urinary cotinine levels were not significantly different at baseline and week 4 (574.8 versus 440.8 ng/mg creatinine). This suggests that the second-generation e-cigarette used in the study provided adequate nicotine replacement from combustible tobacco cigarettes.

In a study by Strasser and colleagues (2016), 28 combustible tobacco cigarette smokers were randomized to use one of 5 popular brands of first-generation e-cigarettes. Participants smoked their usual brand of combustible tobacco cigarette on day 1 and switched to the e-cigarette thereafter, with visits to the lab on days 5 and 10. Saliva cotinine was collected during each visit. Saliva cotinine decreased significantly from day 1 to day 10 for all e-cigarette brands. Relative to baseline, percentage change at day 10 ranged from 23.4–56.3 percent. This indicated significant reduction in nicotine exposure during e-cigarette use compared with combustible tobacco cigarette use. Furthermore, saliva cotinine did not differ between day 5 and day 10, indicating that nicotine exposure during e-cigarette use remained constant, albeit at levels lower than combustible tobacco cigarette use.

Goniewicz and colleagues (2017) enrolled 20 smokers (60 percent female) in a 2-week study and provided them with M201 (first generation, 11-mg nicotine/cartridge). Participants were given 20 tobacco-flavored cartridges per week and were encouraged to substitute their usual cigarettes with the e-cigarettes. Biomarkers were measured at baseline, week 1, and week 2. Total nicotine equivalents did not change from baseline (50 nmol/mg creatinine) to week 1 (45 nmol/mg creatinine) to week 2 (43 nmol/mg creatinine), indicating that the e-cigarettes can be used to sustain daily nicotine intake.

An important limitation of studies conducted in the users' naturalistic settings (real world) is the potential for noncompliance with the study regimen. Compliance was either assessed with expired carbon monoxide (Adriaens et al., 2014; Goniewicz et al., 2017) and/or self-reported combustible tobacco cigarette or e-cigarette consumption (Cravo et al., 2016; Goniewicz et al., 2017; Strasser et al., 2016). All five studies that measured expired carbon monoxide in participants who switched from combustible tobacco cigarettes to e-cigarettes reported significantly lower expired carbon monoxide after switching, indicating fewer combustible tobacco cigarettes were smoked when assigned to use e-cigarettes. However, complete abstinence from combustible tobacco cigarettes could not be guaranteed. Studies done in research facilities enforced compliance (D'Ruiz et al., 2016; O'Connell et al., 2016). Of the seven longitudinal studies involving smokers switching to e-cigarettes, three reported no significant change in nicotine exposure from baseline to follow-up with complete or partial replacement of combustible tobacco cigarettes with e-cigarettes (Adriaens et al., 2014; Goniewicz et al., 2017; Pulvers et al., 2016). These studies suggest that some smokers are able to completely replace their daily nicotine intake from combustible tobacco cigarettes with e-cigarettes. On the other hand, the other four studies suggest that some e-cigarettes are ineffective nicotine delivery devices compared with combustible tobacco cigarettes.

Other Studies of Nicotine Exposure

A few other studies have measured nicotine exposure in long-term e-cigarette users to address the question of whether nicotine exposure from e-cigarettes matches that of combustible tobacco cigarettes. Shahab and colleagues (2017) compared exposure to nicotine and other compounds between long-term users (n = 181) of a variety of nicotine/tobacco products in a cross-sectional study. Combustible tobacco cigarette smokers (n = 37), dual cigarette and NRT users (n = 36), dual combustible tobacco cigarette and e-cigarette users (n = 36), NRT-only users (n = 36), and e-cigarette–only users (n = 36) in the United Kingdom were purposively recruited into the study. Daily nicotine intake was measured using saliva nicotine and cotinine and urinary total nicotine equivalents. While there was greater variability in saliva nicotine and cotinine between product groups than urine total nicotine equivalents, none of the nicotine exposure biomarkers showed clear differences among groups. The following values indicate the urine total nicotine equivalent levels as a percentage of the levels from combustible tobacco cigarette–only smokers: dual cigarette + NRT = 104.2, 95% CI = 64.3–168.9; dual cigarette + e-cigarette = 156.8, 95% CI = 105.1–233.8; NRT-only = 121.6, 95% CI = 62.5–236.8, e-cigarette–only, 126.9, 95% CI = 82.1–196.2. This study was the first to suggest that long-term use of e-cigarettes (and also NRT-only use) is associated with roughly similar daily nicotine intake compared with combustible tobacco cigarette–only use.

Some studies have measured cotinine as a biomarker of nicotine intake and exposure in long-term e-cigarette users. A study by Etter and Bullen (2011) reported saliva cotinine in the saliva of experienced e-cigarette users contacted in real-life settings. Participants visiting a smoking cessation website were recruited to complete an online questionnaire and current e-cigarette users provided a saliva sample (31 of 196 posted vials). Median cotinine of e-cigarette users who had not smoked combustible tobacco cigarettes in the previous 48 hours (n = 30) was 322 ng/ml. In another study by Etter (2016), saliva cotinine levels were measured longitudinally in e-cigarette users. Ninety-eight exclusive e-cigarette users were recruited online to provide saliva samples by mail at baseline and 8 months later. The median cotinine level was 307 ng/ml (interquartile range [IQR] = 114–466 ng/ml) at follow-up and was not significantly different from baseline levels, 252 ng/ml (IQR = 124–421 ng/ml). During that same time, the median nicotine concentration of the e-liquid used had decreased from 11 mg/ml to 6 mg/ml and median volume of e-liquid consumed per month increased from 80 to 100 ml. This study indicated that while e-cigarette users decrease the nicotine concentration of their e-liquids over time, they consume more e-liquid and maintain a relatively constant daily nicotine intake. The authors concluded that in experienced e-cigarette users enrolled online, cotinine levels were similar to levels usually observed in combustible tobacco cigarette smokers.

Hecht and colleagues (2015) measured cotinine and nicotine in the urine of e-cigarette users and smokers enrolled in two separate studies. Average urinary cotinine and nicotine in a group of 28 e-cigarette users who had not smoked combustible tobacco cigarettes for at least 2 months were 1,880 ng/ml (95% CI = 1,420–2,480 ng/ml), and 869 ng/ml (95% CI = 604–1,250 ng/ml), respectively, which were significantly lower than urinary cotinine 3,930 ng/ml (95% CI = 3,500–4,400 ng/ml), and nicotine 1,380 ng/ml (95% CI = 1,190–1,600 ng/ml) from a group of 165 smokers. Urinary cotinine and nicotine from the e-cigarette users were not significantly different when compared with a second group of smokers (n = 40): 1,930 ng/ml (95% CI = 1,530–2,440 ng/ml) and 1,270 ng/ml (95% CI = 834–1,710 ng/ml), respectively.

Goney and colleagues (2016) also measured cotinine in the urine of combustible tobacco smokers (n = 33), e-cigarette users (n = 32), and non-smokers exposed to secondhand smoke (n = 33). Mean urinary cotinine (SD) in e-cigarette users was 1,755 (1,848) ng/g; creatinine; it was not significantly different from that of smokers, 1,720 (1,335) ng/g. Urinary cotinine of those exposed to secondhand smoke was much lower, 81.4 (97.9) ng/g creatinine.

In general, these studies which measured nicotine and/or its metabolites in long-term users of e-cigarettes indicate that nicotine intake in these users match that of combustible tobacco cigarette smokers.

RELATIONSHIP BETWEEN E-CIGARETTE TOPOGRAPHY AND NICOTINE EXPOSURE

Vaping machine studies have demonstrated that puffing topography influences e-cigarette nicotine yields (Talih et al., 2015). Namely, longer puff durations are associated with higher nicotine yields. Therefore, it is worthwhile to examine whether e-cigarette puffing topography is associated with systemic exposure to nicotine among users. Three human studies that addressed this question were identified. For a general discussion of e-cigarette puffing topography, see Chapter 3.

Farsalinos and colleagues (2015) assessed the relationship between puff topography and plasma nicotine in a study with 24 experienced e-cigarette users and 23 e-cigarette–naïve users. Participants were involved in a 10-puff bout over 5 minutes followed by 60 minutes of ad lib use. Number of puffs and puff duration were measured by the e-cigarette (eVic). The study found statistically significant but weak positive correlations between puff duration and plasma nicotine levels after 5 minutes and after 65 minutes. These results are consistent with the vaping machine study (Talih et al., 2015).

In another study, St.Helen and colleagues (2016b) characterized puffing behavior in experienced adult e-cigarette users during 90 minutes of ad lib access to their usual e-cigarette in a hospital research ward. Thirteen participants (seven men, six women) were enrolled. Puff topography (puff duration, interpuff interval, and number of puffs taken) were obtained from video analysis. When all participants were considered (i.e., users of all three generations of e-cigarettes), vaping topography parameters were not significantly correlated with the amount of e-liquid consumed, amount of nicotine inhaled, and nicotine pharmacokinetic parameters. However, when only second-generation (tank) device users (eight participants) were included in the analysis, the number of puffs taken during the session was positively correlated with the amount of nicotine inhaled and plasma nicotine AUC while interpuff interval was negatively correlated with plasma nicotine C_{max}. Puff duration was not significantly correlated with systemic nicotine exposure. The findings suggest that the relationship between puff topography and nicotine exposure may be device-specific (correlations were significant only when one type of device was analyzed). This study had a relatively small sample size, which limits the reliability of the observations made.

Dawkins and colleagues (2016) enrolled 11 e-cigarette users into a crossover study in which study participants used e-liquids with low nicotine (6 mg/ml) and high nicotine (24 mg/ml) during a 60-minute ad lib session. The study found that puff number and puff duration were positively correlated with nicotine boost at each time point under both the high and low nicotine conditions. Interestingly, the correlations were larger at the high nicotine condition, suggesting that device characteristics can moderate the relationship between puff topography and systemic exposure to nicotine.

In summary, these three studies are consistent with the vaping machine study, showing that puffing topography is correlated with systemic exposure to nicotine. More research is needed to understand how the relationship between puffing topography and nicotine exposure differs across device characteristics.

SYNTHESIS

This chapter reviews the literature on nicotine content in e-cigarette liquids and aerosols, e-liquid pH, nicotine pharmacokinetics and pharmacology, and nicotine exposure from e-cigarettes. The nicotine content of e-cigarettes varies widely among products, with varying degrees of agreement between nicotine content on the label and what is chemically measured. The choice of nicotine strength is influenced, in part, by e-cigarette characteristics, such as electrical power. Nicotine concentration in e-cigarette aerosol is also variable among e-cigarettes. The concentration of nicotine in e-cigarette aerosol is a product of device characteristics and user behavior. Nicotine yield increases with e-cigarette power and e-liquid nicotine concentration, and with increasing puff duration. The pH of e-liquids is also variable, with a few studies reporting a range of pH from about 4.3 to 9.9. The committee did not find any study that has systematically assessed the effect of e-liquid pH on e-cigarette pharmacology.

The committee summarized the known pharmacokinetics and pharmacodynamics of nicotine based on reports of the Surgeon General and other authoritative reviews. The potential carcinogenicity and cardiovascular effects of nicotine were discussed. Other potential effects of nicotine, such as developmental and respiratory effects, are discussed in Section II of this report. It is important to note that this chapter does not make conclusions on the health effects of e-cigarettes per se, as these are reviewed in later chapters. However, the potential carcinogenicity and cardiovascular effects of nicotine have implications for the health effects of e-cigarettes. As discussed, there is no evidence to indicate that nicotine is a carcinogen. While it is biologically plausible that nicotine can act as a tumor promoter, there is no evidence from studies of long-term NRT users and users of smokeless tobacco products that nicotine increases human cancer risks. Given this evidence, nicotine exposure from e-cigarette use will likely pose minimal cancer risk to users. Based on known cardiovascular effects of nicotine, exposure to nicotine from e-cigarettes likely elevates the cardiovascular disease risk in people with preexisting cardiovascular disease(s) but the cardiovascular risks in people without cardiovascular disease(s) is uncertain.

Finally, the committee reviewed human studies to examine the nicotine exposure profile of e-cigarettes. Clinical studies of acute nicotine exposure from e-cigarette use in e-cigarette–naïve smokers and experienced e-cigarette users were reviewed, as well as studies of long-term e-cigarette use in combustible tobacco cigarette smokers who switch to e-cigarettes over a study period.

> *Conclusion 4-1. There is* ***conclusive evidence*** *that exposure to nicotine from e-cigarettes is highly variable and depends on product characteristics (including device and e-liquid characteristics) and how the device is operated.*

> *Conclusion 4-2. There is* ***substantial evidence*** *that nicotine intake from e-cigarette devices among experienced adult e-cigarette users can be comparable to that from combustible tobacco cigarettes.*

REFERENCES

Adamson, J., D. Thorne, B. Zainuddin, A. Baxter, J. McAughey, and M. Gaça. 2016. Application of dosimetry tools for the assessment of e-cigarette aerosol and cigarette smoke generated on two different in vitro exposure systems. *Chemistry Central Journal* 10(74):1–16.

Adriaens, K., D. Van Gucht, P. Declerck, and F. Baeyens. 2014. Effectiveness of the electronic cigarette: An eight-week Flemish study with six-month follow-up on smoking reduction, craving and experienced benefits and complaints. *International Journal of Environmental Research & Public Health* 11(11):11220–11248.

Antoniewicz, L., J. A. Bosson, J. Kuhl, S. M. Abdel-Halim, A. Kiessling, F. Mobarrez, and M. Lundback. 2016. Electronic cigarettes increase endothelial progenitor cells in the blood of healthy volunteers. *Atherosclerosis* 255:179–185.

Armitage, A. K., C. T. Dollery, C. F. George, T. H. Houseman, P. J. Lewis, and D. M. Turner. 1975. Absorption and metabolism of nicotine from cigarettes. *BMJ* 4(5992):313–316.

Armitage, A., C. Dollery, T. Houseman, E. Kohner, P. J. Lewis, and D. Turner. 1978. Absorption of nicotine from small cigars. *Clinical Pharmacology & Therapeutics* 23(2):143–151.

Benowitz, N. L. 2008. Neurobiology of nicotine addiction: Implications for smoking cessation treatment. *American Journal of Medicine* 121(4 Supplement 1):S3–S10.

Benowitz, N. L. 2009. Pharmacology of nicotine: Addiction, smoking-induced disease, and therapeutics. *Annual Review of Pharmacology and Toxicology* 49:57–71.

Benowitz, N. L., and A. D. Burbank. 2016. Cardiovascular toxicity of nicotine: Implications for electronic cigarette use. *Trends in Cardiovascular Medicine* 26(6):515–523.

Benowitz, N. L., and J. B. Fraiman. 2017. Cardiovascular effects of electronic cigarettes. *Nature Reviews Cardiology* 14(8):447–456.

Benowitz, N. L., E. J. Perez-Stable, I. Fong, G. Modin, B. Herrera, and P. Jacob, 3rd. 1999. Ethnic differences in *N*-glucuronidation of nicotine and cotinine. *Journal of Pharmacology and Experimental Therapeutics* 291(3):1196–1203.

Benowitz, N. L., E. J. Perez-Stable, B. Herrera, and P. Jacob, 3rd. 2002. Slower metabolism and reduced intake of nicotine from cigarette smoking in Chinese-Americans. *Journal of the National Cancer Institute* 94(2):108–115.

Benowitz, N. L., O. F. Pomerleau, C. S. Pomerleau, and P. Jacob, 3rd. 2003. Nicotine metabolite ratio as a predictor of cigarette consumption. *Nicotine & Tobacco Research* 5(5):621–624.

Benowitz, N. L., B. Herrera, and P. Jacob, 3rd. 2004. Mentholated cigarette smoking inhibits nicotine metabolism. *Journal of Pharmacology and Experimental Therapeutics* 310(3): 1208–1215.

Benowitz, N. L., J. Hukkanen, and P. Jacob, 3rd. 2009. Nicotine chemistry, metabolism, kinetics and biomarkers. *Handbook of Experimental Pharmacology* (192):29–60.

Berg, J. Z., J. Mason, A. J. Boettcher, D. K. Hatsukami, and S. E. Murphy. 2010a. Nicotine metabolism in African Americans and European Americans: Variation in glucuronidation by ethnicity and UGT2B10 haplotype. *Journal of Pharmacology and Experimental Therapeutics* 332(1):202–209.

Berg, J. Z., L. B. von Weymarn, E. A. Thompson, K. M. Wickham, N. A. Weisensel, D. K. Hatsukami, and S. E. Murphy. 2010b. UGT2B10 genotype influences nicotine glucuronidation, oxidation, and consumption. *Cancer Epidemiology, Biomarkers and Prevention* 19(6):1423–1431.

Bergstrom, M., A. Nordberg, E. Lunell, G. Antoni, and B. Langstrom. 1995. Regional deposition of inhaled ^{11}C-nicotine vapor in the human airway as visualized by positron emission tomography. *Clinical Pharmacology & Therapeutics* 57(3):309–317.

Berridge, M. S., S. M. Apana, K. K. Nagano, C. E. Berridge, G. P. Leisure, and M. V. Boswell. 2010. Smoking produces rapid rise of [^{11}C]nicotine in human brain. *Psychopharmacology (Berl)* 209(4):383–394.

Bhatnagar, A. 2016. E-cigarettes and cardiovascular disease risk: Evaluation of evidence, policy implications, and recommendations. *Current Cardiovascular Risk Reports* 10(7):24.

Bullen, C., H. McRobbie, S. Thornley, M. Glover, R. Lin, and M. Laugesen. 2010. Effect of an electronic nicotine delivery device (e cigarette) on desire to smoke and withdrawal, user preferences and nicotine delivery: Randomised cross-over trial. *Tobacco Control* 19(2):98–103.

Cameron, J. M., D. N. Howell, J. R. White, D. M. Andrenyak, M. E. Layton, and J. M. Roll. 2014. Variable and potentially fatal amounts of nicotine in e-cigarette nicotine solutions. *Tobacco Control* 23(1):77–78.

Carmella, S. G., A. Borukhova, D. Desai, and S. S. Hecht. 1997. Evidence for endogenous formation of tobacco-specific nitrosamines in rats treated with tobacco alkaloids and sodium nitrite. *Carcinogenesis* 18(3):587–592.

Chen, G., A. S. Blevins-Primeau, R. W. Dellinger, J. E. Muscat, and P. Lazarus. 2007. Glucuronidation of nicotine and cotinine by UGT2B10: Loss of function by the *UGT2B10* codon 67 (Asp>Tyr) polymorphism. *Cancer Research* 67(19):9024–9029.

Chen, G., N. E. Giambrone, and P. Lazarus. 2012. Glucuronidation of *trans*-3′-hydroxycotinine by UGT2B17 and UGT2B10. *Pharmacogenetics and Genomics* 22(3):183–190.

Chen, J., R. Higby, D. Tian, D. Tan, M. D. Johnson, Y. Xiao, K. J. Kellar, S. Feng, and P. G. Shields. 2008. Toxicological analysis of low-nicotine and nicotine-free cigarettes. *Toxicology* 249(2–3):194–203.

Cheng, T. R. 2014. Chemical evaluation of electronic cigarettes. *Tobacco Control* 23:11–17.

Cobb, N. K., M. J. Byron, D. B. Abrams, and P. G. Shields. 2010. Novel nicotine delivery systems and public health: The rise of the "e-cigarette." *American Journal of Public Health* 100(12):2340–2342.

Cravo, A. S., J. Bush, G. Sharma, R. Savioz, C. Martin, S. Craige, and T. Walele. 2016. A randomised, parallel group study to evaluate the safety profile of an electronic vapour product over 12 weeks. *Regulatory Toxicology and Pharmacology* 81:S1–S14.

Dawkins, L., and O. Corcoran. 2014. Acute electronic cigarette use: Nicotine delivery and subjective effects in regular users. *Psychopharmacology* 231(2):401–407.

Dawkins, L. E., C. F. Kimber, M. Doig, C. Feyerabend, and O. Corcoran. 2016. Self-titration by experienced e-cigarette users: Blood nicotine delivery and subjective effects. *Psychopharmacology (Berl)* 233(15–16):2933–2941.

Dempsey, D., P. Tutka, P. Jacob, 3rd, F. Allen, K. Schoedel, R. F. Tyndale, and N. L. Benowitz. 2004. Nicotine metabolite ratio as an index of cytochrome P450 2A6 metabolic activity. *Clinical Pharmacology & Therapeutics* 76(1):64–72.

Denton, T. T., X. Zhang, and J. R. Cashman. 2004. Nicotine-related alkaloids and metabolites as inhibitors of human cytochrome P-450 2A6. *Biochemical Pharmacology* 67(4):751–756.

Derby, K. S., K. Cuthrell, C. Caberto, S. G. Carmella, A. A. Franke, S. S. Hecht, S. E. Murphy, and L. Le Marchand. 2008. Nicotine metabolism in three ethnic/racial groups with different risks of lung cancer. *Cancer Epidemiology, Biomarker & Prevention* 17(12):3526–3535.

Digard, H., C. Proctor, A. Kulasekaran, U. Malmqvist, and A. Richter. 2013. Determination of nicotine absorption from multiple tobacco products and nicotine gum. *Nicotine & Tobacco Research* 15(1):255–261.

Djordjevic, M. V., and K. A. Doran. 2009. Nicotine content and delivery across tobacco products. *Handbook of Experimental Pharmacology* (192):61–82.

D'Ruiz, C. D., D. W. Graff, and X. S. Yan. 2015. Nicotine delivery, tolerability and reduction of smoking urge in smokers following short-term use of one brand of electronic cigarettes. *BMC Public Health* 15:991. https://doi.org/10.1186/s12889-015-2349-2 (accessed February 5, 2018).

D'Ruiz, C. D., D. W. Graff, and E. Robinson. 2016. Reductions in biomarkers of exposure, impacts on smoking urge and assessment of product use and tolerability in adult smokers following partial or complete substitution of cigarettes with electronic cigarettes. *BMC Public Health* 16:543. https://doi.org/10.1186/s12889-016-3236-1 (accessed February 5, 2018).

Ehmer, U., A. Vogel, J. K. Schutte, B. Krone, M. P. Manns, and C. P. Strassburg. 2004. Variation of hepatic glucuronidation: Novel functional polymorphisms of the UDP-glucuronosyltransferase UGT1A4. *Hepatology* 39(4):970–977.

Eissenberg, T. 2010. Electronic nicotine delivery devices: Ineffective nicotine delivery and craving suppression after acute administration. *Tobacco Control* 19(1):87–88.

El-Hellani, A., R. El-Hage, R. Baalbaki, R. Salman, S. Talih, A. Shihadeh, and N. A. Saliba. 2015. Free-base and protonated nicotine in electronic cigarette liquids and aerosols. *Chemical Research in Toxicology* 28(8):1532–1537.

England, L. J., K. Aagaard, M. Bloch, K. Conway, K. Cosgrove, R. Grana, T. J. Gould, D. Hatsukami, F. Jensen, D. Kandel, B. Lanphear, F. Leslie, J. R. Pauly, J. Neiderhiser, M. Rubinstein, T. A. Slotkin, E. Spindel, L. Stroud, and L. Wakschlag. 2017. Developmental toxicity of nicotine: A transdisciplinary synthesis and implications for emerging tobacco products. *Neuroscience & Biobehavioral Reviews* 72(Supplement C):176–189.

Etter, J. F. 2016. A longitudinal study of cotinine in long-term daily users of e-cigarettes. *Drug and Alcohol Dependence* 160:218–221.

Etter, J. F., and A. Bugey. 2017. E-cigarette liquids: Constancy of content across batches and accuracy of labeling. *Addictive Behaviors* 73:137–143.

Etter, J. F., and C. Bullen. 2011. Saliva cotinine levels in users of electronic cigarettes. *European Respiratory Journal* 38(5):1219–1220.

Etter, J. F., E. Zather, and S. Svensson. 2013. Analysis of refill liquids for electronic cigarettes. *Addiction* 108(9):1671–1679.

Farsalinos, K. E., A. Spyrou, C. Stefopoulos, K. Tsimopoulou, P. Kourkoveli, D. Tsiapras, S. Kyrzopoulos, K. Poulas, and V. Voudris. 2015. Nicotine absorption from electronic cigarette use: Comparison between experienced consumers (vapers) and naïve users (smokers). *Scientific Reports*. https://www.nature.com/articles/srep11269 (accessed February 5, 2018).

Fearon, I. M., A. Eldridge, N. Gale, C. J. Shepperd, M. McEwan, O. M. Camacho, M. Nides, K. McAdam, and C. J. Proctor. 2017. E-cigarette nicotine delivery: Data and learnings from pharmacokinetic studies. *American Journal of Health Behavior* 41(1):16–32.

Flouris, A. D., M. S. Chorti, K. P. Poulianiti, A. Z. Jamurtas, K. Kostikas, M. N. Tzatzarakis, A. W. Hayes, A. M. Tsatsakis, and Y. Koutedakis. 2013. Acute impact of active and passive electronic cigarette smoking on serum cotinine and lung function. *Inhalation Toxicology* 25(2):91–101.

Galitovskiy, V., A. I. Chernyavsky, R. A. Edwards, and S. A. Grando. 2012. Muscle sarcomas and alopecia in A/J mice chronically treated with nicotine. *Life Sciences* 91(21–22): 1109–1112.

Ghosheh, O., and E. M. Hawes. 2002. *N*-Glucuronidation of nicotine and cotinine in humans: Formation of cotinine glucuronide in liver microsomes and lack of catalysis by 10 examined UDP-glucuronosyltransferases. *Drug Metabolism & Disposition* 30(9):991–996.

Goney, G., I. Cok, U. Tamer, S. Burgaz, and T. Sengezer. 2016. Urinary cotinine levels of electronic cigarette (e-cigarette) users. *Toxicology Mechanisms and Methods* 26(6):414–418.

Goniewicz, M. L., T. Kuma, M. Gawron, J. Knysak, and L. Kosmider. 2013. Nicotine levels in electronic cigarettes. *Nicotine & Tobacco Research* 15(1):158–166.

Goniewicz, M. L., P. Hajek, and H. McRobbie. 2014. Nicotine content of electronic cigarettes, its release in vapour and its consistency across batches: Regulatory implications. *Addiction* 109(3):500–507.

Goniewicz, M. L., R. Gupta, Y. H. Lee, S. Reinhardt, S. Kim, B. Kim, L. Kosmider, and A. Sobczak. 2015. Nicotine levels in electronic cigarette refill solutions: A comparative analysis of products from the U.S., Korea, and Poland. *International Journal of Drug Policy* 26(6):583–588.

Goniewicz, M. L., M. Gawron, D. M. Smith, M. Peng, P. Jacob, 3rd, and N. L. Benowitz. 2017. Exposure to nicotine and selected toxicants in cigarette smokers who switched to electronic cigarettes: A longitudinal within-subjects observational study. *Nicotine & Tobacco Research* 19(2):160–167.

Gori, G. B., N. L. Benowitz, and C. J. Lynch. 1986. Mouth versus deep airways absorption of nicotine in cigarette smokers. *Pharmacology Biochemistry and Behavior* 25(6):1181–1184.

Gotti, C., L. Riganti, S. Vailati, and F. Clementi. 2006. Brain neuronal nicotinic receptors as new targets for drug discovery. *Current Pharmaceutical Design* 12(4):407–428.

Grando, S. A. 2014. Connections of nicotine to cancer. *Nature Reviews Cancer* 14(6):419–429.

Gundisch, D. 2000. Nicotinic acetylcholine receptors and imaging. *Current Pharmaceutical Design* 6(11):1143–1157.

Hajek, P., M. L. Goniewicz, A. Phillips, K. Myers Smith, O. West, and H. McRobbie. 2015. Nicotine intake from electronic cigarettes on initial use and after 4 weeks of regular use. *Nicotine & Tobacco Research* 17(2):175–179.

Hajek, P., D. Przulj, A. Phillips, R. Anderson, and H. McRobbie. 2017. Nicotine delivery to users from cigarettes and from different types of e-cigarettes. *Psychopharmacology* 234(5):773–779.

Haussmann, H. J., and M. W. Fariss. 2016. Comprehensive review of epidemiological and animal studies on the potential carcinogenic effects of nicotine per se. *Critical Reviews in Toxicology* 46(8):701–734.

Hecht, S. S. 1998. Biochemistry, biology, and carcinogenicity of tobacco-specific N-nitrosamines. *Chemical Research in Toxicology* 11(6):559–603.

Hecht, S. S., S. G. Carmella, D. Kotandeniya, M. E. Pillsbury, M. Chen, B. W. Ransom, R. I. Vogel, E. Thompson, S. E. Murphy, and D. K. Hatsukami. 2015. Evaluation of toxicant and carcinogen metabolites in the urine of e-cigarette users versus cigarette smokers. *Nicotine & Tobacco Research* 17(6):704–709.

Henningfield, J., J. Pankow, and B. Garrett. 2004. Ammonia and other chemical base tobacco additives and cigarette nicotine delivery: Issues and research needs. *Nicotine & Tobacco Research* 6(2):199–205.

HHS (U.S. Department of Health and Human Services). 1988. *The health consequences of smoking: Nicotine addiction: A report of the Surgeon General.* Atlanta, GA: U.S. Department of Health and Human Services, Centers for Disease Control and Prevention, National Center for Chronic Disease Prevention and Health Promotion, Office on Smoking and Health.

HHS. 2010a. *How tobacco smoke causes disease: The biology and behavioral basis for smoking-attributable disease: A report of the Surgeon General.* Atlanta, GA: U.S. Department of Health and Human Services, Centers for Disease Control and Prevention, National Center for Chronic Disease Prevention and Health Promotion, Office on Smoking and Health.

HHS. 2010b. *How tobacco smoke causes disease: What it means to you: A report of the Surgeon General.* Atlanta, GA: U.S. Department of Health and Human Services, Centers for Disease Control and Prevention, National Center for Chronic Disease Prevention and Health Promotion, Office on Smoking and Health.

HHS. 2014. *The health consequences of smoking—50 years of progress: A report of the Surgeon General.* Atlanta, GA: U.S. Department of Health and Human Services, Centers for Disease Control and Prevention, National Center for Chronic Disease Prevention and Health Promotion, Office on Smoking and Health.

Hukkanen, J., P. Jacob, 3rd, and N. L. Benowitz. 2005. Metabolism and disposition kinetics of nicotine. *Pharmacological Reviews* 57(1):79–115.

IARC (International Agency for Research on Cancer). 2012. *Chromium(VI) compounds.* https://monographs.iarc.fr/ENG/Monographs/vol100C/mono100C-9.pdf (accessed September 29, 2017).

IOM (Institute of Medicine). 2001. *Clearing the smoke: Assessing the science base for tobacco harm reduction.* Washington, DC: National Academy Press.

Kaivosaari, S., P. Toivonen, L. M. Hesse, M. Koskinen, M. H. Court, and M. Finel. 2007. Nicotine glucuronidation and the human UDP-glucuronosyltransferase UGT2B10. *Molecular Pharmacology* 72(3):761–768.

Klaassen, C. D., and J. B. Watkins, eds. 2015. *Casarett & Doull's essentials of toxicology*, third edition. New York: McGraw-Hill Medical.

Knezevich, A., J. Muzic, D. K. Hatsukami, S. S. Hecht, and I. Stepanov. 2013. Nornicotine nitrosation in saliva and its relation to endogenous synthesis of *N*′-nitrosonornicotine in humans. *Nicotine & Tobacco Research* 15(2):591–595.

Leon, M. E., A. Lugo, P. Boffetta, A. Gilmore, H. Ross, J. Schuz, C. La Vecchia, and S. Gallus. 2016. Smokeless tobacco use in Sweden and other 17 European countries. *European Journal of Public Health* 26(5):817–821.

Lerman, C., R. Tyndale, F. Patterson, E. P. Wileyto, P. G. Shields, A. Pinto, and N. Benowitz. 2006. Nicotine metabolite ratio predicts efficacy of transdermal nicotine for smoking cessation. *Clinical Pharmacology & Therapeutics* 79(6):600–608.

Lerman, C., C. Jepson, E. P. Wileyto, F. Patterson, R. Schnoll, M. Mroziewicz, N. Benowitz, and R. F. Tyndale. 2010. Genetic variation in nicotine metabolism predicts the efficacy of extended-duration transdermal nicotine therapy. *Clinical Pharmacology & Therapeutics* 87(5):553–557.

Lisko, J. G., H. Tran, S. B. Stanfill, B. C. Blount, and C. H. Watson. 2015. Chemical composition and evaluation of nicotine, tobacco alkaloids, pH, and selected flavors in e-cigarette cartridges and refill solutions. *Nicotine & Tobacco Research* 17(10):1270–1278.

Lopez, A. A., M. M. Hiler, E. K. Soule, C. P. Ramoa, N. V. Karaoghlanian, T. Lipato, A. B. Breland, A. L. Shihadeh, and T. Eissenberg. 2016. Effects of electronic cigarette liquid nicotine concentration on plasma nicotine and puff topography in tobacco cigarette smokers: A preliminary report. *Nicotine & Tobacco Research* 18(5):720–723.

Luo, J., W. Ye, K. Zendehdel, J. Adami, H. O. Adami, P. Boffetta, and O. Nyren. 2007. Oral use of Swedish moist snuff (snus) and risk for cancer of the mouth, lung, and pancreas in male construction workers: A retrospective cohort study. *Lancet* 369(9578):2015–2020.

Margham, J., K. McAdam, M. Forster, C. Liu, C. Wright, D. Mariner, and C. Proctor. 2016. Chemical composition of aerosol from an e-cigarette: A quantitative comparison with cigarette smoke. *Chemical Research in Toxicology* 29(10):1662–1678.

Maskos, U., B. E. Molles, S. Pons, M. Besson, B. P. Guiard, J. P. Guilloux, A. Evrard, P. Cazala, A. Cormier, M. Mameli-Engvall, N. Dufour, I. Cloez-Tayarani, A. P. Bemelmans, J. Mallet, A. M. Gardier, V. David, P. Faure, S. Granon, and J. P. Changeux. 2005. Nicotine reinforcement and cognition restored by targeted expression of nicotinic receptors. *Nature* 436(7047):103–107.

McRobbie, H., A. Phillips, M. L. Goniewicz, K. M. Smith, O. Knight-West, D. Przulj, and P. Hajek. 2015. Effects of switching to electronic cigarettes with and without concurrent smoking on exposure to nicotine, carbon monoxide, and acrolein. *Cancer Prevention Research* 8(9):873–878.

Mobarrez, F., L. Antoniewicz, J. A. Bosson, J. Kuhl, D. S. Pisetsky, and M. Lundback. 2014. The effects of smoking on levels of endothelial progenitor cells and microparticles in the blood of healthy volunteers. *PLoS ONE* 9(2):e90314. https://doi.org/10.1371/journal.pone.0090314 (accessed February 5, 2018).

Murray, R. P., W. C. Bailey, K. Daniels, W. M. Bjornson, K. Kurnow, J. E. Connett, M. A. Nides, and J. P. Kiley. 1996. Safety of nicotine polacrilex gum used by 3,094 participants in the Lung Health Study. *Chest* 109(2):438–445.

Murray, R. P., J. E. Connett, and L. M. Zapawa. 2009. Does nicotine replacement therapy cause cancer? Evidence from the Lung Health Study. *Nicotine & Tobacco Research* 11(9):1076–1082.

Neunteufl, T., S. Heher, K. Kostner, G. Mitulovic, S. Lehr, G. Khoschsorur, R. W. Schmid, G. Maurer, and T. Stefenelli. 2002. Contribution of nicotine to acute endothelial dysfunction in long-term smokers. *Journal of the American College of Cardiology* 39(2):251–256.

Nides, M. A., S. J. Leischow, M. Bhatter, and M. Simmons. 2014. Nicotine blood levels and short-term smoking reduction with an electronic nicotine delivery system. *American Journal of Health Behavior* 38(2):265–274.

O'Connell, G., D. W. Graff, and C. D. D'Ruiz. 2016. Reductions in biomarkers of exposure (BOE) to harmful or potentially harmful constituents (HPHCs) following partial or complete substitution of cigarettes with electronic cigarettes in adult smokers. *Toxicology Mechanisms and Methods* 26(6):453–464.

Oncken, C. A., M. D. Litt, L. D. McLaughlin, and N. A. Burki. 2015. Nicotine concentrations with electronic cigarette use: Effects of sex and flavor. *Nicotine & Tobacco Research* 17(4):473–478.

Pankow, J. F. 2001. A consideration of the role of gas/particle partitioning in the deposition of nicotine and other tobacco smoke compounds in the respiratory tract. *Chemical Research in Toxicology* 14(11):1465–1481.

Pankow, J. F., B. T. Mader, L. M. Isabelle, W. Luo, A. Pavlick, and C. Liang. 1997. Conversion of nicotine in tobacco smoke to its volatile and available free-base form through the action of gaseous ammonia. *Environmental Science & Technology* 31(8):2428–2433.

Pankow, J. F., K. Kim, K. J. McWhirter, W. Luo, J. O. Escobedo, R. M. Strongin, A. K. Duell, and D. H. Peyton. 2017. Benzene formation in electronic cigarettes. *PLoS ONE* 12(3):e0173055. https://doi.org/10.1371/journal.pone.0173055 (accessed February 5, 2018).

Papaseit, E., M. Farre, S. Graziano, R. Pacifici, C. Perez-Mana, O. Garcia-Algar, and S. Pichini. 2016. Monitoring nicotine intake from e-cigarettes: Measurement of parent drug and metabolites in oral fluid and plasma. *Clinical Chemistry and Laboratory Medicine* 55(3): 415–423.

Pellegrino, R. M., B. Tinghino, G. Mangiaracina, A. Marani, M. Vitali, C. Protano, J. F. Osborn, and M. S. Cattaruzza. 2012. Electronic cigarettes: An evaluation of exposure to chemicals and fine particulate matter (PM). *Annali di Igiene* 24(4):279–288.

Perez-Stable, E. J., B. Herrera, P. Jacob, 3rd, and N. L. Benowitz. 1998. Nicotine metabolism and intake in black and white smokers. *Journal of the American Medical Association* 280(2):152–156.

Picciotto, M. R. 1998. Common aspects of the action of nicotine and other drugs of abuse. *Drug and Alcohol Dependence* 51(1–2):165–172.

Pitarque, M., O. von Richter, B. Oke, H. Berkkan, M. Oscarson, and M. Ingelman-Sundberg. 2001. Identification of a single nucleotide polymorphism in the TATA box of the *CYP2A6* gene: Impairment of its promoter activity. *Biochemical and Biophysical Research Commununications* 284(2):455–460.

Pulvers, K., A. S. Emami, N. L. Nollen, D. R. Romero, D. R. Strong, N. L. Benowitz, and J. S. Ahluwalia. 2016. Tobacco consumption and toxicant exposure of cigarette smokers using electronic cigarettes. *Nicotine & Tobacco Research* 20(2):206–214.

Ramoa, C. P., M. M. Hiler, T. R. Spindle, A. A. Lopez, N. Karaoghlanian, T. Lipato, A. B. Breland, A. Shihadeh, and T. Eissenberg. 2016. Electronic cigarette nicotine delivery can exceed that of combustible cigarettes: A preliminary report. *Tobacco Control* 25(e1):e6–e9. http://dx.doi.org/10.1136/tobaccocontrol-2015-052447 (accessed February 5, 2018).

Rivenson, A., D. Hoffmann, B. Prokopczyk, S. Amin, and S. S. Hecht. 1988. Induction of lung and exocrine pancreas tumors in F344 rats by tobacco-specific and areca-derived *N*-nitrosamines. *Cancer Research* 48(23):6912–6917.

Rose, J. E., S. D. Rose, J. E. Turner, and T. Murugesan. 2008. *Device and method for delivery of a medicament*. U.S. Patent US20080241255 A1, filed March 25, 2008, and issued October 2, 2008.

Schnoll, R. A., F. Patterson, E. P. Wileyto, R. F. Tyndale, N. Benowitz, and C. Lerman. 2009. Nicotine metabolic rate predicts successful smoking cessation with transdermal nicotine: A validation study. *Pharmacology Biochemistry and Behavior* 92(1):6–11.

Schoedel, K. A., E. B. Hoffmann, Y. Rao, E. M. Sellers, and R. F. Tyndale. 2004. Ethnic variation in CYP2A6 and association of genetically slow nicotine metabolism and smoking in adult Caucasians. *Pharmacogenetics* 14(9):615–626.

Shahab, L., M. L. Goniewicz, B. C. Blount, J. Brown, A. McNeill, K. U. Alwis, J. Feng, L. Wang, and R. West. 2017. Nicotine, carcinogen, and toxin exposure in long-term e-cigarette and nicotine replacement therapy users: A cross-sectional study. *Annals of Internal Medicine* 166(6):390–400.

Spindle, T. R., A. B. Breland, N. V. Karaoghlanian, A. L. Shihadeh, and T. Eissenberg. 2015. Preliminary results of an examination of electronic cigarette user puff topography: The effect of a mouthpiece-based topography measurement device on plasma nicotine and subjective effects. *Nicotine & Tobacco Research* 17(2):142–149.

Spindle, T. R., M. M. Hiler, A. B. Breland, N. V. Karaoghlanian, A. L. Shihadeh, and T. Eissenberg. 2017. The influence of a mouthpiece-based topography measurement device on electronic cigarette user's plasma nicotine concentration, heart rate, and subjective effects under directed and ad libitum use conditions. *Nicotine & Tobacco Research* 19(4):469–476.

St.Helen, G., C. Havel, D. A. Dempsey, P. Jacob, 3rd, and N. L. Benowitz. 2016a. Nicotine delivery, retention and pharmacokinetics from various electronic cigarettes. *Addiction* 111(3):535–544.

St.Helen, G., K. C. Ross, D. A. Dempsey, C. M. Havel, P. Jacob, 3rd, and N. L. Benowitz. 2016b. Nicotine delivery and vaping behavior during ad libitum e-cigarette access. *Tobacco Regulatory Science* 2(4):363–376.

St.Helen, G., D. A. Dempsey, C. M. Havel, P. Jacob, 3rd, and N. L. Benowitz. 2017. Impact of e-liquid flavors on nicotine intake and pharmacology of e-cigarettes. *Drug and Alcohol Dependence* 178:391–398.

Stepanov, I., J. Jensen, D. Hatsukami, and S. S. Hecht. 2006. Tobacco-specific nitrosamines in new tobacco products. *Nicotine & Tobacco Research* 8(2):309–313.

Stepanov, I., S. G. Carmella, A. Briggs, L. Hertsgaard, B. Lindgren, D. Hatsukami, and S. S. Hecht. 2009a. Presence of the carcinogen *N'*-nitrosonornicotine in the urine of some users of oral nicotine replacement therapy products. *Cancer Research* 69(21):8236–8240.

Stepanov, I., S. G. Carmella, S. Han, A. Pinto, A. A. Strasser, C. Lerman, and S. S. Hecht. 2009b. Evidence for endogenous formation of *N'*-nitrosonornicotine in some long-term nicotine patch users. *Nicotine & Tobacco Research* 11(1):99–105.

Stiles, M. F., L. R. Campbell, D. W. Graff, B. A. Jones, R. V. Fant, and J. E. Henningfield. 2017. Pharmacodynamic and pharmacokinetic assessment of electronic cigarettes, combustible cigarettes, and nicotine gum: Implications for abuse liability. *Psychopharmacology (Berl)* 234(17):2643–2655.

Strasser, A. A., V. Souprountchouk, A. Kaufmann, S. Blazekovic, F. Leone, N. L. Benowitz, and R. A. Schnoll. 2016. Nicotine replacement, topography, and smoking phenotypes of e-cigarettes. *Tobacco Regulatory Science* 2(4):352–362.

Talih, S., Z. Balhas, T. Eissenberg, R. Salman, N. Karaoghlanian, A. El Hellani, R. Baalbaki, N. Saliba, and A. Shihadeh. 2015. Effects of user puff topography, device voltage, and liquid nicotine concentration on electronic cigarette nicotine yield: Measurements and model predictions. *Nicotine & Tobacco Research* 17(2):150–157.

Teichert, A., P. Brossard, L. Felber Medlin, L. Sandalic, M. Franzon, C. Wynne, M. Laugesen, and F. Ludicke. 2017. Evaluation of nicotine pharmacokinetics and subjective effects following use of a novel nicotine delivery system. *Nicotine & Tobacco Research*. https://doi.org/10.1093/ntr/ntx093 (accessed February 5, 2018).

Tierney, P. A., C. D. Karpinski, J. E. Brown, W. Luo, and J. F. Pankow. 2016. Flavour chemicals in electronic cigarette fluids. *Tobacco Control* 25(e1):e10–e15. http://dx.doi.org/10.1136/tobaccocontrol-2014-052175 (accessed February 5, 2018).

Timberlake, D. S., D. Nikitin, N. J. Johnson, and S. F. Altekruse. 2017. A longitudinal study of smokeless tobacco use and mortality in the United States. *International Journal of Cancer* 141(2):264–270.

Trehy, M. L., W. Ye, M. E. Hadwiger, T. W. Moore, J. F. Allgire, J. T. Woodruff, S. S. Ahadi, J. C. Black, and B. J. Westenberger. 2011. Analysis of electronic cigarette cartridges, refill solutions, and smoke for nicotine and nicotine related impurities. *Journal of Liquid Chromatography and Related Technologies* 34(14):1442–1458.

Vansickel, A. R., and T. Eissenberg. 2013. Electronic cigarettes: Effective nicotine delivery after acute administration. *Nicotine & Tobacco Research* 15(1):267–270.

Vansickel, A. R., C. O. Cobb, M. F. Weaver, and T. E. Eissenberg. 2010. A clinical laboratory model for evaluating the acute effects of electronic "cigarettes": Nicotine delivery profile and cardiovascular and subjective effects. *Cancer Epidemiology, Biomarkers & Prevention* 19(8):1945–1953.

Vansickel, A. R., M. F. Weaver, and T. Eissenberg. 2012. Clinical laboratory assessment of the abuse liability of an electronic cigarette. *Addiction* 107(8):1493–1500.

Wagener, T. L., E. L. Floyd, I. Stepanov, L. M. Driskill, S. G. Frank, E. Meier, E. L. Leavens, A. P. Tackett, N. Molina, and L. Queimado. 2017. Have combustible cigarettes met their match? The nicotine delivery profiles and harmful constituent exposures of second-generation and third-generation electronic cigarette users. *Tobacco Control* 26(e1):e23–e28. http://tobaccocontrol.bmj.com/content/26/e1/e23 (accessed February 5, 2018).

Walele, T., G. Sharma, R. Savioz, C. Martin, and J. Williams. 2016. A randomised, cross-over study on an electronic vapour product, a nicotine inhalator and a conventional cigarette. Part B: Safety and subjective effects. *Regulatory Toxicology and Pharmacology* 74:193–199.

Wang, H., W. Tan, B. Hao, X. Miao, G. Zhou, F. He, and D. Lin. 2003. Substantial reduction in risk of lung adenocarcinoma associated with genetic polymorphism in CYP2A13, the most active cytochrome P450 for the metabolic activation of tobacco-specific carcinogen NNK. *Cancer Research* 63(22):8057–8061.

Westenberger, B. 2009. *Evaluation of e-cigarettes*. http://web.archive.org/web/20170210071043/fda.gov/downloads/drugs/scienceresearch/ucm173250.pdf (accessed February 13, 2018).

Wickholm, S., A. Lahtinen, A. Ainamo, and M. Rautalahti. 2012. [Adverse effects of Swedish smokeless tobacco "snus"]. *Duodecim* 128(10):1089–1096.

Yan, X. S., and C. D'Ruiz. 2015. Effects of using electronic cigarettes on nicotine delivery and cardiovascular function in comparison with regular cigarettes. *Regulatory Toxicology and Pharmacology* 71(1):24–34.

Yuan, J. M., A. D. Knezevich, R. Wang, Y. T. Gao, S. S. Hecht, and I. Stepanov. 2011. Urinary levels of the tobacco-specific carcinogen *N'*-nitrosonornicotine and its glucuronide are strongly associated with esophageal cancer risk in smokers. *Carcinogenesis* 32(9):1366–1371.

5

Toxicology of E-Cigarette Constituents

In general, e-cigarettes often contain ingredients such as propylene glycol (PG) and glycerol, mixed with concentrated flavors and, optionally, a variable percentage of nicotine. Quantitative and qualitative studies have identified a wide variety of chemical components in the cartridges, refill solutions, and aerosols of e-cigarettes. Herrington and Myers (2015) have detected approximately 60 to 70 compounds (unidentified and identified) in each liquid tested, only varying by several constituents throughout the liquid. Kucharska and colleagues (2016) have identified 113 chemicals in 50 brands of liquids. Even more compounds are observed in the aerosol over their respective solution because some chemicals are generated during the vaporization process. An aerosol generated from a single product tested by Herrington and Myers (2015) showed 18 additional compounds observed in the solution.

Substances identified in e-cigarette liquids and aerosols include nicotine, solvent carriers (PG and glycerol), tobacco-specific nitrosamines (TSNAs), aldehydes, metals, volatile organic compounds (VOCs), phenolic compounds, polycyclic aromatic hydrocarbons (PAHs), flavorings, tobacco alkaloids, and drugs. Most reviewed studies have evaluated nicotine and impurities in the liquids such as TSNAs and nicotine-related impurities, while other studies have focused on identifying potentially harmful chemicals in the aerosol, such as carbonyl compounds, VOCs, TSNAs, metals, and silicates. Various chemical substances and ultrafine particles known to be toxic, carcinogenic, and/or to cause respiratory and cardiac disease have been identified in e-cigarette aerosols, cartridges, refill liquids, and environmental emissions. Some of the identified TSNAs, aldehydes, metals, VOCs, phenolic compounds, PAHs, and tobacco alkaloids are harmful or potentially harmful constituents, and their general health risks are described below.

HUMECTANTS (DELIVERY SOLVENTS)

E-cigarettes use humectants as solvent carriers in e-liquids to produce aerosols that simulate combustible tobacco cigarette smoke. In addition to these humectants, water is a common ingredient of e-liquids. PG and glycerol (commonly referred to as a "vegetable glycerin" in liquid formulations) are the most common vaporizing solvents used in e-cigarettes. Hutzler and colleagues (2014) analyzed 28 liquids of 7 manufacturers purchased in Germany and detected both PG and glycerol in all samples. Both PG and glycerol are also commonly used as humectant ingredients in manufactured cigarettes to control and maintain the moisture content of the cut tobacco filler (Uryupin et al., 2013). Users of e-cigarettes often report that PG produces better "throat hit" and carries flavor better than glycerol while glycerol is much smoother than PG. PG is physically much thinner than glycerol (Cheng, 2014; Etter, 2016; Li et al., 2016). Outside of usage in e-cigarette liquids, dermal exposure to PG and glycerol is more common than exposure via inhalation, as most consumer products containing PG and glycerol are liquids or creams. Thus, there are few animal or human studies providing evidence of the possible toxicity of inhaled PG or glycerol. Studies identifying PG and glycerol in e-liquids are described below, and toxicological evidence is described in the following sections.

Hahn and colleagues (2014) used nuclear magnetic resonance methodology for analysis of 54 commercially available liquids for use in e-cigarettes. The study looked at several types of humectants, including dihydroxy (diols, glycols) and polyhydroxy alcohols. PG and glycerol were detected in all samples at concentrations ranging from 0.4 to 98 g/100 g (average 57 g/100 g) and from 0.3 to 95 g/100 g (average 37 g/100 g), respectively. Generally, lower levels of another solvent, ethylene glycol (average 10 g/100 g), were detected. 1,3-Propanediol was detected only in seven samples in the concentration range of 3.3–10 g/100 g. 1,3-Butanediol and diethylene glycol were negative in all samples. The presence of the major compounds glycerol and PG corresponded to the labeling in the majority of cases, except three products contained no labeling information at all. Glycerol was not labeled on five products despite being present. PG was not labeled in two products despite being present. In one case, "vegetal glycol" was labeled without specifying the exact chemical compound. Hutzler and colleagues (2014) analyzed 28 liquids purchased from 7 manufacturers in Germany and, like Hahn and colleagues, detected both PG and glycerol in all samples. Geiss and colleagues (2016) extrapolated lung concentration of PG and glycerol emitted from e-cigarettes using a smoking machine by measuring the average amounts condensed on the filter pad. The estimated lung concentrations were 160 and 220 mg/m^3 for PG and glycerol, respectively.

The most common symptom reported by e-cigarette users is a dry mouth and throat, which is considered to originate from the water-absorbing property of PG and glycerol. However, the health consequences of long-term exposure to PG and glycerol from e-cigarettes have not been investigated. Both compounds might pyrolyze, leading to the formation of carbonyl compounds (aldehydes), which contribute to potential health risks in e-cigarette users (for discussion about carbonyl compounds, see the subsequent section in this chapter).

Propylene Glycol

PG (also known as 1,2-dihydroxypropane, 1,2-propanediol, methyl glycol, and trimethyl glycol) is a clear, colorless, slightly syrupy liquid at room temperature. It is practically odorless and tasteless. It is used by the chemical, food, and pharmaceutical industries as a humectant to absorb extra water and maintain moisture in certain medicines, cosmetics, or food products. It is also used as a solvent for food colors and flavors, and in the paint and plastics industries. PG has been widely used for decades as a solvent for many intravenous drugs, and in some oral preparations such as cough syrups. PG was listed as generally recognized as safe (GRAS) by the Food and Drug Administration (FDA) in 1973 (HHS, 2015). Substances listed as GRAS are deemed as generally safe under conditions of intended use as a food additive. Thus, GRAS substances are safe for ingestion, but not necessarily for other routes of administration like inhalation. PG may exist in air in the aerosol form, but must be heated or briskly shaken to produce a mist. PG is also used to create artificial smoke or fog used in firefighter training and in theatrical productions.

Human Studies and Case Reports on PG Toxicity

Some people have reported having an allergic reaction to PG. Some people have reported upper respiratory irritation after inhaling aerosolized PG for 1 minute (Wieslander et al., 2001), but the longer term health effects in humans are not well defined. Though some preclinical studies showed inhalation of PG and glycerol can be safe up to 28 days (Werley et al., 2011) or 18 months (Robertson et al., 1947), breathing aerosolized PG can also affect the risk of asthma development (Choi et al., 2010). For example, one woman exhibited signs of exogenous lipoid pneumonia (e.g., fever, productive cough, and labored breathing) after using e-cigarettes for half a year (McCauley et al., 2012). The e-cigarette's oil-based humectants likely caused her pneumonia, as her symptoms improved when she quit the device (McCauley et al., 2012).

PG is frequently used as a vehicle for intravenous delivery of antiseizure medications in pediatric populations, typically at concentrations of 40 to 80 percent v:v with saline (Lim et al., 2014). Thus, there have been numerous human studies on the toxicity of relatively large doses of both oral and intravenously administered PG. Lim and colleagues (2014) conducted a systematic literature review of case reports and other clinical studies on the toxicity of PG in pediatric populations. They identified numerous case reports and several small studies that identified a "toxidrome" for PG toxicity that can result following repeated, relatively high-dose intravenous administration of PG. The adverse effects include hyperosmolarity, lactic acidosis, hemolysis, central nervous system (CNS) toxicity, and cardiac arrhythmia. In one particularly striking case study, an 11-year-old was given 2–4 ml per day of PG containing vitamin D for 13 months. Estimated daily dose for this subject was 114 mg (2-ml dose) to 228 mg (4-ml dose) of PG/kg body weight (Arulanantham and Genel, 1978; LaKind et al., 1999). After 13 months of repeated exposures, the child began to have seizures and lapsed into unconsciousness. Once the PG/vitamin D preparation was stopped, the child recovered (LaKind et al., 1999). In another example, a 15-month-old infant receiving large doses of a vitamin C suspension in PG orally had episodes of unresponsiveness, diaphoresis, tachycardia, tachypnea, and hypoglycemia (Martin and Finberg, 1970).

Based on analyses of case reports, Lim and colleagues (2014) attempted to arrive at a "safe" dose of PG for repeated administration of antiseizure drugs that are routinely compounded in 40 percent PG (see Table 5-1). They suggested maximum cumulative dose of 69 g/day in a pediatric population. Although such clinical studies on relatively high doses of orally and intravenously administered PG in pediatric populations is clinically relevant for those populations, it is perhaps of modest relevance to potential health consequence of inhalation of PG vapors from repeated vaping. However, diagnostic procedures, such as characterization of anion gap (or osmolal gap, defined as the discrepancy between the measured and calculated osmolalities) (Lim et al., 2014), and evaluation for the presence of lactic acidosis, could be of potential value in suspected cases of high-dose PG toxicity from extensive vaping.

TABLE 5-1 Dose Limits of Commonly Used Drugs to Avoid Propylene Glycol Intoxication Based on a Maximum Amount of PG Equal to 69 g/day

Drug	Amount of PG (mg/ml)	Maximum Daily Dose	
		Adult	Pediatric
Lorazepam 2 mg/ml	828	166 mg/day (7 mg/hour)	2.4 mg/kg/day (0.01 mg/kg/hour)
Phenobarbital 130 mg/ml	702	12.8 g/day (533 mg/hour)	183 mg/kg/day (7.6 mg/kg/hour)
Pentobarbital 50 mg/ml	414.4	8.3 g/day (346 mg/hour)	119 mg/kg/day (4.9/kg/hour)
Diazepam 5 mg/ml	414.4	832 mg/day (34.7 mg/hour)	12 mg/kg/day (0.5 mg/kg/hour)
Phenytoin 50 mg/ml	414.4	8.3 g/day (346 mg/hour)	119 mg/kg/day (4.9 mg/kg/hour)
TMP/SMX 16:80 mg/ml	414.4	2.7:13.3 g/day	39 mg/kg/day TMP component (1.6 mg/kg/hour)
Etomidate 2 mg/ml	362.6	381 mg/day (16 mg/hour)	5.4 mg/kg/day (0.2 mg/kg/hour)

NOTE: PG = propylene glycol; SMX = sulfamethoxazole; TMP = trimethoprim.
SOURCE: Adapted from Lim et al., 2014.

Pharmacokinetics of PG

PG is well-absorbed orally and can also be absorbed through skin or mucous membranes from topical preparations. Following absorption, the kidneys eliminate 45 percent of the PG, and the liver metabolizes the remainder to lactic acid, pyruvic acid, or acetone. Thus, patients with impaired liver and/or kidney function are generally thought to be at increased risk for developing PG toxicity following high-dose oral or intravenous administration.

Speth and colleagues (1987) conducted a relatively detailed pharmacokinetic analysis of PG following intravenous administration of PG at different dose rates, administered over 4 hours. The elimination half-life of PG was dose dependent; at doses of either 3 or 4.5 g/m^2 (over 4 hours) the terminal half-life was approximately 1.8 hour. However, at a dose rate of 7.5 g/m^2 over 4 hours the half-life increased to approximately 3.1 hours, suggesting saturable elimination at dose rates above about 5 g/m^2 (see Table 5-2).

TABLE 5-2 Plasma Pharmacokinetics of Propylene Glycol Given as a 4-Hour Intravenous Infusion

Patient Initials	Dose MTQ (mg/m^2)	Dose PG (g/m^2)	Dose PG (g/day)	Maximum Plasma Concentration (µg/ml)	$t_{1/2}$ (hour)	V_d (L)	Cl (ml/minute/1.73 m^2)	AUC (µg × hour/ml/1.73 m^2)
KR	120	3	5.1	60	1.8	36	305	261
KR	120	3	5.1	58	1.4	58	390	318
LI	120	3	5.1	48	1.5	41	321	279
KR	180	4.5	7.7	102	2.1	40	196	762
LI	180	4.5	7.7	131	1.8	52	339	390
RI	180	4.5	7.2	116	1.9	41	269	518
JW	300	7.5	12.6	218	3.1	58	206	1,080
BE	300	7.5	13.5	168	3.3	62	221	938
RB	600	15	21.0	425	3.3	40	144	3,719
Mean					2.3 ± 0.7			

NOTE: AUC = area under the plasma concentration–time curve, relative to 1.73 m^2 body surface; Cl = clearance, relative to 1.73 m^2 body surface; MTQ = mitoquidone; PG = propylene glycol; $t_{1/2}$ = half-life; V_d = apparent volume of distribution.
SOURCE: Adapted from Speth et al., 1987.

Yu and colleagues (1985) also reported elimination half-lives of PG following multiple large oral doses (20.7 g three times per day, or 41.4 g two times per day) of PG, with terminal half-lives of 3.8 ± 0.8 hours, with relatively large interpatient variability in plasma concentration. Blood concentrations of PG associated with hyperosmolality and anion gap have been reported, ranging from 177 to 1,520 µg/ml (Fligner et al., 1985; Kelner and Bailey, 1985). However, Yu and colleagues (1985) did not observe any evidence of toxicity (hyperosmolality or lactic acidosis) in subjects with plasma concentrations as high as 425 µg/ml. No studies have evaluated blood concentrations of PG in subjects using e-cigarettes or other vaping devices with PG as the humectant.

Evidence of Health Effects from Occupational Exposures to PG

There is relatively limited evidence of toxicity from occupational exposures to PG. However, glycols are used in theatrical fogs, so actors and performers in the entertainment industry may have routine exposures to relatively high concentrations of PG, as it is often a major component of these fogs. Varughese and colleagues (2005) studied 101 employees in 19 different locations who were routinely exposed to such fogs. They measured the levels of exposure, lung function, and acute and chronic symptoms. The mean concentration of exposure for employees exposed only to PG-based fog on the testing day was 0.49 mg/m^3 (maximum 3.22 mg/m^3). They reported that theatrical fog exposures were significantly associated with chronic work-related wheezing and chest tightness. Although these acute effects appeared to be specific to PG-based fogs, most of the workers were also exposed to mineral oil. Thus, the authors were unable to distinguish the role of PG or mineral oil fogs in the development of chronic effects and work-related symptoms from increasing chronic exposure.

Another study addressed the same general issue regarding the safety of PG used in theatrical fog (Moline et al., 2000). Based on their analysis of symptoms reported by 218 theatrical actors, detailed integrated PG dose and peak exposure estimates were available. They found statistically significant associations between peak PG exposure and reported symptoms of mucous membrane irritation. They also found other respiratory symptoms, including throat and nasal symptoms associated with peak exposure but not integrated dose. The measured peak concentrations during "fogging" at on-stage locations ranged from less than 1 to 16 mg/m^3. Estimates of actors' "per performance" exposures to PG ranged from 0.1 to ~8 µg/show (Moline et al., 2000).

Wieslander and colleagues (2001) conducted a study to examine the effects of PG mist in aviation emergency training. Twenty-seven nonasthmatic volunteers were exposed in an aircraft simulator to a mist of PG at 309 mg/m^3 (176–851 mg/m^3 range) for 1 minute. Subjects were then evaluated for a range of pulmonary function tests and symptoms assessment. Although measures of pulmonary function (FEV1, vital capacity) were not significantly affected, symptoms reported included eye and throat irritation in some of the subjects. Four subjects also reported development of an irritating cough. The reported symptom of eye irritation was supported by measurement of tear film stability, which was decreased following PG exposure.

The Occupational Safety and Health Administration (OSHA, 2006) established an interim 8-hour threshold limit value (TLV) of 10 mg/m^3 for all organic mists (applicable to PG and glycerol) with no specific exposure limits or identified toxicity. The Health Council of the Netherlands (2007) recommends an exposure limit for PG of 50 mg/m^3 over 8 hours. Although they noted a concern about short-term respiratory effects, the proposed limit was not based on observed adverse effects from workplace exposures. Thus, although occupational exposure limits have been proposed for PG, it is important to note that neither of these proposed exposure limits are based on evidence of adverse effects, but rather are "precautionary" in nature. Nevertheless, studies in some workplace populations relate symptoms of eye and throat irritation to acute, and possibly chronic, exposures to PG mist in the low milligram per cubic meter concentrations.

Relevance of Occupational Exposures and Clinical Case Reports of Pharmaceutical Exposures of PG to Exposures from E-Cigarettes

Although the clinical case reports of PG exposures demonstrate that high-dose oral and intravenous exposure to PG can induce toxicity, the relevance of those studies to potential health effects of PG from e-cigarettes depends on the dose and pharmacokinetics of PG following inhalation exposure through e-cigarettes. Burstyn (2014) estimated the potential levels of exposure to PG from e-cigarettes, "assuming extreme consumption of the liquid per day via vaping (5 to 25 ml/day and 50–95 percent propylene glycol in the liquid)" and concluded that "levels of propylene glycol in inhaled air can reach 1–6 mg/m^3." With an assumption of complete absorption via inhalation, Burstyn concluded that "estimated levels of exposure to propylene glycol and glycerin are close enough to TLV to warrant concern." However, putting these values in perspective with the clinical data from intravenous administration of PG in adults may be useful. Speth and colleagues (1987) reported that doses from 5 to 21 g/day (see Table 5-2), which are comparable to the 5 to 25 ml/day calculated by Burstyn (2014), were not associated with any evidence of any adverse effects. In the Speth and colleagues (1987) study, peak plasma concentrations of PG ranged from 48 μg/ml (5.1 g/day; ~88 mg/kg/day) to 425 μg/ml (21 g/day; ~488 mg/kg/day). In one clinical report in a 60-year-old male showing toxicity and for whom blood concentrations were measured, serum levels of PG greater than 180 μg/ml were reported to be associated with toxicity (Arbour and Esparis, 2000). Other investigators found clinical evidence of toxicity at serum PG concentrations that exceeded 250 μg/ml (Hansen et al., 2015), although it is important to note that these are following intravenous administration. Nevertheless, absorption of PG via inhalation theoretically could be very rapid and largely complete, so the comparison of blood levels between patients administered PG intravenously over 4 hours and individuals with extensive vaping may not be unreasonable.

In 1974, the World Health Organization recommended a maximum dose of 25 mg/kg/day of PG when ingested as a food additive. Thus, for a typical young adult with a body weight of 60 kg, this would be equivalent to 1.5 g/day, which is considerably less than the 5–25 ml/day "worst case" exposure to PG from vaping estimated by Burstyn (2014).

There are no studies of clinical measures of potential PG toxicity (e.g., anion gap, lactic acidosis) among heavy users of e-cigarettes, or which have measured blood/serum levels of PG following use of vaping devices containing PG-based liquids.

Allergic Reactions to PG

It has been known for years that some individuals can develop allergic reactions to PG following repeated dermal applications (Aberer et al., 1993; Catanzaro and Smith, 1991; Funk and Maibach, 1994; Lessmann et al., 2005; Warshaw et al., 2009). Although most dermal reactions to PG are the result of irritation, true immunological reactions have been confirmed through patch testing. For example, in a patch test of 1,226 patients who received an application of 5 percent PG in Vaseline, or 10, 30, or 50 percent in water, 208 (17 percent) of the subjects had evidence of irritation and/or allergic dermatitis. Of those showing some dermal reaction, 195 were from irritation, but 13 exhibited an allergic reaction (Aberer et al., 1993). However, a more recent analysis of allergic dermatitis found an incidence of only 2.1 percent in a large sample (5,083 subjects in 2007–2008), and this was significantly decreased from previous years (3.8 percent of 4,095 subjects in 1996–1998) (Fransway et al., 2013). Whether PG could induce allergic reactions via inhalation from e-cigarettes has not been studied.

In Vivo Animal Toxicology Studies of PG

Because of its widespread use as a food additive and other industrial uses, PG was subjected to standard in vivo toxicological assays many years ago, and these studies, coupled with the relative lack of human evidence of toxicity of PG from its use as a food additive, form the basis for FDA's listing of PG as GRAS. A study of male and female Sprague-Dawley rats found that larynx, trachea, and lung tissues were not affected by nose-only exposure to different levels of PG for 90 days (Suber et al., 1989). Additional studies of aerosolized PG found no effects on rat or monkey gross pathology, respiratory tract function, histology, or hematology and clinical chemistry (Robertson et al., 1947). LaKind and colleagues (1999) provide a comprehensive review of the animal toxicology data for PG prior to that date.

Acute Toxicity

PG is considered "practically non-toxic" orally, with acute lethal dose (LD_{50}) values of 20 g/kg or greater (see Table 5-3). Signs and symptoms of acute toxicity included increased respiratory rate, loss of equilibrium, CNS depression, analgesia, coma, and death in 18 to 36 hours. Of more relevance are animal studies using inhalation exposures to PG. Konradova and colleagues (1978) evaluated the effects on airway epithelia of exposure of rabbits to a 10 percent aerosol of PG for 20 and 120 minutes. The 20-minute exposure had no visible effect on ciliated cells in the tracheal epithelium, but did produce alterations in goblet cells.

TABLE 5-3 Acute Lethal Dose (LD_{50}) of Propylene Glycol in Rats, Mice, Guinea Pigs, and Rabbits

Species	Propylene Glycol LD_{50} (g/kg)	Reference
Rats	21.7 26.4 33.5	Laug et al., 1939; Smyth et al., 1941; Weatherby and Haag, 1938
Mice	24.8 31.9	Bornmann, 1954; Laug et al., 1939
Guinea Pigs	18.35 19.6	Laug et al., 1939; Smyth et al., 1941
Rabbits	19.3	Weatherby and Haag, 1938 (based on data by Braun and Cartland, 1936)

SOURCE: Adapted from LaKind et al., 1999.

Longer exposure, for 120 minutes, altered goblet cells and induced some visible alterations in ciliated epithelial cells. Another study examined the results of 15-minute inhalation exposure of dogs to either 10 or 20 percent aerosol of PG on hemodynamic effects and hemolysis (effects seen following large oral doses of PG). No effects on either endpoint were reported (MacCannell, 1969; Renne et al., 1992).

Repeated Dose Exposures to PG to Evaluate Potential Reproductive Effects in Animals

Three standard reproductive assays of PG have been performed, all in male and female mice, using repeated doses and multigeneration assessment for reproductive outcomes (Kavlock et al., 1987; Morrissey et al., 1989; OECD, 2001). None of these studies reported any statistically significant effects of PG exposure on measures of reproductive outcome in different strains of mice given 10,100 mg/kg/day for 14 weeks.

Repeated Dose Exposures to PG to Assess Developmental/Teratogenic Effects in Animals

Several animal studies using standard teratogenicity protocols have been completed for PG. An FDA-sponsored study in pregnant CD-1 mice, Wistar rats, golden hamsters, and Dutch-belted rabbits found no evidence of teratogenicity at the highest doses tested (1,600, 1,600, 1,550, and 1,250 mg/kg/day for 10 days, respectively) (FDRL, 1973).

Long-Term (Chronic Exposure) Bioassays on PG for Assessment of Organ System Function

Because of the well-documented nephrotoxic effects of ethylene glycol, early studies on the toxicity of PG focused on potential effects of chronic PG exposure on kidney functions. Van Winkle and Newman (1941) administered PG in drinking water to female (5 percent PG, twice daily) and male dogs (600 ml of 10 percent PG, once daily) for up to 9 months. Animals were evaluated for liver and kidney function and by histopathology at the end of the experiment. No effects on liver or kidney were observed in any of the animals. A 2-year chronic bioassay in albino rats given PG in the diet at doses approximately equivalent to 1,225 or 2,450 mg/kg/day found no evidence of any organ system toxicity (LaKind et al., 1999; Morris et al., 1942). A 2-year feeding study in dogs given up to 2,000 mg/kg/day also found no significant effects on renal weight. However, a dose of 5,000 mg/kg/day was associated with increased urinary output and decreased water consumption, suggestive of adverse effects on kidney function (LaKind et al., 1999). Other chronic studies of PG in mice and dogs reported in *Patty's Industrial Hygiene and Toxicology* (Clayton and Clayton, 1995) found no significant effects of PG on any organ system.

Inhalation Exposure Levels of PG from E-Cigarette Use

Of importance to the question of the potential health effects of PG in the context of e-cigarette use are the actual concentrations and doses inhaled during a puff. Kienhuis and colleagues (2015) evaluated exposures to both PG and glycerol from a "shisha-pen" device. The authors define a shisha-pen as "an electronic cigarette (e-cigarette) variant that is advertised to mimic the taste of a water pipe, or shisha. . . . The shisha-pen operates in the same manner as an e-cigarette, it can be disposable or rechargeable and refillable, and it is available with and without nicotine" (Kienhuis et al., 2015). They estimated that the PG exposure from one 50- to 70-mL puff would be from 430 to 603 mg/m^3, and noted that "These exposure concentrations were higher than the points of departure for airway irritation based on a human study (propylene glycol, mean concentration of 309 mg/m^3) and a rat study (glycerol, no-observed adverse effect level of 165 mg/m^3)" (Kienhuis et al., 2015, p. 1). As discussed above, Wieslander and colleagues (2001) exposed healthy human subjects in an aircraft simulator to a mist of PG at 309 mg/m^3 (176–851 mg/m^3 range) for 1 minute. This is similar to the range of PG concentrations in puffs of e-liquid from a shisha-pen device. No effects on lung function were noted by Wieslander and colleagues, although some subjects did complain of eye and throat irritation. This is consistent with Web-based literature from vaping groups.[1]

Summary of Toxicological Effects of PG

PG has long been considered "practically non-toxic," consistent with FDA's inclusion of PG on the GRAS list. Animal studies, including chronic studies at very high levels, have consistently failed to identify any target organ, or other evidence of toxicity at doses less than several grams per kilogram per day. Although most of these studies were done decades ago and would not generally meet today's "good laboratory practices" standards, the large doses used, coupled with the consistent lack of any

[1] See, for example, http://www.whitecloudelectroniccigarettes.com/blog/vaping-throat-irritation (accessed January 5, 2018); http://ecigarettereviewed.com/allergies-conditions-and-e-liquid (accessed January 5, 2018); and http://www.ecigarette-politics.com/pg-sensitivity.html (accessed January 5, 2018).

evidence of organ system effect or reproductive or developmental toxicity, provides strong support for the general lack of toxic effects of PG in humans from dietary or occupational exposures. However, there is limited, but consistent evidence from case reports that very high doses of PG administered orally or intravenously to humans can produce toxic effects that appear to be related to osmolar changes in the blood and lactic acid formation secondary to the metabolism of PG.

Finding: Substantial toxicological data indicate that oral exposure to propylene glycol is not likely to be associated with adverse health effects. However, the data from inhalation exposure to propylene glycol are limited. In some individuals, exposure to propylene glycol aerosols in concentrations found in e-cigarettes has been shown to cause irritation to the eyes and throat.

Glycerol

Glycerol (also known as glycerin) is an oily, hygroscopic liquid with a warm, sweet taste. Although glycerol can be derived from naturally occurring fats and oils ("vegetable glycerin"), synthetic glycerol is produced from petrochemical products in a multistep process. Glycerol is used in food products, nutritional supplements, pharmaceutical products, personal care products, and oral care products.

As discussed above, most liquids used in e-cigarettes and other vaping devices contain a mixture of PG and glycerol. Typically, the mixtures are somewhere in the range of 30–50 percent glycerol, with the balance as PG. Among the vaping community, there is a perception, which is supported by acute toxicology studies, that PG is more irritating to upper respiratory airways than glycerol.[2] FDA considers glycerol GRAS.[3]

Human Toxicology Studies

The toxicology of glycerol was reviewed by the Organisation for Economic Co-operation and Development (OECD, 2002). A study of 10 male and 4 female volunteers who were administered glycerol in orange juice with each meal at a dose of 1.3 to 2.2 g/kg/day for 50 days reported no evidence of toxicity or adverse effects on blood or urine production. Based on the highest administered dose, they estimated a no observed adverse

---

[2] See, for example, https://www.misthub.com/blogs/vape-tutorials/76788613-tutorial-propylene-glycol-pg-vs-vegetable-glycerin-vg-e-juice (accessed January 5, 2018); https://vapingdaily.com/best-vape-juices-and-e-liquids/pg-vs-vg (accessed January 5, 2018).

[3] 21 CFR § 182.1320.

effect level (NOAEL) for glycerol greater than or equal to 2.2 g/kg/day (CIR, 2014; OECD, 2002; Tourtellotte et al., 1972).

When used as a drug, reported adverse effects following the oral administration of glycerol at unspecified doses included mild headache, dizziness, nausea, vomiting, thirst, and diarrhea. Headache is likely a result from dehydration (CIR, 2014). Venable and colleagues (CIR, 2015; Venable et al., 1980) evaluated 64 male employees involved in the manufacture of synthetic glycerol for potential effects on reproductive function. They found no differences in sperm counts and percentage of normal forms compared with a similar size control group (n = 63) that had no known occupational exposures to glycerol.

Absorption, distribution, metabolism, and excretion Glycerol is a natural product and endogenous component in the body, largely as triglycerides with fatty acids, but free glycerol is also naturally present in human plasma. Typical serum levels of glycerol in adult humans range from 0.05 to 0.1 mmol/L (Nelson et al., 2011). Exogenous glycerol is rapidly absorbed from the stomach and intestine, with distribution occurring throughout the extracellular space (CIR, 2015). The primary pathway of biotransformation is via glycerol kinase-mediated phosphorylation to α-glycerophosphate in the liver (80 to 90 percent) and kidneys (10 to 20 percent). α-Glycerophosphate is then transformed to form glucose (gluconeogenesis) and glycogen through intermediary metabolic pathways (Lin, 1977). Most of the dose of orally administered glycerol is metabolized in about 2.5 hours, with 7 to 14 percent of eliminated glycerol unchanged in urine. In the liver, exogenously administered glycerol can undergo lipogenesis (combining with free fatty acids to form triglycerides), and these fats can be distributed to adipose tissues. The turnover rate for glycerol is proportional to plasma concentration of glycerol (Bortz et al., 1972).

Glycerol has been used clinically because of its ability to increase the osmotic pressure in plasma. Orally administered glycerol can reduce the volume of intraocular fluids in order to decrease intraocular pressure (IOP). The extent of IOP reduction depends on both the etiology and magnitude of the increased pressure and the glycerol dose. Glycerol's osmotic effect has also been used to decrease in cerebrospinal fluid pressure (Tourtellotte et al., 1972).

In Vivo Animal Toxicological Studies

Acute toxicity As summarized in the Cosmetic Ingredients Review for glycerol (CIR, 2015), oral LD_{50} values of glycerol ranged from 2.53 to 58.4 g/kg in rats. The highest dose used in one study was 24 g/kg, and no deaths were reported. Oral LD_{50} values reported for glycerol were 4.1 to greater than 38 g/kg in mice, 27 g/kg in rabbits, and 77.5 g/kg in guinea pigs (CIR, 2015). The dermal LD_{50} value of glycerol in rats was reported to be greater than 21.9 g/kg, and in rabbits, greater than 18.7 g/kg. The approximate value for the time to death for 50 percent of the rats (LT_{50}) was 423 minutes for exposure to glycerol aerosols at 11.0 mg/L (CIR, 2015). Reported intraperitoneal LD_{50} values of glycerol were 4.42–10.1 g/kg in rats and 8.6–9.5 g/kg in mice. LD_{50} values of glycerol via subcutaneous administration were 100 mg/kg in rats and 91–100 mg/kg in mice (CIR, 2015).

Repeated dose toxicity studies Because glycerol has been used extensively as a vehicle for drug delivery in many drug toxicology studies, Gad and colleagues (2006) surveyed four laboratories on their use of glycerol and other vehicles for in vivo experiments. They found the highest NOAEL was 500 mg/kg for guinea pigs and 15 g/kg for rats for 1 month of oral administration. A study in mice also reported a NOAEL for glycerol of 500 mg/kg for 90 days.

Numerous repeated dose studies, ranging from a few days to 2 years, have been conducted. Glycerol was administered in the diet of rats for 2 years at 5 percent and 10 percent of the diet. There were no pathological or toxicological effects noted, although food consumption increased in males (CIR, 2015).

Undiluted glycerol caused a variety of irritant-related effects, including petechial hemorrhage and erosions in the small intestine that were dose dependent. In several short-term feeding experiments, 20 percent glycerol administered in the diet for 4 weeks had no adverse effects, although an increase in kidney weights and increased liver enzymes were observed in more than half of the animals. Renne and colleagues (1992) established a NOAEL for glycerol of between 115 and 2,300 mg/kg when administered in drinking water to rats for 44 days. In another short-term drinking water study, calcification in kidney tubules between the cortex and medulla was observed in 3 of 5 rats administered 3,335 mg/kg/day glycerol in drinking water for 6 months (CIR, 2014).

A 3-day oral dosing study of glycerol in mixed-breed dogs established a NOAEL of 950 mg/kg/day. At the highest dose of 3,800 mg/kg/day, the stomach mucosa was severely hyperemic with petechial hemorrhages (Latven and Molitor, 1939). Another longer term feeding study in dogs using 35 percent glycerol in the diet found weight loss after 36 weeks. The weight loss continued after reduction of glycerol by 50 to 80 percent for the remainder of a 50-week study (CIR, 2015). Guinea pigs given 6,300 mg/kg/day of glycerol orally for 30–40 days showed no observable pathological changes (CIR, 2015; Ostwald, 1962).

Inhalation—non-human One study exposed rats for 6 hours per day, 5 days per week for 2 weeks to concentrations of 0, 1,000, 1,930 and 3,910 mg/m^3 of aerosolized glycerol (Renne et al., 1992). The authors reported minimal squamous metaplasia of the epiglottis in 2/25, 1/19, 4/20, and 10/21 rats at 0, 33, 167, and 662 mg/L, respectively; one male in the high-dose group showed mild squamous metaplasia. The authors did not observe macroscopic or systemic effects, or changes in organ weights (Renne et al., 1992). They determined a lowest observed adverse effect level for local irritant effects on the upper respiratory tract of 1,000 mg/m^3.

In another study by the same researchers, 11 rats exposed to the highest concentration of respirable glycerol for 13 weeks (6 hours per day, 5 days per week) similarly exhibited mild squamous metaplasia but did not display macroscopic changes or differences in organ weights (Renne et al., 1992). Male rats in the study showed reduced triglyceride levels, but there was no dose–response relationship (Renne et al., 1992). Based on this study, the inhalation NOAEL was 0.167 mg/L (Renne et al., 1992).

Reproductive and developmental toxicity A two-generation reproductive study of 10 rats administered glycerol (0, 20 percent; ~2,000 mg/kg/day in drinking water) for 8 weeks before mating until weaning of pups (CIR, 2015). The researchers observed no adverse effects on the reproductive efficiency of the parents (F0 generation), or the growth, fertility, or reproductive performance of the untreated F1 generation offspring. In the F0 generation, all 10 females became pregnant with similar litter size as the controls (9.0 versus 8.1). In the F1 generation, 9 of 10 females became pregnant. Additionally, there were no significant differences in the onset of estrus cycles, weight gain, and microscopic observations of the endocrine organs between the F1 and the F2 generations and the controls. Tissues from both the F1 and F2 generations showed no histological changes.

Another study administered glycerol (13.1, 60.8, 282, and 1,310 mg/kg/day) by gavage to Wistar rats (n = 25–28) on days 6 through 15 of gestation (CIR, 2015). No adverse effects were observed in the dams (NTIS, 1974). The number of pregnancies, implantations, resorptions, litter sizes, weights, and sex ratio, and the incidences of external, visceral, and skeletal abnormalities were similar among treatment groups compared with controls. The NOAEL for maternal toxicity and teratogenicity was 1,310 mg/kg/day.

A similar study administered glycerol (12.8, 59.4, 276, and 1,280 mg/kg/day) by gavage to CD-1 mice (n = 25) on days 6 through 15 of gestation. As with the study of Wistar rats, the researchers found no adverse effects in the dams (CIR, 2015), and the number of pregnancies, implantations, resorptions, litter sizes, weights, and sex ratio and incidences of external, visceral, and skeletal abnormalities were similar among treated mice compared with controls. The NOAEL for maternal toxicity and teratogenicity was 1,280 mg/kg/day.

A study of Dutch-belted rabbits (n = 25) administered glycerol (11.8, 54.8, 254.5, and 1,180 mg/kg/day) by gavage on days 6 through 18 of gestation, and also reported no adverse effects in the dams (CIR, 2015). Again, the number of pregnancies, implantations, resorptions, litter sizes, weights, sex ratio, and external, visceral, and skeletal abnormalities were similar among treated rabbits compared with controls. The NOAEL for maternal toxicity and teratogenicity was 1,180 mg/kg/day.

Male Fertility

One study found that glycerol injected into the testes of rats (50–200 μL and 862 mg/kg body weight) and monkeys (119 mg/kg body weight) suppressed spermatogenesis (CIR, 2015; Wiebe and Barr, 1984a,b; Wiebe et al., 1989).

Genotoxicity and carcinogenicity Numerous studies have examined the mutagenic potential of glycerol in the Ames *Salmonella* assay, in dose ranges from 0.2 to 50 mg/plate, and using a variety of strains of *S. typhimurium*, with and without metabolic activation, and all reported negative results (CIR, 2015; Clark et al., 1979; Doolittle et al., 1988; Haworth et al., 1983; Ishidate et al., 1984; Stolzenberg and Hine, 1979; Yamaguchi, 1982). Carmines and Gaworski (2005) measured the mutagenicity of mainstream tobacco smoke condensate in the presence and absence of various concentrations of glycerol (5, 10, and 15 percent) and found no difference in mutagenicity in the presence or absence of glycerol.

Glycerol also tested negative in the hypoxanthine-guanine phosphoribosyl transferase mutagenicity assay, sister chromatid exchange assay in Chinese hamster ovary cells, and unscheduled DNA synthesis in rat hepatocytes, at concentrations up to 1 mg/ml (CIR, 2015). Another study looking at interlaboratory comparisons of the DNA damage assay in rat hepatocytes evaluated glycerol as one of three "negative" vehicles for administration of other carcinogens, and confirmed the lack of any effect on DNA damage in rat hepatocytes (CIR, 2015). An in vivo bone marrow chromosome aberration assay tested negative following intraperitoneal injection administration of 1,000 mg/kg glycerol (CIR, 2015).

A chronic bioassay in rats, with glycerol administered at concentrations up to 20 percent for 1 year or up to 10 g/kg for 2 years, failed to increase tumor incidence (CIR, 2015). Thus, there is substantial evidence indicating that glycerol itself is not mutagenic. However, when combusted, glycerol can form thermal decomposition products (see the

Carbonyl Compounds section for discussion of thermal decomposition products).

Ethylene Glycol

In addition to PG and glycerol, studies have also identified ethylene glycol as a solvent used in e-liquids. Ethylene glycol is an odorless, clear, slightly viscous liquid that is commonly used as antifreeze in cooling and heating systems, in hydraulic brake fluids, and as an industrial solvent. Hahn and colleagues (2014) identified ethylene glycol in samples even though it was not listed on any labels. Hutzler and colleagues (2014) found that ethylene glycol replaced PG and glycerol as the dominant compound in five products. In an e-liquid from one particular manufacturer, the ethylene glycol content was as high as 76 percent. Four out of five products from this particular manufacturer revealed more than 70 percent ethylene glycol, whereas only 2 percent was detectable in the fifth. Seven products from three manufacturers contained 1 to 6 percent ethylene glycol, and in one additional sample again more than 30 percent was detected. Conversely, altogether 15 samples produced by three other manufacturers tested negative. Most e-cigarette liquids do not contain ethylene glycol and, where present, it is at levels that are not likely to contribute significantly to adverse health effects. Nonetheless, ethylene glycol is a respiratory irritant and is associated with markedly enhanced toxicological hazards when compared with conventionally used glycerol and PG (Gomes et al., 2002).

FLAVORINGS

There are more than 7,000 unique e-liquid flavors available to e-cigarette users (Zhu et al., 2014), and yet, little is known about them as there are few studies examining exposure to flavorings. Furthermore, flavoring components are often not included in e-cigarette products' ingredient lists. For example, one study of 54 e-liquids found many products labeled with "natural or artificial flavors," and just four samples listed specific flavoring substances (Hahn et al., 2014).

While the Flavor and Extracts Manufacturers Association considers many flavors to be GRAS in food products, at their levels of intended use, these chemicals could still be harmful when they are aerosolized and inhaled, as such ingredients are not safety tested for exposure routes other than ingestion (Barrington-Trimis et al., 2016; FEMA, 2015). For instance, saccharides, which are used to make sweet e-liquid flavors that can appeal to children (Farley et al., 2014; King et al., 2014; Villanti et al., 2013), degrade and produce furans and aldehydes when heated (Soussy et al., 2016). Aldehydes may cause irritation to the respiratory tract (Tierney et al., 2016). One study of 28 e-liquids identified more than 140 volatile flavoring components at concentrations varying from 1 to 5 percent (10 to 50 mg/ml), and detected the formation of aldehydes (Hutzler et al., 2014). Another study that tested multiple flavors in two brands of single-use cigarettes found a similar concentration of flavor chemicals and identified aldehydes such as vanillin and ethyl vanillin (Tierney et al., 2016). Hahn and colleagues (2014) analyzed 54 e-liquids and distinguished ethyl vanillin in 13 samples and thujone in 2 samples.

Other flavoring chemicals have been measured in e-liquids as well. For example, pulegone and eucalyptol were identified in menthol-flavored e-cigarettes (Lisko et al., 2015). Similar to combustible tobacco cigarettes, concentrations of menthol in this study varied from 3,700 to 12,000 μg/g. Additionally, 40 percent of non-menthol products tested in the study had low levels of menthol (Lisko et al., 2015). Menthol's properties include cooling and local anesthesia, as well as effects on drug absorption and metabolism, bronchodilation and respiration changes, and electrophysiology (Ahijevych and Garrett, 2004). Although little is known about the role of menthol in e-cigarettes, the effects of menthol on increasing the reinforcing effects of nicotine on tobacco smoking behavior were evidenced in both qualitative and quantitative empirical studies (Ahijevych and Garrett, 2010). For the menthol smokers, a greater exposure to nicotine and the particulate matter (tar) of the smoked cigarette was observed and can result in increased nicotine dependence and a greater chance of tobacco-attributable disease (Garten and Falkner, 2004).

Exposure to Flavorings

Broadly speaking, flavored tobacco use is associated with younger age; consumers perceive flavored tobacco products more favorably. Flavoring in tobacco products is considered an attractive characteristic and is associated with temporary experimentation and/or initiation of tobacco product use (Feirman et al., 2016; Kowitt et al., 2017). Flavors are extremely common among e-cigarette users, and are often named as a primary reason for e-cigarette use. For example, about 75 percent of regular e-cigarette users report using some non-tobacco flavor (Wang et al., 2015; Yingst et al., 2017). Despite the increasing popularity of e-cigarettes, little is known about users' preferences, selection, and switching among various flavors. Farsalinos and colleagues (2013) conducted an online survey of more than 4,000 e-cigarette users and found that flavors, especially flavor variety, were an important factor in the maintenance of e-cigarette use by current and former smokers. Specifically, nearly half of the study subjects reported that limiting the range of available e-cigarette flavors would increase cravings for combustible tobacco cigarettes and would decrease their likelihood of reducing or quitting smoking. The results also indicated that smokers tended to start with tobacco-flavored products, and then would switch to multiple flavors as they transitioned from dual use to complete (or nearly complete) substitution of e-cigarettes for their usual combustible tobacco cigarettes. Berg (2016) recruited 1,567 adults, ages 18 to 34 years, through Facebook ads targeting tobacco users and non-users. Fruity e-cigarette flavors were the most preferred among both smokers and non-smokers.

Flavors appear to hold value to users. In a willingness-to-pay (WTP) study, removing flavors resulted in an 18 percent drop in WTP among exclusive e-cigarette users, compared with a 1 percent drop for dual users (Nonnemaker et al., 2016). In a discrete-choice experiment context, flavor (cherry in particular) significantly increased intentions to purchase (Czoli et al., 2016). In the laboratory, participants worked harder for flavored puffs, meaning that flavors appear to enhance the reward/reinforcement value of nicotine (Audrain-McGovern et al., 2016). In a concept mapping study among vapers, five statement clusters around flavor use were identified: increased satisfaction and enjoyment, variety and customization, better feel and taste than cigarettes, food craving suppression, and social impacts (Soule et al., 2016). At the same time, data from novice users indicated that non-menthol flavorings were not associated with decreased cigarette consumption over 6 weeks of use (Litt et al., 2016).

In e-liquids, flavor combinations are common and their classification is not straightforward. This has been a limitation in determining preferred flavors among e-cigarette users, as common measures have not been used, resulting in widely divergent estimates across studies. A classification system with transparent decision rules that can be applied across product classes may yield more consistent findings to inform regulatory science (Yingst et al., 2017).

The role of menthol in e-cigarette users has not been studied. However, for combustible tobacco cigarettes, African American smokers report substantially greater preference for menthol cigarettes relative to smokers of European ancestry. This had led some to speculate that menthol may contribute to the greater incidence and severity of certain smoking-related diseases among African Americans. Certain studies also suggest that menthol may influence the rates of smoking initiation and cessation (TPSAC, 2011).

Although studies have dealt with flavoring chemicals in e-cigarette products, there is little information on how these chemicals affect health during long-term exposures by inhalation. Studies have shown that users switch among flavors frequently. Additionally, the choice of flavor may change over the course of a smoker's substitution of combustible tobacco with e-cigarettes, such that tobacco flavors are more popular when users start using e-cigarettes (Farsalinos et al., 2013). Flavoring compounds might also include substances of sensitizing, toxic, or irritating potency. Although few studies have examined the effects of flavoring substances administered by inhalation, there are some chemicals that, although approved for ingestion, have established adverse health effects when inhaled. Table 5-4 presents an overview of common flavorings and their inhalation toxicity. Examples of such chemicals include diacetyl, acetylpropionyl, acetoin, cinnamaldehyde, and benzaldehyde; these are reviewed in details below.

Diacetyl, acetylpropionyl (also known as 2,3-pentanedione), and acetoin are chemicals used by food manufactures to add creamy flavors like butter, caramel, butterscotch, piña colada, and strawberry to food products. Acetylpropionyl is structurally similar to diacetyl and therefore can be used as a flavoring substitute. However, these ingredients have been associated with adverse respiratory health outcomes. For example, investigations in microwave popcorn manufacturing plants found increased incidences of chronic cough and bronchitis, asthma, and bronchiolitis obliterans, a severe lung condition that can result in permanent pulmonary scarring and obstruction (Kreiss et al., 2002; NIOSH, 2016). Workers in these facilities inhaled diacetyl and acetoin when butter flavoring containing these chemicals was heated and became aerosolized (Kreiss et al., 2002; NIOSH, 2016). Workers with bronchiolitis obliterans have also been found in flavoring production companies (NIOSH, 2016).

These flavoring ingredients have also been measured in e-cigarette liquids. For instance, a study of flavored e-cigarettes available in the United States identified at least one of these three chemicals in more than 90 percent of the tested e-cigarettes (Allen et al., 2016). Of the 51 samples, 46 flavors had acetoin (concentration ranging up to 529 μg per e-cigarette), 39 contained diacetyl (up to 239 μg per e-cigarette), and 23 flavors included acetylpropionyl (up to 64 μg per e-cigarette) (Allen et al., 2016). Another study of 159 sweet-flavored liquids from 36 American and European manufacturers found diacetyl and/or acetylpropionyl in nearly three-quarters of sampled liquids and their aerosols (Farsalinos et al., 2015c). These samples indicated a median daily exposure of 56 μg of diacetyl per day (interquartile range [IQR] = 26–278 μg/day); the median daily exposure to acetylpropionyl was 91 μg/day (IQR = 20–432 μg/day) (Farsalinos et al., 2015c).

Several studies examined the cinnamaldehyde-containing e-liquids and e-cigarette aerosols. Cinnamaldehyde is the major chemical in cinnamon-flavored e-cigarette products, but also has been found in tobacco-, sweet- (including caramel), and fruit-flavored e-liquids (Behar et al., 2016). Behar and colleagues (2016) evaluated the distribution, concentration, and

TABLE 5-4 Overview of Common Flavorings and Their Inhalation Toxicity

Chemical Group	Flavoring Chemical	CAS Number	Flavor Type
Nature Identical			
Alcohols	Geraniol	106-24-1	Floral
	Menthol	2216-51-5	Mentholic
	Thymol	89-83-8	Herbal
	Eugenol	97-53-0	Spicy
Acids	Butyric acid	107-92-6	Cheesy
	Valeric acid	109-52-4	Cheesy
	2-Methylbutyric acid	116-53-0	Acidic
Esters	Ethyl butyrate	105-54-4	Fruity
	2-Methylbutyrate	105-37-3	Fruity
	Methyl cinnamate	103-26-4	Balsamic
	Methyl salicylate	119-36-8	Minty
Lactones	γ-nonalactone	104-61-0	Coconut
	δ-decalactone	705-86-2	Coconut
Aldehydes	Geranial	141-27-5	Citrus
	Benzaldehyde	100-52-7	Fruity
	Cinnamaldehyde	104-55-2	Spicy
	Vanilin	121-33-5	Vanilla

Flavor Descriptor	Respiratory Irritant	Inhalation Toxicity
Sweet, floral, fruity, rose, waxy, citrus		
Peppermint, cooling, mentholic, minty		
Herbal, thyme, phenolic, medicinal camphor	✓	
Sweet, spicy, clove, woody	✓	
Sharp, dairy-like, cheesy, buttery, with a fruity nuance		Mouse LC > 500 mg/m^3
Acidic and sharp, cheesy, sour milky, tobacco, with fruity nuances		Mouse LC_{50} > 4,100 mg/m^3/2 hours
Acidic, fruity, dirty, cheesy with a fermented nuance		
Fruity, juicy fruit, pineapple, cognac		
Sweet, ethereal, rummy, grape, winey		
Sweet, balsam, strawberry, cherry, cinnamon		
Wintergreen, mint		
Coconut, creamy, waxy, sweet, buttery, oily		
Coconut, creamy, fatty, buttery, milky, and nutty with a slightly fruity nuance		
Citrus, lemon		
Almond, fruity, powdery, nutty, and benzaldehyde-like	✓	Mouse LC > 500 mg/m^3 Rat LC > 500 mg/m^3
Sweet, spice, cinnamon red hots, warm	✓	
Sweet, vanilla, creamy, chocolate		Mouse LC > 41,700 µg/kg/2 hours Rat LC > 41,700 µg/kg/4 hours

continued

TABLE 5-4 Continued

Chemical Group	Flavoring Chemical	CAS Number	Flavor Type
Ketones	Diacetyl	431-03-8	Buttery
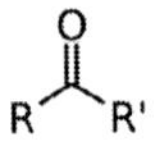	Acetyl propionyl	600-14-6	Buttery
	Raspberry ketone	5471-51-2	Fruity
Heterocycles			
Oxygen containing	Furfural	98-01-1	Bready
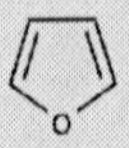	5-Methylfurfural	620-02-0	Caramellic
	Maltol	118-71-8	Caramellic
Nitrogen containing	2-Acetylpyrazine	22047-25-2	Popcorn
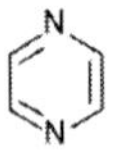	2,3,5-Trimethylpyrazine	14667-55-1	Nutty
	2-Acetylpyrrole	1072-83-9	Musty
Sulfur containing	2-Isopropyl-4-methylthiazole	15679-13-7	Fruity
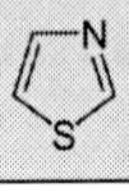	2-Isobuthylthiazole	18640-74-9	Green
Sulfur Compounds			
Mercaptans	Furfuryl mercaptan	98-02-2	Coffee
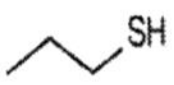	Thiomenthone	38462-22-5	Sulfurous
	p-Menthene-8-thiol	71159-90-5	Citrus

Flavor Descriptor	Respiratory Irritant	Inhalation Toxicity
Sweet, creamy, buttery, pungent, with a pungent caramellic nuance	✓	
Buttery, nutty, toasted, caramellic, diacetyl and acetoin notes	✓	
Sweet, berry jam, raspberry, ripe, floral		
Brown, sweet, woody, bready, nutty, caramellic with a burnt astringent nuance	✓	Human TC_{LO} 310 µg/m^3 Rat LC_{50} 175 ppm/6 hours
Sweet, caramellic, bready, brown, coffee-like	✓	
Sweet, caramel, cotton candy, jam, fruity, baked bread	✓	
Musty, roasted, corn chip, popcorn, nutty, potato-like	✓	
Nutty, musty, powdery cocoa, potato, musty	✓	
Musty, nutty-like with a coumarin nuance	✓	
Musty alliaceous, earthy sulfury, slight fruity, coffee, meaty		
Green, vegetable, tomato-like with raw musty nuances	✓	
Roasted coffee, sulfurous, with a burnt match note	✓	
Fruity, berry, and tropical with a raspberry, minty nuance		
Grapefruit, fresh, tropical, juicy, mango		

continued

TABLE 5-4 Continued

Chemical Group	Flavoring Chemical	CAS Number	Flavor Type
Sulfides	Dimethyl sulfide (DMS)	75-18-3	Sulfurous
R–S–R'	Tropathiane	67715-80-4	Tropical
Flavor Synthetic			
	Ethyl vanillin	121-32-4	Vanilla
	Ethyl maltol	4940-11-8	Caramel
	Ethyl 3-methyl-3-phenylglycidate	77-83-8	Fruity

toxicity of cinnamaldehyde in 39 e-liquids and aerosols generated from e-cigarettes. The study used the gas chromatography–mass spectrometry method and found that 20 of the 39 refill fluids contained cinnamaldehyde at concentrations that were cytotoxic to human embryonic and lung cells in the cell viability assay. The study also revealed that aerosol generated from a single product (cinnamon Ceylon) from a cartomizer-style e-cigarette was cytotoxic. The same product has been shown to be more cytotoxic when aerosol is generated with battery output voltage settings of 5 V than with 3 V, potentially due to additional chemicals released at higher voltage settings, including 2,3-butandione (diacetyl) as confirmed in the study. Cinnamaldehyde depolymerized microtubules in human pulmonary fibroblasts. At concentrations that produced no effect in the cytotoxicity assay, cinnamaldehyde decreased cell growth, attachment, and spreading; altered cell morphology and motility; increased DNA strand breaks; and increased cell death. In general, studies described above have shown that, even at low concentrations, cinnamaldehyde in e-cigarette products is cytotoxic and genotoxic and adversely affects cell processes and survival. These studies also indicate that cinnamaldehyde in e-cigarettes may impair homeostasis in the respiratory system.

Benzaldehyde, which imparts a fruity taste, is an aromatic aldehyde commonly used in food and cosmetics. Studies suggest that oral and dermal exposure to benzaldehyde produces little to no toxicity; however, occupational exposure has been linked to irritation of the eyes and mucous membranes of the respiratory passages (MAK Commission, 2002). One study measured benzaldehyde in aerosol generated from an e-cigarette

Flavor Descriptor	Respiratory Irritant	Inhalation Toxicity
Sulfurous, creamy, tomato, scallop, berry fruity, vegetative nuances	✓	Rat LC_{50} 40,250 ppm Mouse LC_{50} 3,1620 µg/m^3
Green, tropical, galbanum, pineapple	✓	
Sweet, creamy, vanilla, caramel	✓	
Sweet, caramel, jam, strawberry, cotton candy		
Sweet, fruity, strawberry, floral, honey, fatty		

refilled with 145 flavored nicotine-containing solutions purchased from international online retailers (Kosmider et al., 2016). The solutions were classified into groups according to labeled flavor characteristics: berry/tropical fruit (n = 40), tobacco (n = 37), alcohol-related/drink (n = 15), chocolate/sweet flavor (n = 11), coffee/tea (n = 11), mint/menthol (n = 10), cherry (n = 10), and other, non-identifiable flavor varieties (e.g, Indian summer and cosmopolitan) (n = 11). Benzaldehyde was present in 75 percent of 145 e-cigarette refill fluids, with the highest concentrations in cherry flavors. The benzaldehyde doses inhaled using 30 puffs from flavored e-cigarettes were often higher than doses inhaled from a combustible tobacco cigarette. The estimated median daily inhaled dose of benzaldehyde from cherry-flavored e-cigarettes was 70.3 µg, a level of exposure more than 1,000 times lower than the permissible exposure limit (PEL) of benzaldehyde as defined by the workplace environmental exposure level guides.

CARBONYL COMPOUNDS

It is important to evaluate the health effects of e-cigarettes when e-liquid is heated and aerosolized; under such conditions, chemical reactions may result in the formation of new compounds. For example, although refill liquids can contain carbonyl compounds such as reactive aldehydes, heating can enhance the concentrations of these compounds in the aerosol.

Several studies have shown that e-cigarettes emit toxic carbonyl compounds, generated from thermal decomposition of e-liquid ingredients. Carbonyl compounds such as formaldehyde, acetaldehyde, acrolein, and glyoxal, which have been found in e-cigarette aerosols, are potentially hazardous and may induce various health effects in users. Formaldehyde is classified as a human carcinogen (Group 1) by the International Agency for Research on Cancer (IARC), and acetaldehyde is classified as possibly carcinogenic to humans (Group 2B) (Bekki et al., 2014). Glycidol is a probable carcinogen and acrolein causes irritation of the nasal cavity and damages the lining of the lungs (ATSDR, 2007; NTP, 2007). How formaldehyde-releasing agents (hemiacetals) behave in the respiratory tract is currently unknown. Glyoxal and methylglyoxal show mutagenicity. The amount of carbonyl compounds in e-cigarettes varied significantly not only among different brands but also among different samples of the same products. Although, in most cases, detected levels of carbonyl compounds were lower than those in combustible tobacco cigarette smoke, very high levels of formaldehyde were also reported in e-cigarette aerosols (a comparison of toxicants from combustible tobacco cigarette smoke and e-cigarette aerosols is discussed in Chapter 18) (Canistro et al., 2017; Gillman et al., 2016).

Uchiyama and colleagues (2010, 2013) measured carbonyl compounds in e-cigarette aerosols using high-performance liquid chromatography (see also Bekki et al., 2014; Ohta et al., 2011). The authors tested 13 brands of Japanese e-cigarettes and detected several derivative peaks of carbonyl compounds, including formaldehyde, acetaldehyde, acetone, acrolein, propanal, crotonaldehyde, butanal, glyoxal, and methylglyoxal (Bekki et al., 2014; Ohta et al., 2011; Uchiyama et al., 2013). Four out of the 13 e-cigarette brands did not generate any carbonyl compounds. The other nine e-cigarette brands generated various carbonyl compounds. The maximum concentrations of formaldehyde, acetaldehyde, acrolein, propanal, glyoxal, and methylglyoxal were 140, 120, 40, 46, 23, and 21 μg/10 puffs, respectively.

Goniewicz and colleagues (2014) measured 15 carbonyl compounds in aerosol generated from 12 e-cigarette brands. Only four carbonyl compounds (formaldehyde, acetaldehyde, acrolein, and *o*-methylbenzaldehyde) were found in aerosols and these compounds were identified in nearly all examined e-cigarettes. The content of formaldehyde ranged from 2.0 mg to 56.1 mg, acetaldehyde from 1.1 mg to 13.6 mg, and acrolein from 0.7 mg to 41.9 mg per e-cigarette (150 puffs).

Kosmider and colleagues (2014) tested 13 samples of aerosol generated from Polish e-cigarettes and detected formaldehyde and acetaldehyde in 8 of them. The amounts of formaldehyde and acetaldehyde in e-cigarette aerosols at a lower voltage were on average 13- and 807-fold lower than those in combustible tobacco cigarette smoke, respectively.

E-cigarette aerosols generated from PG-based e-liquids were found to have the highest levels of carbonyls. Furthermore, different e-cigarettes showed large variations in carbonyl levels.

Hutzler and colleagues (2014) measured formaldehyde in e-cigarette aerosol and estimated that exposure to formaldehyde can be comparable with combustible tobacco cigarettes. They measured 20 to 50 μg of formaldehyde per 10 puffs in the final fractions, which roughly corresponds to the expected exposure from smoking one combustible tobacco cigarette.

Flora and colleagues (2016) tested the aerosols of four MarkTen® e-cigarettes (rechargeable with disposable cartridges) for potential degradation products. They found formaldehyde levels that varied from 0.09 to 0.33 μg/puff. The same research team found formaldehyde residues in both the gas (approximately 30 percent) and liquid (approximately 70 percent) phases of an aerosol (Flora et al., 2017).

Blair and colleagues (2015) measured acrolein in aerosol from e-cigarettes and tobacco smoke and found that five puffs of an e-cigarette emitted 0.290 ± 0.018 μg of acrolein while nine puffs on a combustible tobacco cigarette emitted 2.61 ± 0.16 μg of this toxicant. There was a substantial range in the relative standard deviations reported for all mean value measurements, suggesting inconsistencies across products in the release of these chemicals.

Papousek and colleagues (2014) measured acrylamide and acrolein in tobacco smoke and three e-cigarette aerosol samples. The e-cigarette aerosol samples contained no detectable levels of acrylamide. Acrolein levels in combustible tobacco cigarette smoke varied from 4.48 to 8.27 μg per cigarette while levels detected in an equivalent sample of e-cigarette aerosol varied from 0.17 to 3.70 μg.

Sleiman and colleagues (2016) detected up to 31 compounds, including formaldehyde, acetaldehyde, glycidol, acrolein, acetol, and diacetyl, in e-cigarette aerosols from different devices. Emission rates were significantly higher for a single-coil versus a double-coil device, ranging from tens to thousands of nanograms of toxicants per milligram of e-liquid aerosol.

Tayyarah and Long (2014) tested 55 harmful and potentially harmful constituents in e-cigarette aerosol (blu and SKYCIG brands) and quantified three carbonyls (acrolein, acetaldehyde, and propionaldehyde) at levels 86 to 544 times lower than combustible tobacco cigarette smoke.

Table 5-5 summarizes experimental studies to determine carbonyl compounds in e-cigarette aerosols, their setups (i.e., methods to trap and analyze carbonyls, e-liquids used), and results. Because carbonyl compounds were primarily detected in aerosol and only traces have been reported in e-liquids, it has been suggested that these compounds are generated when e-liquid ingredients are heated. Figure 5-1 illustrates the

TABLE 5-5 Summary of Experimental Studies Determining Carbonyl Compounds in E-Cigarette Aerosols

Reference	Methodology for Carbonyl Trapping/ Analysis	Type of E-Cigarette(s)	Liquid(s) Used	Determined Carbonyl Emissions
Geiss et al., 2016	Machine smoking (puff volume: 50 ml, puff duration: 3.0 seconds, puff frequency: 20 seconds, 10 puffs), direct trapping on DNPH-sorbent, HPLC	Third-generation e-cigarette with variable voltage/wattage (5 W, 10 W, 15 W, 20 W, 25 W tested). Heating element with 1.6-Ω resistance, 2,200-mAh battery	Glycerol (50%), PG (40%), water, fragrance, nicotine	Formaldehyde: 24–2,559 ng/puff Acetaldehyde: 13–350 ng/puff Acrolein: 2.5 ng/puff (at 20 W)
Tayyarah and Long, 2014	Machine smoking (puff volume: 55 ml every 30 seconds, 99 puffs), smoke/aerosol collected in two DNPH-containing impingers, HPLC	Two disposable and three rechargeable e-cigarettes; no detailed information on e-cigarette properties available	(1) Glycerol/PG (20/70%), water, nicotine, fragrance; (2) Glycerol (80%), water, nicotine, fragrances	Expressed as total carbonyls: <900 ng/puff Acetaldehyde: 320 ng/puff Acrolein: 150 ng/puff Propionaldehyde: 110 ng/puff
Kosmider et al., 2014	Machine smoking (puff volume: 70 ml, puff duration: 1.8 seconds, puff interval: 17 seconds, 30 puffs), direct trapping on DNPH-sorbent tubes, HPLC	Second-generation e-cigarette with variable voltage (3.2 V/4.3 W, 4 V/6.7 W, and 4.8 V/9.6 W tested); heating element with 2.4-Ω resistance, 900-mAh battery	(1) primarily glycerol; (2) glycerol and PG; (3) primarily PG	Formaldehyde: 3.2–3.9 ng/puff Acetaldehyde: 1.3–7.1 ng/puff Acetone: 3.9–19.7 ng/puff Acrolein: <DL Propionaldehyde: <DL

Bekki et al., 2014	Machine smoking (puff volume: 55 ml, puff duration: 2 seconds, puff interval: 30 seconds, 10 puffs), direct trapping on cartridges (hydroquinone and DNPH), HPLC	13 Japanese e-cigarette brands; no detailed information on e-cigarette properties available	No detailed information available	Formaldehyde: 660–3,400 ng/puff Acetaldehyde: 20–2,600 ng/puff Acrolein: 110–2,000 ng/puff (at 20 W) Propionaldehyde: 40–1,500 ng/puff
Goniewicz et al., 2014	Machine smoking (puff volume: 70 ml, puff duration: 1.8 seconds, puff interval: 10 seconds, 15 puffs), sorbent trapping, HPLC	11 popular Polish brands; no detailed information on e-cigarette properties available	No detailed information available	Formaldehyde: 21–374 ng/puff Acetaldehyde: 13–91 ng/puff Acrolein: 4.6–201 ng/puff (at 20 W)
Hutzler et al., 2014	Machine smoking (puff volume: 55 ml, puff duration: 3 seconds, puff interval: 30 seconds, puffing until no vapors observable), collected in two DNPH-containing impingers, HPLC	First-generation e-cigarette; no detailed information on e-cigarette properties available	Prefilled cartridges; no detailed information available	Formaldehyde: ~300 ng/puff Acetaldehyde: ~500 ng/puff Acrolein: 500–2,500 ng/puff (only when overheating) Propionaldehyde: 100–1,100 ng/puff (only when overheating)

NOTE: DL = detectable level; DNPH = 2,4-dinitrophenylhydrazine; HPLC = high-performance liquid chromatography; PG = propylene glycol.
SOURCE: Adapted from Geiss et al., 2016.

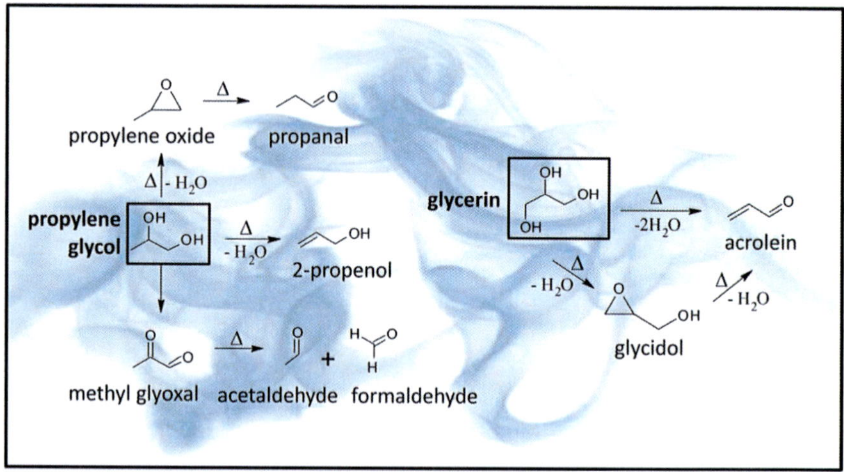

FIGURE 5-1 Postulated pathways and by-products formed during thermal dehydration of propylene glycol and glycerol.
SOURCE: Sleiman et al., 2016.

pathways and by-products formed during thermal dehydration of PG and glycerol as postulated by Sleiman and colleagues (2016). Hutzler and colleagues (2014) incubated e-cigarette liquids at various temperatures and found levels of acetaldehyde and formaldehyde from 10-fold to 20-fold higher at the temperature of 150°C compared with ambient temperatures for samples containing PG. They did not observe this effect at 100°C.

Several studies looked at the potential mechanisms for generating carbonyl compounds in e-cigarettes. In addition to temperature and effects from potential overheating, airflow and catalytic properties of metal heating coils may influence the occurrence of decomposition products. As described in the section on humectants, PG and glycerol can be a source of carbonyl compounds. It has been shown that the oxidation and fragmentation of PG and glycerol contained in e-liquids when they come in contact with the heating coil generates carbonyl compounds (Bekki et al., 2014; Geiss et al., 2016; Goniewicz et al., 2014; Ohta et al., 2011; Uchiyama et al., 2013). Lower liquid levels within the cartridges or tanks also seem to be associated with the occurrence of carbonyls, because low liquid levels may increase airflow and could therefore promote overheating of the wire if no safety features are incorporated to maintain a constant and lower temperature. Results reported by Geiss and colleagues (2016) confirmed that the PG oxidation is involved primarily in the formation of acetaldehyde, while the oxidation of glycerol typically generates acrolein. Oxidation of both PG and glycerol can generate formaldehyde, although a predominance of glycerol can be observed. Glycerol forms acrolein and acetaldehyde as oxidation by-products only at higher coil temperatures.

Gillman and colleagues (2016) demonstrated that glycerol can undergo thermal decomposition to form reactive aldehydes, including formaldehyde, acetaldehyde, and acrolein. The extent of formation is dependent upon both the power (watts) of the coil and the design of the device itself. Estimated exposures to total aldehydes from daily consumption of 3 grams of e-liquid ranged from less than 0.1 to 41 mg/day. Formaldehyde was the predominant aldehyde present, with the highest estimated exposure to be 22 mg/day. The authors reported a 750-fold difference in total aldehyde production between different devices, using the same e-liquid. For the device that generated the highest levels of aldehydes, the estimated daily doses exceed the OSHA occupational health PEL for formaldehyde by 10-fold.

Canistro and colleagues (2017) also found that heating of glycerol produces temperature-dependent amounts of formaldehyde, acetaldehyde, and acrolein (see Table 5-6). When rats were exposed via inhalation to e-cigarette aerosols (11 cycles/day, 5 days/week for 4 weeks), a statistically significant fourfold increase in the formation of 8-hydroxy-deoxyguanosine was found in the lungs, along with other evidence of oxidative stress in these animals. Thus, it is likely that glycerol in e-liquids, under some circumstances that are both device- and power (watt)-dependent, can undergo thermal decomposition to generate reactive aldehydes capable of contributing to oxidative tissue injury, including potential DNA damage. However, for other devices, the levels of aldehyde were very low, relative to both typical indoor air and the levels found in combustible tobacco cigarette smoke. It should be noted that the conditions that resulted in very high levels of aldehydes were extreme and not typically attained during normal consumer use. Nevertheless, the potential exists for e-cigarette devices to form very high levels of aldehydes under extreme conditions.

Some e-cigarette devices allow users to change the power of the device or output voltage of the battery to increase aerosol production and nicotine delivery. The battery output voltage, and consequently the heat generated on the coil, has been reported to affect the quantity of carbonyls formed. Kosmider and colleagues (2014) showed that increasing the voltage from 3.2 V to 4.8 V resulted in an increase from 4 to more than 200 times in the levels of formaldehyde, acetaldehyde, and acetone. The levels of formaldehyde in aerosol generated from high-voltage devices were nearly identical to those in combustible tobacco cigarette smoke (1.6–52 μg per cigarette) (see Figure 5-2).

Increasing levels of carbonyl compounds were observed for a voltage over 3 V (Bekki et al., 2014; Ohta et al., 2011). Thus, commercial

TABLE 5-6 Volatile Compounds Detected in E-Cigarette Aerosol

	Chamber 1		Chamber 5		
	Mean	Standard Deviation	Mean	Standard Deviation	Statistical Significance
1,2-Propanediamine	0.83	0.08	1.09	0.11	ns
Acrolein	0.02	0.00	0.03	0.02	ns
Indole	0.19	0.24	0.18	0.02	ns
Acetole*	0.07	0.03	0.07	0.00	ns
3-Hexen-1-ol*	0.05	0.00	0.06	0.02	ns
Diacetyl*	0.03	0.01	0.08	0.01	ns
PG	87.71	1.03	88.66	0.19	ns
1-Methoxy-2-propyl acetate	0.07	0.04	0.05	0.01	ns
Methyl propionate*	0.20	0.01	0.21	0.06	ns
Propanoic acid, 1-Methylpropyl ester	0.09	0.00	0.09	0.02	ns
Nicotine	6.36	0.62	6.54	0.18	ns
Glycerol	4.36	1.68	2.98	0.05	ns
PG/Glycerol	21.80	8.63	29.80	0.43	ns

NOTES: Volatile organic compounds (VOCs) detected in the first and last treatment chambers during exposure to e-cigarette vapor. Values are expressed as a percentage (%) of total peak area of VOCs; factorial analysis of variance (ANOVA) was performed to study the effect of exposure cycling on the formation of VOCs. Statistically different means were investigated (Tukey's test, $p < 0.05$); * = flavor compounds; PG = propylene glycol; VOC = volatile organic compound.
SOURCE: Canistro et al., 2017.

e-cigarettes with 4- to 5-V batteries may generate carbonyl compounds. The battery output voltage significantly affects the concentration of carbonyl compounds in the e-cigarette aerosol, and high-voltage e-cigarettes may expose users to high levels of carbonyl compounds.

Formaldehyde also reacts with PG and glycerol during aerosolization to produce hemiacetals. Jensen and colleagues (2015) analyzed commercial e-liquid aerosolized with the use of a tank system e-cigarette featuring a variable-voltage battery. They detected no formation of any formaldehyde-releasing agents at 3.3 V. However, at 5.0 V, they detected a mean ± SE of 380 ± 90 μg/sample (10 puffs) of formaldehyde as hemiacetals. Similarly, Sleiman and colleagues (2016) found that when they increased the voltage applied to a single-coil device from 3.3 to 4.8 V, the mass of e-liquid consumed doubled from 3.7 to 7.5 mg/puff and the total aldehyde emission rates tripled from 53 to 165 μg/puff, with acrolein rates growing by a factor of 10.

Flora and colleagues (2017) evaluated the effect of e-cigarette heating coil temperature on formaldehyde formation. Using an infrared camera to measure the maximum heat coil temperature and Fourier-transform infrared spectrometer to measure gas-phase formaldehyde, the authors found that, in some of the commercial e-cigarettes tested, the levels of formaldehyde were greater than those detected in combustible tobacco cigarettes, and as high as 14.1 μg/puff. The study found that e-cigarettes produce low amounts of formaldehyde at temperatures below 350°C, but as the temperature increases, the levels of formaldehyde also rise steeply. The authors concluded that the high levels of formaldehyde observed in some e-cigarettes tested in the study were likely due to heating coil temperatures above 350°C.

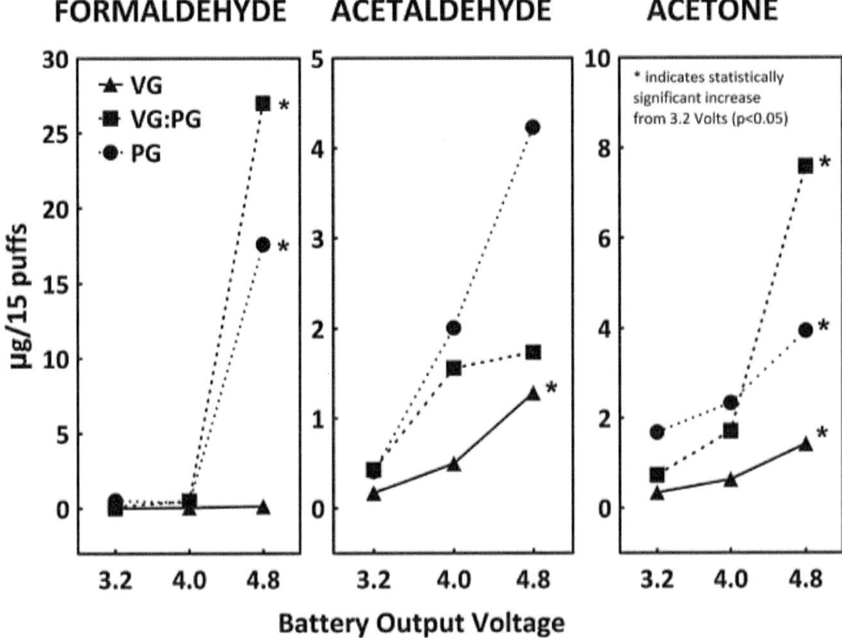

FIGURE 5-2 Effects of nicotine solvent and battery output voltage on levels of carbonyl compounds released from e-cigarettes (μg/15 puffs; n = 3; puff duration = 1.8 seconds, puff volume = 70 ml, puff intervals = 17 seconds).
NOTES: * = statistically significant increase from 3.2 Volts ($p < 0.05$). PG = propylene glycol; VG = glycerol.
SOURCE: Kosmider et al., 2014.

Geiss and colleagues (2016) also reported correlation between the amounts of carbonyl compounds emitted by e-cigarettes with the temperature of the heating coil. The authors used infrared thermography to determine the temperature of the heating coil and had an experienced e-cigarette user conduct a subjective sensorial quality evaluation of the aerosol generated at each temperature. The study found a steep increase in the generated carbonyls when applying a battery output of at least 15 W corresponding to 200°–250°C on the heating coil. At 20 W, the e-cigarette user provided a negative sensorial quality evaluation, suggesting that an e-cigarette user would be unlikely to apply such wattage in real-world use.

Wang and colleagues (2017) investigated how PG and glycerol influence carbonyl compound formation under precisely controlled temperatures in the absence of nicotine and flavor additives. At reactor temperatures equal to or greater than 215°C for both PG and glycerol, the authors detected significant amounts of formaldehyde and acetaldehyde. Only e-liquids containing glycerol at temperatures exceeding 270°C produced acrolein. At 318°C, 2.03 ± 0.80 μg of formaldehyde, 2.35 ± 0.87 μg of acetaldehyde, and a trace amount of acetone were generated per milligram of PG; at the same temperature, 21.1 ± 3.80 μg of formaldehyde, 2.40 ± 0.99 μg of acetaldehyde, and 0.80 ± 0.50 μg of acrolein were detected per milligram of glycerol.

Other factors causing elevated carbonyl levels should also be considered. It is expected that both the heating element and wicking material will deteriorate with use, which could lead to more thermal degradation (Guthery, 2016). Sleiman and colleagues (2016) found that, after an e-cigarette device was used several times, carbonyl emissions increased by more than 60 percent, and they attributed this effect to the buildup of polymerization by-products that degraded upon heating. Flavoring compounds may also play a role. Using three popular brands of e-cigarettes filled with both flavored and unflavored e-liquids, Khlystov and Samburova (2016) measured several toxic aldehydes and showed that the formation of aldehydes during e-cigarette use comes primarily from thermal decomposition of flavoring compounds. They also found that the production of aldehydes was exponentially dependent on concentration of flavoring compounds. Sucrose, a sweetener and flavor enhancer detected in e-liquids in concentrations from 0.76 to 72.93 μg/g, also has been suggested as a potential ingredient that may thermally degrade to produce carbonyl compounds (Kubica et al., 2014).

Several studies have examined the potential exposure to carbonyl compounds from e-cigarettes. Using American Conference of Governmental Industrial Hygienists (ACGIH) standards, Khlystov and Samburova (2016) assessed e-cigarette users' carbonyls exposure risk from e-cigarettes. ACGIH defines the threshold limit value–ceiling (TLV–C) as the concentration that should not be exceeded during any part of the working exposure; the TLV-C for formaldehyde is 0.3 mg m^3, and, for acrolein, is 0.23 mg/m^3. To compare exposure to these aldehydes from one puff, the authors divided the amount per puff by 500 ml, the average tidal volume of a healthy adult, and found that all flavored products of a single brand exceeded the ACGIH formaldehyde ceiling level by factors of 190–270 and the acrolein ceiling level by factors of 11–24, depending on the flavor used. Three of five liquids of the second brand tested exceeded the formaldehyde ceiling level by 2.0-fold to 13-fold, depending on the liquid flavor. No acrolein was detected in the second brand tested. All flavored products of the third brand tested exceeded the formaldehyde ceiling level by 2.9-fold to 66-fold and four products of the same brand exceeded the acrolein ceiling by 1.5-fold to 6.0-fold. The authors concluded that one puff of any of the tested flavored e-cigarette liquids exposes the smoker to dangerous levels of these two aldehydes.

Jensen and colleagues (2015) extrapolated the formaldehyde dose from levels of formaldehyde-releasing agents (hemiacetals) detected in aerosol generated at high voltage. The high battery output voltage setting (5 V) used by Jensen and colleagues resulted in excessive breakdown of PG to formaldehyde. The estimated daily dose of formaldehyde-releasing agent for an e-cigarette user vaping at a rate of 3 ml/day would be as high as 14.4 ± 3.3 mg. This dose is much higher than the estimated daily dose of formaldehyde from combustible tobacco cigarettes, which is approximately 3 mg/pack of 20 combustible tobacco cigarettes (150 µg/cigarette). Under the assumption that the risk per unit associated with inhaling formaldehyde-releasing agents is the same as the risk associated with inhaling gaseous formaldehyde, the authors estimated that long-term e-cigarette use is associated with an incremental lifetime cancer risk from inhaling formaldehyde of 4.2×10^{-3}. This risk is from 5 to 15 times higher than the risk associated with inhaling formaldehyde during long-term combustible tobacco smoking.

Wang and colleagues (2017) estimated that the daily exposure to formaldehyde and acetaldehyde for an e-cigarette user vaping at 215°C could reach 105 ± 117 µg and 36 ± 42 µg, respectively. This estimated daily formaldehyde exposure is above the "no significant risk level" of 40 µg/day from the California Office of Environmental Health Hazard Assessment (OEHHA, 2013). Same authors estimated that if the e-cigarette heating temperature exceeds 270°C, the formaldehyde generated from 10 50-ml puffs could reach levels similar to those from combustible tobacco smoking (comparisons of exposure to potentially toxic substances from e-cigarettes with combustible tobacco cigarette smoking are described in more detail in Chapter 18 on harm reduction).

In summary, when e-liquids are heated and aerosolized, they can produce chemical reactions that could form carbonyl compounds such as reactive aldehydes, which are considered to have toxic effects on human health. At temperatures within the range of most e-cigarette products (150°–350°C), formaldehyde, acetaldehyde, and acrolein have been detected at levels that have raised concerns about chronic health endpoints (Jensen et al., 2015).

MINOR TOBACCO ALKALOIDS

Although the main alkaloid found in tobacco-derived products, including e-liquids, is nicotine, several minor tobacco alkaloids have been identified. The process by which nicotine in e-liquids is extracted from tobacco may produce some impurities including minor alkaloids: nornicotine, anatabine, anabasine, cotinine, nicotine *N*-oxides, myosmine, β-nicotyrine, and β-nornicotyrine. These minor alkaloids may arise from biosynthetic processes in the living plant or by bacterial action or oxidation during tobacco processing (Gorrod and Jacob, 1999).

Etter and colleagues (2013) analyzed samples of e-liquids from 20 bottles of 10 different brands using ultra-high-performance liquid chromatography, and found that minor tobacco alkaloids constituted 1–2 percent of the nicotine content in most samples. The most common substances found were *cis*-*N*-oxide, *trans*-*N*-oxide, myosmine, anatabine, and anabasine. The authors hypothesized that oxidative degradation of nicotine during the manufacturing of the ingredient or of the final liquids, interactions with packaging material, inadequate handling and storage, or an unstable formulation could have resulted in the high amounts of nicotine-related impurities measured.

Testing nicotine-containing e-liquids, Lisko and colleagues (2015) found minor tobacco alkaloids in all samples, and observed that their relative concentrations varied widely among manufacturers. eSmoke brand e-liquids had the highest concentrations of the minor tobacco alkaloids (6.3–48.2 μg/g nornicotine, 8.7–62.7 μg/g myosmine, 21.2–152 μg/g anabasine, 63.1–485 μg/g anatabine, and 2.4–20.7 μg/g isonicoteine). Other products tested contained considerably lower concentrations of minor tobacco alkaloids. These variations could be due to use of purer nicotine extract or minimization of nicotine oxidation. These minor tobacco alkaloid concentrations in e-liquids are much lower when compared with combustible tobacco cigarettes, which have minor tobacco alkaloid concentrations in the range of 659–986 μg/g for nornicotine, 8.6–17.3 μg/g for myosmine, 127–185 μg/g for anabasine, 927–1,390 μg/g for anatabine and 23.4–45.5 μg/g for isonicoteine (comparisons between e-cigarettes and combustible tobacco cigarettes are described in more detail in Chapter 18 on harm reduction).

Flora and colleagues (2016) tested the liquids and aerosols of four MarkTen® e-cigarettes (rechargeable with disposable cartridges) for potential impurities and degradation products. They found that liquids contained 11–19 µg/g of nicotine *N*-oxides, undetectable levels to 9.4 µg/g of cotinine, 14–31 µg/g of nornicotine, and 7.4–13.0 µg/g of myosmine. Regueiro and colleagues (2016) tested 12 e-cigarette liquids purchased from different vendors in the European Union. Among the nicotine-related compounds studied, the authors detected only anatabine, cotinine, myosmine, and nornicotine in any of the samples, and at concentrations in the microgram-per-milliliter level.

Nicotine dehydrogenation also results in another alkaloid: nicotyrine. Considerable quantities of this nicotine analogue have been measured in an analysis of various e-cigarette aerosols (Martinez et al., 2014). Nicotyrine has been shown to hinder nicotine metabolism in mice (Stålhandske and Slanina, 1982). Therefore, its presence in e-cigarette aerosols could diminish smoking cravings by aiding nicotine absorption in the lungs, restraining metabolism, and consequently maintaining nicotine levels (Martinez et al., 2014).

Nicotine purity varies by grade and manufacturer. The American E-Liquid Manufacturing Standards Association requires members to use U.S. Pharmacopeia (USP)-certified nicotine in e-liquids, although the group does not have regulatory authority (AEMSA, 2014). According to USP standards, nicotine solutions cannot exceed 0.5 percent (5 mg/g) of a single impurity or 1 percent (10 mg/g) of total impurities (U.S. Pharmacopeia, n.d.). Nicotine-related impurities are less toxic than nicotine, but the health effects of these minor tobacco alkaloids to e-cigarette users, especially at high levels, is unknown.

TOBACCO-SPECIFIC NITROSAMINES

TSNAs are potent carcinogenic chemicals (Hecht, 1998; Hecht and Hoffmann, 1988), which are derived from tobacco leaves and formed during the curing process via nitrosation of amines. Low levels of TSNAs have been reported in e-cigarette liquids and aerosol, typically at levels similar to those found in pharmaceutical nicotine products. This is probably attributed to the use of pharmaceutical-grade nicotine that most manufacturers claim to use. This grade of nicotine is highly purified to remove the majority of impurities, including TSNAs.

Using liquid chromatography–tandem mass spectrometry, Kim and Shin (2013) detected TSNAs in 105 refill liquid brands purchased from 11 e-cigarette companies in the Korean market. They measured

TSNAs in concentration ranges of 0.34–60.08 µg/L (64.8 percent detection frequency) for *N′*-nitrosonornicotine (NNN), 0.22–9.84 µg/L (88.6 percent detection frequency) for 4-(methylnitrosamino)-1-(3-pyridyl)-1-butanone (NNK), 0.11–11.11 µg/L (54.3 percent detection frequency) for *N′*-nitrosoanabasine (NAB), and 0.09–62.19 µg/L (75.2 percent detection frequency) for *N′*-nitrosoanatabine. Farsalinos and colleagues (2015b) evaluated the presence of selected tobacco-derived chemicals in liquids produced by extracting flavor from cured tobacco leaves and found that total nitrosamine concentrations varied from 2.5 to 38.5 ng/ml. In another study, Farsalinos and colleagues (2015a) also compared the levels of TSNAs in three commercial e-liquids and the aerosol from three 100-puff sets from each liquid trapped in filter pads. In two of the liquids, NAB was found at trace levels (1.2 and 2.3 ng/g); the third contained 1.5 ng/g NAB and 7.7 ng/g NNN (Farsalinos et al., 2015a). The authors found no TSNAs in the aerosol from the 100-puff sets. Finally, Goniewicz and colleagues (2014) analyzed aerosol generated from 12 brands of e-cigarette and identified two nitrosamines (NNN and NNK) in all but three products. The NNN yields ranged from 0.8 ng to 4.3 ng and the NNK yields from 1.1 ng to 28.3 ng per 150 puffs.

FREE RADICALS AND REACTIVE OXYGEN SPECIES

Reactive oxygen species (ROS), including free radicals, can stem from normal biological processes as well as from external sources, such as tobacco smoke. ROS cause oxidative stress, which damages cellular proliferation, metabolism, and health, and can be involved in the development of several cardiovascular (e.g., atherosclerosis), respiratory (e.g., chronic obstructive pulmonary disease, asthma), and neurodegenerative disorders (e.g., Parkinson's disease, multiple sclerosis) as well as diabetes, rheumatoid arthritis, and some types of cancers (e.g., lung, colorectal) (Domej et al., 2014; HHS, 2010; Kehrer and Klotz, 2015; Kirkham and Rahman, 2006; Messner and Bernhard, 2014; Phaniendra et al., 2015; Prescott and Bottle, 2017; Pryor, 1997).

E-cigarette users may be exposed to both highly reactive and more stable ROS during use. Activating the e-cigarette's heating element and aerosolizing the e-liquid produce ROS; these species are drawn into the lungs directly from the device (Lerner et al., 2015b). This process is affected by the age of the heating element (Lerner et al., 2015a). Oxidants are also derived from a device's lithium ion battery, similar to that used in combustible tobacco cigarette filters and e-cigarette cartomizers (Lerner et al., 2015a). Goel and colleagues (2015) identified free radicals from all e-cigarettes and e-liquids tested (at 3.3 V, 2.5×10^{13} to 10.3×10^{13} radicals per puff), as well from glycerol and PG and during dry-puff scenarios.

Sussan and colleagues (2015) found 7×10^{11} free radicals per puff. In their mouse model, these free radicals caused oxidative stress and airway inflammation and disrupted antibacterial and antiviral responses. Lerner and colleagues (2015b) similarly detected free radicals in a popular e-cigarette brand. In examining unaerosolized e-liquids, the authors found tobacco flavors were weaker oxidizers than sweet or fruity flavors (Lerner et al., 2015b).

OTHER TOXICANTS

Volatile Organic Compounds and Phenols

Lim and Shin (2017) tested flavored e-liquids (n = 283), nicotine liquids (n = 21), and disposable cartridges (n = 12) and detected 14 VOCs, including alcohols. Specifically, they detected VOCs in the following concentration ranges: benzene (0.008–2.28 mg/L), toluene (0.006–0.687 mg/L), ethylbenzene (0.01–1.21 mg/L), *m*-xylene (0.002–1.13 mg/L), *p*-xylene (0.007–2.8 mg/L), *o*-xylene (0.004–2.27 mg/L), styrene (0.011–0.339 mg/L), ethyl acetate (0.3–669.9 mg/L), ethanol (16–38,742 mg/L), methanol (66–3,375 mg/L), pyridine (0.077–99.7 mg/L), acetylpyrazine (0.077–147 mg/L), 2,3,5-trimethylpyrazine (0.008–96.8 mg/L), and octamethylcyclotetrasiloxane (0.1–57.2 mg/L). According to the authors, the use of petrogenic hydrocarbons as a solvent in the extraction of flavor compounds and nicotine from natural plants may have produced benzene (classified as a Group 1 carcinogen by IARC), toluene, ethylbenzene, *m*-xylene, *p*-xylene, and *o*-xylene. The maximum detected concentrations of benzene, methanol, and ethanol in the samples were higher than their authorized maximum limits as residual solvents in pharmaceutical products. Farsalinos and colleagues (2015b) evaluated the presence of selected tobacco-derived chemicals in liquids produced by extracting flavor from cured tobacco leaves and found nitrate (levels varied from undetectable to 317.9 μg/ml) and small amounts of phenols (total average 1.5 μg/ml), including catechol, *m*-cresol and *o*-cresol, and phenol. Goniewicz and colleagues (2014) measured 11 VOCs in aerosol generated from 12 brands of e-cigarettes. Among 11 VOCs analyzed, only two (toluene and *m*- and *p*-xylene) were found in almost all examined e-cigarettes. The yields of toluene ranged from 0.2 mg to 6.3 mg per one e-cigarette (150 puffs). Although the *m*- and *p*-xylene levels found in analyzed samples of e-cigarette aerosol ranged from 0.1 mg to 0.2 mg/150 puffs, it was also found at the same level in blank samples.

Microorganisms and Residual Solvents

Varlet and colleagues (2015) analyzed 42 models from 14 brands of refill liquids for e-cigarettes for the presence of microorganisms, diethylene glycol, ethylene glycol, hydrocarbons, ethanol, and solvents. All of the products tested contained some potentially toxic compounds. The authors detected diethylene glycol, ethylene glycol, and ethanol at levels within limits permitted for food and pharmaceutical products. The authors also found terpenic compounds and residual solvents such as 1,3-butadiene, cyclohexane, and acetone in some products. In compliance with norms, none of the liquids contained yeast, mold, aerobic microbes, *Staphylococcus aureus*, or *Pseudomonas aeruginosa*.

Furans

The thermal degradation of sugars can produce toxic furans, such as 5-hydroxymethylfurfural and furfural. Furfural is known to cause irritation to the upper respiratory tract in humans (Arts et al., 2004), and both furanic compounds show tumorigenic activity in mice (Irwin, 1990; Surh and Tannenbaum, 1994; Surh et al., 1994). Soussy and colleagues (2016) investigated the formation of furanic compounds in e-cigarette aerosols using e-liquids of varying sweetener concentrations and devices under different power settings and puff durations. The authors detected both 5-hydroxymethylfurfural and furfural in the aerosols of sweet-flavored e-liquids. Levels of furans in the e-cigarette emissions were significantly correlated with power of the device and sweetener concentration, but not puff duration. The formation of furanic compounds from a sugar alcohol was negligible.

Phthalates

A recent study found diethyl phthalate (DEP) and diethylhexyl phthalate (DEHP) in e-liquids, although the quantified levels in the study's sample were below phthalate exposure limits (Oh and Shin, 2015). DEP can be a solvent or plasticizer and is found in variety of consumer products, including fragrances, cosmetics, and detergent bases. DEHP is a plasticizer often used in making polyvinyl chloride products. These antiandrogenic, estrogen-like compounds have been shown to initiate early breast development; IARC classifies DEHP as "possibly carcinogenic to humans" (IARC, 2000, p. 529). Researchers hypothesize that DEP and DEHP originated from the e-liquid packaging or during the e-liquid production process (Oh and Shin, 2015).

Caffeine

E-liquid flavors like coffee, tea, chocolate, and energy drinks, which are associated with having caffeine, often contain caffeine at concentrations significantly lower than their dietary counterparts. Lisko and colleagues (2015) measured caffeine concentrations in 44 flavored e-liquids from cartridges, disposables, and refill solutions. The researchers chose flavors traditionally associated with caffeine, marketed as energy boosters, or labeled as containing caffeine by the manufacturer. They detected caffeine in 42 percent of coffee-flavored products, 66 percent of tea-flavored products, and 50 percent of chocolate-flavored e-liquids in concentrations ranging from 3.3 µg/g to 703 µg/g. They did not detect caffeine in energy drink–flavored e-liquids. Eleven of 12 products marketed as energy enhancers contained caffeine in concentrations that varied substantially, ranging from 31.7 µg/g to 9,290 µg/g. Although the estimated caffeine exposures from e-cigarettes are at levels significantly lower than those from drinking caffeinated beverages, very little is known about the effects of caffeine inhalation, and health risks cannot be estimated.

Pharmaceutical Drugs

In addition to the toxicants described above, although rare, e-cigarette users may also be exposed to pharmacological components in their devices' e-liquids. For example, one study found evidence of a weight-loss medication (rimonabant), originally approved in Europe, in an analysis of e-liquids (Hadwiger et al., 2010). This treatment has been associated with adverse neurological events such as seizures and suicide, and is not approved by FDA (2007). Furthermore, this study also found e-liquid can contain an analogue (amino tadalafil) to the active ingredient in Cialis, an erectile dysfunction drug (Hadwiger et al., 2010). The potential exposure to medicinal compounds in some e-liquids places users at risk of experiencing undetermined or harmful health effects.

SYNTHESIS

- Many chemicals other than nicotine have been identified in liquids and aerosols generated from e-cigarettes.
- Compounds not listed on labels also have been identified in e-liquids.
- Several hazardous compounds have been found in liquids and in the heated aerosol produced by e-cigarettes, including formaldehyde, acetaldehyde, and acrolein, which are known carcinogenic toxicants.

- Of greater concern are the added flavorings that are considered safe for use in food, but have not been widely tested for sensitizing, toxic, or irritating potency.
- E-cigarettes are a source of extremely high particulate doses in the human respiratory system. Fine particles are emitted when humectants (mostly PG and glycerol) are aerosolized.[4]

Conclusion 5-1. There is ***conclusive evidence*** *that in addition to nicotine, most e-cigarette products contain and emit numerous potentially toxic substances.*

Conclusion 5-2. There is ***conclusive evidence*** *that, other than nicotine, the number, quantity, and characteristics of potentially toxic substances emitted from e-cigarettes are highly variable and depend on product characteristics (including device and e-liquid characteristics) and how the device is operated.*

Conclusion 5-3. There is ***substantial evidence*** *that except for nicotine, under typical conditions of use, exposure to potentially toxic substances from e-cigarettes is significantly lower compared with combustible tobacco cigarettes.*

METALS

As discussed above, research on the chemical constituents of e-cigarettes has generally focused on nicotine, the carcinogens formaldehyde and acetaldehyde, flavoring compounds, and particles. An increasing number of studies have also found toxic metals such as lead, nickel, and chromium in e-liquid emissions (Aherrera et al., 2017; Farsalinos et al., 2015b; Goniewicz et al., 2014; Hess et al., 2017; Lerner et al., 2015a; Mikheev et al., 2016; Williams et al., 2013, 2017). Metal exposure may originate from several parts of the device, including the metallic coil, a complex alloy that heats the e-liquid to produce the aerosol that is inhaled by the user (Aherrera et al., 2017; Hess et al., 2017; Olmedo et al., 2018; Williams et al., 2017). Other parts of the device, such as the joints and wires, could also contribute. For example, Kanthal, an alloy frequently used in e-cigarettes, contains aluminum, chromium, and iron. Other com-

[4] As described in Chapter 3, the particle count in e-cigarette aerosols may not be substantially different than mainstream combustible tobacco smoke. However, whereas e-cigarette aerosol particulate consists largely of aqueous droplets and vapors of humectants, particulate matter in combustible tobacco smoke are complex, largely organic constituents that include known or suspected carcinogens. Thus, it would be incorrect to assume that the long-term health risks of the two aerosols were similar just because particle count was similar.

mon alloys are Ni-200, which is made of nickel, and nichrome, which includes chromium and nickel. Furthermore, metals such as tin have been found in the joints (Williams et al., 2017). E-liquids may also contain metals at varying concentrations. For instance, some e-liquid solutions contain arsenic (Beauval et al., 2016; Mikheev et al., 2016).

A small number of studies have investigated the role of e-cigarette aerosols in metal exposure. Most of these studies have evaluated one or two devices to measure metals in e-cigarette emissions and assess which metals are in higher concentrations compared with other metals, as well as to compare metals found in e-cigarette emissions and tobacco smoke. For example, Saffari and colleagues (2014) used quartz filters to study emission rates of a European tank-style device and found evidence of several metals. The authors detected boron (mean emission rate, ng/h: 964), cadmium (0.480), chromium (28.1), lanthanum (3.21), lead (96.2), nickel (131), potassium (7,765), silver (20.9), titanium (50.2), and zinc (1,142), but did not identify aluminum, copper, iron, or tin. However, the particle-sampling method the authors used in this study could have failed to distinguish metals during the aerosol phase. A study by Goniewicz and colleagues (2014) assessed metal concentrations in aerosols from a pharmaceutical nicotine inhaler and 12 e-cigarettes. Metals, including cadmium (concentrations varied from undetectable to 0.22 µg/150 puffs), lead (0.03 to 0.57 µg/150 puffs), and nickel (0.11 to 0.29 µg/150 puffs), were found in most of the samples tested. Mikheev and colleagues (2016) used quartz filters and inductively coupled plasma mass spectrometry to study metals in aerosols from a tank-style device and cigalike products. The authors measured antimony (0.05 to 0.50 ng/mg), arsenic (0.01 to 0.70 ng/mg), chromium (0.40 to 5.0 ng/mg), copper (0.05 to 5.0 ng/mg), nickel (0.05 to 5.0 ng/mg), tin (0.02 to 0.50 ng/mg), and zinc (1.50 to 50.0 ng/mg) in most samples, but did not measure lead. In another study, Williams and colleagues (2013) detected aluminum, iron, nickel, silver, and tin in particles greater than 1 µm from one brand's 22 cigalike cartomizers; nanoparticles (less than 100 nm) had chromium, nickel, and tin. The authors also used inductively coupled plasma optical emission spectrometry to identify lead (0.017 µg/10 puffs).

One of the key hypotheses is that metals in the coil leach during the heating process into the generated aerosol. For instance, Williams and colleagues (2013) describe the coil in their study of 22 cartomizers as a nickel-chromium filament soldered with tin to a thicker, silver-coated copper wire. The thick, copper-silver wire was also attached to the air tube and mouthpiece at tin solder joints. The same study group detected 35 of 36 selected elements in electronic hookahs and disposable e-cigarettes; in comparison, the authors found 15 of these elements in combustible tobacco cigarette smoke (Williams et al., 2017). Some metals, like copper, lead, nickel, and tin, were quantified at significantly higher concentrations in e-cigarette aerosols than combustible tobacco smoke, while levels of cadmium were lower. In an analysis of disposable e-cigarette wires and joints using electron microscopy and energy-dispersive X-ray spectroscopy, nickel, chromium, copper, silver, zinc, iron, aluminum, tin, calcium, and lead were clearly detected in different parts of the device (see Figure 5-3).

While many of the studies on e-cigarettes and metals have been done with first- or second-generation devices, a recent study has compared metal concentrations in e-liquid before being in contact with the device to metal concentrations in the aerosol generated after heating the coil of 56 modified e-cigarette devices from daily e-cigarette users (Olmedo et al., 2018). In the study, major increases in metal concentrations were found in aerosol samples compared with e-liquid samples for lead and zinc (increases greater than 2,000 percent) and chromium, nickel, and tin (increases greater than 600 percent). The finding of lead in e-cigarette aerosol samples, a metal not listed among the components of heating coils but that can be present in metal alloys or may be in some other parts of the device, can be of concern. Aerosol mass concentrations for the detected metals (nickel, chromium, lead, and manganese) spanned several orders of magnitude and exceeded current occupational or environmental standards for 50 percent of samples or more. In that study, 10 percent of the e-liquid samples had detectable arsenic concentrations, and the levels remained similar in the aerosol (Olmedo et al., 2018).

FIGURE 5-3 Scanning electron microscopy and energy dispersive X-ray spectroscopy analysis of disposable e-cigarette/e-hookah wires and joints.

NOTES: (A) Scanning electron micrograph of the clamp joining thick and thin wires (red arrow) in BluCig. The filaments (0.13 mm) were usually comprised of nickel (B) and chromium (C) as shown for BluCig. For all brands, the thick wire (0.33 mm) was comprised of copper (D) and silver (E). The clamps in all brands were comprised of copper (D) and zinc (F) (2.4 mm). The filament (0.11 mm) from Square 82 was unusual in that it was comprised of chromium (G), iron (H), and aluminum (I). In some brands, the thick wire and filament were joined by tin solder. The solder joint (J) (1 mm) in Square 82 was comprised of tin (K) and calcium (L). The solder joint (M) (1.8 mm) between the thick wire and filament in Imperial Hookah was comprised of tin (N) and lead (O). The solder joint (P) (2 mm) between the thick wire and filament in Luxury Lites was comprised of tin (Q) and lead (R). (S) Example of poorly manufactured solder joints, comprised of tin (T) (0.78 mm) in most e-cigarette/e-hookah brands. White arrow = filament (thin wire); Orange arrow = thick wire; Red arrow = joints between the thick and thin wires.

SOURCE: Williams et al., 2017.

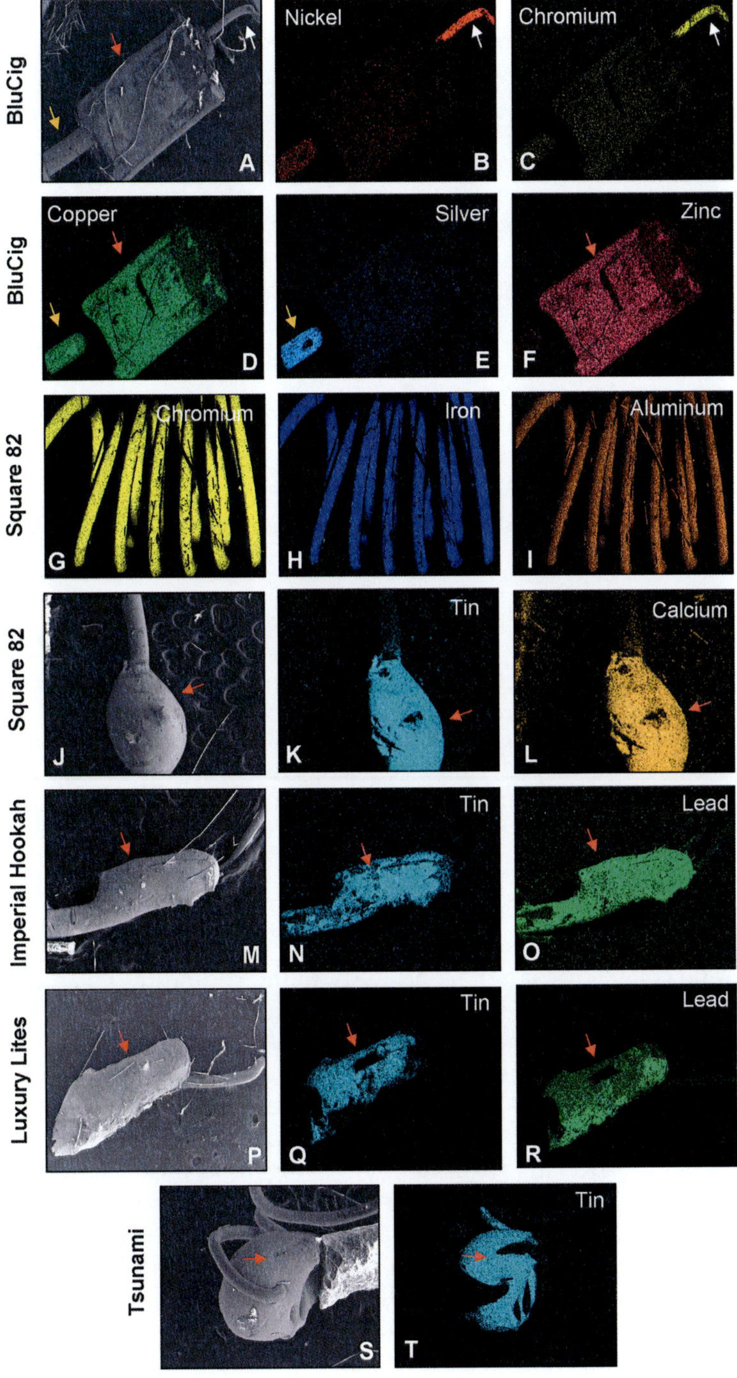
BluCig
A
Nickel
B
Chromium
C
BluCig
Copper
D
Silver
E
Zinc
F
Square 82
Chromium
G
Iron
H
Aluminum
I
Square 82
J
Tin
K
Calcium
L
Imperial Hookah
M
Tin
N
Lead
O
Luxury Lites
P
Tin
Q
Lead
R
Tsunami
S
Tin
T

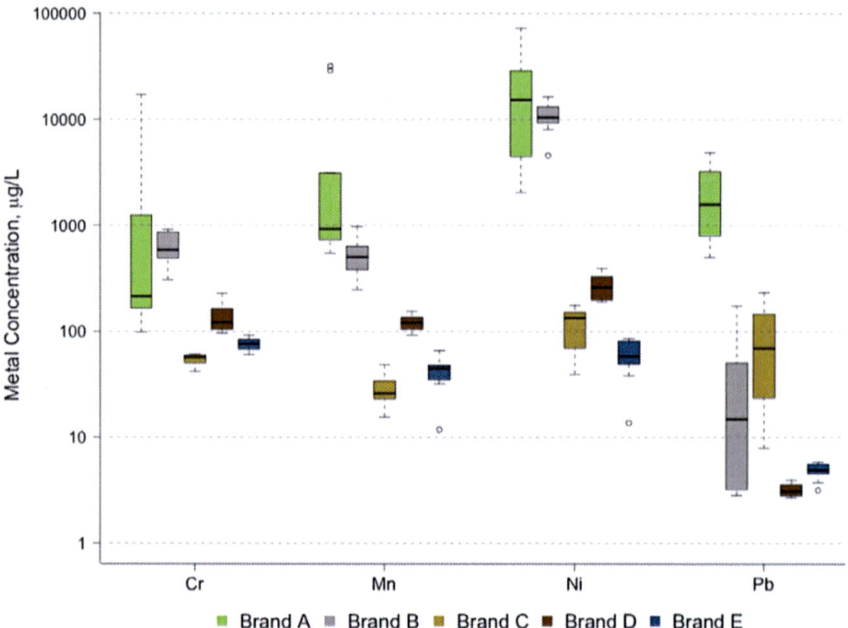

FIGURE 5-4 Distribution of metal concentrations within and across brands of disposable e-cigalike devices.
NOTES: Horizontal lines within boxes indicate medians; boxes, interquartile ranges; error bars, values within 1.5 times the interquartile range; solid circles, outlying data points. Cr = chromium; Mn = manganese; Ni = nickel; Pb = lead.
SOURCE: Hess et al., 2017.

E-liquids may also acquire metals after they come in contact with e-cigarette coils. For example, one study found cadmium (mean concentration varied from 0.42 to 205 μg/L), chromium (53.9 to 2,110 μg/L), lead (4.89 to 1,970 μg/L), manganese (28.7 to 6,910 μg/L), and nickel (0.059 to 22.6 μg/L) in e-liquids touching unused cartomizer coils from five different cigalike brands (Hess et al., 2017). By measuring five devices of each of five brands, this study illustrates the substantial variability within and across brands, especially for chromium, manganese, nickel, and lead (see Figure 5-4). Beauval and colleagues (2016) found generally low concentrations of metals in a study of e-liquids, with the exceptions of copper, nickel, and zinc (20, 16, and 200 μ/L, respectively). Furthermore, arsenic was measured in 57 percent of samples (mean concentration of 1.57 μg/L).

So far, only one published study has compared metal concentrations in e-cigarette emissions to metal biomarker concentrations in an e-cigarette study. In that study, conducted among 64 daily e-cigarette users (59 using second- and third-generation devices and 5 using first-generation cigalikes), the levels of chromium and nickel were measured in several samples collected from the e-cigarette device (dispenser, aerosol, and tank) used by the participant, as well as in several biomarkers collected non-invasively: urine, saliva, and exhaled breath condensate (EBC); and data on e-cigarette use (Aherrera et al., 2017). Median nickel and chromium levels were 0.73 and 0.39 μg/g creatinine, respectively, in urine; 2.25 and 1.53 μg/L in saliva; and 1.25 and 0.29 μg/L in EBC. In adjusted models, tertiles 2 and 3 of aerosol nickel concentrations were associated with 16 percent and 72 percent higher urine nickel and 202 percent and 321 percent higher saliva nickel compared with the lowest tertile. Tertile 3 of aerosol chromium levels was associated with 193 percent higher saliva chromium. An earlier time to first vape in the morning and more frequent coil change were associated with higher urine nickel. Tertile 2 of e-liquid consumption per week and voltage were associated with higher saliva nickel levels than tertile 1. Therefore, this study presents evidence that participants' internal doses of chromium and nickel were positively associated with e-cigarette aerosol concentrations. Additional research is needed to evaluate the association between metal levels in e-cigarette emissions and metal biomarkers, as well as comparing metal biomarker levels in e-cigarette users and a comparable group of non-users.

Exposure to metals through e-cigarettes is relevant as certain metals can cause serious health effects. For example, lead exposure is associated with neurotoxicity (Garza et al., 2006) and cardiovascular disease (Navas-Acien et al., 2007), and chromium(VI) and nickel have been associated with respiratory diseases such as lung cancer (IARC, 2012, 2017; Jaishankar et al., 2014). Nickel can also induce an allergic response in some individuals. Several cases of nickel-induced allergic dermatitis have been related to e-cigarette use (Maridet et al., 2015; Ormerod and Stone, 2017). Another concern is that metal absorption is markedly higher through inhalation, as compared with ingestion, and that while some of the metals found in e-cigarette aerosol are essential elements when ingested (zinc, manganese, copper, and chromium[III]), exposure to these metals through inhalation tends to be toxic (Goyer and Lavoie, 2001; Tchounwou et al., 2012). For chromium, no study has measured the valence state and it is currently unknown if the form of chromium in the aerosol is chromium(III) or chromium(VI). The implications could be major as chromium(VI) is an established carcinogen.

Few studies have measured the toxic characteristics of metals in e-cigarette aerosols, although in principle, metal toxicity would not necessarily change compared with metal exposure from other sources. In one of the few studies testing this metal e-cigarette toxicity, an in vitro study of copper nanoparticles from e-cigarette aerosols, it was found that copper nanoparticles increased mitochondrial oxidative stress and DNA fragmentation, supporting their critical toxic role (Lerner et al., 2016). Metals have also been involved as one possible reason explaining cellular damage, generation of ROS, and activation of global defense systems observed in vitro experiments (Bharadwaj et al., 2017; Lerner et al., 2015a).

Limitations of the current research include the small number of studies, the small sample size, the evaluation mostly of first-generation devices, the limited investigation on which characteristics of the device and patterns of use (e.g., wattage, temperature) could be major contributors of exposure, and the evaluation of devices that are selected by the investigators but which do not necessarily reflect what the consumers are using. Only one study has measured metal biomarkers in e-cigarette users, comparing chromium and nickel concentrations in e-liquid and e-cigarettes aerosols obtained from the participant's devices (mostly tank-style and mod devices) to the corresponding metal biomarker (Aherrera et al., 2017).

Synthesis

An increasing but still limited number of studies have detected metals in e-liquid and aerosol samples generated by e-cigarette devices. Some of the key metals include chromium, nickel, lead, manganese, aluminum, tin, and iron. The coils and other parts of the device could be a source of metals, which could be leaking to the aerosol. Cadmium, which is a metal typically found in e-cigarettes, is found at a markedly lower level than in combustible tobacco cigarettes. However, the number of metals appears to be large, even larger than for combustible tobacco cigarettes. There is also substantial variability in metal levels, which can be substantially high in some instances. Overall the number of studies is small and the relevance for tank-style and mod devices is limited, as most studies have assessed first- and second-generation devices. One biomarker study evaluating e-cigarette devices actually used by the users supports that metals can be inhaled, contributing to metal internal dose, at least for chromium and nickel. While it is well established that metals are highly toxic for multiple organs and systems through inhalation, no studies have evaluated the specific health effects of metals in e-cigarettes, except in the study of copper nanoparticles from e-cigarettes and mitochondrial oxidative stress and DNA fragmentation.

> *Conclusion 5-4. There is* ***substantial evidence*** *that e-cigarette aerosol contains metals. The origin of the metals could be the metallic coil used to heat the e-liquid, other parts of the e-cigarette device, or e-liquids.*

Product characteristics and use patterns may contribute to differences in the actual metals and metal concentrations measured in e-cigarette aerosol.

*Conclusion 5-5. There is **limited evidence** that the number of metals in e-cigarette aerosol could be greater than the number of metals in combustible tobacco cigarettes, except for cadmium, which is markedly lower in e-cigarettes compared with combustible tobacco cigarettes.*

REFERENCES

Aberer, W., T. Fuchs, K. P. Peters, and P. J. Frosch. 1993. Propylene glycol: Cutaneous side effects and test methods. Literature and results of a multicenter study of the German contact allergy group (DKG). *Dermatosen in Beruf und Unwelt* 41:25–27.

AEMSA (American E-Liquid Manufacturing Standards Association). 2014. *E-liquid manufacturing standards*. http://www.aemsa.org/wp-content/uploads/2014/02/AEMSA-Standards_Version-1-8.pdf (accessed October 9, 2017).

Aherrera, A., P. Olmedo, M. Grau-Perez, S. Tanda, W. Goessler, S. Jarmul, R. Chen, J. E. Cohen, A. M. Rule, and A. Navas-Acien. 2017. The association of e-cigarette use with exposure to nickel and chromium: A preliminary study of non-invasive biomarkers. *Environmental Research* 159:313–320.

Ahijevych, K., and B. E. Garrett. 2004. Menthol pharmacology and its potential impact on cigarette smoking behavior. *Nicotine & Tobacco Research* 6(Supplement 1):S17–S28. https://doi.org/10.1080/14622200310001649469 (accessed February 6, 2018).

Ahijevych, K., and B. E. Garrett. 2010. The role of menthol in cigarettes as a reinforcer of smoking behavior. *Nicotine & Tobacco Research* 12(Supplement 2):S110–S116. https://doi.org/10.1093/ntr/ntq203 (accessed February 6, 2018).

Allen, J. G., S. S. Flanigan, M. LeBlanc, J. Vallarino, P. MacNaughton, J. H. Stewart, and D. C. Christiani. 2016. Flavoring chemicals in e-cigarettes: Diacetyl, 2,3-pentanedione, and acetoin in a sample of 51 products, including fruit-, candy-, and cocktail-flavored e-cigarettes. *Environmental Health Perspectives* 124(6):733–739.

Arbour, R., and B. Esparis. 2000. Osmolar gap metabolic acidosis in a 60-year-old man treated for hypoxemic respiratory failure. *Chest* 118(2):545–546.

Arts, J. H., H. Muijser, M. J. Appel, C. Frieke Kuper, J. G. Bessems, and R. A. Woutersen. 2004. Subacute (28-day) toxicity of furfural in Fischer 344 rats: A comparison of the oral and inhalation route. *Food and Chemical Toxicology* 42(9):1389–1399.

Arulanantham, K., and M. Genel. 1978. Central nervous system toxicity associated with ingestion of propylene glycol. *Journal of Pediatrics* 93(3):515–516.

ATSDR (Agency for Toxic Substances and Disease Registry). 2007. *Acrolein*. https://www.atsdr.cdc.gov/toxfaqs/tfacts124.pdf (accessed December 22, 2017).

Audrain-McGovern, J., A. A. Strasser, and E. P. Wileyto. 2016. The impact of flavoring on the rewarding and reinforcing value of e-cigarettes with nicotine among young adult smokers. *Drug and Alcohol Dependence* 166:263–267.

Barrington-Trimis, J. L., R. Urman, A. M. Leventhal, W. J. Gauderman, T. B. Cruz, T. D. Gilreath, S. Howland, J. B. Unger, K. Berhane, J. M. Samet, and R. McConnell. 2016. E-cigarettes, cigarettes, and the prevalence of adolescent tobacco use. *Pediatrics* 138(2):e20153983. http://pediatrics.aappublications.org/content/138/2/e20153983 (accessed February 6, 2018).

Beauval, N., M. Howsam, S. Anthérieu, D. Allorge, M. Soyez, G. Garçon, J. F. Goossens, J. M. Lo-Guidice, and A. Garat. 2016. Trace elements in e-liquids—Development and validation of an ICP-MS method for the analysis of electronic cigarette refills. *Regulatory Toxicology and Pharmacology* 79:144–148.

Behar, R. Z., W. T. Luo, S. C. Lin, Y. H. Wang, J. Valle, J. F. Pankow, and P. Talbot. 2016. Distribution, quantification and toxicity of cinnamaldehyde in electronic cigarette refill fluids and aerosols. *Tobacco Control* 25:ii94–ii102. http://dx.doi.org/10.1136/tobaccocontrol-2016-053224 (February 6, 2018).

Bekki, K., S. Uchiyama, K. Ohta, Y. Inaba, H. Nakagome, and N. Kunugita. 2014. Carbonyl compounds generated from electronic cigarettes. *International Journal of Environmental Research and Public Health* 11(11):11192–11200.

Berg, C. J. 2016. Preferred flavors and reasons for e-cigarette use and discontinued use among never, current, and former smokers. *International Journal of Public Health* 61(2):225–236.

Bharadwaj, S., R. J. Mitchell, A. Qureshi, and J. H. Niazi. 2017. Toxicity evaluation of e-juice and its soluble aerosols generated by electronic cigarettes using recombinant bioluminescent bacteria responsive to specific cellular damages. *Biosensors and Bioelectronics* 90:53–60.

Blair, S. L., S. A. Epstein, S. A. Nizkorodov, and N. Staimer. 2015. A real-time fast-flow tube study of VOC and particulate emissions from electronic, potentially reduced-harm, conventional, and reference cigarettes. *Aerosol Science and Technology* 49(9):816–827.

Bornmann, G. 1954. Grundwirkungen der glykile und ihre bedeutung für die toxizatät. *Arzneimittelforschung* 4:643–646.

Bortz, W. M., P. Paul, A. C. Haff, and W. L. Holmes. 1972. Glycerol turnover and oxidation in man. *Journal of Clinical Investigation* 51(6):1537–1546.

Braun, H. A., and G. F. Cartland. 1936. The toxicity of propylene glycol. *Journal of the American Pharmacists Association* 25(9):746–749.

Burstyn, I. 2014. Peering through the mist: Systematic review of what the chemistry of contaminants in electronic cigarettes tells us about health risks. *BMC Public Health* 14:18. https://doi.org/10.1186/1471-2458-14-18 (accessed February 6, 2018).

Canistro, D., F. Vivarelli, S. Cirillo, C. Babot Marquillas, A. Buschini, M. Lazzaretti, L. Marchi, V. Cardenia, M. T. Rodriguez-Estrada, M. Lodovici, C. Cipriani, A. Lorenzini, E. Croco, S. Marchionni, P. Franchi, M. Lucarini, V. Longo, C. M. Della Croce, A. Vornoli, A. Colacci, M. Vaccari, A. Sapone, and M. Paolini. 2017. E-cigarettes induce toxicological effects that can raise the cancer risk. *Scientific Reports* 7(1):2028.

Carmines, E. L., and C. L. Gaworski. 2005. Toxicological evaluation of glycerin as a cigarette ingredient. *Food and Chemical Toxicology* 43(10):1521–1539.

Catanzaro, J. M., and J. G. Smith, Jr. 1991. Propylene glycol dermatitis. *Journal of the American Academy of Dermatology* 24(1):90–95.

Cheng, T. R. 2014. Chemical evaluation of electronic cigarettes. *Tobacco Control* 23:11–17.

Choi, H., N. Schmidbauer, J. Spengler, and C. G. Bornehag. 2010. Sources of propylene glycol and glycol ethers in air at home. *International Journal of Environmental Research and Public Health* 7(12):4213–4237.

CIR (Cosmetic Ingredient Review). 2014. *Safety assessment of glycerin as used in cosmetics: Draft report for panel review*. https://www.cir-safety.org/sites/default/files/glycerin.pdf (accessed January 2, 2018).

CIR. 2015. *Safety assessment of glycerin as used in cosmetics: Final report*. http://www.cir-safety.org/sites/default/files/glycer_122014_FR.pdf (accessed September 29, 2017).

Clark, C. R., T. C. Marshall, B. S. Merickel, A. Sanchez, D. G. Brownstein, and C. H. Hobbs. 1979. Toxicological assessment of heat transfer fluids proposed for use in solar energy applications. *Toxicology and Applied Pharmacology* 51(3):529–535.

Clayton, G. E., and F. E. Clayton, eds. 1995. *Patty's industrial hygiene and toxicology. Volume 2E: Toxicology*, 4th edition. New York: Wiley.

Czoli, C. D., M. Goniewicz, T. Islam, K. Kotnowski, and D. Hammond. 2016. Consumer preferences for electronic cigarettes: Results from a discrete choice experiment. *Tobacco Control* 25(e1):e30–e36. http://tobaccocontrol.bmj.com/content/25/e1/e30 (accessed February 6, 2018).

Domej, W., K. Oettl, and W. Renner. 2014. Oxidative stress and free radicals in COPD—Implications and relevance for treatment. *International Journal of Chronic Obstructive Pulmonary Disease* 9:1207–1224.

Doolittle, D. J., D. A. Lee, and C. K. Lee. 1988. The genotoxic activity of glycerol in an in vitro test battery. *Food and Chemical Toxicology* 26(7):631–635.

Etter, J. F. 2016. Throat hit in users of the electronic cigarette: An exploratory study. *Psychology of Addictive Behaviors* 30(1):93–100.

Etter, J. F., E. Zather, and S. Svensson. 2013. Analysis of refill liquids for electronic cigarettes. *Addiction* 108(9):1671–1679.

Farley, S. M., H. Seoh, R. Sacks, and M. Johns. 2014. Teen use of flavored tobacco products in New York City. *Nicotine & Tobacco Research* 16(11):1518–1521.

Farsalinos, K. E., G. Romagna, D. Tsiapras, S. Kyrzopoulos, A. Spyrou, and V. Voudris. 2013. Impact of flavour variability on electronic cigarette use experience: An Internet survey. *International Journal of Environmental Research and Public Health* 10(12):7272–7282.

Farsalinos, E. K., G. Gillman, K. Poulas, and V. Voudris. 2015a. Tobacco-specific nitrosamines in electronic cigarettes: Comparison between liquid and aerosol levels. *International Journal of Environmental Research and Public Health* 12(8):9046–9053.

Farsalinos, K. E., I. G. Gillman, M. S. Melvin, A. R. Paolantonio, W. J. Gardow, K. E. Humphries, S. E. Brown, K. Poulas, and V. Voudris. 2015b. Nicotine levels and presence of selected tobacco-derived toxins in tobacco flavoured electronic cigarette refill liquids. *International Journal of Environmental Research and Public Health* 12(4):3439–3452.

Farsalinos, K. E., K. A. Kistler, G. Gillman, and V. Voudris. 2015c. Evaluation of electronic cigarette liquids and aerosol for the presence of selected inhalation toxins. *Nicotine & Tobacco Research* 17(2):168–174.

FDA (Food and Drug Administration). 2007. *FDA briefing document: NDA 21-888 Zimulti (rimonabant) tablets, 20 mg*. https://www.fda.gov/ohrms/dockets/ac/07/briefing/2007-4306b1-fda-backgrounder.pdf (accessed October 9, 2017).

FDRL (Food and Drug Research Laboratories, Inc.). 1973. *Teratologic evaluation of FDA 71-56 (propylene glycol) in mice, rats, hamsters and rabbits*. Waverly, NY: FDRL.

Feirman, S. P., D. Lock, J. E. Cohen, D. R. Holtgrave, and T. J. Li. 2016. Flavored tobacco products in the United States: A systematic review assessing use and attitudes. *Nicotine & Tobacco Research* 18(5):739–749.

FEMA (Flavor and Extract Manufacturers Association of the United States). 2015. *The safety assessment and regulatory authority to use flavors—Focus on e-cigarettes*. https://www.femaflavor.org/sites/default/files/FEMAGRAS_Ecig_March_3_2015.pdf (accessed October 4, 2017).

Fligner, C. L., R. Jack, G. A. Twiggs, and V. A. Raisys. 1985. Hyperosmolality induced by propylene glycol. A complication of silver sulfadiazine therapy. *Journal of the American Medical Association* 253(11):1606–1609.

Flora, J. W., N. Meruva, C. B. Huang, C. T. Wilkinson, R. Ballentine, D. C. Smith, M. S. Werley, and W. J. McKinney. 2016. Characterization of potential impurities and degradation products in electronic cigarette formulations and aerosols. *Regulatory Toxicology and Pharmacology* 74:1–11.

Flora, J. W., C. T. Wilkinson, J. W. Wilkinson, P. J. Lipowicz, J. A. Skapars, A. Anderson, and J. H. Miller. 2017. Method for the determination of carbonyl compounds in e-cigarette aerosols. *Journal of Chromatographic Science* 55(2):142–148.

Fransway, A. F., K. A. Zug, D. V. Belsito, V. A. Deleo, J. F. Fowler, Jr., H. I. Maibach, J. G. Marks, C. G. Mathias, M. D. Pratt, R. L. Rietschel, D. Sasseville, F. J. Storrs, J. S. Taylor, E. M. Warshaw, J. Dekoven, and M. Zirwas. 2013. North American Contact Dermatitis Group patch test results for 2007–2008. *Dermatitis* 24(1):10–21.

Funk, J. O., and H. I. Maibach. 1994. Propylene glycol dermatitis: Re-evaluation of an old problem. *Contact Dermatitis* 31(4):236–241.

Gad, S. C., C. D. Cassidy, N. Aubert, B. Spainhour, and H. Robbe. 2006. Nonclinical vehicle use in studies by multiple routes in multiple species. *International Journal of Toxicology* 25(6):499–521.

Garten, S., and R. V. Falkner. 2004. Role of mentholated cigarettes in increased nicotine dependence and greater risk of tobacco-attributable disease. *Preventive Medicine* 38(6): 793–798.

Garza, A., R. Vega, and E. Soto. 2006. Cellular mechanisms of lead neurotoxicity. *Medical Science Monitor* 12(3):RA57–RA65.

Geiss, O., I. Bianchi, and J. Barrero-Moreno. 2016. Correlation of volatile carbonyl yields emitted by e-cigarettes with the temperature of the heating coil and the perceived sensorial quality of the generated vapours. *International Journal of Hygiene and Environmental Health* 219(3):268–277.

Gillman, I. G., K. A. Kistler, E. W. Stewart, and A. R. Paolantonio. 2016. Effect of variable power levels on the yield of total aerosol mass and formation of aldehydes in e-cigarette aerosols. *Regulatory Toxicology and Pharmacology* 75:58–65.

Goel, R., E. Durand, N. Trushin, B. Prokopczyk, J. Foulds, R. J. Elias, and J. P. Richie, Jr. 2015. Highly reactive free radicals in electronic cigarette aerosols. *Chemical Research in Toxicology* 28(9):1675-1677.

Gomes, R., R. Liteplo, and M. E. Meek. 2002. *Concise International Chemical Assessment Document #45: Ethylene glycol: Human health aspects*. Geneva, Switzerland: World Health Organization.

Goniewicz, M. L., J. Knysak, M. Gawron, L. Kosmider, A. Sobczak, J. Kurek, A. Prokopowicz, M. Jablonska-Czapla, C. Rosik-Dulewska, C. Havel, I. P. Jacob, and N. Benowitz. 2014. Levels of selected carcinogens and toxicants in vapour from electronic cigarettes. *Tobacco Control* 23(2):133–139.

Gorrod, J. W., and P. Jacob. 1999. *Analytical determination of nicotine and related compounds and their metabolites*, 1st edition. Amsterdam, The Netherlands, and New York: Elsevier.

Goyer, N., and J. Lavoie. 2001. Emissions of chemical compounds and bioaerosols during the secondary treatment of paper mill effluents. *American Industrial Hygiene Association Journal* 62(3):330–341.

Guthery, W. 2016. Emissions of toxic carbonyls in an electronic cigarette. *Beitrage zur Tabakforschung International/Contributions to Tobacco Research* 27(1):30–37.

Hadwiger, M. E., M. L. Trehy, W. Ye, T. Moore, J. Allgire, and B. Westenberger. 2010. Identification of amino-tadalafil and rimonabant in electronic cigarette products using high pressure liquid chromatography with diode array and tandem mass spectrometric detection. *Journal of Chromatography A* 1217(48):7547–7555.

Hahn, J., Y. B. Monakhova, J. Hengen, M. Kohl-Himmelseher, J. Schössler, H. Hahn, T. Kuballa, and D. W. Lachenmeier. 2014. Electronic cigarettes: Overview of chemical composition and exposure estimation. *Tobacco Induced Diseases* 12(1):23.

Hansen, L., R. Lange, and S. Gupta. 2015. Development and evaluation of a guideline for monitoring propylene glycol toxicity in pediatric intensive care unit patients receiving continuous infusion lorazepam. *Journal of Pediatric Pharmacology and Therapeutics* 20(5):367–372.

Haworth, S., T. Lawlor, K. Mortelmans, W. Speck, and E. Zeiger. 1983. *Salmonella* mutagenicity test results for 250 chemicals. *Environmental Mutagenesis* 5(Supplement 1):1–142. https://doi.org/10.1002/em.2860050703 (accessed February 6, 2018).

Health Council of the Netherlands. 2007. *Propylene glycol (1,2-propanediol): Health-based recommended occupational exposure limit.* https://www.gezondheidsraad.nl/sites/default/files/200702osh_propylene_glycol.pdf (accessed October 3, 2017).

Hecht, S. S. 1998. Biochemistry, biology, and carcinogenicity of tobacco-specific *N*-nitrosamines. *Chemical Research in Toxicology* 11(6):559–603.

Hecht, S. S., and D. Hoffmann. 1988. Tobacco-specific nitrosamines, an important group of carcinogens in tobacco and tobacco smoke. *Carcinogenesis* 9(6):875–884.

Herrington, J. S., and C. Myers. 2015. Electronic cigarette solutions and resultant aerosol profiles. *Journal of Chromatography A* 1418:192–199.

Hess, C. A., P. Olmedo, A. Navas-Acien, W. Goessler, J. E. Cohen, and A. M. Rule. 2017. E-cigarettes as a source of toxic and potentially carcinogenic metals. *Environmental Research* 152:221–225.

HHS (U.S. Department of Health and Human Services). 2010. *How tobacco smoke causes disease: The biology and behavioral basis for smoking-attributable disease: A report of the Surgeon General.* Atlanta, GA: U.S. Department of Health and Human Services, Centers for Disease Control and Prevention, National Center for Chronic Disease Prevention and Health Promotion, Office on Smoking and Health.

HHS. 2015. *Select committee on GRAS substances (SCOGS) opinion: Propylene glycol and propylene glycol monostearate.* https://www.fda.gov/food/ingredientspackaginglabeling/gras/scogs/ucm261045.htm (accessed September 28, 2017).

Hutzler, C., M. Paschke, S. Kruschinski, F. Henkler, J. Hahn, and A. Luch. 2014. Chemical hazards present in liquids and vapors of electronic cigarettes. *Archives of Toxicology* 88(7):1295–1308.

IARC (International Agency for Research on Cancer). 2000. *IARC monographs on the evaluation of carcinogenic risks to humans, Volume 77: Some industrial chemicals.* http://publications.iarc.fr/Book-And-Report-Series/Iarc-Monographs-On-The-Evaluation-Of-Carcinogenic-Risks-To-Humans/Some-Industrial-Chemicals-2000 (accessed October 19, 2017).

IARC. 2012. *Chromium(VI) compounds.* https://monographs.iarc.fr/ENG/Monographs/vol100C/mono100C-9.pdf (accessed September 29, 2017).

IARC. 2017. *Nickel and nickel compounds.* http://monographs.iarc.fr/ENG/Monographs/vol100C/mono100C-10.pdf (accessed September 29, 2017).

Irwin, R. 1990. *Toxicology and carcinogenesis: Studies of furfural (CAS no. 98-01-1) in F344/N rats and B6C3F1 mice (gavage studies).* Research Triangle Park, NC: National Toxicology Program. https://ntp.niehs.nih.gov/ntp/htdocs/lt_rpts/tr382.pdf (accessed February 6, 2018).

Ishidate, M., Jr., T. Sofuni, K. Yoshikawa, M. Hayashi, T. Nohmi, M. Sawada, and A. Matsuoka. 1984. Primary mutagenicity screening of food additives currently used in Japan. *Food and Chemical Toxicology* 22(8):623–636.

Jaishankar, M., T. Tseten, N. Anbalagan, B. B. Mathew, and K. N. Beeregowda. 2014. Toxicity, mechanism and health effects of some heavy metals. *Interdisciplinary Toxicology* 7(2):60–72.

Jensen, R. P., W. Luo, J. F. Pankow, R. M. Strongin, and D. H. Peyton. 2015. Hidden formaldehyde in e-cigarette aerosols. *New England Journal of Medicine* 372(4):392–394.

Kavlock, R. J., R. D. Short, Jr., and N. Chernoff. 1987. Further evaluation of an in vivo teratology screen. *Teratogenesis, Carcinogenesis, and Mutagenesis* 7(1):7–16.

Kehrer, J. P., and L.-O. Klotz. 2015. Free radicals and related reactive species as mediators of tissue injury and disease: Implications for health. *Critical Reviews in Toxicology* 45(9):765–798.

Kelner, M. J., and D. N. Bailey. 1985. Propylene glycol as a cause of lactic acidosis. *Journal of Analytical Toxicology* 9(1):40–42.

Khlystov, A., and V. Samburova. 2016. Flavoring compounds dominate toxic aldehyde production during e-cigarette vaping. *Environmental Science & Technology* 50(23):13080–13085.

Kienhuis, A. S., L. G. Soeteman-Hernandez, P. M. Bos, H. W. Cremers, W. N. Klerx, and R. Talhout. 2015. Potential harmful health effects of inhaling nicotine-free shisha-pen vapor: A chemical risk assessment of the main components propylene glycol and glycerol. *Tobacco Induced Diseases* 13(1):15. https://doi.org/10.1186/s12971-015-0038-7 (accessed March 1, 2018).

Kim, H. J., and H. S. Shin. 2013. Determination of tobacco-specific nitrosamines in replacement liquids of electronic cigarettes by liquid chromatography–tandem mass spectrometry. *Journal of Chromatography A* 1291:48–55.

King, B. A., M. A. Tynan, S. R. Dube, and R. Arrazola. 2014. Flavored-little-cigar and flavored-cigarette use among U.S. middle and high school students. *Journal of Adolescent Health* 54(1):40–46.

Kirkham, P., and I. Rahman. 2006. Oxidative stress in asthma and COPD: Antioxidants as a therapeutic strategy. *Pharmacology & Therapeutics* 111(2):476–494.

Konradova, V., V. Vavrova, and J. Janota. 1978. Effect of the inhalation of a surface tension-reducing substance (propylene glycol) on the ultrastructure of epithelium of the respiratory passages in rabbits. *Folia Morphologica (Praha)* 26(1):28–34.

Kosmider, L., A. Sobczak, M. Fik, J. Knysak, M. Zaciera, J. Kurek, and M. L. Goniewicz. 2014. Carbonyl compounds in electronic cigarette vapors: Effects of nicotine solvent and battery output voltage. *Nicotine & Tobacco Research* 16(10):1319–1326.

Kosmider, L., A. Sobczak, A. Prokopowicz, J. Kurek, M. Zaciera, J. Knysak, D. Smith, and M. L. Goniewicz. 2016. Cherry-flavoured electronic cigarettes expose users to the inhalation irritant, benzaldehyde. *Thorax* 71(4):376–377.

Kowitt, S. D., C. Meernik, H. M. Baker, A. Osman, L. L. Huang, and A. O. Goldstein. 2017. Perceptions and experiences with flavored non-menthol tobacco products: A systematic review of qualitative studies. *International Journal of Environmental Research and Public Health* 14(4):338.

Kreiss, K., A. Gomaa, G. Kullman, K. Fedan, E. J. Simoes, and P. L. Enright. 2002. Clinical bronchiolitis obliterans in workers at a microwave-popcorn plant. *New England Journal of Medicine* 347(5):330–338.

Kubica, P., A. Wasik, A. Kot-Wasik, and J. Namiesnik. 2014. An evaluation of sucrose as a possible contaminant in e-liquids for electronic cigarettes by hydrophilic interaction liquid chromatography–tandem mass spectrometry. *Analytical and Bioanalytical Chemistry* 406(13):3013–3018.

Kucharska, M., W. Wesołowski, S. Czerczak, and R. Soćko. 2016. Testing of the composition of e-cigarette liquids—Manufacturer-declared vs. true contents in a selected series of products. *Medycyna Pracy* 67(2):239–253.

LaKind, J. S., E. A. McKenna, R. P. Hubner, and R. G. Tardiff. 1999. A review of the comparative mammalian toxicity of ethylene glycol and propylene glycol. *Critical Reviews in Toxicolology* 29(4):331–365.

Latven, A. R., and H. Molitor. 1939. Comparison of the toxic, hypnotic and irritating properties of eight organic solvents. *Journal of Pharmacology and Experimental Therapeutics* 65(1):89.

Laug, E. P., H. O. Calvery, H. J. Morris, and G. Woodard. 1939. The toxicology of some glycols and derivatives. *Journal of Industrial Hygiene and Toxicology* 21(6):173–201.

Lerner, C. A., I. K. Sundar, R. M. Watson, A. Elder, R. Jones, D. Done, R. Kurtzman, D. J. Ossip, R. Robinson, S. McIntosh, and I. Rahman. 2015a. Environmental health hazards of e-cigarettes and their components: Oxidants and copper in e-cigarette aerosols. *Environmental Pollution* 198:100–107.

Lerner, C. A., I. K. Sundar, H. Yao, J. Gerloff, D. J. Ossip, S. McIntosh, R. Robinson, and I. Rahman. 2015b. Vapors produced by electronic cigarettes and e-juices with flavorings induce toxicity, oxidative stress, and inflammatory response in lung epithelial cells and in mouse lung. *PLoS ONE* 10(2):e0116732. https://doi.org/10.1371/journal.pone.0116732 (accessed February 6, 2018).

Lerner, C. A., P. Rutagarama, T. Ahmad, I. K. Sundar, A. Elder, and I. Rahman. 2016. Electronic cigarette aerosols and copper nanoparticles induce mitochondrial stress and promote DNA fragmentation in lung fibroblasts. *Biochemical and Biophysical Research Communications* 477(4):620–625.

Lessmann, H., A. Schnuch, J. Geier, and W. Uter. 2005. Skin-sensitizing and irritant properties of propylene glycol. *Contact Dermatitis* 53(5):247–259.

Li, Q. D., Y. C. Zhan, L. Wang, S. J. Leischow, and D. D. Zeng. 2016. Analysis of symptoms and their potential associations with e-liquids' components: A social media study. *BMC Public Health* 16:674. https://doi.org/10.1186/s12889-016-3326-0 (accessed February 6, 2018).

Lim, H. H., and H. S. Shin. 2017. Determination of volatile organic compounds including alcohols in refill fluids and cartridges of electronic cigarettes by headspace solid-phase micro extraction and gas chromatography–mass spectrometry. *Analytical and Bioanalytical Chemistry* 409(5):1247–1256.

Lim, T. Y., R. L. Poole, and N. M. Pageler. 2014. Propylene glycol toxicity in children. *Journal of Pediatric Pharmacology and Therapeutics* 19(4):277–282.

Lin, E. C. 1977. Glycerol utilization and its regulation in mammals. *Annual Review of Biochemistry* 46:765–795.

Lisko, J. G., H. Tran, S. B. Stanfill, B. C. Blount, and C. H. Watson. 2015. Chemical composition and evaluation of nicotine, tobacco alkaloids, pH, and selected flavors in e-cigarette cartridges and refill solutions. *Nicotine & Tobacco Research* 17(10):1270–1278.

Litt, M. D., V. Duffy, and C. Oncken. 2016. Cigarette smoking and electronic cigarette vaping patterns as a function of e-cigarette flavourings. *Tobacco Control* 25:ii67–ii72. http://tobaccocontrol.bmj.com/content/25/Suppl_2/ii67 (accessed February 6, 2018).

MacCannell, K. L. 1969. Hemodynamic responses to glycols and to hemolysis. *Canadian Journal of Physiology and Pharmacology* 47(6):563–569.

MAK Commission. 2002. Benzaldehyde [MAK value documentation, 2002]. In *The MAK collection for occupational health and safety*. Weinheim, Germany: Wiley-VCH Verlag GmbH & Co. KGaA, Pp.14–36.

Maridet, C., B. Atge, J. M. Amici, A. Taieb, and B. Milpied. 2015. The electronic cigarette: The new source of nickel contact allergy of the 21st century? *Contact Dermatitis* 73(1):49–50.

Martin, G., and L. Finberg. 1970. Propylene glycol: A potentially toxic vehicle in liquid dosage form. *Journal of Pediatrics* 77(5):877–888.

Martinez, R. E., S. Dhawan, W. Sumner, and B. Williams. 2014. On-line chemical composition analysis of refillable electronic cigarette aerosol—Measurement of nicotine and nicotyrine. *Nicotine & Tobacco Research* 17(10):1263–1269.

McCauley, L., C. Markin, and D. Hosmer. 2012. An unexpected consequence of electronic cigarette use. *Chest* 141(4):1110–1113.

Messner, B., and D. Bernhard. 2014. Smoking and cardiovascular disease: Mechanisms of endothelial dysfunction and early atherogenesis. *Arteriosclerosis, Thrombosis, and Vascular Biology* 34(3):509–515.

Mikheev, V. B., M. C. Brinkman, C. A. Granville, S. M. Gordon, and P. I. Clark. 2016. Real-time measurement of electronic cigarette aerosol size distribution and metals content analysis. *Nicotine & Tobacco Research* 18(9):1895–1902.

Moline, J. M., A. L. Golden, J. H. Highland, K. R. Wilmarth, and A. S. Kao. 2000. *Health effects evaluation of theatrical smoke, haze, and pyrotechnics*. http://www.actorsequity.org/docs/safesan/finalreport.pdf (accessed September 28, 2017).

Morris, H. J., A. A. Nelson, and H. O. Calvery. 1942. Observations on the chronic toxicities of propylene glycol, ethylene glycol, diethylene glycol, ethylene glycol mono-ethyl-ether, and diethylene glycol mono-ethyl-ether. *Journal of Pharmacology and Experimental Therapeutics* 74(3):266–273.

Morrissey, R. E., J. C. Lamb, 4th, R. W. Morris, R. E. Chapin, D. K. Gulati, and J. J. Heindel. 1989. Results and evaluations of 48 continuous breeding reproduction studies conducted in mice. *Fundamental and Applied Toxicology* 13(4):747–777.

Navas-Acien, A., E. Guallar, E. K. Silbergeld, and S. J. Rothenberg. 2007. Lead exposure and cardiovascular disease—A systematic review. *Environmental Health Perspectives* 115(3):472–482.

Nelson, J. L., M. E. Harmon, and R. A. Robergs. 2011. Identifying plasma glycerol concentration associated with urinary glycerol excretion in trained humans. *Journal of Analytical Toxicology* 35(9):617–623.

NIOSH (National Institute for Occupational Safety and Health). 2016. *Exposures to flavoring chemicals: How and where exposures may occur.* https://www.cdc.gov/niosh/topics/flavorings/exposure.html (accessed October 11, 2017).

Nonnemaker, J., A. E. Kim, Y. O. Lee, and A. MacMonegle. 2016. Quantifying how smokers value attributes of electronic cigarettes. *Tobacco Control* 25(e1):e37–e43. http://dx.doi.org/10.1136/tobaccocontrol-2015-052511 (accessed February 6, 2018).

NTIS (National Technical Information Service). 1974. *Teratological evaluation of glycerin in mice, rats and rabbits.* Rockville, MD: U.S. Department of Commerce.

NTP (National Toxicology Program). 2007. *Study of glycidol in genetically modified haploinsufficient $p16^{Ink4a}/p19^{Arf}$ mice.* https://ntp.niehs.nih.gov/ntp/htdocs/gmm_rpts/gmm13.pdf (accessed December 22, 2017).

OECD (Organisation for Economic Co-operation and Development). 2001. *Dipropylene glycol (mixed isomers and dominant isomer): CAS no: 25265-71-8 & 110-98-5.* http://www.inchem.org/documents/sids/sids/25265-71-8.pdf (accessed December 22, 2017).

OECD. 2002. *Screening information data set (SIDS): SIDS initial assessment report for SIAM 14; glycerol: CAS no: 56-81-5.* http://www.inchem.org/documents/sids/sids/56815.pdf (accessed February 6, 2018).

OEHHA (Office of Environmental Health Hazard Assessment). 2013. *Proposition 65: No significant risk levels (NSRLs) for carcinogens and maximum allowable dose levels (MADLs) for chemicals causing reproductive toxicity.* http://oehha.ca.gov/media/downloads/proposition-65/chemicals/safeharbor081513_0.pdf (accessed August 18, 2017).

Oh, J. A., and H. S. Shin. 2015. Identification and quantification of several contaminated compounds in replacement liquids of electronic cigarettes by gas chromatography–mass spectrometry. *Journal of Chromatography B* 53(6):841–848.

Ohta, K., S. Uchiyama, Y. Inaba, H. Nakagome, and N. Kunugita. 2011. Determination of carbonyl compounds generated from the electronic cigarette using coupled silica cartridges impregnated with hydroquinone and 2,4-dinitrophenylhydrazine. *Bunseki Kagaku* 60(10):791–797.

Olmedo, P., W. Goessler, S. Tanda, M. Grau-Perez, S. Jarmul, A. Aherrera, R. Chen, M. Hilpert, J. E. Cohen, A. Navas-Acien, and A. M. Rule. 2018. Metal concentrations in e-cigarette liquid and aerosol samples: The contribution of metallic coils. *Environmental Health Perspectives* 126(2):027010. https://doi.org/10.1289/EHP2175 (accessed March 1, 2018).

Ormerod, E., and N. Stone. 2017. Contact allergy and electronic cigarettes (and eyelash curlers). *Clinical and Experimental Dermatology* 42(6):682–683.

OSHA (Occupational Safety and Health Administration). 2006. *Glycerin mist (total dust).* https://www.osha.gov/dts/chemicalsampling/data/CH_243600.html (accessed September 7, 2017).

Ostwald, R. 1962. Glycerol intake, blood cholesterol level and anemia in the guinea pig and rabbit. *Proceedings of the Society for Experimental Biology and Medicine* 111:632–634.

Papousek, R., Z. Pataj, P. Novakova, K. Lemr, and P. Bartak. 2014. Determination of acrylamide and acrolein in smoke from tobacco and e-cigarettes. *Chromatographia* 77(17-18): 1145–1151.

Phaniendra, A., D. B. Jestadi, and L. Periyasamy. 2015. Free radicals: Properties, sources, targets, and their implication in various diseases. *Indian Journal of Clinical Biochemistry* 30(1):11–26.

Prescott, C., and S. E. Bottle. 2017. Biological relevance of free radicals and nitroxides. *Cell Biochemistry and Biophysics* 75(2):227–240.

Pryor, W. A. 1997. Cigarette smoke radicals and the role of free radicals in chemical carcinogenicity. *Environmental Health Perspectives* 105(Supplement 4):875–882.

Regueiro, J., A. Giri, and T. Wenzl. 2016. Optimization of a differential ion mobility spectrometry–tandem mass spectrometry method for high-throughput analysis of nicotine and related compounds: Application to electronic cigarette refill liquids. *Analytical Chemistry* 88(12):6500–6508.

Renne, R. A., A. P. Wehner, B. J. Greenspan, H. S. Deford, H. A. Ragan, R. B. Westerberg, R. L. Buschbom, G. T. Burger, A. W. Hayes, R. L. Suber, and A. T. Mosberg. 1992. 2-Week and 13-week inhalation studies of aerosolized glycerol in rats. *Inhalation Toxicology* 4(2):95–111.

Robertson, O. H., C. G. Loosli, T. T. Puck, H. Wise, H. M. Lemon, and W. Lester. 1947. Tests for the chronic toxicity of propylene glycol and triethylene glycol on monkeys and rats by vapor inhalation and oral administration. *Journal of Pharmacology and Experimental Therapeutics* 91(1):52–76.

Saffari, A., N. Daher, A. Ruprecht, C. De Marco, P. Pozzi, R. Boffi, S. H. Hamad, M. M. Shafer, J. J. Schauer, D. Westerdahl, and C. Sioutas. 2014. Particulate metals and organic compounds from electronic and tobacco-containing cigarettes: Comparison of emission rates and secondhand exposure. *Environmental Sciences: Processes and Impacts* 16(10):2259–2267.

Sleiman, M., J. M. Logue, V. N. Montesinos, M. L. Russell, M. I. Litter, L. A. Gundel, and H. Destaillats. 2016. Emissions from electronic cigarettes: Key parameters affecting the release of harmful chemicals. *Environmental Science & Technology* 50(17):9644–9651.

Smyth, H. F., Jr., J. Seaton, and L. Fischer. 1941. The single dose toxicity of some glycols and derivatives. *Journal of Industrial Hygiene and Toxicology* 23:259–268.

Soule, E. K., A. Nasim, and S. Rosas. 2016. Adverse effects of electronic cigarette use: A concept mapping approach. *Nicotine & Tobacco Research* 18(5):678–685.

Soussy, S., A. El-Hellani, R. Baalbaki, R. Salman, A. Shihadeh, and N. A. Saliba. 2016. Detection of 5-hydroxymethylfurfural and furfural in the aerosol of electronic cigarettes. *Tobacco Control* 25(Supplement 2):ii88–ii93. http://tobaccocontrol.bmj.com/content/25/Suppl_2/ii88.long (February 6, 2018).

Speth, P. A., T. B. Vree, N. F. Neilen, P. H. de Mulder, D. R. Newell, M. E. Gore, and B. E. de Pauw. 1987. Propylene glycol pharmacokinetics and effects after intravenous infusion in humans. *Therapeutic Drug Monitoring* 9(3):255–258.

Stålhandske, T., and P. Slanina. 1982. Nicotyrine inhibits in vivo metabolism of nicotine without increasing its toxicity. *Toxicology and Applied Pharmacology* 65(3):366–372.

Stolzenberg, S. J., and C. H. Hine. 1979. Mutagenicity of halogenated and oxygenated three-carbon compounds. *Journal of Toxicology and Environmental Health* 5(6):1149–1158.

Suber, R. L., R. Deskin, I. Nikiforov, X. Fouillet, and C. R. Coggins. 1989. Subchronic nose-only inhalation study of propylene glycol in Sprague-Dawley rats. *Food & Chemical Toxicology* 27(9):573–583.

Surh, Y. J., and S. R. Tannenbaum. 1994. Activation of the Maillard reaction product 5-(hydroxymethyl)furfural to strong mutagens via allylic sulfonation and chlorination. *Chemical Research in Toxicology* 7(3):313–318.

Surh, Y. J., A. Liem, J. A. Miller, and S. R. Tannenbaum. 1994. 5-sulfooxymethylfurfural as a possible ultimate mutagenic and carcinogenic metabolite of the Maillard reaction product, 5-hydroxymethylfurfural. *Carcinogenesis* 15(10):2375–2377.

Sussan, T. E., S. Gajghate, R. K. Thimmulappa, J. Ma, J. H. Kim, K. Sudini, N. Consolini, S. A. Cormier, S. Lomnicki, F. Hasan, A. Pekosz, and S. Biswal. 2015. Exposure to electronic cigarettes impairs pulmonary anti-bacterial and anti-viral defenses in a mouse model. *PLoS ONE* 10(2):e0116861. https://doi.org/10.1371/journal.pone.0116861 (accessed February 6, 2018).

Tayyarah, R., and G. A. Long. 2014. Comparison of select analytes in aerosol from e-cigarettes with smoke from conventional cigarettes and with ambient air. *Regulatory Toxicology and Pharmacology* 70(3):704–710.

Tchounwou, P. B., C. G. Yedjou, A. K. Patlolla, and D. J. Sutton. 2012. Heavy metals toxicity and the environment. *EXS* 101:133–164.

Tierney, P. A., C. D. Karpinski, J. E. Brown, W. Luo, and J. F. Pankow. 2016. Flavour chemicals in electronic cigarette fluids. *Tobacco Control* 25(e1):e10–e15. http://dx.doi.org/10.1136/tobaccocontrol-2014-052175 (accessed February 6, 2018).

Tourtellotte, W. W., J. L. Reinglass, and T. A. Newkirk. 1972. Cerebral dehydration action of glycerol. I. Historical aspects with emphasis on the toxicity and intravenous administration. *Clinical Pharmacology & Therapeutics* 13(2):159–171.

TPSAC (Tobacco Products Scientific Advisory Committee). 2011. *Menthol cigarettes and public health: Review of the scientific evidence and recommendations.*Silver Spring, MD: Center for Tobacco Products, Food and Drug Administration.

Uchiyama, S., Y. Inaba, and N. Kunugita. 2010. Determination of acrolein and other carbonyls in cigarette smoke using coupled silica cartridges impregnated with hydroquinone and 2,4-dinitrophenylhydrazine. *Journal of Chromatography A* 1217(26):4383–4388.

Uchiyama, S., K. Ohta, Y. Inaba, and N. Kunugita. 2013. Determination of carbonyl compounds generated from the e-cigarette using coupled silica cartridges impregnated with hydroquinone and 2,4-dinitrophenylhydrazine, followed by high-performance liquid chromatography. *Analytical Sciences* 29(12):1219–1222.

Uryupin, A. B., A. S. Peregudov, K. A. Kochetkov, L. N. Bulatnikova, S. S. Kiselev, and Y. S. Nekrasov. 2013. Qualitative and quantitative compositions of fluids for electronic cigarettes. *Pharmaceutical Chemistry Journal* 46(11):687–692.

USP (U.S. Pharmacopeia). n.d. *Nicotine.* http://www.pharmacopeia.cn/v29240/usp29nf24s0_m56620.html (accessed October 9, 2017).

Van Winkle, W., Jr., and H. W. Newman. 1941. Further results of continued administration of propylene glycol. *Journal of Food Science* 6(5):509–516.

Varlet, V., K. Farsalinos, M. Augsburger, A. Thomas, and J. F. Etter. 2015. Toxicity assessment of refill liquids for electronic cigarettes. *International Journal of Environmental Research and Public Health* 12(5):4796–4815.

Varughese, S., K. Teschke, M. Brauer, Y. Chow, C. van Netten, and S. M. Kennedy. 2005. Effects of theatrical smokes and fogs on respiratory health in the entertainment industry. *American Journal of Industrial Medicine* 47(5):411–418.

Venable, J. R., C. D. McClimans, R. E. Flake, and D. B. Dimick. 1980. A fertility study of male employees engaged in the manufacture of glycerine. *Journal of Occupational and Environmental Medicine* 22(2):87–91.

Villanti, A. C., A. Richardson, D. M. Vallone, and J. M. Rath. 2013. Flavored tobacco product use among U.S. young adults. *American Journal of Preventive Medicine* 44(4):388–391.

Wang, L., Y. C. Zhan, Q. D. Li, D. D. Zeng, S. J. Leischow, and J. Okamoto. 2015. An examination of electronic cigarette content on social media: Analysis of e-cigarette flavor content on Reddit. *International Journal of Environmental Research and Public Health* 12(11):14916–14935.

Wang, P., W. Chen, J. Liao, T. Matsuo, K. Ito, J. Fowles, D. Shusterman, M. Mendell, and K. Kumagai. 2017. A device-independent evaluation of carbonyl emissions from heated electronic cigarette solvents. *PLoS ONE* 12(1):e0169811. https://doi.org/10.1371/journal.pone.0169811 (accessed February 6, 2018).

Warshaw, E. M., N. C. Botto, H. I. Maibach, J. F. Fowler, Jr., R. L. Rietschel, K. A. Zug, D. V. Belsito, J. S. Taylor, V. A. DeLeo, M. D. Pratt, D. Sasseville, F. J. Storrs, J. G. Marks, Jr., and C. G. Mathias. 2009. Positive patch-test reactions to propylene glycol: A retrospective cross-sectional analysis from the North American Contact Dermatitis Group, 1996 to 2006. *Dermatitis* 20(1):14–20.

Weatherby, J. H., and H. B. Haag. 1938. Toxicity of propylene glycol. *Journal of the American Pharmacists Association* 27(6):466–471.

Werley, M. S., P. McDonald, P. Lilly, D. Kirkpatrick, J. Wallery, P. Byron, and J. Venitz. 2011. Non-clinical safety and pharmacokinetic evaluations of propylene glycol aerosol in Sprague-Dawley rats and beagle dogs. *Toxicology* 287(1–3):76–90.

Wiebe, J. P., and K. J. Barr. 1984a. The control of male fertility by 1,2,3-trihydroxypropane (THP; glycerol): Rapid arrest of spermatogenesis without altering libido, accessory organs, gonadal steroidogenesis, and serum testosterone, LH and FSH. *Contraception* 29(3):291–302.

Wiebe, J. P., and K. J. Barr. 1984b. Suppression of spermatogenesis without inhibition of steroidogenesis by a 1,2,3-trihydroxypropane solution. *Life Sciences* 34(18):1747–1754.

Wiebe, J. P., K. J. Barr, and K. D. Buckingham. 1989. Sustained azoospermia in squirrel monkey, *Saimiri sciureus*, resulting from a single intratesticular glycerol injection. *Contraception* 39(4):447–457.

Wieslander, G., D. Norback, and T. Lindgren. 2001. Experimental exposure to propylene glycol mist in aviation emergency training: Acute ocular and respiratory effects. *Occupational and Environmental Medicine* 58(10):649–655.

Williams, M., A. Villarreal, K. Bozhilov, S. Lin, and P. Talbot. 2013. Metal and silicate particles including nanoparticles are present in electronic cigarette cartomizer fluid and aerosol. *PLoS ONE* 8(3):e57987. https://doi.org/10.1371/journal.pone.0057987 (accessed February 6, 2018).

Williams, M., K. Bozhilov, S. Ghai, and P. Talbot. 2017. Elements including metals in the atomizer and aerosol of disposable electronic cigarettes and electronic hookahs. *PLoS ONE* 12(4):e0175430. https://doi.org/10.1371/journal.pone.0175430 (accessed February 6, 2018).

Yamaguchi, T. 1982. Mutagenicity of trioses and methyl glyoxal on *Salmonella typhimurium*. *Agricultural and Biological Chemistry* 46(3):849–851.

Yingst, J. M., S. Veldheer, E. Hammett, S. Hrabovsky, and J. Foulds. 2017. A method for classifying user-reported electronic cigarette liquid flavors. *Nicotine & Tobacco Research* 19(11):1381–1385.

Yu, D. K., W. F. Elmquist, and R. J. Sawchuk. 1985. Pharmacokinetics of propylene glycol in humans during multiple dosing regimens. *Journal of Pharmaceutical Sciences* 74(8):876–879.

Zhu, S. H., J. Y. Sun, E. Bonnevie, S. E. Cummins, A. Gamst, L. Yin, and M. Lee. 2014. Four hundred and sixty brands of e-cigarettes and counting: Implications for product regulation. *Tobacco Control* 23(Supplement 3):iii3–iii9. http://dx.doi.org/10.1136/tobaccocontrol-2014-051670 (accessed February 6, 2018).

6

Research Needs: E-Cigarette Devices, Constituents, and Exposures

The committee was tasked to provide a list of research needs to inform the Food and Drug Administration (FDA) and e-cigarette regulation that will be prioritized with respect to

- Research to gather information of most importance for the regulation of e-cigarettes to protect the population health
- Research that should be a priority for federal funding

Given the relatively short time that e-cigarettes have been in use, it is understandable that the evidence base regarding their effects is limited. There is a great need for more evidence, as other research groups have documented (Walton et al., 2015). Manufacturers will need to produce this research in a short amount of time if current statutory deadlines remain in place. Researchers from academia will also be involved directly (in contracts with manufacturers and in grants from government and others) in the generation of these data. Some types of research involve a long-term horizon; other important and informative research requires much less time to conduct. One type of research does not substitute for the other; a complete portfolio of research is needed. The committee understands that, in any new field, researchers struggle to conduct optimal research due to limitations of knowledge. Also, researchers feel the urgency to study a new important question and adapt what they know, without complete adjustments in research design or methods sufficient to address the nuances of the problem. Finally, the rapidly changing nature of the devices has made comparisons among studies difficult.

The committee identified many gaps in the literature during its review and identified dozens of specific research needs that are important for understanding the effects of e-cigarettes and for FDA regulatory action. The committee identified two overarching research needs: addressing gaps in substantive knowledge and improving research methods and quality. Specific items for consideration identified by the committee are noted for each of these and are not listed in any priority order.

ADDRESSING GAPS IN SUBSTANTIVE KNOWLEDGE

Recommendation 6-1: The committee recommends that the Food and Drug Administration and other federal research sponsors and/or device manufacturers prioritize e-cigarette research that addresses key gaps regarding knowledge about e-cigarette devices, constituents, and exposures. This might include rapid response funding opportunities. Specific items for consideration follow.

- Study the effects of carrier solvents and additives, including flavor ingredients and device characteristics (including the type of coil and power), on aerosol generation, aerosol physical properties, and the chemical profile of e-cigarette emissions.
- Study the stability of e-liquid ingredients when heated, identify potential by-products of thermal degradation and of compounds that were not initially present in the e-liquid, and ascertain determinants of change in aerosol composition.
- Study the impact of e-cigarette use on indoor air quality and biomarkers of secondhand e-cigarette exposure in scenarios and exposure surveys that are relevant for the populations exposed, including workers in vape shops and vaping convention attendees, children, pregnant women, and patients with cardiorespiratory disease who live with adults who use e-cigarettes.
- Conduct research that would inform product standards regarding ingredient purity, batteries and chargers, and priority and novel emissions.
- Establish procedures to rapidly evaluate changes to products currently on the U.S. market, focusing on device designs, design evolution (initiated by both manufacturers and users) and the corresponding alteration of chemical substance release patterns.

IMPROVING RESEARCH METHODS AND QUALITY

Recommendation 6-2: The committee recommends that the Food and Drug Administration and other federal research sponsors and/or device manufacturers prioritize research that improves the quality of e-cigarette research to better understand the devices, constituents, and exposures. This includes protocol and methods validation and development and use of appropriate study design, including the use of the appropriate control groups. Specific examples are given below.

- Develop one or more standardized puffing protocols that are different from the standard puffing protocol for combustible tobacco cigarettes and reflect a range of how e-cigarettes are used in real-life settings, including extreme use.
- Develop and validate methods to produce aerosols and to analyze target constituents in e-cigarettes; the standardized method should reflect not only the average puffing conditions observed among the users in real-life settings, but also intensive puffing behaviors.
- Develop and validate a standardized method to measure particle size distribution and respiratory deposition of e-cigarette aerosols.
- Develop analytical methods to test chemicals in e-cigarette liquids and aerosols with a focus on screening and identifying potentially toxic compounds, including study of the effects of power and temperature and other device characteristics that generate such compounds.
- Use exposure conditions and animal models that are relevant to real-life inhalation exposure in humans.
- Evaluate potentially biologically relevant interactions between nicotine and other constituents, such as flavorings, in in vitro and in vivo bioassays.

REFERENCE

Walton, K. M., D. B. Abrams, W. C. Bailey, D. Clark, G. N. Connolly, M. V. Djordjevic, T. E. Eissenberg, M. C. Fiore, M. L. Goniewicz, L. Haverkos, S. S. Hecht, J. E. Henningfield, J. R. Hughes, C. A. Oncken, L. Postow, J. E. Rose, K. L. Wanke, L. Yang, and D. K. Hatsukami. 2015. NIH electronic cigarette workshop: Developing a research agenda. *Nicotine & Tobacco Research* 17(2):259–269.

Section II

Effects of E-Cigarettes on Health

Although laboratory tests of e-cigarette ingredients, in vitro toxicological tests, and short-term human studies suggest that e-cigarettes are likely less harmful than combustible tobacco cigarettes, due to lack of long-term epidemiological studies and large clinical trials, the implications for long-term effects on morbidity and mortality are not yet clear and the absolute safety of the products cannot be unambiguously assessed at this time. Use of e-cigarettes instead of combustible tobacco cigarettes by those with existing respiratory disease might be less harmful.

7

Modes of Action

Although the use of electronic cigarettes has increased steadily since their introduction into the market about a decade ago, much is unknown about their safety profile. As concluded in Chapter 5, the number of chemicals and their content in combustible tobacco cigarette smoke is much higher than emissions from most e-cigarette products, yet there are still concerns about the toxic properties of the variable combination of chemicals present in e-liquids and the additional chemicals generated during the aerosolization of e-liquids. The toxicology of e-cigarettes is a fertile area of investigation and one of current vigorous activity. Whereas previous chapters discussed toxicology of individual constituents, this section discusses toxicology of e-cigarette aerosols as a whole. The majority of the published work on the subject is in the form of acute in vivo studies, along with multiple in vitro studies using various human- and animal-derived cell lines, including endothelial, fibroblast, and cardiomyocytes, to name a few. Figure 7-1 shows the trend in publications per year on e-cigarettes and in vitro systems. The first publications (n = 5) appeared in 2013. Since then, there has been a steady increase in the number of publications, with a cumulative total of 124 as of September 2017. This section discusses two modes of action—endothelial cell dysfunction and oxidative stress—that are associated with the development of a range of health outcomes. Appendix D contains a summary of in vitro studies in which cytotoxicity is assessed.

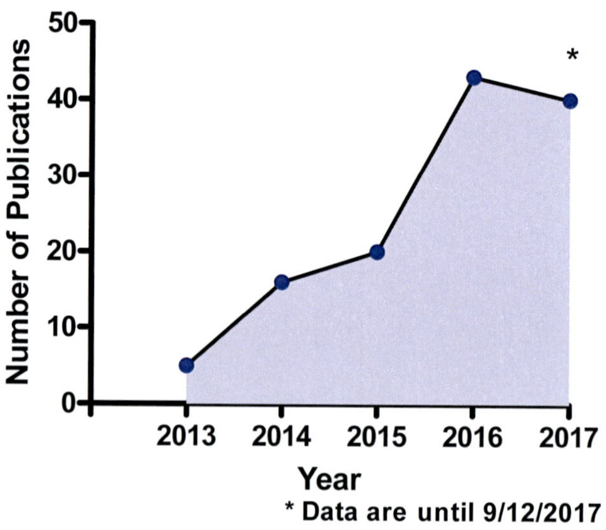

FIGURE 7-1 Publications by year on e-cigarettes and in vitro systems.

ENDOTHELIAL CELL DYSFUNCTION

Smoking is among the most prominent preventable contributing risk factors for the development of various diseases, primarily cancers and cardiovascular diseases. The role of chemicals generated from traditional tobacco smoke on endothelial cell function has been well documented. With the introduction and recent use of electronic cigarettes, a key question is whether e-cigarette use and the chemicals present in e-liquids as well as those generated during use produce similar effects on endothelial cell function. The two emerging questions are whether such effects are seen with e-cigarette use and what the magnitude of these effects is compared with traditional combustible tobacco cigarette smoke or to neither e-cigarette nor combustible tobacco use. It is well accepted that endothelial cell dysfunction produced by traditional tobacco burning involves various key initiating events, including a reduction in nitric oxide (NO) net availability, increased reactive oxygen species (ROS) generation, and increased expression of adhesion molecules that facilitate trans-endothelial movement and deposition of activated complement components. More details on the effect of tobacco smoking on endothelial cell activation and dysfunction, and the molecular mechanisms involved can be found in the review by Morris and colleagues (2015). Figure 7-2,

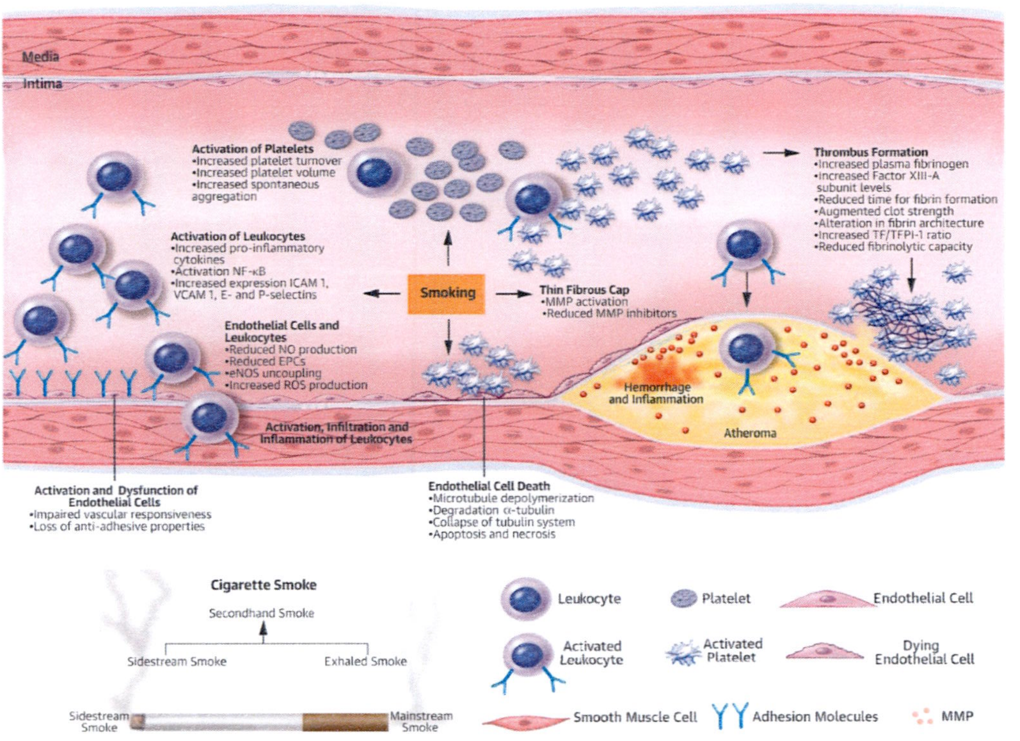

FIGURE 7-2 Endothelial cell dysfunction by tobacco smoke.
SOURCE: Morris et al., 2015.

from this review, highlights the key events associated with endothelial cell dysfunction by tobacco smoke.

Evidence Review

In a study by Antoniewicz and colleagues (2016), the effect of e-cigarette inhalation on vascular function was evaluated in healthy sporadic smokers (10 combustible tobacco cigarettes or fewer per month). Circulating endothelial progenitor cells (EPCs) and microvesicles (MVs) in blood were the two endpoints measured. Elevation in circulating levels of EPCs in blood is indicative of and a commonly used marker of vascular endothelial injury. EPCs are stem cells produced primarily in the bone marrow. Their increased presence in blood reflects regeneration of endothelial cells following vascular injury. MVs of endothelial origin can also be used as a biomarker of endothelial cell activation and/or death via apoptosis. Both biomarkers are used when assessing the risk of cardiovascular complications and are also implicated in pulmonary disease (chronic obstructive pulmonary disease [COPD] and emphysema). Their results show that levels of circulating EPCs increased significantly with short-term exposure to e-cigarette inhalation, while MV remained unchanged. The authors concluded that the effect of e-cigarette use on EPCs is similar in magnitude to that produced by combustible tobacco cigarette smoking, and is indicative of vascular injury. They attributed the unaffected MV values to insufficient exposure time because cotinine levels were much lower in their e-cigarette subjects compared with combustible tobacco cigarette users (Antoniewicz et al., 2016). The question of which of these two biomarkers (EPCs versus endothelial-derived MVs) is a more sensitive and earlier indicator of endothelial dysfunction well in advance of detection of ultrastructural changes in endothelial cells in response to e-cigarette use warrants further scrutiny.[1]

Another study, by Putzhammer and colleagues (2016), investigated the effect of e-cigarette aerosol extracts in human umbilical vein endothelial cells (HUVECs). Cells were exposed to hydrophilic fractions from aerosols obtained from various types of e-cigarette devices. Cell death was measured, as well as generation of ROS, cell proliferation rates, and cell morphology. ROS was assessed by measuring the oxidation of 2′,7′-dichlorodihydrofluorescein diacetate. Their results showed that 5 of the 11 e-cigarette aerosols analyzed produced acute cytotoxicity. Similarly, 5 of the 11 aerosols tested reduced cell proliferation rates, while only 1 of

[1] Chapter 9 also includes the Antoniewicz et al. (2016) study in its review and focuses on the effects of e-cigarette exposure on E-selectin MVs. The committee finds no conflict between the evidence presented in this chapter and the evidence presented in Chapter 9.

the aerosol extracts led to the generation of ROS. The aerosols generated from different liquids using the same e-cigarette show substantial differences, pointing to the liquids as an important source of toxicity. As previously demonstrated with combustible tobacco cigarette smoke extracts, exposure of HUVECs to e-cigarette aerosols produces prominent changes in cell morphology and alters the functional endothelial monolayer. The authors clearly demonstrated that the source of the e-liquid and type of device used are determining factors in the cytotoxic potency of e-cigarette aerosols and the capacity to change endothelial cell morphology. Equally important, some e-cigarette products showed toxic effects similar to those of combustible, high-nicotine, tobacco cigarettes. Of note, formation of ROS by the e-cigarette extracts tested in this study did not always correlate with their toxic potential, which is an intriguing observation due to the well-proven role of ROS in the cytotoxicity of combustible tobacco cigarette smoke. The authors suggest that the mechanisms of toxicity of certain e-cigarette vapors in endothelial cells may be distinct from those of combustible tobacco cigarettes, where ROS are central to disease etiology. Additionally, two of the three highly toxic e-liquids did not contain nicotine, but contained flavoring or herbal constituents (Putzhammer et al., 2016).

Another study on HUVECs exposed to extracts from e-cigarette aerosol or combustible tobacco cigarette smoke showed that both exposures produced apoptotic and necrotic cell death and that this cytotoxicity is associated with the generation of ROS and DNA damage (Anderson et al., 2016). Not surprisingly, the cytotoxicity was dose dependent for both treatments. The study also addressed the question of what level of oxidative stress is produced in the HUVECs exposed to the extract from e-cigarette aerosol in comparison to that produced by combustible tobacco cigarette smoke exposure. A concentration of 500 μM was used for both types of extracts. This treatment concentration was selected based on the results of their initial cytotoxicity assay with the e-cigarette aerosol extract. The results of the ROS generation fluorescence-based assay indicate that the e-cigarette aerosol extract produces a significant 4.5-fold increase in ROS levels over control values. However, this value is lower than the 7.8-fold increase produced by combustible tobacco cigarette smoke (relative to controls). The role of oxidative stress in the toxic response of these endothelial cells to e-cigarette aerosol exposure was further documented by the use of the antioxidants α-tocopherol and *N*-acetyl-L-cysteine. Although antioxidant treatment was capable of preventing necrotic cell death, it only afforded partial protection against e-cigarette aerosol-induced apoptotic cell death. This indicates that ROS indeed play a role, in part, in e-cigarette-induced cytotoxicity (Anderson et al., 2016). The lack of complete blockade of endothelial cell apoptosis by antioxidants, in contrast to the prevention of necrotic cell death, indicates that components other than ROS in extracts from e-cigarette aerosol are also contributing to cytotoxicity of endothelial cells.

A study by Barber and colleagues (2016) goes further in identifying the specific components of e-cigarettes responsible for alterations in endothelial cell function and viability. Again, HUVECs were used as an in vitro model of endothelial cell function/dysfunction. HUVECs were exposed to extracts from combustible tobacco cigarettes and e-cigarettes. In some experiments, pure nicotine was used at a concentration that approximates the blood concentration of someone who smokes one combustible tobacco cigarette. The endpoints analyzed for all exposures included inflammatory response, cell viability and density, and metabolic activity, the latter determined by the 3-(4,5-dimethylthiazol-2-yl)-2,5-diphenyltetrazolium bromide (MTT) assay.

The results indicate that endothelial cells exposed to tobacco or e-cigarette products, but not nicotine, experienced a significant decrease in viability. By contrast, all forms of exposures (including pure nicotine at a final concentration of 50 nM) reduced cell density by approximately 25 percent. Interestingly, the responsiveness of endothelial cells to changes in cell density was not dependent on the concentration of nicotine present in the formulations tested, or apparently the composition of the "toxic" gases generated from these formulations, because no differences in magnitude of changes in cell density were detected between tobacco smoke extracts and e-cigarette aerosol extracts. The five e-cigarette products tested contained nicotine concentrations ranging from 0 to 18 mg/ml.

The results of the MTT assay revealed that for the majority of e-cigarette aerosol extracts and for all tobacco smoke extracts, metabolic activity is significantly reduced to comparable levels. Moreover, pure nicotine exposure did not change endothelial cell metabolic activity in comparison to control exposures. The authors emphasize observations indicating that endothelial cell metabolic activity was sensitive to the presence of the extracts, but not to the exact formulation of each extract. Worth also noting is that pure nicotine did not change endothelial cell metabolic activity (Barber et al., 2016).

Lastly, enhanced deposition of various components of complement onto endothelial cells was detected with exposure to both tobacco smoke and e-cigarette aerosol extracts. This was typically independent of the exact formulation. Specifically, deposition of the complement component C4d was of a lesser magnitude as a result of exposure to e-cigarette aerosol than to tobacco smoke. From these studies, the authors conclude that fine particulate matter from both e-cigarette aerosol and tobacco smoke extracts, and not nicotine or toxic combustion products, may be responsible for alterations in complement deposition that might be pivotal for the inflammatory response in endothelial cells produced by tobacco and e-cigarette use. Of note, what is referred to as "toxic combustion product" in this article is rather broad and unclear. Nevertheless, the strength of the paper is that it addresses and/or attempts to define the specific components of combustible tobacco smoke and e-cigarette aerosols mediating detrimental effects on endothelial function. The evidence here is strongly suggestive of particulate matter as the main culprit responsible for endothelial cell dysfunction with e-cigarette aerosol (Barber et al., 2016).

The British American Tobacco Investments Ltd. recently developed a novel hybrid tobacco product consisting of a warm aerosol stream generated by electronic aerosolization and tobacco flavor produced by passing the aerosol through a bed of blended cut tobacco (Breheny et al., 2017; Poynton et al., 2017). In vitro studies addressed toxicological responses from this novel hybrid tobacco product in comparison with those from commercially available and prototype tobacco heating products, as well as a 3R4F reference combustible tobacco cigarette. Exposure matrices consisted of total particulate matter, whole aerosol, and aqueous aerosol extracts for all products tested. Endothelial dysfunction was among a battery of toxicological endpoints measured. The scratch wound assay using HUVECs was employed to measure rates of endothelial cell migration upon in vitro exposure to aqueous aerosol extracts from all test products. The results showed that wound repair after exposure to aqueous extract from the hybrid tobacco product and the commercial tobacco heating product was not significantly impaired, in contrast with the 3R4F reference combustible tobacco cigarette extract, which significantly impaired wound repair. This process was also inhibited by the aqueous extract from the prototype tobacco heating product tested, but at a lesser magnitude than that produced by the 3R4F reference combustible tobacco cigarette exposure. Similarly, outcomes of other toxicological endpoints such as mutagenicity, oxidative stress, and cytotoxicity were negative with the hybrid tobacco product. The study also measured carbonyls and nicotine levels in the aqueous aerosol extracts from these tobacco heating products. The carbonyls analyzed were acetaldehyde, acetone, acrolein, butyraldehyde, crotonaldehyde, formaldehyde, methyl ethyl ketone, and propionaldehyde. Overall, the most abundant carbonyls in the products tested (and in the 3R4F cigarette) were acetaldehyde and formaldehyde. Approximately 80 percent to 90 percent reductions in yield of total carbonyls were observed for extracts from tobacco heating and the novel hybrid tobacco products, by comparison with levels of carbonyls present in 3R4F and 3R4F-derived extract samples.

Interestingly, these reductions in yields of carbonyls with these devices correlated well with the significantly lower in vitro cytotoxicity responses obtained and the largely negative results from most of the endpoints measured, such as mutagenicity, genotoxicity, tumor promotion, oxidative stress, and endothelial cell dysfunction.

Flow-mediated dilation (FMD) is a non-invasive, ultrasound-based test to measure endothelial function (Raitakari and Celermajer, 2000). In this test, the arterial diameter is measured in response to an increase in sheer stress, causing endothelium-dependent dilatation. It is well documented that traditional tobacco smokers develop endothelial dysfunction, as evidenced by lower FMD values. Abnormal performance in this test is an early indicator of atherogenesis and closely associated with coronary artery disease (Carnevale et al., 2016).

In a crossover, single-blind study by Carnevale and colleagues (2016), 40 healthy subjects without cardiovascular disease (20 smokers and 20 non-smokers) smoked combustible tobacco cigarettes for a week. In the second phase of the study, all subjects were switched to smoking a tobacco-flavored e-cigarette product with a mean nicotine content of 16 mg per cartridge (equivalent to 250 puffs of tobacco cigarettes), which is approximately the same nominal nicotine content of combustible tobacco cigarettes. The overall goal of this study was to evaluate the differences between combustible tobacco cigarette and e-cigarette smoking in oxidative stress and endothelial dysfunction. For this purpose, ultrasound assessment of basal brachial diameter and endothelial-dependent FMD of the brachial artery were investigated according to established guidelines. Other parameters measured included blood levels of 8-*iso*-prostaglandin $F_2\alpha$, nitric oxide, soluble NOX2-derived peptide, and vitamin E (Carnevale et al., 2016).

Both combustible tobacco cigarette smoking and/or e-cigarette use resulted in a significant increase in soluble NOX2-derived peptide and 8-*iso*-prostaglandin $F_2\alpha$, while nitric oxide and vitamin E values were significantly decreased. Furthermore, the outcome of the FMD test showed that the brachial artery was significantly altered by both traditional and e-cigarette smoking, indicative that endothelial dysfunction occurs with both forms of smoking. E-cigarette use also appears to produce a less pronounced effect on levels of soluble NOX2-derived peptide, 8-*iso*-prostaglandin $F_2\alpha$, and nitric oxide content than combustible tobacco cigarette smoking. Future studies are warranted to clarify the chronic vascular effects of e-cigarette smoking. Although the authors are right to conclude that their results raise some degree of concern about the potential adverse vascular effect of e-cigarettes, they also acknowledged some of the limitations of the work, including the lack of assessment of chronic effects of e-cigarettes on endothelial function and no measurements of blood nicotine levels (Carnevale et al., 2016).

Reactive toxic aldehydes are commonly generated during combustion processes, including tobacco burning. In fact, a plethora of reactive aldehydes can be found at high concentrations in tobacco smoke. Acrolein is a prominent tobacco-generated aldehyde and a well-known risk factor for cardiovascular diseases and pulmonary disease (COPD and emphysema) in smokers (Bein and Leikauf, 2011; Moghe et al., 2015). Although the impact of high levels of exposure to acrolein on cardiovascular health has been well studied, the systemic effects of exposure to lower levels of acrolein such as those found in combustible tobacco smoke and also in some electronic cigarettes are not known. In this context, Conklin and colleagues (2017) investigated the effect of exposing mice to 0.5 or 1 ppm acrolein for 12 weeks. This inhalation dosing regimen resulted in a significant increase in the primary urinary metabolite of acrolein 3-hydroxypropyl mercapturic acid. Concurrently, acrolein-protein adducts, expression of acrolein-metabolizing enzymes, and Nrf2-dependent gene products were all increased in the lungs of acrolein-treated mice.

Although exposure to acrolein reduced circulating levels of EPCs by 40 percent to 50 percent, there was no evidence of a lung inflammatory response or endoplasmic reticulum stress. Neither were elevations in circulating levels of endothelial-derived microparticles (MPs; referred to in other articles as endothelial-derived MVs) detected. From these findings, the authors suggest that circulating levels of specific EPCs could be used as sensitive biomarkers of inhaled acrolein-induced lung injury and that low-level acrolein exposure, such as that reported in e-cigarettes, poses a risk for cardiovascular diseases by hampering repair of endothelial cells (Conklin et al., 2017). Although proposing EPC changes as a sensitive and early biomarker of endothelial cell dysfunction for acrolein and other carbonyl compounds known to be generated in some e-cigarette aerosols is justifiable based on the evidence in this article, no remarkable changes in MPs were observed (as reported by others investigating e-cigarette exposures), and other key events associated with endothelial cell dysfunction, such as NO bioavailability, were not measured. Overall, what distinguishes this from other in vivo studies is the use of acrolein as a single toxicant in a chronic inhalation exposure regimen and at a concentration likely to be found in aerosols of combusted or heated tobacco products, including some e-cigarettes.

In another in vitro study, Teasdale and colleagues (2016) investigated the capacity of combustible tobacco cigarette smoke and electronic cigarette aerosol extracts to induce a stress response in endothelial cells. This study is distinguished from other in vitro studies because it used human coronary artery endothelial cells (HCAECs) instead of the more commonly used HUVECs. In this study, mainstream smoke from a single Marlboro Gold combustible tobacco cigarette was drawn through 10 ml of endothelial cell growth media MV2 to generate the combustible tobacco cigarette smoke extract. The e-cigarette aerosol extract was created using the same apparatus, an iStick battery at 10.8-W (4.3-V) constant power output with an Aerotank Mini atomizer with Haven fluid USA Mix 18 mg/ml nicotine solution (80 percent glycerol/20 percent propylene glycol). A higher power output was selected with this e-cigarette unit to generate an e-cigarette aerosol extract expected to contain a greater proportion of potentially harmful chemicals. Any particulate matter from both combustible tobacco cigarette smoke and e-cigarette aerosol extracts was removed by filtration. The final samples applied to the cultured media contained the same nicotine concentration. Nicotine only (350 ng/ml) in media was used as an additional control.

Endpoints analyzed included Nrf2 nuclear localization by immunohistochemistry (indicative of an antioxidant stress response) and qPCR analysis of Nrf2-dependent and other genes. The genes selected were *HMOX1*, *GCLM*, *OSGIN1*, *PAR4*, *CYP1A1*, and *CYP1B1*. Their selection criteria were based on clear evidence that the expression of these genes changes in response to combustible tobacco cigarette smoke extract exposure to values greater than twofold (relative to controls). Not all these genes are Nrf2-dependent. For example, the CYP450 isoforms *CYP1A1* and *CYP1B1* were included in the analysis because of the previous evidence of their regulation by combustible tobacco cigarette smoke extract. The results demonstrated that exposure of HCAECs to combustible tobacco cigarette smoke extract resulted in Nrf2 activation, nuclear translocation, and transcriptional regulation of its target genes. In addition, the expression of the Nrf2-independent genes *CYP1A1* and *CYP1B1* was also upregulated by combustible tobacco cigarette smoke extract. In contrast, e-cigarette aerosol extracts did not affect expression of any of the genes analyzed, nor did it result in Nrf2 activation or changes in nuclear translocation levels. They also assessed interleukin 8 (*IL8*) and neuronal pentraxin-I (*NTPX1*) expression because both genes are known to be regulated by combustible tobacco cigarette smoke extract (observations from their unpublished data). Combustible tobacco cigarette smoke extract similarly upregulated the expression of both *IL8* and *NTPX1*, but e-cigarette aerosol extract did not. Interestingly, *IL8* expression was reduced and *NTPX1* was increased by nicotine. Based on the responsiveness of human coronary artery endothelial cells, the authors concluded that the use of e-cigarettes as a substitute for combustible tobacco cigarettes is likely to reduce harm to the cardiovascular system (Teasdale et al., 2016).

Rubenstein and colleagues (2015) proposed a novel concept in which hepatic Kupffer cell function and activation can be a contributing factor to cardiovascular disease initiation and/or progression associated with tobacco use. In addition to the well-known role of Kupffer cells as resident macrophages in the liver, primarily responsible for the clearance of pathogens and other foreign particles from portal blood, Kupffer cells recently have been shown to interact with platelets and leukocytes via an adhesion process—an interaction that results in inflammatory processes. Then, the reentry of platelets and leukocytes into the systemic circulation after interacting with Kupffer cells could lead to changes in the systemic circulation, producing adverse effects on the cardiovascular system, including vascular endothelial cell function. For these studies, the authors hypothesized that upon exposure to tobacco smoke or e-cigarette aerosol extracts, Kupffer cells would initiate inflammatory responses that would subsequently contribute to cardiovascular disease initiation and/or progression. In these in vitro studies, Kupffer cells were incubated with tobacco smoke extracts, e-cigarette aerosol extracts, or pure nicotine. An immortalized Kupffer cell line derived from Sprague-Dawley rats was employed. Exposure to both tobacco smoke and e-cigarette aerosol extracts were at a final concentration of 1 cigarette/5 L, while pure nicotine exposure was at a concentration of 50 nM, with all exposures lasting 48 hours. Endpoints measured included complement deposition, complement receptor expression, oxidative stress production, cytokine release, and cell viability and density. Their results conclusively showed that both tobacco and e-cigarette extracts induced a pronounced inflammatory response. Markers of oxidative stress, production and release of cytokines from Kupffer cells, were also significantly increased by both exposures with no notable differences between tobacco and e-cigarette extracts.

Complement C1q and C4d deposition onto Kupffer cells, which is indicative of classical complement pathway activation, was increased significantly by exposure to tobacco and e-cigarette extracts. Deposition of other components of the complement pathways (classical as well as alternative) was also enhanced significantly by both types of exposures. The effects on cell viability were less pronounced (about 80 percent) than on cell density (reductions by approximately 50 percent) for both tobacco and e-cigarette extracts compared with control exposures. Their overall conclusion is that by releasing cytokines and oxidative stress–mediator molecules, altered Kupffer cell function in the liver by e-cigarette aerosol and tobacco smoke exposure can affect the functionality of other cardiovascular cells, such as platelets, endothelial cells, and leukocytes (Rubenstein et al., 2015).

Schweitzer and colleagues (2011, 2015) conducted two studies examining effects of e-cigarettes on endothelial cells. The earlier study showed that in addition to damaging the pulmonary epithelium, soluble components of combustible tobacco cigarette smoke can directly damage lung endothelial cells by disrupting endothelial barrier function (Schweitzer et al., 2011). What is not entirely known is whether nicotine itself or exposure to aerosols released by electronic cigarettes have similar effects to those of combustible tobacco cigarettes on lung endothelia. In one of their more recent studies (Schweitzer et al., 2015), the researchers investigated the effect of nicotine itself or an e-cigarette on lung endothelial cell injury and the mechanism(s). These studies employed primary rat lung endothelial cells (RLECs) and the human bronchial epithelial cell line BEAS-2B. Cell monolayers were exposed to nicotine, e-cigarette solution, or condensed e-cigarette aerosol (1–20 mM nicotine) or to nicotine-free combustible tobacco cigarette smoke extract or e-cigarette solutions.

Reductions in endothelial monolayer permeability as determined by transcellular electrical resistance (TER) measurements are indicative of endothelial cell monolayer disruption. As expected, exposure of primary RLECs to nicotine-containing combustible tobacco cigarette smoke extract (10 percent vol:vol) results in increased monolayer permeability in a time-dependent manner, a reduction of approximately 40 percent at 5 hours and 50 percent at 20 hours. A significantly diminished effect was observed with nicotine-free combustible tobacco cigarette smoke extract at the same time points. This indicates that nicotine itself is an important contributor to the damaging effects of soluble combustible tobacco cigarette smoke extract on the endothelial barrier. To confirm this, RLECs were then incubated with increasing concentrations of nicotine (up to 50 mM for up to 15 hours). They noted a significant time- and dose-dependent decrease in TER. The use of both mouse- and human-derived cells produced the same results, indicating that nicotine's effects on endothelial monolayer disruption are not species specific (Schweitzer et al., 2015).

Two separate nicotine-containing solutions used in commercially available e-cigarettes also induced barrier dysfunction in RLECs, with the dysfuction proportional to the nicotine concentration in the e-liquid. Furthermore, barrier dysfunction was also observed with exposures to similar volumes of an e-cigarette solution without nicotine. However, the effect of an aerosol condensate from the non-nicotine–containing e-cigarette solution in altering the RLEC barrier was less potent.

Of note, the nicotine-free e-cigarette 2 was marketed as having the same flavor as nicotine-containing e-cigarette 2 and shared the same manufacturer. Because aerosolization of e-cigarette solutions may generate different metabolites than the original solution due to heating, the authors investigated whether the condensed aerosol isolated from an e-cigarette affected endothelial function. Overall, the in vitro studies showed that the endothelial barrier–disruptive effect of e-cigarette solutions is nicotine dose dependent and of a comparable magnitude to that produced by 3 percent combustible tobacco cigarette smoke extract exposure (a concentration known not to cause cell death). Furthermore, they concluded that the effects of e-cigarette solutions and aerosols on endothelial function are only in part dependent on nicotine (Schweitzer et al., 2015).

In addition, animal experiments were carried out in which C57BL/6 mice were nebulized using either one dose of nicotine (2 μg) and harvested immediately, or two doses of e-cigarette solution (1 μg each) and harvested 30 minutes or 24 hours later. The results showed a trend toward a rapid increase in polymorphonuclear cells in bronchoalveolar lavage fluid, indicative of higher extravasation of inflammatory cells by the endothelial barrier dysfunction. In addition, systemic oxidative and nitroxidative stress, as evidenced by increased levels of 8-hydroxy-2′-deoxyguanosine (8-OHdG) and nitrotyrosine levels in plasma, was observed in response to inhalation of analytical-grade nicotine. A similar in vivo experiment was done with an e-cigarette liquid, but the data were not shown. The authors state that oxidative stress tended to increase by approximately 10–15 percent compared with a saline vehicle in mice exposed to e-cigarette solutions, as indicated by measured levels of 8-OHdG in plasma.

Lastly, mechanistic studies showed that the endothelial barrier–disruptive effects of cigarette smoke are associated with increased intracellular ceramides, p38 mitogen-activated protein kinase (MAPK) activation, and myosin light-chain phosphorylation. Furthermore, they showed that this signaling cascade is dependent on the function of Rho-associated kinase. The remaining question is whether the same is true for e-cigarettes. Figure 7-3, obtained from Schweitzer and colleagues (2015), depicts the proposed signaling cascade triggered by nicotine that partially overlaps with that used by combustible tobacco cigarette smoke extracts to disrupt the endothelial cell barriers and cell proliferation. A recent microRNA (miRNA) profiling study was conducted using normal human bronchial epithelial (NHBE) cells to determine the global effects of e-cigarette exposure on the miRNA transcriptome in lung epithelia (Solleti et al., 2017). The study first determined whether exposure to an e-cigarette induces oxidative stress in NHBE. They analyzed expression of various oxidative stress response genes by qPCR. NHBE were exposed to 2 percent non-aerosolized or aerosolized and condensed e-cigarette liquid that either contained or lacked nicotine. Their analysis showed that exposure of NHBE to any e-liquid resulted in induction of various oxidative stress–response genes, including *GCLM*, *GCLC*, *GPX2*, *NQO1*, and *HO-1*. Most of these are Nrf2-responsive genes. Of note, aerosolized e-liquid and the presence of nicotine in the exposure regimens resulted in a greater oxidative stress response. Their genome-wide transcriptional analysis of miRNAs identified 578 miRNAs with altered expression from e-cigarette exposure. Nicotine-containing e-cigarette aerosol produced the most profound changes in miRNA expression. They further validated the differential expression of eight miRNAs predicted to be affected significantly by treatment with any e-cigarette liquid by qPCR. While the expression of multiple miRNAs was increased, reduced expression of others was also noted. Overall, these results indicate that e-cigarette exposure has the

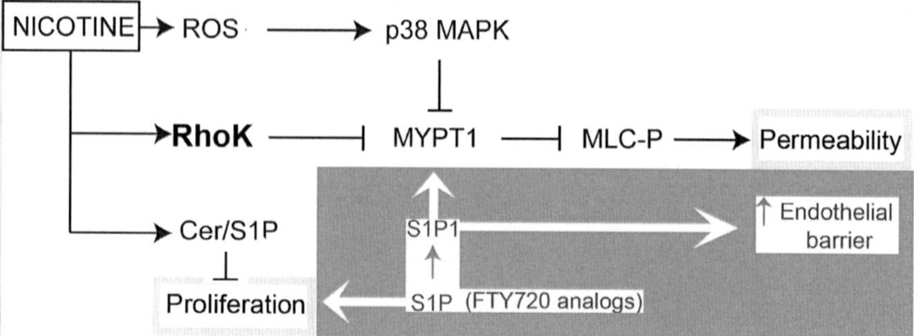

FIGURE 7-3 Proposed signaling cascade triggered by nicotine that partially overlaps with that used by combustible tobacco cigarette smoke extracts to disrupt the endothelial cell barriers and cell proliferation.
NOTES: Arrows indicate activation, and blocked lines indicate inhibition. Nicotine activates Rho-kinase, which in turn inhibits the myosin phosphatase target subunit 1, MYPT1, enhancing phosphorylation of myosin light chains (MLC-P) to increase endothelial permeability. Rho-kinase may have other targets in the cell to increase endothelial permeability because nicotine-induced oxidative stress-dependent p38 MAPK activation also contributed to MLC-P, but not sufficiently to alone increase permeability. Nicotine also increases the ceramide/sphingosine-1-phosphate (S1P) ratios, which may inhibit lung endothelial cell proliferation. Enhancing S1P signaling opposes the decreased cell proliferation and the increase in permeability induced by nicotine in part by inhibiting MLC-P and restoring the lung endothelial barrier function. ROS = reactive oxygen species.
SOURCE: Schweitzer et al., 2015.

capacity to alter the miRNA transcriptome of an endothelial cell line. The importance of these changes and potential role in endothelial dysfunction is yet to be determined.

Previous studies by Fearon and colleagues (2012) reported the development and use of a "scratch wound" assay to measure the rate of HUVEC migration in vitro following artificial wound infliction. In those studies, wounding was inflicted to HUVEC with or without exposure to combustible tobacco cigarette smoke extracts. The results show that rates of HUVEC migration are reduced by combustible tobacco cigarette smoke extracts. In a more recent publication, Taylor and colleagues (2016) compared the effects of e-cigarette aqueous extracts generated from two commercial products to e-cigarette aqueous extracts from the 3R4F reference combustible tobacco cigarette on human bronchial epithelial cell (HBEC) migration. A "cig-a-like" cartomizer style (Vype eStick) and a closed modular (Vype ePen) device were used with blended tobacco–flavored variant containing 36 mg/ml nicotine (cartomizer style; operated at 3.7 V) and

18 mg/ml nicotine (closed modular; operated at 4.0 V). Aqueous aerosol extracts from the e-cigarette devices and the 3R4F reference cigarette were generated by procedures standard to this laboratory.

In the study by Fearon and colleagues (2012), 20 hours of exposure of HUVEC to the 3R4F extract produced a concentration-dependent inhibition of cell migration. This inhibition was complete with concentrations of 3R4F extract greater than 20 percent. As a point of reference, the aqueous extract from 3R4F at concentrations ranging from 0 to 30 percent provides nicotine exposure values of 0.09 to 1.98 μg/ml. By contrast, extracts from the e-cigarette devices at concentrations between 40 percent and 100 percent (equivalent to 1.56 and 1.90 to 4.76 μg/ml nicotine exposure) did not produce any significant reductions in cell migration rates, even when the concentration of nicotine was twice as high as that found in the 3R4F extract. Based on the conditions employed, the authors concluded that the commercial e-cigarette units used in this study do not inhibit endothelial cell migration in vitro. Clearly, analysis of other types of e-cigarette products and e-liquids are required to determine this in in vitro systems.

OXIDATIVE STRESS

Oxidative stress is the cornerstone of many chronic inflammatory diseases. Because there is a large body of evidence on the damage from oxidative stress due to cigarette smoking (both acutely and chronically), evaluation of oxidative stress with e-cigarette use is essential to identify and understand the potential biological and toxicological consequences of any pro-oxidant state produced by chemicals present and/or generated during e-cigarette use. The emerging in vitro literature investigating oxidative stress from e-cigarette use employs either immortalized cell lines, tumor cell lines, or primary cells in culture. Not surprisingly, the publication trend for in vitro oxidative stress by e-cigarettes parallels that presented previously for e-cigarettes and in vitro systems. This publication trend is captured in Figure 7-4, showing numbers of studies on e-cigarettes and oxidative stress.

The type of cell culture system used to study chemical-induced oxidative stress is a very important consideration because major differences in study outcomes can be explained by cell-type selection and the predictive value of the model. To better illustrate this, primary hepatocytes differ widely from commonly used hepatoma cell lines, such as HepG2, in that they are metabolically poor (e.g., biotransformation and disposition capacity) compared with hepatocytes. This is particularly important because chemicals may act directly as toxicants on cells and organs or following bioactivation into reactive intermediates by drug-metabolizing enzymes. However, it must be acknowledged that immortalized cell lines do offer

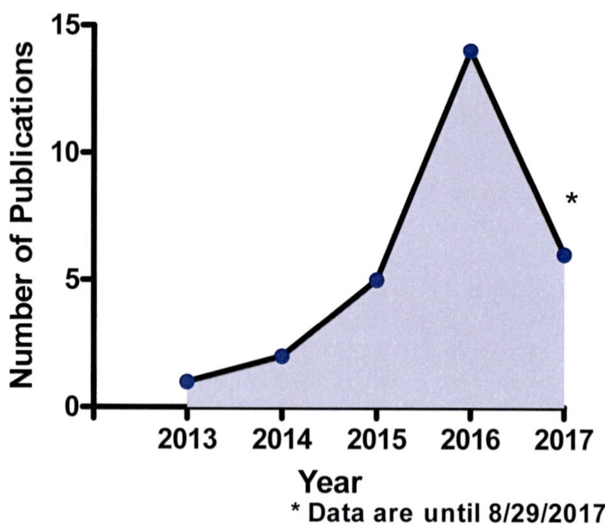

FIGURE 7-4 Publications by year on e-cigarettes and oxidative stress.

various advantages over primary cells, such as unlimited life span, lack of interindividual (or donor) variability, ease of use, and availability, making them popular and useful for in vitro toxicological screening. The selection of different in vitro systems with a wide range of metabolic competencies to study oxidative stress in response to exposure to e-cigarette constituents is one of multiple variables responsible for the wide spectrum of responses reported in the literature to date. Direct addition of e-liquids to cells in culture, as opposed to exposure to either the aerosolized form of or extracts from e-liquid aerosols, adds further variability to the oxidative stress responses measured in cell culture systems. This section will summarize the relevant literature on oxidative stress induced by e-cigarettes into in vitro systems. Establishing comparisons among different studies is somewhat challenging because of the multiple cell types used (primary versus immortalized cells), type and length of exposure (e-liquids versus aerosols and extracts), type of e-cigarette device, and e-liquid selection and composition. In addition, selected in vivo studies assessing the capacity of e-cigarettes to produce oxidative stress also will be discussed in support of and/or complimentary to in vitro studies.

Evidence Review

In a study by Anthérieu and colleagues (2017), human bronchial epithelial BEAS-2B cells, a commonly used bronchial epithelial cell line for respiratory toxicology studies, were exposed to e-cigarette aerosols and combustible tobacco cigarette smoke generated by a smoking machine. Specifically, samples were applied to air–liquid interface cultures of BEAS-2B cells. The puffing frequency/intervals used for cigarette smoke are recognized as the gold standard procedure for smoking machine use of cigarettes, while high puff volume and frequency were selected for e-cigarette aerosols because no standard regimens of exposure are defined and because it has been suggested that the e-cigarette use profile is more intense than the International Organization for Standardization combustible tobacco cigarette smoking profile. The time of exposure to both combustible tobacco cigarette smoke and e-cigarette aerosols ranged from 8 to 288 minutes. Effects on BEAS-2B cells analyzed were cytotoxicity, oxidative stress, and inflammatory response. Additionally, transcriptomic studies were carried out to identify changes in gene expression and potential mechanistic pathways linked to any adverse outcome from these exposures. As expected, exposure to cigarette smoke produced a strong time-dependent decrease in cell viability. However, no cytotoxicity was noted with e-aerosols up to 288 minutes of exposure. Oxidative stress was evaluated by measuring reduced glutathione (GSH) and oxidized glutathione (GSSG) levels. In agreement with the cytotoxicity studies, GSSG/GSH ratios were significantly elevated at both 8- and 48-minute exposure time points relative to controls, with no alterations detected for e-aerosols at any of the time points examined. This indicates, based on a single assay (or endpoint), that the e-aerosol exposure regimen employed in this study does not produce oxidative stress. The authors also analyzed the secretion of 10 inflammatory mediators from BEAS-2B cells in culture media, employing a Luminex-based assay. Exposure to e-cigarette aerosols induced secretion of only IL-6. Exposure to cigarette smoke (8 minutes) similarly induced IL-6 secretion, while also increasing IL-8 secretion. In contrast, secretion of GRO-α, MCP-1 in culture media was decreased by cigarette smoke. A longer exposure to cigarette smoke (48 minutes) reduced the expression of GRO-α, MCP-1, and IL-8. These effects were not seen with exposure to e-cigarette aerosols. Lastly, and as expected, the transcriptomic data showed dysregulation of a large number of genes by cigarette smoke, including genes mediating oxidative stress and/or responses to oxidative stress (e.g., heme oxygenase, superoxide dismutase), cell death (e.g., caspase 10, tumor necrosis factor), and cell signaling pathways associated with cytotoxic responses (e.g., FOS, JUN, STAT1). In contrast, no to very small numbers of genes were found to be differentially regulated by e-cigarette aerosols. Overall, the results of this study strongly suggest lower oxidative stress and cytotoxicity of e-cigarette aerosols in comparison to cigarette smoke in the BEAS-2B cell line. The accompanying gene ontology analysis supports these findings.

Although the respiratory and cardiovascular systems are major targets in tobacco-related pathologies, cigarette smoking apparently accelerates the progression of chronic kidney disease, with nicotine being a proven exacerbator of ischemia-mediated renal injury via oxidative stress. Although the in vitro cytotoxicity of e-liquids has been investigated in various cardiovascular-derived cell lines, the effects of e-cigarettes in the renal system are unknown. A study by El Golli and colleagues (2016) determined whether or not e-cigarette liquid produces renal oxidative stress by generating free radicals or by altering antioxidant responses. In this in vivo study, four groups of rats were injected intraperitoneally with either vehicle saline, e-liquid without nicotine, e-liquid containing nicotine (0.5 mg of nicotine/kg of body weight/day), or nicotine alone (0.5 mg of nicotine/kg of body weight/day). Blood urea, creatinine, and uric acid were measured as endpoints of renal function. The results indicate that there are no significant differences in creatinine values between the e-liquid and vehicle control treated groups, whereas nicotine alone produced a significant increase in creatinine. However, urea and uric acid levels were significantly reduced in both the nicotine and the e-liquid without nicotine groups in comparison to vehicle controls. The e-liquid with nicotine produced a less pronounced decrease in these two endpoints. Total renal sulfhydryl content was increased in all three groups in comparison to vehicle controls, whereas superoxide dismutase and catalase activities were decreased. Renal glutathione-*S*-transferase activity was also decreased with e-liquid treatment. However, no evidence of lipid peroxidation (as evidenced by lack of changes in malondialdehyde levels) was found with e-liquid exposure. Tissue histology also showed the presence of ultrastructural changes, primarily in collecting ducts, that are consistent with an oxidative stress–mediated event by e-liquid treatment. Lastly, the strong correlation observed between superoxide dismutase activity and the renal biomarkers uric acid and urea is also indicative of the presence of oxidative stress/antioxidant response. Although the outcome of this study supports a renal oxidative stress/antioxidant response by e-liquid exposure, the overall relevance of this finding must be interpreted in the context of the route (intraperitoneal) and form of exposure (e-liquid as opposed to aerosol) selected for this study.

In a study that combines both in vivo and in vitro approaches, Husari and colleagues (2016) examined and compared the effect of cigarette smoke to electronic cigarette aerosol generated from a commercially available prefilled cartomizer that contained a propylene glycol/glycerol (80/20) solution of nicotine (18 mg/ml). The in vivo study consisted of three groups of mice: control, e-cigarette, and cigarette smoke. The exposure regimen was 6 hours per day for 3 days, using smoke generator "nose-only" exposure chambers. A characterization of total particulate matter, nicotine, and aldehyde concentration produced by the smoke generation was also carried out in association with this in vivo study. Total particulate matter exposure for the e-cigarette was set at higher levels than for cigarette smoke. Lung injury was determined by measuring wet-to-dry tissue ratio, albumin concentration in bronchoalveolar lavage fluid, gene expression of selected inflammatory mediators, oxidative stress, and histopathological analysis. Oxidative stress was evaluated by confocal microscopy of dihydroethidium fluorescence. This is a commonly used indicator probe of reactive oxygen species production.

For in vitro studies, the human alveolar basal epithelial cell line A549 was selected. Cells were exposed to e-cigarette extract (0–64 mg/ml) or cigarette smoke extract (0–8 mg/ml) for 24 hours. Cytotoxicity and cell morphology were evaluated.

The in vivo studies showed that exposure to e-cigarette aerosol does not result in any increases in lung tissue oxidative stress in comparison to control mice, even when significantly higher concentrations of several chemicals (e.g., various volatile aldehydes, nicotine) and total particulate matter were detected in e-cigarette aerosol in comparison to cigarette smoke. Concurrently, a significant number of TUNEL-positive cells and apoptotic nuclei were detected in lung tissues of cigarette smoke–exposed mice. This was not observed in the lungs of e-cigarette–exposed animals. The other endpoints of lung injury analyzed were similarly unaffected by exposure to e-cigarette aerosol, with the exception of a significant increase in IL-1β. Alterations in these parameters and endpoints are commonly associated with the ability of xenobiotics and their metabolites to generate ROS and induction of oxidative stress.

The outcome of the in vitro studies was also similar. Cytotoxicity and cell morphology changes were evident in A549 cells exposed to combustible tobacco cigarette smoke, but not to the e-cigarette extract. Although oxidative stress in A549 cells was not assessed, it is safe to assume based on cytotoxicity and cell morphology that oxidative stress most likely occurred with cigarette smoke, but not e-cigarette exposure. Overall, the authors concluded that despite higher exposure conditions, exposure to e-cigarette aerosol produces less oxidative stress and less toxic effects both in vivo and in vitro in comparison to exposure to cigarette smoke (Husari et al., 2016).

Ji and colleagues (2016) evaluated the effect of e-cigarette aerosols on oral epithelial cells in vitro. Various e-liquids with different nicotine content and flavors were used to generate aerosols using a homemade puffing machine as described in the article. Particle number concentration and size distribution in e-cigarette aerosols were measured. Furthermore, the physiochemical characteristics of e-cigarette aerosol particles in liquid were also analyzed, determining their size and distribution in water and cell culture media. Technologies such as transmission electron microscopy, X-ray spectroscopy, and dynamic light scattering analysis were employed for particle characterization.

In both water and culture media liquid phases, the size of nanoparticles was significantly larger than those found in the gas phase, which is most likely due to the aggregation of nanoparticles in the liquid phase. The cytotoxicity of e-cigarette aerosols was assessed using normal human oral keratinocytes (NHOKs) in culture. In vitro analysis of e-cigarette aerosol-treated NHOKs show that these aerosols are able to induce oxidative stress as reflected by the significantly lower levels of intracellular GSH. Exposure to fumed silica as a positive control produce similar reductions in GSH as e-cigarette aerosols in NHOKs. This reduction in GSH by e-cigarette aerosol was dose dependent. Oxidative stress represents a dynamic equilibrium between antioxidant defense that acts to restore redox equilibrium and oxidant injury responses that can result in toxicological outcomes. The combined reduction in GSH content, the significant cytotoxicity reflected by drastic reductions in NHOK ATP levels (to approximately 20 percent of control values), and the increased expression of the Nrf2-dependent gene heme oxygenase is suggestive of induction of oxidative stress. Overall, the results of this in vitro study suggest that e-cigarette aerosols could produce cytotoxicity to the oral cavity epithelium through a mechanism that potentially involves oxidative stress induced by nanoparticles and chemicals present in these aerosols. However, the magnitude of these effects by e-cigarette aerosols on NHOKs in relation to traditional tobacco smoke is uncertain because tobacco smoke exposures were not included in this study (Ji et al., 2016).

There is ample evidence indicating that cigarette smoke promotes cerebrovascular conditions that can lead to cerebral ischemia and stroke via generation of ROS, inflammation, and impairment of blood–brain barrier functions. Furthermore, the role of cigarette smoke in promoting vascular endothelial dysfunction and the role of oxidative stress are also well documented. More recent findings support an additive effect on the release and/or formation of angiogenic, oxidative, and inflammatory factors by endothelial cells in the blood–brain barrier in response to hyperglycemia and/or stroke conditions with simultaneous exposure to extracts from cigarette smoke (Prasad et al., 2015, 2017). From these studies, the authors suggested that the blood–brain barrier dysfunction and increased risk for stroke from combustible tobacco smoke resembles the cerebrovascular diseases seen in pathogenic stages of type 2 diabetes that also involve some of the same mediators, such as oxidative stress, inflammation, and changes in antioxidant responses regulated by the transcription factor Nrf2.

In a recent study by the same group, brain ischemic injury was induced by transient middle artery occlusion in groups of mice previously exposed chronically (for 2 weeks total) to either combustible tobacco cigarette smoke (3R4F reference cigarette) or e-cigarette aerosol (blu brand e-cig) via direct inhalation using standard inhalation protocols (Kaisar et al., 2017). The combustible tobacco cigarette smoke and e-cigarette aerosol groups of mice were subdivided and treated with either metformin or saline. Metformin treatment was included because previous studies have shown that this antidiabetic drug has the capacity to reduce oxidative stress and inflammatory responses associated with stroke injury via an Nrf2- and AMP-activated protein kinase (AMPK)-dependent mechanism(s) (Ashabi et al., 2015). In addition to the in vivo studies, C57BL/6 mouse primary brain microvascular endothelial cell (mBMEC) cultures were exposed to 5 percent soluble cigarette smoke or e-cigarette extracts for 24 hours. These extracts were prepared using a standard smoking protocol with a Single Cigarette Smoking Machine. In addition, transwell cultures of mBMEC cells were set up to measure changes in transendothelial electrical resistance (TEER) as an indicator of cell monolayer integrity to measure potential endothelial dysfunction by exposure to extracts.

The results showed that the levels of oxidative stress produced by e-cigarette aerosol and combustible tobacco cigarette smoke in mBMEC cells were not dissimilar and significantly greater than in control cultures. Oxidative stress was measured using the fluorogenic probe CellROX. Correspondingly, strong activation of the transcription factor Nrf2, master sensor and regulator of genes responsive to oxidative stress, was observed with both exposures. Induction of NAD(P)H:quinone oxidoreductase-1 protein, an Nrf2-dependent target, was of very similar magnitude with e-cigarette aerosol and combustible tobacco cigarette smoke exposure. Similarly, nicotine-only exposure of mBMEC cells produced a time- and concentration-dependent Nrf2 activation, as evidenced by its nuclear accumulation. Overall, the in vitro data led the authors to suggest that from a functional perspective, e-cigarette exposure is as damaging as that of combustible tobacco smoke, both eliciting similar levels of oxidative stress and thus oxidative stress–mediated inflammation. Similar correlative results were obtained in the in vivo studies. Interestingly, the in vivo studies show that metformin treatment confers partial support against the detrimental effects of both combustible tobacco cigarette smoke and e-cigarettes in stroke injury by reducing oxidative stress and inflammation (Kaisar et al., 2017).

A study by Moses and colleagues (2017) investigated the impact of electronic cigarette aerosols on the global gene expression profile of primary HBECs, compared with the effect of combustible tobacco cigarette smoke. Cells were isolated from the lungs of a 23-year-old man with no history of smoking or lung disease. Gene expression analysis was carried out in cells grown at the air–liquid interface and exposed to one of four different e-cigarette aerosols, combustible tobacco cigarette smoke (3R4F reference cigarette), and clean air. The authors studied the blu brand of e-cigarettes. The blu e-cigarettes used were labeled as either menthol or tobacco flavored and with or without nicotine (24 mg/cartridge).

The authors first measured cytotoxicity via cell viability and TEER. Although HBECs exposed to combustible tobacco cigarette smoke (six 3R4F cigarettes) exhibited cytotoxicity, no significant effect was observed with up to 400 puffs of electronic cigarette exposure. Furthermore, no significant cytotoxicity was detected when HBECs were exposed to 400 puffs of electronic cigarette aerosols from the four different blu products tested. The gene expression profiling was then carried out under the same conditions (six 3R4F cigarettes or 400 blu electronic cigarette puffs).

Principal component analysis of gene expression data was carried out to examine the effect of all exposures. This is depicted in Figure 7-5. This type of analysis compares how gene expression patterns for combustible tobacco cigarette smoke, e-cigarette aerosols, and air are organized (and whether there is clustering) relative to each other. Of note, the gene expression pattern for the four groups of cells exposed to different blu products clustered together (ECIGs cluster in upper right quadrant). A total of 546 genes were determined to be differentially expressed among the three exposure groups. Gene ontology was also performed to identify gene expression patterns with roles in specific biological processes or signaling pathways highly enriched within the different clusters. Among the genes upregulated by e-cigarette aerosol and combustible tobacco cigarette smoke, they found enrichment for genes involved in oxidative stress, apoptosis, and DNA damage. However, relative to air control, the magnitude of changes in gene expression was greater for combustible tobacco cigarette smoke than for e-cigarettes. The studies also showed that these changes in gene expression are more pronounced in the nicotine-containing e-cigarette than the product without nicotine and that the induction of genes supportive of greater ROS production appears to be dose dependent. It is worth noting that even at the high exposure levels of e-cigarette aerosols (400 puffs) used, induction and/or activation of oxidative stress signaling and xenobiotic metabolism pathways is only a fraction of the magnitude of change produced by cigarette smoke exposures. The genomics data were validated for a selected number of genes by qPCR and also with an immunoassay that detects generation of reactive oxygen species.

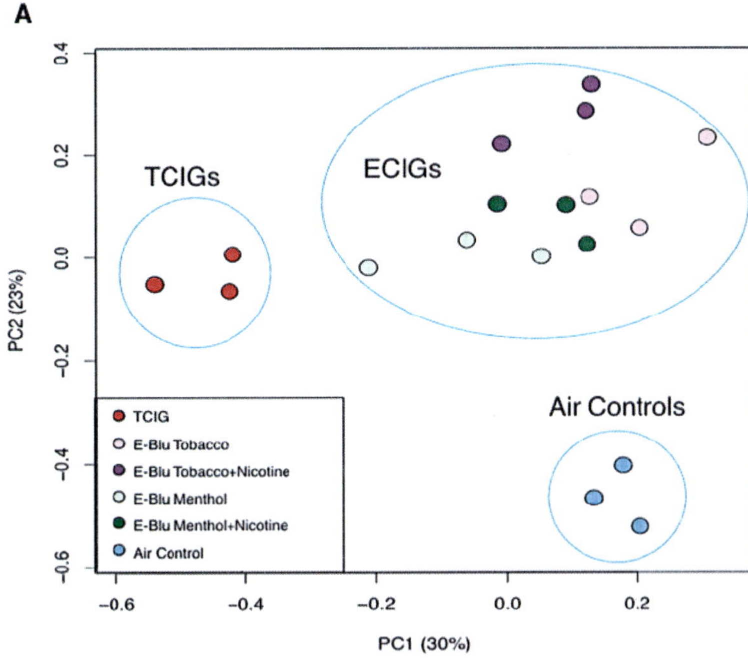

FIGURE 7-5 Principal component analysis of top 2,000 genes by median absolute deviation.
NOTE: ECIG = e-cigarette; TCIG = combustible tobacco cigarette.
SOURCE: Moses et al., 2017.

An intriguing component of this study is that the authors compared the results of the gene expression profiles between bronchial epithelial samples obtained from former cigarette smokers and former smokers who switched to e-cigarette use. The authors justify the importance of this new genomics analysis with e-cigarette exposure based on their past evidence documenting alterations in airway epithelial gene expression patterns by combustible tobacco cigarette smoke that can serve as a biomarker of pulmonary diseases in smokers, including the early detection of cancer (Beane et al., 2007; Silvestri et al., 2015). By gene enrichment analysis, the authors compared gene expression signatures from the in vitro e-cigarette exposures to those generated from bronchial epithelial brushings of current cigarette smokers and former smokers who switched to e-cigarettes. Interestingly, the gene expression differences observed in vitro were concordant with differences observed in airway epithelium collected from e-cigarette users. Overall, e-cigarette aerosols can induce changes in gene expression in vitro, in the bronchial airway epithelium, with a subset of these changes in common with regular cigarette smoke, but of a much lesser magnitude. This study also demonstrates commonalities between in vitro responses and what is observed in individuals who are e-cigarette users (Moses et al., 2017).

A comparative study by Scheffler and colleagues (2015) analyzed the sensitivity of various cell lines, along with primary NHBE cells, to e-liquid aerosol and cigarette smoke. NHBE cells were obtained from healthy tissue from a 75-year-old patient with non-small cell lung cancer. The cells were named NHBE48. For immortalization, the cells underwent transfection with well-defined immortalization genes. The immortalized cells were named CL-1548. In addition, the widely used adenocarcinomic human alveolar basal epithelial cells A549 were selected for analysis. NHBE, NHBE48, and A549 cells were then exposed at the air–liquid interface to e-liquid aerosol, cigarette mainstream smoke, or clean air in a CULTEX RFS compact module.

For e-cigarette aerosol exposure, 200 puffs from a Reevo Mini-S e-cigarette were taken, while for mainstream cigarette smoke, 10 K3R4F cigarettes were used (each puffed six times). Details of puff volume, duration, and blow-out time are described in the article. The tested refill e-liquids were propylene glycol–based (75 percent propylene glycol, 25 percent glycerol) with nicotine concentrations of 0.0 percent and 2.4 percent (24 mg/ml).

Viability data showed that primary NHBE48 cells are the most sensitive cells, showing decreases in viability by 60 percent and 52 percent for nicotine- and non-nicotine–containing e-liquid aerosol exposure, respectively, compared with clean air controls. This is a much smaller response than that seen in combustible tobacco cigarette smoke–exposed cells, where 7 percent viability was measured. The A549 cells were least sensitive to both combustible tobacco cigarette smoke (21 percent viability compared with control air) and both e-liquid aerosols (88 percent viability relative to control air). The immortalized CL-1548 cells were less sensitive to e-liquid aerosols and combustible tobacco cigarette smoke exposure compared with the NHBE48 cells, but significantly more sensitive than A549 cells to both e-liquid aerosols (75 percent and 70 percent viability) and combustible tobacco cigarette smoke (10 percent viability). For all cell types, the presence or absence of nicotine did not significantly affect cell viability values for e-liquid aerosols.

To also analyze oxidative stress, samples from all the different cell types exposed to e-liquid aerosols, combustible tobacco cigarette smoke, and clear air were analyzed using the ROS-Glo™ H_2O_2 fluorescence-based assay. The results were in complete agreement with the cell viability data.

The levels of oxidative stress are highest in primary NHBE48 cells, followed by those in CL-1548 cells, and finally in A549 cells, with both e-liquid aerosols and combustible tobacco cigarette smoke. Also in agreement with the cell viability data, accumulation of oxidative stress with either e-liquid aerosol is only a fraction of that seen with combustible tobacco cigarette smoke. Not only does this study document the use of a new immortalized HBEC cell line for in vitro toxicity testing of e-cigarettes, but it also adds further evidence that e-cigarette aerosols are cytotoxic and produce oxidative stress at levels that are significantly lower than those produced by combustible tobacco cigarette smoke (Scheffler et al., 2015).

A study by Taylor and colleagues (2016) investigated whether a human bronchial epithelial cell line can be employed as a reliable in vitro model of airway epithelium to differentiate cellular stress responses to aqueous aerosol extracts obtained from traditional cigarette smoke and e-cigarette aerosols. The human bronchial epithelial cell line (NCI-H292) was selected as in vitro model. For endpoints, the authors analyzed cellular ratios of reduced GSH to the oxidized form (GSSG), generation of ROS, and transcriptional activation of gene antioxidant response element (ARE) as an indirect indicator of Nrf2 activation and nuclear translocation.

In addition, caspase 3/7 activity was analyzed as a marker of initiation of apoptotic responses to oxidative stress. To generate extracts from both combustible tobacco cigarettes and e-cigarettes, reference 3R4F cigarettes and two Vype e-cigarettes (cigarette-like, cartomizer style; and a closed modular product) were used, respectively. Nicotine and total carbonyl concentrations in the aqueous extracts were quantified to ensure batch-to-batch consistency among extracts used in this study.

As expected, a concentration-dependent induction of cytotoxicity was observed following exposure to cigarette smoke aqueous extract. By contrast, no cytotoxicity was detected with either type of e-cigarette aerosol extracts. Similarly, activation of caspase 3/7 was detected (up to a maximum of 40 percent compared with control exposure), with no changes detected with e-cigarette extracts, even when applied to cells undiluted. Intracellular generation of reactive oxygen species increased by up to 83 percent, while the GSH/GSSG ratios were lowered by more than 90 percent with cigarette smoke aqueous extract. Changes in GSH status and generation of reactive oxygen species are shown in Figure 7-6.

Also, activation of the ARE luciferase reporter gene increased by approximately 300 percent. None of these endpoints of oxidative stress and ROS generation were affected by any of the e-cigarette extracts. The methodology employed was of suitable sensitivity for comparative studies of traditional tobacco and e-cigarettes. Collectively, these results led the authors to conclude that aqueous extracts from the e-cigarettes

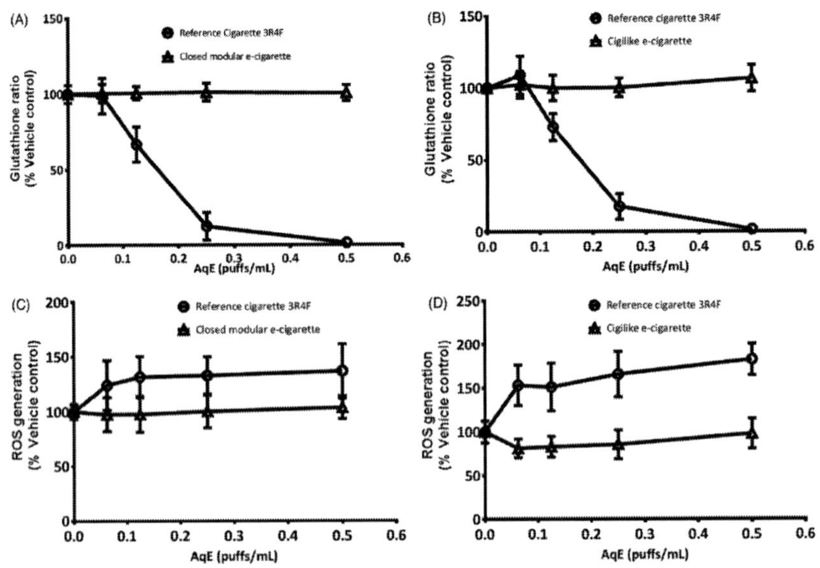

FIGURE 7-6 Changes in glutathione status and generation of reactive oxygen species.
NOTE: AqE = aqueous extract; ROS = reactive oxygen species.
SOURCE: Taylor et al., 2016.

tested in the NCI-H292 human bronchial epithelial cells do not contain either the chemical drivers or the sufficient concentrations to produce oxidative stress or cytotoxicity.

Recent studies by Tran and colleagues (2015) documented that proteostasis and autophagy impairment is a novel mechanism for promoting aggresome formation and apoptosis in COPD–emphysema induced by cigarette smoke. Furthermore, it is well established that oxidative stress is an important mediator of autophagy impairment, which in turn is correlated with induction of proteostasis imbalance and accumulation of ubiquitinated proteins (Korovila et al., 2017). The role of oxidative stress in this response is further supported by the effects of promising new drug candidates for treating COPD, such as a cysteamine-based drug with antioxidant properties that are able to restore autophagy while inhibiting and/or neutralizing reactive oxygen species.

A more recent study by the same group (Shivalingappa et al., 2015) evaluated whether exposure to e-cigarette aerosols modulates proteostasis and autophagy as a potential mechanism for inflammatory and oxidative stress induced by nicotine and/or other chemical components in e-cigarettes. This study also evaluated whether chemical modulation of autophagy can alleviate e-cigarette aerosol–mediated inflammatory and oxidative stress responses.

The study evaluated the effects of e-cigarette aerosol exposure (2.5 or 7.5 mg) on the accumulation of total polyubiquitinated proteins in BEAS-2B cells, an immortalized human bronchial epithelial cell line. Cell treatments with e-cigarette aerosol–exposed culture media lasted 1, 3, or 6 hours. The results showed a time-dependent increase in ubiquitin, primarily in the insoluble protein fractions. Then, autophagy activity in BEAS-2B cells was investigated by immunoblot analysis of the aberrant autophagy marker p62. Significant increases of p62 translocation and accumulation in the insoluble protein fractions at 6 hours were observed, suggesting an impairment of autophagy by exposure to e-cigarette aerosol. Aggresome formation, a cytoplasmic structure containing misfolded proteins, was similarly induced by e-cigarette aerosol.

In order to determine if e-cigarette aerosol induces inflammatory and oxidative stress via autophagy impairment, activation of the transcription factor NFκB and nitrotyrosine protein adduct formation were measured in the presence or absence of the autophagy inducers carbamazepine and cysteamine; the latter has also been an antioxidant. NFκB activation and nitrotyrosine protein adducts were used as markers of inflammation and oxidative stress, respectively. The results showed that BEAS-2B cells preincubated with carbamazepine for 6 hours and then exposed to e-cigarette aerosol for 1 hour showed an attenuation in the normal increases in total protein NFκB levels and nitrotyrosine protein adduct formation induced by e-cigarette aerosol–only exposure, confirming that this autophagy inducer ameliorates the oxidative and inflammatory stress produced by e-cigarette aerosols. The capacity of cysteamine to alter e-cigarette aerosol–induced oxidative stress in BEAS-2B cells was also assessed. E-cigarette aerosol by itself produced a significant increase in levels of intracellular ROS, which were significantly reduced by preincubation with cysteamine. Similarly, cysteamine treatment was capable of rescuing e-cigarette aerosol–induced aggresome formation and aberrant autophagy.

Collectively, this study demonstrated for the first time that exposure to e-cigarette aeosols impairs proteostasis and autophagy, which cascades into accumulation of ubiquitinated proteins, oxidative stress, apoptosis, and cell senescence (Shivalingappa et al., 2015). All these events can be reduced by autophagy inducers, such as carbamazepine and cysteamine. However, in the absence of comparative experiments that include exposure to cigarette smoke, the magnitude and physiological relevance of the effects observed with e-cigarette relative to combustible tobacco cigarette smoke remain uncertain.

CONCLUSIONS

*Conclusion 7-1. There is **substantial evidence** that e-cigarette aerosols can induce acute endothelial cell dysfunction, although the long-term consequences and outcomes on these parameters with long-term exposure to e-cigarette aerosol are uncertain.*

*Conclusion 7-2. There is **substantial evidence** that components of e-cigarette aerosols can promote formation of reactive oxygen species/ oxidative stress. Although this supports the biological plausibility of tissue injury and disease from long-term exposure to e-cigarette aerosols, generation of reactive oxygen species and oxidative stress induction are generally lower from e-cigarettes than from combustible tobacco cigarette smoke.*

Adverse outcome pathway (AOP) is a relatively new, knowledge-driven concept that provides a framework that organizes in a sequential fashion molecular initiating events, intermediate key events, and an adverse outcome spanning layers of biological organization. Various AOPs have been developed for chemical-induced pathologies, such as cholestasis, liver fibrosis, and steatosis. The other use of AOPs is their potential for predicting disease risk. Pertinent to the health effects and risk analysis of e-cigarette use is a recently developed AOP for the onset of hypertension by oxidative stress–mediated perturbation of endothelial function. This AOP specifically describes how vascular endothelial peptide oxidation leads to hypertension through perturbation of endothelial nitric oxide bioavailability, resulting in impaired vasodilation (Lowe et al., 2017). The authors proposed that this and related AOPs can serve as a tool for the regulatory assessment of the harm reduction potential of e-cigarettes relative to combustible tobacco products. Another use of this or related AOPs is the assessment of harm associated with individual or combined components in e-cigarette products as well as device characteristic and mode of use. Lastly, as new biomarkers are identified and/ or validated that can distinguish harm and magnitude of e-cigarette use from traditional cigarette smoking, they can be integrated with AOPs to better assess health risks associated with e-cigarettes and related nicotine products.

REFERENCES

Anderson, C., A. Majeste, J. Hanus, and S. Wang. 2016. E-cigarette aerosol exposure induces reactive oxygen species, DNA damage, and cell death in vascular endothelial cells. *Toxicological Sciences* 154(2):332–340.

Anthérieu, S., A. Garat, N. Beauval, M. Soyez, D. Allorge, G. Garçon, and J. M. Lo-Guidice. 2017. Comparison of cellular and transcriptomic effects between electronic cigarette vapor and cigarette smoke in human bronchial epithelial cells. *Toxicology in Vitro* 45(Part 3):417–425.

Antoniewicz, L., J. A. Bosson, J. Kuhl, S. M. Abdel-Halim, A. Kiessling, F. Mobarrez, and M. Lundback. 2016. Electronic cigarettes increase endothelial progenitor cells in the blood of healthy volunteers. *Atherosclerosis* 255:179–185.

Ashabi, G., L. Khalaj, F. Khodagholi, M. Goudarzvand, and A. Sarkaki. 2015. Pre-treatment with metformin activates Nrf2 antioxidant pathways and inhibits inflammatory responses through induction of AMPK after transient global cerebral ischemia. *Metabolic Brain Disease* 30(3):747–754.

Barber, K. E., B. Ghebrehiwet, W. Yin, and D. A. Rubenstein. 2016. Endothelial cell inflammatory reactions are altered in the presence of e-cigarette extracts of variable nicotine. *Cellular and Molecular Bioengineering* 10(1):124–133.

Beane, J., P. Sebastiani, G. Liu, J. S. Brody, M. E. Lenburg, and A. Spira. 2007. Reversible and permanent effects of tobacco smoke exposure on airway epithelial gene expression. *Genome Biology* 8(9):R201.

Bein, K., and G. D. Leikauf. 2011. Acrolein—A pulmonary hazard. *Molecular Nutrition & Food Research* 55(9):1342–1360.

Breheny, D., J. Adamson, D. Azzopardi, A. Baxter, E. Bishop, T. Carr, I. Crooks, K. Hewitt, T. Jaunky, S. Larard, F. Lowe, O. Oke, M. Taylor, S. Santopietro, D. Thorne, B. Zainuddin, M. Gaça, C. Liu, J. Murphy, and C. Proctor. 2017. A novel hybrid tobacco product that delivers a tobacco flavour note with vapour aerosol (part 2): In vitro biological assessment and comparison with different tobacco-heating products. *Food and Chemical Toxicology* 106(Part A):533–546.

Carnevale, R., S. Sciarretta, F. Violi, C. Nocella, L. Loffredo, L. Perri, M. Peruzzi, A. G. M. Marullo, E. De Falco, I. Chimenti, V. Valenti, G. Biondi-Zoccai, and G. Frati. 2016. Acute impact of tobacco vs. electronic cigarette smoking on oxidative stress and vascular function. *Chest* 150(3):606–612.

Conklin, D. J., M. V. Malovichko, I. Zeller, T. P. Das, T. V. Krivokhizhina, B. H. Lynch, P. Lorkiewicz, A. Agarwal, N. Wickramasinghe, P. Haberzettl, S. D. Sithu, J. Shah, T. E. O'Toole, S. N. Rai, A. Bhatnagar, and S. Srivastava. 2017. Biomarkers of chronic acrolein inhalation exposure in mice: Implications for tobacco product-induced toxicity. *Toxicological Sciences* 158(2):263–274.

El Golli, N. E., A. Jrad-Lamine, H. Neffati, H. Dkhili, D. Rahali, Y. Dallagi, M. V. El May, and S. El Fazaa. 2016. Impact of e-cigarette refill liquid exposure on rat kidney. *Regulatory Toxicology and Pharmacology* 77:109–116.

Fearon, I. M., D. O. Acheampong, and E. Bishop. 2012. Modification of smoke toxicant yields alters the effects of cigarette smoke extracts on endothelial migration: An in vitro study using a cardiovascular disease model. *International Journal of Toxicology* 31(6):572–583.

Husari, A., A. Shihadeh, S. Talih, Y. Hashem, M. El Sabban, and G. Zaatari. 2016. Acute exposure to electronic and combustible cigarette aerosols: Effects in an animal model and in human alveolar cells. *Nicotine & Tobacco Research* 18(5):613–619.

Ji, E. H., B. B. Sun, T. K. Zhao, S. Shu, C. H. Chang, D. Messadi, T. Xia, Y. F. Zhu, and S. Hu. 2016. Characterization of electronic cigarette aerosol and its induction of oxidative stress response in oral keratinocytes. *PLoS ONE* 11(5):e0154447. https://doi.org/10.1371/journal.pone.0154447 (accessed February 6, 2018).

Kaisar, M. A., H. Villalba, S. Prasad, T. Liles, A. E. Sifat, R. K. Sajja, T. J. Abbruscato, and L. Cucullo. 2017. Offsetting the impact of smoking and e-cigarette vaping on the cerebrovascular system and stroke injury: Is metformin a viable countermeasure? *Redox Biology* 13:353–362.

Korovila, I., M. Hugo, J. P. Castro, D. Weber, A. Hohn, T. Grune, and T. Jung. 2017. Proteostasis, oxidative stress and aging. *Redox Biology* 13:550–567.

Lowe, F. J., K. Luettich, M. Talikka, V. Hoang, L. E. Haswell, J. Hoeng, and M. D. Gaça. 2017. Development of an adverse outcome pathway for the onset of hypertension by oxidative stress-mediated perturbation of endothelial nitric oxide bioavailability. *Applied In Vitro Toxicology* 3(1):131–148.

Moghe, A., S. Ghare, B. Lamoreau, M. Mohammad, S. Barve, C. McClain, and S. Joshi-Barve. 2015. Molecular mechanisms of acrolein toxicity: Relevance to human disease. *Toxicological Sciences* 143(2):242–255.

Morris, P. B., B. A. Ference, E. Jahangir, D. N. Feldman, J. J. Ryan, H. Bahrami, M. F. El-Chami, S. Bhakta, D. E. Winchester, M. H. Al-Mallah, M. Sanchez Shields, P. Deedwania, L. S. Mehta, B. A. P. Phan, and N. L. Benowitz. 2015. Cardiovascular effects of exposure to cigarette smoke and electronic cigarettes: Clinical perspectives from the Prevention of Cardiovascular Disease Section Leadership Council and Early Career Councils of the American College of Cardiology. *Journal of the American College of Cardiology* 66(12):1378–1391.

Moses, E., T. Wang, S. Corbett, G. R. Jackson, E. Drizik, C. Perdomo, C. Perdomo, E. Kleerup, D. Brooks, G. O'Connor, S. Dubinett, P. Hayden, M. E. Lenburg, and A. Spira. 2017. Molecular impact of electronic cigarette aerosol exposure in human bronchial epithelium. *Toxicological Sciences* 155(1):248–257.

Poynton, S., J. Sutton, S. Goodall, J. Margham, M. Forster, K. Scott, C. Liu, K. McAdam, J. Murphy, and C. Proctor. 2017. A novel hybrid tobacco product that delivers a tobacco flavour note with vapour aerosol (part 1): Product operation and preliminary aerosol chemistry assessment. *Food & Chemical Toxicology* 106(Part A):522–532.

Prasad, S., R. K. Sajja, J. H. Park, P. Naik, M. A. Kaisar, and L. Cucullo. 2015. Impact of cigarette smoke extract and hyperglycemic conditions on blood-brain barrier endothelial cells. *Fluids Barriers CNS* 12:18. https://doi.org/10.1186/s12987-015-0014-x (accessed February 6, 2018).

Prasad, S., R. K. Sajja, M. A. Kaisar, J. H. Park, H. Villalba, T. Liles, T. Abbruscato, and L. Cucullo. 2017. Role of Nrf2 and protective effects of metformin against tobacco smoke-induced cerebrovascular toxicity. *Redox Biology* 12:58–69.

Putzhammer, R., C. Doppler, T. Jakschitz, K. Heinz, J. Forste, K. Danzl, B. Messner, and D. Bernhard. 2016. Vapours of U.S. and E.U. market leader electronic cigarette brands and liquids are cytotoxic for human vascular endothelial cells. *PLoS ONE* 11(6):e0157337. https://doi.org/10.1371/journal.pone.0157337 (accessed February 6, 2018).

Raitakari, O. T., and D. S. Celermajer. 2000. Flow-mediated dilatation. *British Journal of Clinical Pharmacology* 50(5):397–404.

Rubenstein, D. A., S. Hom, B. Ghebrehiwet, and W. Yin. 2015. Tobacco and e-cigarette products initiate Kupffer cell inflammatory responses. *Molecular Immunology* 67(2):652–660.

Scheffler, S., H. Dieken, O. Krischenowski, and M. Aufderheide. 2015. Cytotoxic evaluation of e-liquid aerosol using different lung-derived cell models. *International Journal of Environmental Research and Public Health* 12(10):12466–12474.

Schweitzer, K. S., H. Hatoum, M. B. Brown, M. Gupta, M. J. Justice, B. Beteck, M. Van Demark, Y. Gu, R. G. Presson, Jr., W. C. Hubbard, and I. Petrache. 2011. Mechanisms of lung endothelial barrier disruption induced by cigarette smoke: Role of oxidative stress and ceramides. *American Journal of Physiology—Lung Cellular and Molecular Physiology* 301(6):L836–L846.

Schweitzer, K. S., S. X. Chen, S. Law, M. Van Demark, C. Poirier, M. J. Justice, W. C. Hubbard, E. S. Kim, X. Lai, M. Wang, W. D. Kranz, C. J. Carroll, B. D. Ray, R. Bittman, J. Goodpaster, and I. Petrache. 2015. Endothelial disruptive proinflammatory effects of nicotine and e-cigarette vapor exposures. *American Journal of Physiology—Lung Cellular and Molecular Physiology* 309(2):L175–L187.

Shivalingappa, P. C., R. Hole, C. V. Westphal, and N. Vij. 2015. Airway exposure to e-cigarette vapors impairs autophagy and induces aggresome formation. *Antioxidants & Redox Signaling* 24(4):186–204.

Silvestri, G. A., A. Vachani, D. Whitney, M. Elashoff, K. Porta Smith, J. S. Ferguson, E. Parsons, N. Mitra, J. Brody, M. E. Lenburg, A. Spira, and A. S. Team. 2015. A bronchial genomic classifier for the diagnostic evaluation of lung cancer. *New England Journal of Medicine* 373(3):243–251.

Solleti, S. K., S. Bhattacharya, A. Ahmad, Q. Wang, J. Mereness, T. Rangasamy, and T. J. Mariani. 2017. MicroRNA expression profiling defines the impact of electronic cigarettes on human airway epithelial cells. *Scientific Reports*. https://doi.org/10.1038/s41598-017-01167-8 (accessed February 6, 2018).

Taylor, M., T. Carr, O. Oke, T. Jaunky, D. Breheny, F. Lowe, and M. Gaça. 2016. E-cigarette aerosols induce lower oxidative stress in vitro when compared to tobacco smoke. *Toxicology Mechanisms and Methods* 26(6):465–476.

Teasdale, J. E., A. C. Newby, N. J. Timpson, M. R. Munafo, and S. J. White. 2016. Cigarette smoke but not electronic cigarette aerosol activates a stress response in human coronary artery endothelial cells in culture. *Drug and Alcohol Dependence* 163:256–260.

Tran, I., C. Ji, I. Ni, T. Min, D. Tang, and N. Vij. 2015. Role of cigarette smoke-induced aggresome formation in chronic obstructive pulmonary disease-emphysema pathogenesis. *American Journal of Respiratory Cell and Molecular Biology* 53(2):159–173.

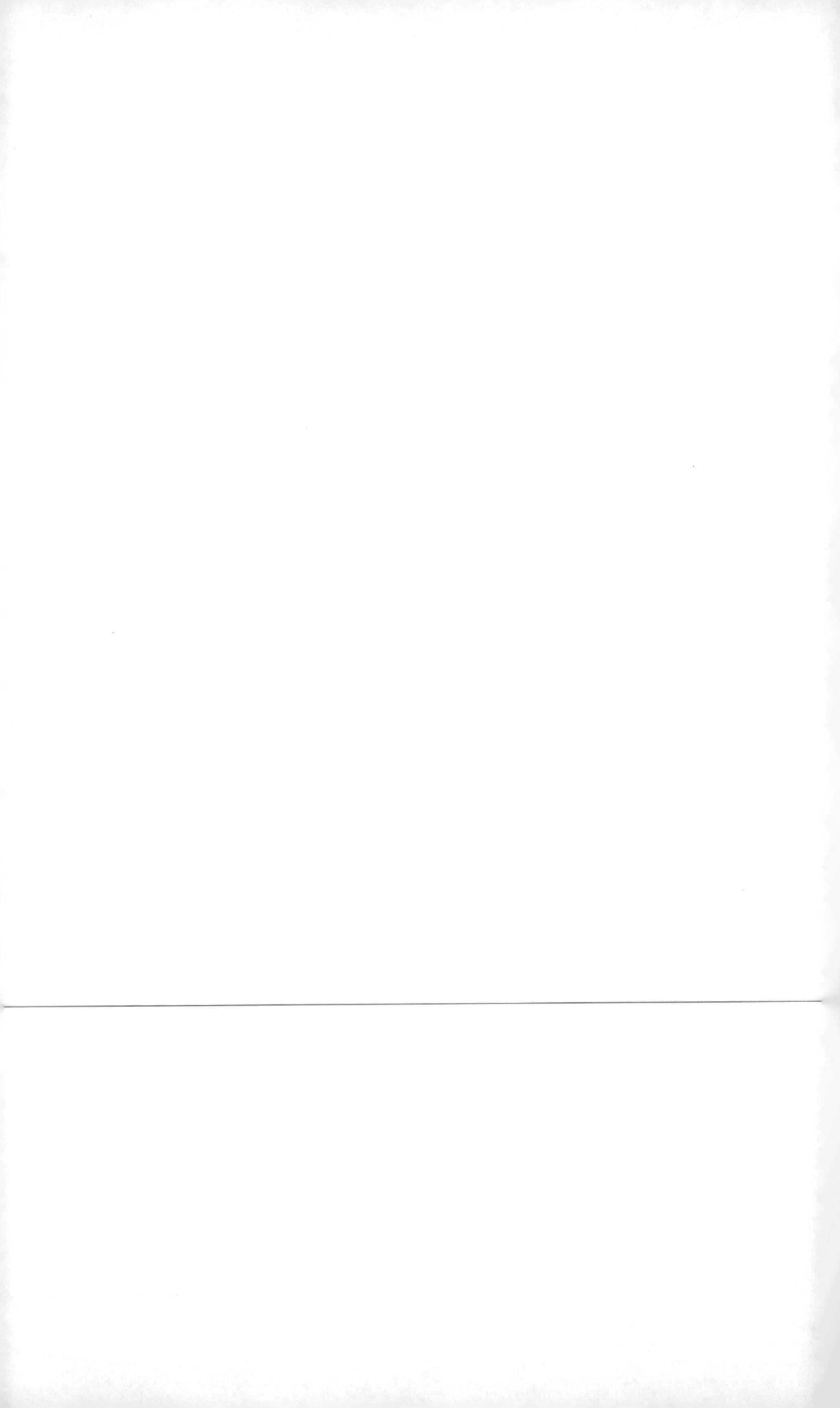

8

Dependence and Abuse Liability

Studies on the health effects of combustible tobacco have focused on physical disease endpoints (e.g., cancer, cardiovascular disease, respiratory disease). However, combustible tobacco use also has important effects on mental health, including tobacco dependence syndrome. Tobacco use disorder, which is a medical condition recognized by the World Health Organization's *International Classification of Diseases* (ICD), had a past-year prevalence of 20 percent among all U.S. adults in 2012–2013 (Chou et al., 2016). It produces clinically significant distress and impairment to those affected. As with other substance use disorders, tobacco dependence[1] is characterized by unpleasant withdrawal symptoms and loss of behavioral control over use, which result in dependent individuals spending considerable time obtaining or using combustible tobacco cigarettes, interfering with the ability to fulfill important social or occupational role obligations and having a variety of other social and physical consequences (Fiore et al., 2008; Volkow et al., 2016). As with other psychiatric disorders, the

[1] The committee uses the term "dependence" to describe the constellation of behavioral symptoms associated with the problematic use of tobacco and nicotine products. While earlier versions of the *Diagnostic and Statistical Manual of Mental Disorders* (DSM) used the term "dependence" to describe the mental health syndrome caused by problematic tobacco use, DSM-5 no longer uses the term dependence and now uses "tobacco use disorder," which includes many of the symptoms previously identified for the DSM-IV nicotine dependence disorder. Much of the field uses the term "dependence" to describe the mental health symptoms caused by the compulsive use of tobacco, which includes but is not limited to the DSM-IV nicotine dependence operationalizations of the construct.

symptoms of tobacco dependence are experienced by the user as subjectively distressing (Hughes, 2006) and are linked to neurobiological adaptations in the brain's circuitry underpinning emotion, motivation, and cognition (Markou, 2008). While the amount of tobacco use is associated with risk and severity of tobacco dependence, the correlation is typically of moderate magnitude, and dependence symptoms are reported by an appreciable portion of infrequent and low-intensity tobacco users (Japuntich et al., 2009; Reyes-Guzman et al., 2017), indicating that dependence is a unique outcome in and of itself that is influenced by a combination of the amount of tobacco exposure and other factors. Overall, the tobacco dependence syndrome is an important primary health endpoint to consider.

Nicotine is the principal pharmacological agent that causes dependence on combustible tobacco cigarettes (Benowitz, 2008). Because nicotine is delivered via a pulmonary route, the speed, efficiency, and magnitude of nicotine delivered in "bolus" form produces a higher addiction potential of nicotine relative to other nicotine-delivery devices with slower pharmacokinetics (see Chapter 4 for a detailed review of nicotine pharmacokinetics). While nicotine is necessary, the pharmacological action of nicotine is not sufficient to account for the high addiction potential of combustible tobacco cigarettes (Rose, 2006). "Non-nicotine factors" associated with tobacco self-administration (e.g., taste, smell, and sensations associated with the act of smoking) are critical to the establishment and maintenance of dependence on combustible tobacco cigarettes (Fagerström, 2012). Habitual combustible tobacco cigarette smokers will continue smoking "denicotinized cigarettes" (i.e., cigarettes made with engineered tobacco leaves that contain only trace amounts of nicotine) or very low nicotine-containing cigarettes (i.e., engineered cigarettes with roughly 2–3 percent of the amount in a normal cigarette) for extended periods of time (Donny et al., 2007, 2015). Like other drugs of abuse, denicotinized cigarette smoking can cause a significant release of dopamine in the brain's reward circuit of regular combustible tobacco cigarette smokers, albeit at lower levels (Domino et al., 2013). Behaviors that have no direct pharmacological effects produce symptoms of addiction (e.g., gambling) and may be associated with dysregulation in brain reward circuits (Quester and Romanczuk-Seiferth, 2015). For these reasons, it is now established that combustible tobacco cigarette dependence is not merely addiction to the nicotine, per se (Rose, 2006). This has prompted experts to call for the reframing and relabeling of the tobacco use disorder concept and measurement away from terms that prioritize nicotine, such as "nicotine dependence," to conceptualizations and terms that acknowledge the role of non-nicotine factors, such as the term "cigarette dependence" or "tobacco dependence" (Fagerström, 2012).

Given this background, this section focuses on "e-cigarette dependence," the constellation of behaviors and symptoms that are distressing to the user and promote the compulsive use of e-cigarettes due to nicotine and non-nicotine factors (Strong et al., 2017). Like combustible tobacco cigarettes, if e-cigarette use were to cause dependence symptoms, the symptoms would be strongly influenced by, but not entirely caused by, nicotine per se. Preclinical researchers attempting to uncover the reasons why combustible tobacco cigarettes have such a high addiction potential struggled for decades because animal models were challenged by the fact that, unlike other drugs of abuse, rodents did not easily acquire habitual self-administration of nicotine intravenously (Caggiula et al., 2009). Ultimately, it was discovered that when intravenous nicotine administration was paired with other non-pharmacological sensory stimuli that are pleasant and rewarding (e.g., a sound paired with sucrose) (Caggiula et al., 2009), rats would more easily acquire habitual nicotine self-administration in a manner similar to other drugs of abuse. Based on such research and other studies, it is now established that addiction potential of tobacco products is dependent on the stimulus context that coincides with nicotine administration. The combination of pleasant stimuli associated with the tobacco self-administration ritual (e.g., the taste, smells, sight, and sensations of inhaling and exhaling as well as the hand-to-mouth movements) and the drug itself synergize to account for the high addiction potential of combustible tobacco cigarettes.

Given what is known about the role of nicotine and non-nicotine factors in tobacco product dependence, it is plausible that e-cigarette use may cause dependence symptoms, and the reason may not be explained merely by the fact the e-cigarettes are a nicotine delivery device. Most e-cigarette products are available in desirable flavors and have other characteristics that generate aerosols with a unique profile of pleasurable sensory stimuli due to the taste, sights, smells, and airway sensations, that (like combustible tobacco cigarettes) could have synergistic effects with nicotine on dependence risk. Such enjoyable sensory stimuli in combination with the delivery of "boluses" of nicotine via a pulmonary route (as in combustible tobacco cigarettes) may produce a dependence potential with e-cigarette use. However, it is also possible that e-cigarettes may not produce symptoms of dependence, or that they produce dependence, but at a risk that is significantly lower than combustible tobacco cigarettes. Unlike these combusitble tobacco cigarettes that reliably and quickly deliver nicotine to the brain, the efficiency, speed, and magnitude of nicotine delivery to the user varies widely across different e-cigarette products and user characteristics (see Chapter 4 for a detailed review of nicotine delivery). Relative to a combustible tobacco cigarette, variations in e-cigarette product characteristics and other conditions have been shown to produce plasma nicotine levels that are below, equal to, or exceed those (Breland et al., 2017). In addition, non-nicotine pharmacological components of combustible tobacco smoke (e.g., monoamine oxidase inhibitors) and other additives may also contribute to the dependence risk caused by combustible tobacco cigarettes (Fagerström, 2012); these compounds may not be present in e-cigarette aerosol. Hence, whether e-cigarettes cause dependence and what the relative magnitude of risk is relative to combustible tobacco cigarettes are questions that cannot be answered solely by the translation of knowledge about nicotine and combustible cigarettes and necessitate a review of the empirical evidence. Furthermore, given the wide variety of products that may alter the nicotine delivery and sensory experience of e-cigarettes, it is plausible that variations in e-cigarette product characteristics affect risk of dependence. Because combustible tobacco cigarette dependence symptoms are known to produce distress as well as social and functional impairment (APA, 2013; Hughes, 2006), independent of the impact of smoking on physical disease, evidence that e-cigarette use causes dependence symptoms would warrant consideration in regulatory policies directed toward e-cigarette manufacture, distribution, and sales.

CHARACTERIZATION OF DISEASE ENDPOINTS AND INTERMEDIATE OUTCOMES

The strongest evidence to characterize the potential association between e-cigarette use and dependence would include methodologically rigorous epidemiological studies with e-cigarette dependence symptoms as an endpoint. While there is no widely agreed-upon method of assessing and diagnosing e-cigarette dependence yet, the initial efforts to operationalize dependence as a health outcome of e-cigarettes have adapted methods of assessing combustible tobacco cigarette dependence to e-cigarettes (Foulds et al., 2015; Strong et al., 2017). Essentially many of the same survey or interview questions aimed at assessing symptom presence or severity are used, but the term "e-cigarettes" is substituted for "cigarettes" on the measure. For instance, the U.S. Population Assessment of Tobacco and Health (PATH) study, a nationally representative survey of tobacco use, adapted dependence measures based on the American Psychiatric Association's (APA's) *Diagnostic and Statistical Manual of Mental Disorders* (DSM) definition of cigarette use disorder. PATH also employed other validated questionnaires that collectively assess various symptoms recognized to be part of the nicotine dependence syndrome, including compulsion to smoke, intensity of smoking (e.g., cigarettes per day), distressing withdrawal symptoms upon abstinence, typical time to first use after awakening each day, and craving for the product. The key manifestations of the DSM and the ICD drug dependence classification system, which are common to tobacco products and all other substances of abuse, and are summarized in Box 8-1.

E-cigarette dependence can be operationalized as a category (e.g., having at least one or more symptoms, surpassing a "clinical" threshold of two symptoms or more [APA, 2013]), or on a continuum with a score

BOX 8-1
Criteria for Tobacco Use Disorder from the American Psychiatric Association's *Diagnostic and Statistical Manual of Mental Disorders*, 5th Edition

A problematic pattern of tobacco use leading to clinically significant impairment or distress, as manifested by at least two of the following factors, occurring within a 12-month period:

1. Tobacco is often taken in larger amounts or over a longer period than was intended.
2. There is a persistent desire or unsuccessful efforts to cut down or control tobacco use.
3. A great deal of time is spent in activities necessary to obtain or use tobacco.
4. Craving, or a strong desire or urge to use tobacco.
5. Recurrent tobacco use resulting in a failure to fulfill major role obligations at work, school, or home.
6. Continued tobacco use despite having persistent or recurrent social or interpersonal problems caused or exacerbated by the effects of tobacco (e.g., arguments with others about tobacco use).
7. Important social, occupational, or recreational activities are given up or reduced because of tobacco use.
8. Recurrent tobacco use in situations in which it is physically hazardous (e.g., smoking in bed).
9. Tobacco use is continued despite knowledge of having a persistent or recurrent physical or psychological problem that is likely to have been caused or exacerbated by tobacco.
10. Tolerance, as defined by either of the following:
    a. A need for markedly increased amounts of tobacco to achieve the desired effect.
    b. A markedly diminished effect with continued use of the same amount of tobacco.
11. Withdrawal, as manifested by either of the following:
    a. The characteristic withdrawal syndrome for tobacco (refer to Criteria A and B of the criteria set for tobacco withdrawal).
    b. Tobacco (or a closely related substance, e.g., nicotine) is taken to relieve or avoid withdrawal symptoms.

SOURCE: APA, 2013.

reflecting a gradient of severity of dependence from none to mild, moderate, or severe. Additional well-established measures of tobacco dependence include the Fagerström Test for Cigarette Dependence (FTCD) (Heatherton et al., 1991), the Heaviness of Smoking Index, the Hooked on Nicotine Checklist (DiFranza et al., 2002), the Nicotine Dependence Syndrome Scale (NDSS) (Shiffman et al., 2004), and the Wisconsin Inventory of Smoking Dependence Motives (Piper et al., 2004). These measures assess symptoms similar to APA and ICD symptoms (e.g., tolerance, withdrawal) and evaluate other domains reflecting other motives for tobacco use or manifestations of habitual smoking (e.g., strong motive to use tobacco to alleviate negative emotions, smoking automatically and instinctually without thinking about it).

Supportive evidence comes from human laboratory investigations that apply "abuse liability" testing methods to e-cigarettes and reflect important intermediate outcomes. Abuse liability tests typically involve human laboratory behavioral pharmacology experiments that test the acute effects of controlled drug administration on indicators that are suspected to be proxies of the likelihood that the drug will produce dependence, including subjective effects (e.g., mood enhancement, drug liking) or behavioral choices indicating the motivational value of the drug (e.g., amount of money willing to trade for the drug, willingness to execute a demanding behavior to obtain the drug) (Henningfield et al., 2011). Abuse liability testing is a long-used paradigm relied on by public health regulatory agencies, such as the Food and Drug Administration (FDA), to indicate whether a novel compound is likely to produce dependence. It is particularly useful for screening the potential for dependence of novel psychoactive compounds (e.g., sedatives, stimulants) prior to obtaining epidemiological data on reports of dependence in the population. Laboratory evidence of abuse liability may not be an exact replication of what occurs in the natural ecology, yet cross-drug differences in laboratory-obtained abuse liability data are in concordance with cross-drug differences in population-level dependence risk among use initiators (Griffiths and Wolf, 1990; Kollins, 2003; Wagner and Anthony, 2002). There is a well-developed literature applying the abuse liability paradigm to combustible tobacco cigarettes and, more recently, emerging literature on the abuse liability of non-traditional tobacco products with specific methodological guidelines put forth from tobacco product abuse liability testing experts (Carter et al., 2009; Henningfield et al., 2011).

OPTIMAL STUDY DESIGN

Primary Endpoint: Epidemiological Evidence of Dependence Symptoms Caused by E-Cigarettes

The optimal epidemiological study would be a longitudinal cohort investigation that follows individuals who initiate e-cigarette use and tracks the development, escalation, and persistence of e-cigarette dependence symptoms in a nationally representative sample. In such a design, descriptive population-level estimates of the speed, likelihood, and duration of dependence symptoms among e-cigarette–ever users would permit inferences regarding the dependence potential of e-cigarettes, with estimates of greater prevalence, speed, and duration of dependence symptoms being indicative of greater dependence risk caused by e-cigarettes. In addition, studies of the association between levels of e-cigarette exposure and likelihood of dependence would also provide key data, with evidence of a dose–response being supportive of greater dependence risk caused by e-cigarette use.

A critical confounder is the use of other tobacco products (namely, combustible tobacco cigarettes), which is strongly associated with e-cigarette use (Kasza et al., 2017; Schoenborn and Gindi, 2015). A large portion of adults in the United States age 25 or older who use e-cigarettes are current or prior combustible tobacco cigarette smokers (CDC, 2016), many of whom have tobacco use disorder (Chou et al., 2016). Individuals with considerable histories of smoking report using e-cigarettes to alleviate nicotine withdrawal caused by their cessation of combustible tobacco cigarettes or to satisfy cravings for such cigarettes (Etter and Bullen, 2014). For current or recent ex-smokers, any behavioral signs or symptoms indicative of dependence on e-cigarettes (e.g., short duration between awakening and time of first e-cigarette) could be attributed merely as an artifact of dependence-like behavior produced by smoking. The confounder of smoking is particularly problematic for dual users; statistical adjustment of smoking behavior may be insufficient for making inferences regarding whether dependence is produced by e-cigarettes. In former smokers who transitioned to using only e-cigarettes, their dependence-like habits with e-cigarettes may be driven by a desire to regulate nicotine levels carried over from when they were smoking. In such cases, statistical adjustment of total combustible tobacco cigarette exposure (e.g., pack-years), age of smoking onset, duration of smoking, and severity and duration of combustible tobacco cigarette dependence could provide some insight into determining whether dependence-like symptoms are the result of e-cigarette use or whether they reflect transference of nicotine dependence from prior combustible tobacco use. Although both reflect forms of dependence, as described above, the committee's interest is in whether e-cigarette use may cause dependence on e-cigarettes apart from dependence on nicotine alone.

The optimal epidemiological design would follow a nationally representative sample of never users of tobacco products who initiate use of e-cigarettes and never go on to start using other tobacco products; it would assess the prevalence and association between e-cigarette exposure and e-cigarette dependence symptoms to determine if there is a dose–response association, and if thresholds of exposure that increase risk are comparable to exposure thresholds for combustible tobacco cigarettes. However, the majority of never smokers who use e-cigarettes are youth and young adults (Jamal et al., 2017; Kasza et al., 2017), and a significant portion of them transition to become combustible tobacco cigarette users within several years of e-cigarette use (Soneji et al., 2017). Thus, the incidence of "pure" cases of e-cigarette dependence in the absence of exposure to other tobacco products is likely to be low even if e-cigarettes were to cause dependence.

Supplementary Intermediate Endpoint: Abuse Liability Evidence

For the abuse liability literature used to provide secondary evidence, the optimal design would involve a within-subject, crossover counterbalanced design in which each participant provides data on abuse liability indexes in response to a laboratory "challenge" of at least two conditions, one involving e-cigarettes. Randomized between-subject designs would also provide strong evidence. For example, designs may involve controlled e-cigarette administration challenges with pre- versus post-measures of subjective pleasant effects, with, ideally, comparison data on these measures with no challenge or a sham challenge (e.g., puffing from an unlit combustible tobacco cigarette; see Vansickel et al., 2010). Additional strong designs have an active comparator, such as the comparison of abuse liability indexes across two e-cigarette products that vary on an important dimension of product diversity (e.g., nicotine concentration, flavoring), the comparison of an e-cigarette to a combustible tobacco cigarette, or the comparison of an e-cigarette to an alternative nicotine delivery product (e.g., nicotine gum). Null findings by studies with active controls (or evidence that e-cigarettes have less abuse liability than combustible tobacco cigarettes) should not be interpreted as evidence that e-cigarettes do not produce dependence. However, positive findings from active control studies would provide supportive evidence that e-cigarettes produce dependence to some degree and can address questions regarding the relative dependence risk caused by e-cigarettes compared with combustible tobacco cigarettes or across e-cigarettes with differing product characteristics. From a practical and scientific perspective, the ideal comparator in an abuse liability study would be a nicotine product known to have low abuse liability (e.g., nicotine lozenge, gum, or transdermal patch).

For the majority of the research, the ideal challenge in laboratory abuse testing involves an experimentally controlled administration whereby the number and pace of puffs is standardized to control the dose administered (e.g., Goldenson et al., 2016). Less ideal (but perhaps more ecologically valid), the participant is permitted to self-administer the product ad libitum (ad lib), which can result in systematic differences in the "dose" of exposure across experimental conditions. For instance, when comparing the pleasant effects of a high- versus low-nicotine e-cigarette, condition challenge involving 5 minutes of ad lib use and the participants self-administering an average of twice as many puffs with the high dose will leave unclear whether differences between conditions are caused by the nicotine level or the number of puffs taken. Thus, how e-cigarettes are used will influence their abuse liability, and patterns of use vary substantially. For example, some users cluster their puffs in cigarette-like sessions or use intermittently throughout the day in short clusters. Large clusters of puffs in relatively quick succession result in a near-bolus dose of nicotine, rapid rise in blood nicotine levels, and likely greater nicotine-related effects (positive reinforcement). This type of use may be associated with greater abuse liability of e-cigarettes. On the other hand, intermittent vaping in short clusters of puffs results in gradual increase in blood nicotine levels throughout the day. This type of use may be done for negative reinforcement (to alleviate nicotine withdrawal symptoms).

Because it is unethical to expose tobacco-product–naïve subjects to e-cigarettes, the majority of research includes either e-cigarette–naïve or inexperienced combustible tobacco cigarette smokers willing to try e-cigarettes or experienced e-cigarette users. E-cigarette–naïve smokers may be unfamiliar with proper use of e-cigarettes, and therefore may produce levels of nicotine exposure that are lower than those of experienced users of the same product (due to differences in puffing topography; see Chapter 3) (Farsalinos et al., 2014; Vansickel and Eissenberg, 2013). Thus, studies using e-cigarette–naïve smokers without proper training in use may result in underestimation of the abuse liability of the product.

An important consideration is the type of outcomes that could be considered evidence of abuse liability in studies that conduct controlled tests of e-cigarette administration. Several controlled laboratory studies of combustible tobacco cigarette smokers who have been acutely deprived of nicotine test the effects of e-cigarette use administration on nicotine withdrawal symptoms, combustible tobacco cigarette craving, and other factors believed to maintain smoking behavior. Such studies are not considered to provide evidence regarding whether e-cigarettes produce dependence. The suppression of withdrawal and combustible tobacco cigarette craving is known to be caused by a number of products with little or no abuse liability, including FDA-approved smoking cessation medications. In contrast, subjective euphoria, liking, sensory satisfaction, and willingness to exert effort to obtain e-cigarettes are considered evidence of abuse liability, consistent with guidelines provided by FDA and the National Institute on Drug Abuse (ADAMHA, 1989). These particular outcomes generally are not affected by FDA-approved smoking cessation medications.

Ancillary Evidence: Clinical Trials Involving Product Exposure Outside a Laboratory

A number of research studies provide participants (usually e-cigarette–naïve smokers) with an e-cigarette product to use ad lib in the natural ecology for a multiday period. At the end of the period, retrospective reports of the rewarding effects of the product are sometimes collected. While these types of clinical trials may have relevant comparison conditions (e.g., e-cigarette products with differing levels of nicotine strength), which strengthens causal inference, the uncontrolled conditions allow for a number of systematic differences in level of exposure to the product, use of other tobacco product, and other factors that may confound comparisons across conditions.

QUESTIONS ADDRESSED BY THE LITERATURE

Given that e-cigarettes have been widely available for only the past several years, long-term data on whether dependence symptoms emerge among never-smoking e-cigarette users is unavailable. Hence, in the epidemiological data, cross-sectional evidence using e-cigarette dependence symptom measures were considered. Such studies were required to report data on e-cigarette dependence symptoms (e.g., craving for e-cigarettes, short time to first e-cigarette after awakening, difficulty refraining from e-cigarette use in situations when vaping is not allowed; see the section on the characterization of disease endpoints, above); mere reporting on the frequency of use was not considered relevant to dependence. The abuse liability literature was used as supportive evidence. Clinical trials were considered ancillary evidence.

Several epidemiological studies report the prevalence, distribution, and correlates of e-cigarette dependence, including whether frequency of e-cigarette use is associated with symptoms of e-cigarette dependence (Dawkins and Corcoran, 2014; Dawkins et al., 2016; Etter, 2015, 2016; Etter and Eissenberg, 2015; Foulds et al., 2015; Goldenson et al., 2016; Gonzalez-

Roz et al., 2017; Hobkirk et al., 2017; Johnson et al., 2017; Liu et al., 2017; Nichols et al., 2016; Rostron et al., 2016; Strong et al., 2017; Yingst et al., 2015). Descriptive epidemiological reports on base rates and the distribution of e-cigarette dependence symptoms that show that a meaningful portion of e-cigarette users report symptoms of e-cigarette dependence provide evidence to address the question: *Does use of e-cigarettes have an effect on e-cigarette dependence risk?* Additional epidemiological evidence that the level of exposure to e-cigarettes has a dose–response association with e-cigarette dependence symptom outcomes further addressed that question. In certain experimental studies, data on the prevalence or severity of e-cigarette dependence scores are presented for the purpose of describing the sample used. Because such studies are typically in smaller and non-representative samples, they were used as additional epidemiological evidence. Human laboratory studies of the effects of e-cigarettes (versus a comparator other than combustible tobacco cigarettes) were also supportive evidence.

Some epidemiological studies compared the dependence severity of e-cigarettes to other tobacco products for the typical user (Strong et al., 2017). Some human laboratory studies compared the effects of e-cigarettes to combustible tobacco cigarettes. Collectively, these two streams of evidence address the question: *Is the effect of e-cigarette use on e-cigarette dependence risk weaker than the effect of combustible tobacco cigarette use on cigarette dependence?*

Finally, there is an emerging epidemiological literature on whether e-cigarette users of products with certain characteristics (e.g., high nicotine concentration) report different levels of e-cigarette dependence than e-cigarette users of products without such characteristics (e.g., low nicotine concentration). Furthermore, there is a human laboratory literature that compares the effects of e-cigarettes with varying product dimensions (e.g., nicotine concentration, flavor) on abuse liability outcomes. Collectively, these streams of evidence address the question: *Do e-cigarettes with certain product characteristics have stronger effects on e-cigarette dependence risk than those with other product characteristics?*

For each study reviewed, the committee took into account the methodological rigor to grade the strength of evidence. As described above in the Optimal Study Design section, for epidemiological data factors such as the representativeness of the sampling strategy, incorporation of particular exclusions (e.g., excluding current smokers) and covariate adjustment, if relevant, were used to grade the weight of evidence provided by each study. For abuse liability studies, issues such as the inclusion of a comparison condition and sample size were considered.

EPIDEMIOLOGY

The search resulted in 15 studies that reported epidemiological data that matched the requirements above. Review of the studies revealed a natural clustering of different types of studies distinguished by their methodology and rigor: three studies that used nationally representative samples; six online survey studies that did not use a systematic sampling method; two in-person studies that used a non-representative sampling (e.g., recruited users at an e-cigarette convention); and four additional laboratory-based studies that incidentally reported data on e-cigarette dependence symptoms to describe the sample. A brief description of each study's finding and whether the result provides evidence that is in support of, against, or inconclusive are reviewed in Tables 8-1 and 8-2.

Nationally Representative Studies

Rostron and colleagues (2016) analyzed reports of dependence symptoms among those who were exclusive daily users of e-cigarettes (n = 124), combustible tobacco cigarettes (n = 3,963), or cigars (n = 131) within the past 30 days as well as dependence symptoms of poly-product users in the past 30 days. Data were drawn from the 2012–2013 National Adult Tobacco Survey (NATS), a nationally representative cross-sectional telephone survey. For each product used and each dependence symptom, participants were asked whether they experienced the symptom within the past 30 days. The questions were worded identically across the different products—a strength of the study, which facilitated cross-product comparisons. Among daily e-cigarette users, there were appreciable prevalence rates of various dependence symptoms, including use within 30 minutes of awakening (46.1 percent; 95% CI = 35.1–57.4), strong cravings (46.2 percent; 95% CI = 35.2–57.5), need to use (46.2 percent; 95% CI = 35.2–57.5), and withdrawal symptoms upon abstinence (22.8 percent; 95% CI = 14.8–33.4). Prevalence rates for each dependence symptom were significantly lower among exclusive daily e-cigarette users as compared with exclusive combustible tobacco cigarette smokers and were not significantly different from symptom prevalence estimates for exclusive daily cigar users. Poly-product users of e-cigarettes and combustible tobacco products reported higher prevalence of most symptoms than exclusive e-cigarette, combustible tobacco cigarette, and cigar smokers.

Given the representative sampling, this study provides strong evidence on dependence symptom prevalence estimates in the United States. The separation of exclusive e-cigarette users from poly-product users facilitates inferences that dependence symptoms are not manifestations of dependence toward use of any form of nicotine or tobacco that are driven by dependence on another tobacco product. A limitation is that comparisons across different groups of users did not statistically adjust for possible confounding factors, such as prior history of tobacco use and demographic factors. In addition, the data were collected from 2012 to 2013 when prevalence of e-cigarette use was low and the marketplace was saturated with early model devices (e.g., cigalikes) and products, which may have had fairly poor nicotine delivery and lacked variety in flavorings (Breland et al., 2017). Modern e-cigarette devices and e-liquids with greater appeal and nicotine delivery effectiveness have become more widely available and more popular within the past few years, but were uncommon when this study was performed. Hence, the generalizability to the current environment is questionable and there is a possibility that e-cigarette prevalence estimates may be different than what would be observed today. In sum, this study provides strong evidence that dependence symptoms are common among daily e-cigarette users and suggestive evidence that the probability of experiencing dependence symptoms is lower for e-cigarettes compared with combustible tobacco cigarettes and not different in comparison to cigars.

Liu and colleagues (2017) analyzed the relative level of dependence among adult participants in the Wave 1 of the PATH study in 2013–2014 who were exclusive everyday users of e-cigarettes (n = 156) and combustible tobacco cigarettes (n = 3,430) in the past 30 days. Four binary dependence symptoms were examined (yes/no), which included identical wording for assessment of e-cigarette and combustible tobacco cigarette dependence:

1. "Do you consider yourself addicted to cigarettes/e-cigarettes?"
2. "Do you ever have strong cravings to smoke cigarettes/use e-cigarettes?"
3. "In the past 12 months, did you find it difficult to keep from smoking cigarettes/using e-cigarettes in places where it was prohibited?"
4. "Have you ever felt like you really needed to smoke cigarettes/use e-cigarettes?"

In addition, time to first product use after awakening was also assessed as a quantitative outcome. Results showed high prevalence for both e-cigarettes and combustible tobacco cigarettes for most dependence symptoms—consider yourself addicted (e-cigarettes = 77.2 percent versus combustible tobacco cigarettes = 94.0 percent), strong cravings (e-cigarettes = 72.8 percent versus combustible tobacco cigarettes = 86.9 percent), difficulty refraining from use where prohibited (e-cigarettes = 5.6 percent versus combustible tobacco cigarettes = 28.6 percent), feel need to use (e-cigarettes = 71.5 percent versus combustible tobacco cigarettes = 88.5 percent), time to first use after awakening (grand mean e-cigarettes = 23.46, 95% CI =

TABLE 8-1 Epidemiological Studies on E-Cigarettes and Dependence

Reference	Study Population	Dependence Measure
Nationally Representative Studies		
Liu et al., 2017	Wave 1 adult interview group of PATH database: 156 e-cigarette users; 3,430 combustible tobacco cigarette users	Self-reported time-to-first-use (minutes), and questionnaire: "Do you consider yourself addicted to cigarettes/e-cigarettes?" "Do you ever have strong cravings to smoke cigarettes/use e-cigarettes?" "In the past 12 months, did you find it difficult to keep from smoking cigarettes/using e-cigarettes in places where it was prohibited?" "Have you ever felt like you really needed to smoke cigarettes/use e-cigarettes?"
Rostron et al., 2016	National Adult Tobacco Survey (2012–2013): 60,192 total respondents, daily single tobacco product users: n = 124 e-cigarettes n = 131 cigars n = 3,963 combustible tobacco cigarettes	Average number of cigarettes smoked per day, time to first tobacco use after waking, whether or not respondents sometimes wake at night to use a tobacco product, have had a strong craving to use any tobacco product in the past 30 days, have felt like they really needed to use a tobacco product in the past 30 days, have had a time when they wanted to use a tobacco product so much that it was difficult to think of anything else in the past 30 days, if the statement that they feel restless or irritable after not using tobacco for a while was "not at all true," "sometimes true," "often true," or "always true."

Results	E-Cigarettes Have Some Dependence Risk?	E-Cigarettes Have Lower Dependence Potential Than Combustible Tobacco Cigarettes?	Product Characteristics Alter Dependence Risk?
Moderate to high endorsement of e-cigarette dependence symptoms.	+	+	
E-cigarette dependence in e-cigarette–exclusive users was lower than combustible tobacco cigarette dependence in combustible tobacco cigarette–exclusive smokers (e.g., after adjusting for potential confounders, combustible tobacco cigarette smokers were significantly more likely to have strong cravings, believe they really needed to use the product, and consider themselves addicted).			
Time-to-first-use: 15% of e-cigarette users said 5 minutes; 24% of combustible tobacco cigarettes users said the same. After adjustment, e-cigarette users had significantly longer time to first use than combustible tobacco cigarette smokers.			
Sizable rates of dependence symptoms endorsed in e-cigarette–only users (23–46%). E-cigarette–users were less likely than users of other products to report withdrawal/craving symptoms, still reported dependence symptoms (e.g., craving for tobacco).	+	+	
Dual combustible tobacco cigarette and e-cigarette users and e-cigarette poly-product users (cigarette, cigar, e-cigarette) were significantly more likely to report strong craving for tobacco in past 30 days compared with exclusive combustible tobacco cigarette smokers.			
Symptoms were less prevalent in users of only e-cigarettes and only cigars than people who used both combustible tobacco cigarettes and cigars (e.g., exclusive e-cigarette users reported longer median time to first use than exclusive combustible tobacco cigarette smokers).			

continued

TABLE 8-1 Continued

Reference	Study Population	Dependence Measure
Strong et al., 2017	Adult, established users of a tobacco product from Wave 1 PATH study: combustible tobacco cigarette–only respondents (n = 8,689), e-cigarette–only respondents (n = 437), cigar-only respondents (n = 706), hookah-only respondents (n = 461), smokeless-only respondents (n = 971)	Used four tools (the Hooked on Nicotine Checklist [3 items], WISDM [12 items], NDSS [4 items], the *Diagnostic and Statistical Manual* criteria [4 items], and Time to First Tobacco Use [1 item]) to obtain 24 tobacco dependence symptoms
Studies Using Non-Representative Sampling		
Gonzalez-Roz et al., 2017	39 experienced e-cigarette users, 36% of whom were dual users	FTND and NDSS, CO and urinary cotinine

Results	E-Cigarettes Have Some Dependence Risk?	E-Cigarettes Have Lower Dependence Potential Than Combustible Tobacco Cigarettes?	Product Characteristics Alter Dependence Risk?
With levels of tobacco dependence anchored at 0.0 (SD = 1.0) among combustible tobacco cigarette–only users, mean tobacco dependence was more than a full standard deviation lower for e-cigarette–only users (mean = −1.37, SD = 2.36), cigar-only users (mean = −1.92, SD = 2.11), and hookah-only users (mean = −1.71, SD = 0.53). Higher level of tobacco dependence among daily groups when compared with non-daily e-cigarette–only users (mean difference = 0.40, SE = 0.07, F(1,10) = 35.1, p < 0.002).	+	+	
E-cigarette users were dependent on e-liquids containing nicotine, but were less nicotine dependent than current tobacco smokers (FTND 4.38 ± 1.93 versus 5.57 ± 1.48 and NDSS-T 26.26 ± 5.29 versus 40.50 ± 8.14, respectively). This trend was true for all NDSS measures (impulsivity, priority, tolerance, continuity, and stereotyping).	+	+	

continued

TABLE 8-1 Continued

Reference	Study Population	Dependence Measure
Johnson et al., 2017	131 current e-cigarette users who attended Orlando Vape Convention (October 17, 2015)	FTND and select questions from PSECDI
Anonymous Web Surveys of E-Cigarette Users		
Dawkins et al., 2013	Never (n = 6, 4%), current (n = 218, 16%), and former (n = 1,123, 83%) combustible tobacco cigarette smokers, and current e-cigarette users	Author-constructed survey

Results	E-Cigarettes Have Some Dependence Risk?	E-Cigarettes Have Lower Dependence Potential Than Combustible Tobacco Cigarettes?	Product Characteristics Alter Dependence Risk?
Most users did not wake up during the night to use their device. One-quarter of users reported time to first use within 5 minutes of waking; another 20% reported within 6–15 minutes. More than two-thirds of users would rather forgo other e-cigarette sessions throughout the day than give up their morning session. 50% of respondents used their product 30 times per day for at least 10 minutes. More than 50% said they had ever experienced moderate to extremely strong cravings and 60% had such urges over the past week. 31% reported irritability and 27% reported anxiety if they could not use their device. 60% of users received an FTND score of at least 5. Presence of nicotine in e-liquid and length of e-cigarette use (less than or more than 1 year) were significantly associated with nicotine dependence scores. More than 70% of those who had used an e-cigarette for more than 1 year were classified as moderately or highly nicotine dependent compared with 45% of those who were users for less than 1 year.	+		+
68% of respondents said "very much so" to "E-cigarette use is as satisfying as tobacco smoking"; 13.3% answered "not at all" to the question "I crave e-cigarettes as much as I do/did tobacco"; 18.4% said "very much so" in response to the same question.	+	+	

continued

TABLE 8-1 Continued

Reference	Study Population	Dependence Measure
Etter, 2015	374 adult daily users of e-cigarettes who had quit smoking in the previous 62 days	Online non-representative survey Used adapted FTND, NDSS, CDS tools to assess dependence on e-cigarettes; also measured urge to use e-cigarette with MPSS (2 items); used modified version item of craving subscale of WSWS
Etter and Eissenberg, 2015	1,284 adult daily users of e-cigarettes	Used adapted FTND, NDSS, CDS tools to assess dependence on e-cigarettes and nicotine gum; also measured unsuccessful attempts to quit product, and perceptions of likeliness to succeed if stopped using product and addiction to e-cigarette or nicotine gum compared with combustible tobacco cigarette

Results	E-Cigarettes Have Some Dependence Risk?	E-Cigarettes Have Lower Dependence Potential Than Combustible Tobacco Cigarettes?	Product Characteristics Alter Dependence Risk?
Median time to first e-cigarette ranged from 15 to 45 minutes. Users who said e-cigarettes "definitely" decreased tobacco cravings were more likely to report e-cigarettes also alleviated withdrawal symptoms such as anxiety, nervousness, anger, irritability, frustration, depressed mood, sadness, restlessness, impatience, mood swings compared with those who said e-cigarettes had a weak effect on craving.	+		
Ex-smokers who used only e-cigarettes reported significantly lower time to first cigarette when smoked combustible tobacco cigarettes versus time to first e-cigarette; time to first e-cigarette less than 30 minutes on average. Lower time to first e-cigarette associated with nicotine versus placebo use. 62% of daily dual users said their current dependence on e-cigarettes was weaker than dependence on combustible tobacco cigarettes.	+	+	+
Daily e-cigarette users who used nicotine-containing devices had higher e-FTND scores than those who used non-nicotine–containing devices.			
Some evidence that gum dependence was more severe (not adjusted for confounding).			

continued

TABLE 8-1 Continued

Reference	Study Population	Dependence Measure
Etter, 2016	1,672 adult current users of e-cigarettes (daily and occasionally)	Online non-representative survey

Results	E-Cigarettes Have Some Dependence Risk?	E-Cigarettes Have Lower Dependence Potential Than Combustible Tobacco Cigarettes?	Product Characteristics Alter Dependence Risk?
Median time to first e-cigarette ranged from 15 to 30 minutes and was lower for those who reported greater throat hit. Strength of throat hit was associated with satisfaction and dependence variables: "Like the taste of the vapor produced by e-cigarette" (% agree: very weak = 75%; rather weak = 78%; average = 88%; rather strong = 90%; very strong = 88%; $\chi^2 = 64.9$; $p < 0.001$). "Likes the sensation when inhales vapor" (% agree: very weak = 60%; rather weak = 81%; average = 86%; rather strong = 92%; very strong = 91%; $\chi^2 = 99.6$; $p < 0.001$). "It feels so good to vape" (% agree: very weak = 59%; rather weak = 68%; average = 75%; rather strong = 81%; very strong = 91%; $\chi^2 = 41.8$; $p < 0.001$). "Addiction to the e-cigarette" (scale of 0 to 100: very weak = 50%; rather weak = 50%; average = 65%; rather strong = 70%; very strong = 65%; KW = 32.9; $p < 0.001$). "I am a prisoner of the electronic cigarette" (% agree: very weak = 17%; rather weak = 21%; average = 26%; rather strong = 28%; very strong = 19%; $\chi^2 = 43.3$; $p < 0.001$). "I am unable to stop vaping" (% agree = average: 25%; $\chi^2 = 41.4$; $p < 0.001$). "If decided to stop using e-cigarette, likely to succeed" (% agree: very weak = 55%; rather weak = 36%; average = 30%; rather strong = 28%; very strong = 42%; $\chi^2 = 51.5$; $p < 0.001$). *(continues on next page)*	+	+	+

continued

TABLE 8-1 Continued

Reference	Study Population	Dependence Measure
Etter, 2016 continued		

Results	E-Cigarettes Have Some Dependence Risk?	E-Cigarettes Have Lower Dependence Potential Than Combustible Tobacco Cigarettes?	Product Characteristics Alter Dependence Risk?
(continued)			
"Stopping using e-cigarette for good would be very difficult" (% agree: very weak = 6%; rather weak = 23%; average = 28%; rather strong = 30%; very strong = 35%; $\chi^2 = 56.7$; $p < 0.001$).			
"Felt the urge to vape today" (% a lot of the time + almost all the time + all the time: very weak = 15%; rather weak = 27%; average = 32%; rather strong = 35%; very strong = 31%; $\chi^2 = 46.5$; $p = 0.001$).			
"Use the e-cigarette because they are addicted to it" (% very true: very weak = 2%; rather weak = 6%; average = 8%; rather strong = 9%; very strong = 9%; $\chi^2 = 31.2$; $p = 0.002$).			
"Former smokers: addiction to e-cigarette compared with former addiction to tobacco cigarette" (% same or stronger: very weak = 12%; rather weak = 15%; average = 25%; rather strong = 25%; very strong = 23%; $\chi^2 = 49.7$; $p < 0.001$).			

continued

TABLE 8-1 Continued

Reference	Study Population	Dependence Measure
Foulds et al., 2015	3,609 adult former combustible tobacco cigarette smokers who currently use e-cigarettes	Penn State Cigarette Dependence Index and PSECDI
Yingst et al., 2015	Current advanced-generation e-cigarette device users (n = 3,373); Current first-generation e-cigarette device users (n = 1,048)	Online survey asking, "Did you switch to your current preferred type of e-cigarette because it gives you a more satisfying "hit" than previous e-cigarettes your tried?" (Yes/No); also PSECDI

Results	E-Cigarettes Have Some Dependence Risk?	E-Cigarettes Have Lower Dependence Potential Than Combustible Tobacco Cigarettes?	Product Characteristics Alter Dependence Risk?
The overall PSECDI for e-cigarette users was significantly lower than their Cigarette Dependence Index, as was the individual score on every other item. More than 90% reported they had experienced strong urges to smoke and withdrawal symptoms when a smoker, but only 25–35% reported experiencing these symptoms of dependence as an e-cigarette user. Those who have used e-cigarettes for a longer time, who have previously tried more e-cigarette models, who currently use an e-cigarette larger than a combustible tobacco cigarette, with a button, with more than one battery, that cost more than $50, and who use a higher concentration of nicotine liquid tend to have a higher e-cigarette dependence index (all $p < 0.05$). Those using zero nicotine liquid had a significantly lower e-cigarette dependence index than those using 1–12 mg/ml ($p < 0.001$), who were significantly lower than those using 13 or greater mg/ml nicotine liquid ($p < 0.001$).	+	+	+
Advanced-generation versus first-generation device users: significantly more dependence on e-cigarettes (despite liquid with lower nicotine concentration) than first-generation device users; also shorter time to first use. Advanced-generation device user was less likely to be a current smoker. Reported switching to current device because it delivered a more satisfying throat hit.	+		+

continued

TABLE 8-1 Continued

Reference	Study Population	Dependence Measure
Descriptive Data on E-Cigarette Dependence Symptoms in Small Laboratory Studies		
Dawkins et al., 2016	11 experienced male e-cigarette users completed 60 minutes of ad lib use under low (6 mg/ml) and high (24 mg/ml) nicotine liquid conditions in two separate sessions	Adapted FTND; CDS
Goldenson et al., 2016	20 e-cigarette users (≥1 day per week for ≥1 month; smoking ≤15 combustible tobacco cigarettes per day; no use of smoking cessation medication)	PSECDI; FTCD
Hobkirk et al., 2017	9 adult past-month (≥20 in the past 28 days) e-cigarette users	PSECDI
Nichols et al., 2016	7 e-cigarette users	PSECDI

NOTES: + = positive evidence; – = no positive evidence; +/– = mixed results (some outcomes or analyses yielded positive evidence and others did not yield positive evidence); 0 = inconclusive evidence to determine whether the results are positive or not; CDS = Cigarette Dependence Scale; FTCD = Fagerström Test for Cigarette Dependence; FTND = Fagerström Test for Nicotine Dependence; MPSS = Mood and Physical Symptoms Scale; NDSS = Nicotine Dependence Syndrome Scale; PSECDI = Penn State Electronic Cigarette Dependence Index; WISDM = Wisconsin Inventory of Smoking Dependence Motives; WSWS = Wisconsin Smoking Withdrawal Scale.

Results	E-Cigarettes Have Some Dependence Risk?	E-Cigarettes Have Lower Dependence Potential Than Combustible Tobacco Cigarettes?	Product Characteristics Alter Dependence Risk?
eFTND: mean = 4.73 (SD = 1.35) (range = 2–7). e-cigarette self-rated addiction item rating: mean = 3.18 (SD = 1.17) (range = 1–5).	+		
PSECDI: mean = 8.4 (95% CI = 6.4–10.4). FTCD in past 30-day smokers: mean = 6.3 (95% CI = 5.8–6.8).	+		
The sample's average self-reported dependence on e-cigarettes was low based on PSECDI total scores, which ranged from 3 to 8 (mean = 6.33, SD = 1.80) out of a possible score range of 0–20.	+		
PSEDCI: low to medium levels of e-cigarette dependence (mean = 7, SD = 3).	+		

TABLE 8-2 Laboratory/Experimental Studies on Dependence and Abuse Liability

Reference	Study Design	Study Population	Device Measure
Studies Testing the Effects of Flavor			
Audrain-McGovern et al., 2016	Laboratory	32 young adult combustible tobacco cigarette smokers who used e-cigarettes at least once	"e-GO" tank-style e-cigarette with a 2.4-ml refillable e-liquid tank 2 flavored e-liquid options: fruit-flavored (green apple), and dessert-flavored (chocolate), with 6, 12, or 18 mg/ml of nicotine depending on the nicotine content of the participant's usual smoking rate

Dependence Measure	Results	E-Cigarettes Have Some Dependence Risk?	E-Cigarettes Have Lower Dependence Potential Than Combustible Tobacco Cigarettes?	Product Characteristics Alter Dependence Risk?
Modified satisfaction subscale of the Cigarette Evaluation Scale for e-cigarette use, relative reinforcing value of flavor, and number of flavored versus unflavored e-cigarette puffs consumed	Fruit- and dessert-flavored e-cigarettes had a significantly higher reward value than unflavored e-cigarettes; fruit flavor preferred. Users took significantly more flavored puffs than unflavored. Menthol combustible tobacco cigarette smokers took significantly more (at least three times as many) e-cigarette puffs as non-menthol combustible tobacco cigarette smokers.	+		+

continued

TABLE 8-2 Continued

Reference	Study Design	Study Population	Device Measure
Goldenson et al., 2016	Laboratory and used epidemiological data	20 e-cigarette users (≥1 day per week for ≥1 month; smoking ≤15 combustible tobacco cigarettes per day; no use of smoking cessation medication)	Joyetech "Delta 23 Atomizer" tanks connected to a Joyetech "eVic Supreme" battery 20 e-cigarette solutions in 10 flavors were either 0 or 6 mg/ml nicotine (10 flavors included 6 sweet-flavored [peach, watermelon, blackberry, cotton candy, cola, and sweet lemon tea], 3 non-sweet-flavored [mint, tobacco, and menthol], and a single flavorless solution)
Rosbrook and Green, 2016, Experiment #1	Laboratory	18–45 years of age (n = 32)	Challenge study, controlled e-cigarette use

Dependence Measure	Results	E-Cigarettes Have Some Dependence Risk?	E-Cigarettes Have Lower Dependence Potential Than Combustible Tobacco Cigarettes?	Product Characteristics Alter Dependence Risk?
Visual analogue scale assessing "How much did you like it?", "Would you use it again?", "How much would you pay for a day's worth of it?", "How sweet was it?", "How strong was the throat hit?", and "What flavor is it?"	Significant effect of flavor on each appeal outcome: sweet-flavored solutions produced higher appeal ratings than non-sweet and flavorless solutions. No significant main effects of nicotine or flavor × nicotine interaction effects. Ratings of sweetness positively associated with each appeal outcome: sweeter associated with increased liking, willingness to use again, and amount willing to pay for a day's worth of solution. Throat hit not associated with willingness to use again and subjective value and were inversely associated with liking.	+		+
General Labeled Magnitude Scale and Labeled Hedonic Scale	No significant effects of menthol or nicotine on liking. Liking was low and did not vary significantly across menthol or nicotine concentrations.	–		–

continued

TABLE 8-2 Continued

Reference	Study Design	Study Population	Device Measure
Rosbrook and Green, 2016, Experiment #2	Laboratory	18–45 years of age (n = 32)	Challenge study, controlled e-cigarette use
St.Helen et al., 2017	Laboratory	14 e-cigarette users	Inpatient crossover study with strawberry, tobacco, and user's usual flavor e-liquid. Nicotine levels were nominally 18 mg/ml in the strawberry (pH = 8.29) and tobacco (pH = 9.10) e-liquids and ranged between 3–18 mg/ml in the usual brands (mean pH = 6.80).

Dependence Measure	Results	E-Cigarettes Have Some Dependence Risk?	E-Cigarettes Have Lower Dependence Potential Than Combustible Tobacco Cigarettes?	Product Characteristics Alter Dependence Risk?
General Labeled Magnitude Scale and Labeled Hedonic Scale	Average liking ratings of the e-liquid flavors did not exceed "like slightly" on the Labeled Hedonic Scale. A trend toward higher ratings for liking of the menthol and menthol–mint flavors over the unflavored e-liquid was supported by a main effect of flavor ($F_{2,60}$ = 8.11, $p < 0.001$).	+/–		+/–
Minnesota Nicotine Withdrawal Scale, Questionnaire for Smoking Urges modified for e-cigarettes, Positive and Negative Affect Schedule, and modified Cigarette Evaluation Questionnaire	No difference in mCEQ reward or satisfaction subscale between strawberry and tobacco e-liquids, except ratings of sensations in throat and chest (significantly higher with tobacco). Usual brand e-liquids had significantly more satisfaction and enjoyment of sensations than experimenter-provided liquids.	+/–		+/–

continued

TABLE 8-2 Continued

Reference	Study Design	Study Population	Device Measure
Studies Testing the Effects of Nicotine Concentration			
Baldassarri et al., 2017	Laboratory and epidemiological	Adult experienced e-cigarette users (n = 4) and cigarette smokers (n = 3)	"e-Go type e-cigarette"; nicotine concentrations with a linear range of 0.5–50 µg/ml
Dawkins et al., 2016	Laboratory	11 experienced male e-cigarette users completed 60 minutes of ad lib use under low (6 mg/ml) and high (24 mg/ml) nicotine liquid conditions in two separate sessions	"eVic™ supreme" e-cigarette from Joyetech, fitted with a "Nautilus Aspire" tank e-cigarette with 6 mg/ml (low) and 24 mg/ml (high) nicotine Halo Smokers' Angels e-liquid

Dependence Measure	Results	E-Cigarettes Have Some Dependence Risk?	E-Cigarettes Have Lower Dependence Potential Than Combustible Tobacco Cigarettes?	Product Characteristics Alter Dependence Risk?
Fagerström Test for Nicotine Dependence adapted for e-cigarettes	Ratings of product liking were similar after each e-cigarette use (0 mg/ml = 80 ± 28; 8 mg/ml = 75 ± 38; 36 mg/ml = 74 ± 26). Liking following use of the combustible tobacco cigarette was (37 ± 40); this did not differ compared with the e-cigarette at either liquid strength (8 mg/ml: 75 ± 38; 36 mg/ml: 74 ± 26).	–		–
Change in craving and withdrawal symptoms (Mood and Physical Symptoms Scale) Visual analogue scale assessing positive (hit and satisfaction) and adverse effects associated with nicotine and e-cigarette use	Mean (SD) percentage hit and satisfaction levels were 61.86 (31.50) and 60.70 (17.30), respectively, in the high condition and 44.73 (23.00) and 46.89 (16.93) in the low condition. These differences did not reach statistical significance (hit: Z = −1.60, p = 0.11; satisfaction: Z = −1.69, p = 0.09).			0

continued

TABLE 8-2 Continued

Reference	Study Design	Study Population	Device Measure
Goldenson et al., 2016	Laboratory and used epidemiological data	20 e-cigarette users (≥1 day per week for ≥1 month; smoking ≤15 combustible tobacco cigarettes per day; no use of smoking cessation medication)	Joyetech "Delta 23 Atomizer" tanks connected to a Joyetech "eVic Supreme" battery; 20 e-cigarette solutions in 10 flavors were either 0 or 6 mg/ml nicotine (10 flavors included 6 sweet-flavored [peach, watermelon, blackberry, cotton candy, cola and sweet lemon tea], 3 non-sweet-flavored [mint, tobacco and menthol] and a single flavorless solution)
Perkins et al., 2015	Laboratory	Adult dependent combustible tobacco cigarette smokers (n = 28) in a fully within-subjects design	E-cigarettes with as much as 36 mg/ml nicotine; "rawhide red (tobacco)" for non-menthol and "Freeport (menthol)" for menthol flavors
Rosbrook and Green, 2016, Experiment #1	Laboratory	18–45 years of age (n = 32)	Challenge study, controlled e-cigarette use

Dependence Measure	Results	E-Cigarettes Have Some Dependence Risk?	E-Cigarettes Have Lower Dependence Potential Than Combustible Tobacco Cigarettes?	Product Characteristics Alter Dependence Risk?
Visual analogue scale assessing "How much did you like it?", "Would you use it again?", "How much would you pay for a day's worth of it?", "How sweet was it?", "How strong was the throat hit?", and "What flavor is it?"	Significant effect of flavor on each appeal outcome. No significant main effects of nicotine or flavor × nicotine interaction effects. Significant effect of nicotine on throat hit: a stronger throat hit in nicotine versus placebo solutions. Throat hit not associated with willingness to use again and subjective value and were inversely associated with liking.	+		+
Reward reinforcement task	Nicotine: significantly greater liking compared with the placebo e-cigarette.	+		+
General Labeled Magnitude Scale and Labeled Hedonic Scale	No significant effects of menthol or nicotine on liking. Liking was low and did not vary significantly across menthol or nicotine concentrations.	–		–

continued

TABLE 8-2 Continued

Reference	Study Design	Study Population	Device Measure
Rosbrook and Green, 2016, Experiment #2	Laboratory	18–45 years of age (n = 32)	Challenge study, controlled e-cigarette use

Dependence Measure	Results	E-Cigarettes Have Some Dependence Risk?	E-Cigarettes Have Lower Dependence Potential Than Combustible Tobacco Cigarettes?	Product Characteristics Alter Dependence Risk?
General Labeled Magnitude Scale and Labeled Hedonic Scale	Average liking ratings of the e-liquid flavors did not exceed "like slightly" on the Labeled Hedonic Scale. A trend toward higher ratings for liking of the menthol and menthol–mint flavors over the unflavored e-liquid was supported by a main effect of flavor ($F_{2,60}$ = 8.11, $p < 0.001$). Significant effect of nicotine on coolness/cold perceptions.	+/–		+/–

continued

TABLE 8-2 Continued

Reference	Study Design	Study Population	Device Measure
Comparison of E-Cigarette to Combustible Tobacco Cigarettes and Other Products			
Stiles et al., 2017	Laboratory	59 e-cigarette–naïve combustible tobacco cigarette smokers	Vuse Solo e-cigarettes were evaluated in this study, containing either 14, 29, or 36 mg of nicotine. Vuse Solo e-cigarettes are composed of a battery, heating element, microchips, sensor, and a cartridge containing propylene glycol, glycerol, nicotine, flavorings, and water. The three devices were presented without brand style information and were visually indistinguishable by subjects.

Dependence Measure	Results	E-Cigarettes Have Some Dependence Risk?	E-Cigarettes Have Lower Dependence Potential Than Combustible Tobacco Cigarettes?	Product Characteristics Alter Dependence Risk?
Questionnaires: Product Liking, Urge to Smoke, Urge for Product, Intent to Use Product Again, Product Effects	The mean maximum scores (E_{max}) on the Product Liking questionnaire were substantially lower for the three Vuse Solo e-cigarettes compared with the combustible tobacco cigarette condition (LS [least square] mean E_{max} scores ranging from 4.13 to 4.57, LS mean E_{max} = 9.06, $p < 0.001$ for all, respectively), and somewhat higher than nicotine gum (LS mean E_{max} = 3.21, $p < 0.05$ for all). A similar pattern was seen with the Intent to Use Again questionnaire. The mean E_{max} intent to use again scores were substantially lower for the three Vuse Solo e-cigarettes (LS mean E_{max} scores ranging from 4.07 to 4.75) compared with the combustible tobacco cigarette condition (LS mean E_{max} = 6.81, $p < 0.001$ for all), and higher than nicotine gum (LS mean E_{max} = 3.29, $p < 0.006$ for all). A similar pattern was also shown for the Liking of Positive Effects measure.	+	+	

continued

TABLE 8-2 Continued

Reference	Study Design	Study Population	Device Measure
Strasser et al., 2016	Trial	28 e-cigarette–naïve current combustible tobacco cigarette smokers	5 first-generation design brands: NJOY, 18 mg nicotine; V2, 18 mg nicotine; Green Smoke, 18.9–20.7 mg nicotine; blu, 20–24 mg nicotine; and White Cloud, 23–24 mg nicotine
Vansickel et al., 2010	Laboratory	32 e-cigarette–naïve combustible tobacco cigarette smokers	16–18 mg/ml first-generation devices that didn't give nicotine yield in blood. Users' own brand of combustible tobacco cigarettes versus sham (unlit combustible tobacco cigarette) versus "NPRO" e-cigarette versus "HYDRO" e-cigarette

Dependence Measure	Results	E-Cigarettes Have Some Dependence Risk?	E-Cigarettes Have Lower Dependence Potential Than Combustible Tobacco Cigarettes?	Product Characteristics Alter Dependence Risk?
Withdrawal Symptom Checklist and questionnaire of Smoking Urges	Compared with combustible tobacco cigarette smoking, e-cigarettes provided significantly lower nicotine levels (25–50%), reduced CO exposure, and lower ratings of liking ($p < 0.05$). No differences by brand detected. E-cigarette use on day 5 significantly reduced levels of craving and withdrawal; similar results at day 10.			+
Questionnaire of Smoking Urges Brief (QSU Brief); visual analogue scale	Significant condition by time interactions were observed for ratings of "satisfying," "pleasant," "taste good," "dizzy," "calm," "concentrate," "awake," and "reduce hunger."		+	

continued

TABLE 8-2 Continued

Reference	Study Design	Study Population	Device Measure
Vansickel et al., 2012	Laboratory	20 e-cigarette–naïve combustible tobacco cigarette smokers	"Vapor King" (KR808 model) automatic e-cigarette, 18 mg
Clinical Trials			
Meier et al., 2017	Laboratory/ Crossover	24 adult combustible tobacco cigarette smokers, no vaping in past 6 months	blu cigarette starter kit with up to seven cartridges prefilled with 16-mg nicotine solution Within a double-blind randomized crossover design, smokers (n = 24; 75% male; mean age = 48.5 years) smoked as usual for 1 week, followed by two counterbalanced naturalistic (i.e., ad lib use) weeks of either placebo or active first-generation e-cigarettes

Dependence Measure	Results	E-Cigarettes Have Some Dependence Risk?	E-Cigarettes Have Lower Dependence Potential Than Combustible Tobacco Cigarettes?	Product Characteristics Alter Dependence Risk?
Questionnaire of Smoking Urges Brief (QSU Brief); visual analogue scale	Effects of the highest magnitude were observed for ratings of "pleasant" ($F_{6,114} = 21.1$, $p < 0.0001$), "satisfying" ($F_{6,114} = 19.5$, $p < 0.0001$), and "taste good" ($F_{6,114} = 20.2$, $p = 0.0001$). Crossover values were greater in the own brand versus money choice condition relative to the e-cigarette versus money choice condition. Collapsed across time, the average crossover value was $1.06 (SD = $0.16) in the e-cigarette versus money choice condition and $1.50 (SD = $0.26) in the own brand versus money choice condition.	+	+	
Minnesota Nicotine Withdrawal Scale; Brief Wisconsin Inventory of Smoking Dependence Motives; Glover-Nilsson Smoking Behavioral Questionnaire; and modified Cigarette Evaluation Scale	Modified Cigarette Evaluation Scale scores for e-cigarette use did not differ between active and placebo e-cigarettes.	–		–

continued

TABLE 8-2 Continued

Reference	Study Design	Study Population	Device Measure
Steinberg et al., 2014	Clinical trial	41 e-cigarette–naïve combustible tobacco cigarette smokers	Device type unknown. Each participant used e-cigarette and nicotine inhaler each for 3 days, in random order, with a washout period between each one.

NOTE: + = positive evidence; – = no positive evidence; +/– = mixed results (some outcomes or analyses yielded positive evidence and others did not yield positive evidence); 0 = inconclusive evidence to determine whether the results are positive or not.

19.47–28.27 minutes versus grand mean combustible tobacco cigarettes = 19.25, 95% CI = 18.25–20.30 minutes). Of note, as described in Chapter 1, overall prevalence of e-cigarette use is low in the PATH study relative to other nationally representative surveys. Regression analyses adjusted for demographics showed that, relative to exclusive daily combustible tobacco cigarette users, exclusive daily e-cigarette users reported lower prevalence for each dependence symptom and longer time to first use.

A strength of this study was the report on the product characteristics used among the e-cigarette users, which provides information generalizability on a key source of potential variability in dependence risk (i.e., device type). Among e-cigarette users, 96.3 percent reported that the

Dependence Measure	Results	E-Cigarettes Have Some Dependence Risk?	E-Cigarettes Have Lower Dependence Potential Than Combustible Tobacco Cigarettes?	Product Characteristics Alter Dependence Risk?
Modified Cigarette Evaluation Questionnaire	The total Psychological Rewards scores were higher for the combustible tobacco cigarette and e-cigarette compared with the inhaler. E-cigarettes scored significantly lower on aversion scores than combustible tobacco cigarettes. Compared with inhaler, e-cigarettes scored higher on measures of perception such as helpful for not smoking and effective for quitting, similar to combustible tobacco cigarettes, acceptable to smokers, and cool image.	+		

e-cigarette they used most of the time was rechargeable, 76.5 percent reported that they were able to refill their e-cigarette or e-cigarette cartridges with e-liquid, and 95.8 percent reported using e-cigarettes that usually contained nicotine. The analyses excluded those who used more than one product in the past 30 days, which reduces the impact of current exposure to other products on reports of e-cigarette dependence symptoms. Comparisons in dependence symptoms between e-cigarette and combustible tobacco cigarette users were adjusted for sociodemographics, which helps to rule out some confounding effects.

Prior tobacco use history characteristics were not adjusted for in the analysis, leaving unclear whether chronicity and level of prior tobacco product exposure, which may directly influence risk of dependence on any tobacco product, may differ between e-cigarette and combustible tobacco cigarette users and explain group differences in dependence. It is possible that one of the groups consumed more tobacco or had greater total exposure to nicotine in their lifetime prior to the past 30 days. The authors reported 92.9 percent of exclusive daily e-cigarette users were former regular combustible tobacco cigarette smokers; hence, both groups had chronic combustible tobacco cigarette exposure. Previous tobacco consumption could produce chronic neurobiological alterations that may increase liability dependency on any product, including e-cigarettes. Consequently, the prevalence estimates reported may be less than what would be observed for e-cigarette users who have little history of use of other tobacco products.

Finally, some the symptoms are likely to be less valid indicators of the underlying addiction to e-cigarettes as compared with combustible tobacco cigarettes. For example, the symptom "difficulty refraining from use in places where prohibited," which is a well-validated symptom of combustible tobacco cigarette dependence, may be less relevant to e-cigarettes because there are fewer restrictions on where e-cigarettes may be used. Indeed, the authors reported that the majority of e-cigarette users reported living in a place that allows the use of their product anywhere and at any time inside their home (61.9 percent), compared with only 26.5 percent of the combustible tobacco cigarette smokers. In sum, this study provides strong evidence that the prevalence and severity of e-cigarette dependence symptoms in exclusive users are fairly high overall in the U.S. population, but not as high as what is found in exclusive combustible tobacco cigarette smokers.

A separate analysis of PATH Wave 1 2013–2014 data looked at whether responses to dependence symptom questions mapped onto a common "latent dimension" of dependence severity for various tobacco products (Strong et al., 2017). Like the other studies, survey questions for each dependence symptom were worded identically across different tobacco products, and a primary goal was to compare results across mutually exclusive past-year tobacco user groups, including combustible tobacco cigarette only (n = 8,689), e-cigarette only (n = 437), cigar only (traditional, cigarillo, or filtered) (n = 706), hookah only (n = 461), smokeless tobacco only (n = 971), combustible tobacco cigarette plus e-cigarette (n = 709), and multiple tobacco product users (n = 2,314). Wording of each symptom interview question is listed in Table 8-3. To satisfy the study inclusion criteria for current established use, for combustible tobacco cigarettes, a current established user is defined as an adult who has smoked at least 100 cigarettes in his/her lifetime and now smokes every day or some days. For all other tobacco products, a current established user is defined as an adult who has ever used the product "fairly regularly" and now uses it every day or some days.

Though both Liu and colleagues (2017) and Strong and colleagues (2017) use PATH Wave 1 data, the samples are only partially overlapping, because Strong and colleagues included both daily and non-daily users, whereas Liu and colleagues included daily users. Hence, the results from the two studies provide results from non-redundant data sources. Another difference between the studies was the data analysis approach. Liu and colleagues used regression modeling. A unique strength of the Strong and colleagues study was the application of item response–based statistical modeling, which permitted assessment of whether the extent to which each symptom was a valid indicator of the underlying latent dependence syndrome and whether its validity differed depending on whether it was being reported for one product versus another (i.e., differential item functioning [DIF]). The latent dimension is empirically estimated upon a common-dimension intersymptom association using factor analytic techniques. Once a common latent dimension is ascribed and only items that are equally valid indicators of the dimension are retained to estimate the dimension, comparisons of the relative "severity" of dependence on the dimension can be made with greater rigor and assurance of a common metric. Without doing so, any differences in the relative prevalence or severity of a particular dependence symptom across different user groups could be ascribed to the symptom being a less valid indicator for use of one product versus another. For example, the study found that reporting difficulty refraining from using the product in places where it was prohibited was less strongly associated with the latent dependence dimension for exclusive e-cigarette users than for combustible tobacco cigarette users. This may be due in part to less comprehensive indoor air quality restrictions against e-cigarette use than combustible tobacco cigarette use, making this particular symptom a less relevant indicator of e-cigarette dependence than of combustible tobacco cigarette dependence. The study then used the empirically validated latent dimension to compare the average severity of dependence across different tobacco product user groups.

DIF analyses supported use of 16 of the 24 examined tobacco dependence (TD) indicators for comparisons across different tobacco product users. Three items were omitted from further analyses because they were invalid indicators of the latent dependence dimension in multiple users (i.e., "most of the people I spend time with are tobacco users"; "tobacco use is causing a health problem"; "giving up activities as tobacco use not allowed"); others were retained or eliminated based on DIF analysis and the authors' judgment, including retaining symptom indicators that may have yielded statistically significant DIF that were not of clinical or practical significance. Using the item response–based model with the

TABLE 8-3 Tobacco Dependence Instruments and Questions Included, Examined in Response Models, and Retained on a Final Common Tobacco Dependence Instrument in the Population Assessment of Tobacco and Health Study Wave 1

Item Number	Original Instrument	Domain	Question Text	Final Common Instrument
1	HONC	Loss of control	Do you consider yourself addicted to [product]?	No
2	HONC	Craving	Do you ever have strong cravings to [product]?	No
3	HONC	Craving	Have you ever felt like you really needed [product]?	No
4	WISDM: Primary	Automaticity	I find myself reaching for [product] without thinking about it.	Yes
5	WISDM: Primary	Craving	I frequently crave [product].	Yes
6	WISDM: Primary	Craving	My urges keep getting stronger if I don't use [product].	Yes
7	WISDM: Primary	Loss of control	Tobacco products control me.	Yes
8	WISDM: Primary	Loss of control	My [product] use is out of control.	Yes
9	WISDM: Primary	Tolerance	I usually want to use [product] right after I wake up.	Yes
10	WISDM: Primary	Craving	I can only go a couple of hours without using [product].	Yes
11	WISDM: Primary	Automaticity	I frequently find myself almost using [product] without thinking about it.	Yes
12	WISDM: Secondary	Negative reinforcement	Using [product] would really help me feel better if I've been feeling down.	Yes
13	WISDM: Secondary	Cognitive enhancement	Using [product] helps me think better.	Yes
14	WISDM: Secondary	Social reinforcement	Most of the people I spend time with are tobacco users.	No
15	WISDM: Secondary	Affiliative attachment	I [would] feel alone without my [product].	Yes
16	NDSS	Loss of control	I would find it really hard to stop using [product].	Yes
17	NDSS	Loss of control	I would find it hard to stop using [product] for a week.	Yes

18	NDSS	Withdrawal	After not using [product] for a while, I need/I would like to use [product] in order to feel less restless and irritable.	Yes
19	NDSS	Withdrawal	After not using [product] for a while, I need to use [product] in order to keep myself from experiencing any discomfort.	Yes
20	DSM: Risky Use	Use despite consequences	Do you believe that [product] is causing a health problem or making it worse?	No
21	DSM: Social impairment	Give up activities	In the past 12 months, did you give up or cut down on activities that were enjoyable or important to you because [product] was not permitted at the activity?	No
22	DSM: Impaired control	Loss of control	In the past 12 months, did you find it difficult to keep from using [product] in places where it was prohibited?	Yes
23	DSM: Withdrawal	Withdrawal	Withdrawal syndrome.	No
24	Time to first tobacco	Tolerance	On days that you smoke, how soon after you wake up do you typically smoke your first cigarette of the day? Please enter the number of minutes or hours.	No

NOTES: The Final Common Instrument identifies as "Yes" the 16 items used to compare levels of tobacco dependence (TD) across product users. Items labeled "No" were set aside due to evidence of poor relation to overall levels of TD or differences in how the items measured TD symptoms across products. DSM = *Diagnostic and Statistical Manual of Mental Disorders*; HONC = Hooked on Nicotine Checklist; NDSS = Nicotine Dependence Syndrome Scale; WISDM = Wisconsin Inventory of Smoking Dependence Motives.
SOURCE: Strong et al., 2017.

validated 16 item cross-product dependence index to estimate the latent dependence severity across all groups, mean tobacco product dependence severity scores were 1.37 standard deviation units lower for e-cigarette–only users than combustible tobacco cigarette–only users (see Figure 8-1). E-cigarette–only users were comparable to cigar-only users and slightly higher than hookah-only users. Poly-product users of e-cigarettes and other products were comparable to combustible tobacco cigarette–only users. Among e-cigarette–only users, the 70.1 percent (SE ± 2.12 percent) of exclusive e-cigarette users who were daily users scored significantly higher on the latent dependence dimension than non-daily exclusive e-cigarette users (mean difference in standard deviation units = 0.40, SE = 0.07). Overall, e-cigarette–only users did have a lower level of TD, but increased frequency of use was significantly associated with increasing levels of TD (Strong et al., 2017).

The results of this study highlight the importance of considering the relative validity of symptom indicators across different tobacco products. Given that certain measurements of dependence symptoms differ in their relative validity, the prevalence and mean severity estimates may be less accurate and perhaps biased for one product versus another. Nonetheless, the bulk of the indicator symptoms (21 of 24) in this study exhibited consistent relationships with the primary dependence dimension for each product, suggesting that any error or bias across products may be modest, and 16 of the 24 were deemed to have minimal or no differential validity across products after substantial empirical scrutiny. The highly rigorous approach of estimating a well-vetted index with a comprehensive set of items is a major strength of the study, as was the use of a large nationally representative sample and separation of multiple mutually exclusive single- and poly-product user groups. In addition to providing precise mean dependence severity estimates of e-cigarette users relative to other user groups, this study shows that frequency of e-cigarette use is significantly associated with severity of dependence. This provides additional evidence that, as with combustible tobacco cigarettes and other drugs of abuse, dependence severity is higher among those who use more frequently. Limitations include the use of a cross-sectional design, which leaves unclear whether the association between level of e-cigarette use and dependence is a result of greater exposure to the product increasing severity of dependence, more frequent use as a consequence of the strong drive to use, or other confounding influences. The omission of other covariates in these analyses and comparisons of dependence severity across different product user groups further leaves unclear the role of alternative explanations for observed associations other than a causal effect. In sum, this study provides robust evidence that the typical level of dependence symptoms among exclusive e-cigarette users is comparable

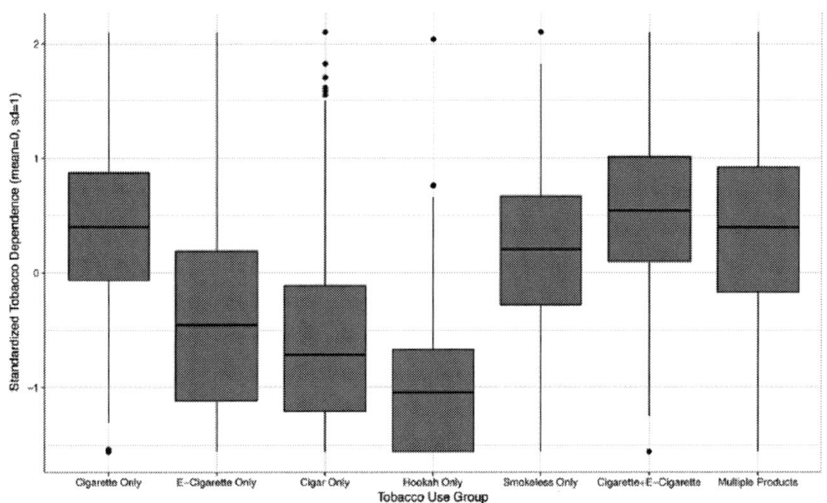

FIGURE 8-1 Distribution of tobacco dependence among each tobacco product use group in the Population Assessment of Tobacco and Health study Wave 1.
SOURCE: Strong et al., 2017.

to cigar users and lower than combustible tobacco cigarette users in the U.S. population. In addition, the association between frequency of use and dependence among exclusive e-cigarette users further suggests that dependence symptoms are directly linked to e-cigarette exposure.

Studies Using Non-Representative Sampling

Johnson and colleagues (2017) surveyed 117 e-cigarette users attending a large southeastern e-cigarette convention in fall 2015. Modified questions from the FTCD adapted for e-cigarette use and other questions were administered via a paper and pencil survey at the convention center lobby. Total scores were then categorized into one of four categories to approximate the clinical cutoffs for the FTCD. These categories were "low dependence" (score = 1–2, n = 20, 17.1 percent of respondents), "low to moderate dependence" (score = 3–4, n = 26, 22.2 percent), "moderate dependence" (score 5–7; n = 53, 45.3 percent), and "high dependence" (score = 8 or higher; n = 18, 15.4 percent of respondents). Hence, a significant proportion of the sample was classified as moderate or high dependence. Of the sample, 10 percent also used combustible tobacco cigarettes. This low prevalence may reflect a selection bias. Although smokers were not removed from the analysis, current or past smoking status were not significantly different across the modified-FTCD e-cigarette dependence severity categories, suggesting that the confounder of current smoking was modest. Length of e-cigarette use was positively associated with e-cigarette dependence category. More than half of respondents who have used e-cigarettes for more than a year were ranked as moderately or highly nicotine dependent (70.5 percent). Fewer than half (45.7 percent) who have used e-cigarettes for less than a year were ranked as moderately to highly nicotine dependent. There is a statistical trend in differences between those who used e-liquid with (versus without) nicotine and modified-FTCD dependence level ($p = 0.054$). Among those who used e-liquid without nicotine, 36.4 percent were classified as low, 22.7 percent were low-to-moderate, 36.4 percent were moderate, and 4.6 percent were highly dependent. In those who used e-liquid with nicotine, the distribution was shifted toward more severe dependence, such that 12.8 percent were low, 22.3 percent were low-to-moderate, 46.8 percent were moderate, and 18.1 percent were high. The idiosyncratic and highly selected sample limits the generalizability of the findings and raises considerable questionability regarding the generalizability of the prevalence estimates. Furthermore, the sample was modest and statistical comparisons did not adjust for confounders. In sum, this study provides weak suggestive evidence that dependence symptoms are of appreciable prevalence, associated with chronicity of use, and are higher among those who use nicotine.

In a letter to the editor, Gonzalez-Roz and colleagues (2017) reported nicotine dependence levels in a sample of "experienced e-cigarette users" (n = 39, men = 77 percent) and current combustible tobacco cigarette smokers (n = 42, men = 57 percent). The authors administered adapted and non-adapted versions of both the FTCD and the NDSS to e-cigarette and combustible tobacco cigarette users, respectively. The authors also collected and analyzed samples for biochemical markers of carbon monoxide and urinary cotinine. Based on the mean scores of each group, the authors concluded that "(1) e-cigarette users were dependent on e-liquids containing nicotine, [and] (2) e-cigarette users were found to be less nicotine dependent than current tobacco cigarette smokers [on all self-reported measures]" (Gonzalez-Roz et al., 2017, pp. 136–137). Cotinine values did not significantly differ between the groups, while CO was higher in smokers than e-cigarette users. This study is subject to the same limitations that all cross-sectional studies using dependence symptom measures that are not psychometrically validated via item-response modeling. Furthermore, because details regarding the recruitment strategy, population, and other variables (e.g., demographics) were not provided nor were adjusted analyses performed, clear conclusions regarding the contribution of this study to the evidence base could not be drawn. This study was judged to provide very weak evidence that e-cigarette dependence symptoms are of appreciable prevalence and severity in e-cigarette users at levels lower than combustible tobacco cigarette users.

Anonymous Web Surveys of E-Cigarette Users

Foulds and colleagues (2015) collected data on the prevalence and correlates of e-cigarette dependence symptoms among e-cigarette users who completed an online survey. Participation in the survey was voluntary and anonymous; data were collected from December 2012 to August 2014. Participants were recruited by following links to the survey, which the investigators posted on a range of medical websites and those popular among e-cigarette users such as http://www.webMD.com and http://www.e-cigaretteforum.com. Visitors to these sites could also send or post a link to the survey to friends and other websites. The analysis was limited to 3,609 respondents who were exclusive current daily e-cigarette users who had not smoked combustible tobacco cigarettes in the past 30 days. Participants were asked to report on 10 dependence symptoms that compose the Penn State Electronic Cigarette Dependence Index (PSECDI), which assesses frequency of use, time to first use after awakening, difficulty refraining from use when prohibited, craving, and other related symptoms. An analogously worded cigarette dependence index was also completed. Because participants were all past smokers, they were asked "Think back to a time when you were primarily a traditional cigarette smoker . . . before you used e-cigs. To the best of your ability, answer the following questions regarding your cigarette smoking at that time." Within-person comparisons of the dependence symptoms showed that for nearly all questions, symptoms were more likely and reported at higher levels when participants were asked to recall their experience with combustible tobacco cigarettes than their current experience with e-cigarettes. The mean (SD) composite dependence score for e-cigarettes was 8.1 (3.5), which would be classified as between "low" and "medium" severity dependence, which was significantly lower than the corresponding mean (SD) dependence score for combustible tobacco cigarettes 14.5 (3.7), which would be classified as "high" severity dependence. The e-cigarette versus combustible tobacco cigarette comparison was a "within-subject" comparison that rules out systematic confounders that occur across different populations. However, given that recall errors and other reporting biases for historical information were present only for e-cigarette use, these results are highly impacted by potential methodological confounding. The authors conducted a regression model in which number of demographic and e-cigarette and combustible tobacco cigarette use characteristics were included as simultaneous predictors of PSECDI score. PSECDI was significantly higher in women (versus men), whites (versus other races), those without (versus with) a college education, those who are older (versus younger), those who have used e-cigarettes for a longer time, those who have previously tried more e-cigarette models, those who currently use a device larger than a combustible tobacco cigarette (versus a cigalike model), those who use a more advanced device with a button (versus other models), those who use a device that costs greater versus less than $50, and those who use a higher concentration of nicotine liquid (see Figure 8-2).

Because participation was anonymous and the recruitment method allowed anyone to complete the survey, the representativeness of the sample is uncertain. The authors note that "those who found out about the survey on specialist websites and took the time to complete the survey are a particularly experienced and likely 'pro-e-cig' sample of e-cig users, and it is possible their answers were designed to make e-cigs look 'good' relative to traditional cigarettes" (Foulds et al., 2015, p. 191). The authors attempted to address this via sensitivity analyses adjusting for and restricting to self-reported public advocacy for e-cigarettes online (which was reported by 42 percent of participants) and being an e-cigarette retailer (3 percent), which did not affect the main results. The non-representative sample is a limitation, but the fairly large sample is a strength. In sum, this study provides suggestive evidence that e-cigarette dependence symptoms are of appreciable severity and lower than for combustible tobacco cigarettes. Higher nicotine concentration and other device characteristics typically associated with greater power and nicotine yield (e.g., newer generation, higher price) are associated with more severe e-cigarette dependence symptoms.

A study by Yingst and colleagues (2015) drew from the same dataset as in Foulds and colleagues (2015), and compared dependence symptoms among participants using "first-generation" devices (n = 1,048; same size as a combustible tobacco cigarette with no button) and "advanced-generation" devices (n = 3,373; larger than a cigarette with a manual button); participants were combustible tobacco cigarette–ever smokers who reported using an e-cigarette at least 30 days in their lifetime. Results showed that participants currently using an advanced- (compared with first-) generation device exhibited higher scores on the PSECDI dependence symptom composite index (mean [SD] = 8.3 [3.3] versus 7.1 [4.0]) and short time to first e-cigarette after wakening (mean [SD] = 38.7 [60.0] versus 67.3 [116.1] minutes) despite using a liquid with a lower nicotine concentration (mean [SD] = 15.1 [6.6] versus 19.1 [12.7] mg/ml). These results were not adjusted for potential confounding covariates, although device type was also associated with dependence scores in the Foulds and colleagues (2015) analysis, which did adjust for many relevant confounding factors. While subject to the same limitations as Foulds and

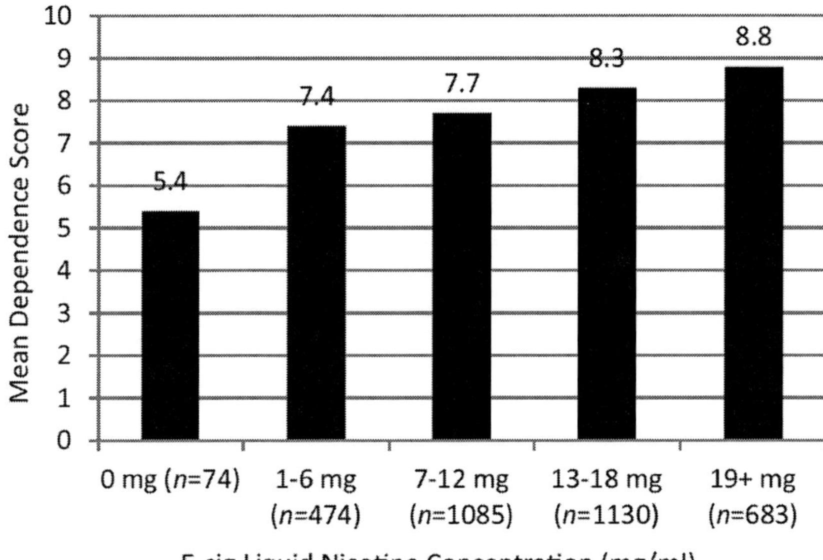

FIGURE 8-2 Dependence score as a function of nicotine concentration.
NOTES: Penn State Electronic Cigarette Dependence Index was adjusted for gender, age, race, education level, days used an e-cigarette, e-cigarette size, e-cigarette button, battery, and number of e-cigarettes. All between-group p values < 0.003 except between (1) 1–6 and 7–12 mg groups, and (2) 13–18 and 19+ mg groups.
SOURCE: Foulds et al., 2015.

colleagues (2015) and providing some replicatory findings, this study provides confirmatory evidence that advanced- (compared with first-) generation devices are associated with higher dependence, and this association is clearly not driven by differences in the nicotine concentration of the liquid. The authors speculate that because advanced-generation devices provide more power and greater nicotine delivery per equivalent nicotine composition in e-liquid (Shihadeh and Eissenberg, 2015), greater nicotine exposure to the user may account for the higher dependence levels in advanced- versus first-generation device users.

Dawkins and colleagues (2013) conducted a study of never (n = 6; 4 percent), current (n = 218; 16 percent); and former (n = 1,123; 83 percent) smokers who were also current e-cigarette users. Participants recruited on e-cigarette retailer websites completed a Web survey on e-cigarette dependence and use characteristics, including several survey questions addressing factors relevant to dependence and abuse liability. In the whole sample, the proportion of survey responses indicating the highest level of endorsement (i.e., "very much so") was 56.2 percent for an item indicative of abuse liability ("I get a definite nicotine hit from the e-cigarette") and 18.4 percent for an item indicative of possible dependence ("crave e-cigarettes as much as I do/did tobacco"). The representativeness of this study is questionable given the recruitment method and the cursory survey. In sum, this study provides weak suggestive evidence in support of dependence symptoms (and abuse liability to some degree) in e-cigarette use that is lower than corresponding dependence in combustible tobacco use.

In a series of three papers reporting on an overlapping sample, Etter (2015, 2016) and Etter and Eissenberg (2015) reported the prevalence and correlates of dependence symptoms among nicotine- and tobacco-product–using respondents in Internet surveys. The investigators posted links to the e-cigarette survey on health-related websites, smoking cessation websites, and websites selling e-cigarettes or with information about them from October 2012 to September 2014. They collected data on nicotine gum users between 2004 and 2007, also on the Internet. The FTCD, the NDSS, the Cigarette Dependence Scale, and adaptations of these scales for e-cigarettes and nicotine gums were used. Additional questions assessing correlates were also included.

In Etter and Eissenberg (2015), users of nicotine-containing e-cigarettes reported higher dependence ratings than users of nicotine-free e-cigarettes. The authors also found that, among former smokers, those who had used e-cigarettes for more than 3 months (long-term users) were less dependent on e-cigarettes than those who had used nicotine gum for more than 3 months were dependent on the gum. Dependence ratings between short-term (3 months or less) users of gums or e-cigarettes had few differences. Cross-product findings were judged to carry little weight given the dramatic difference in sampling, methodology, and time frame (2004–2007 versus 2012–2014) across the gum and e-cigarette use groups. The nicotine strength comparisons among e-cigarette users were judged to provide weak evidence, given the non-representative sample and the lack of adjustment for confounders.

In Etter (2015), 374 daily users of e-cigarettes who had quit smoking in the previous 2 months had a median time to first e-cigarette that ranged from 15 to 45 minutes across groups, depending on whether participants' response to the question "Does e-cigarette relieve desire or craving to smoke?" was definitely (median = 15 min), a lot (median = 20), or somewhat/no/maybe (median = 45). This suggests mild to moderate levels of dependence for this particular symptom in the sample and that dependence is higher among those who report that e-cigarettes alleviate combustible tobacco cigarette cravings. No additional relevant analyses were reported. This provides additional weak suggestive evidence of mild to moderate levels of dependence in a sample of e-cigarette users.

In Etter (2016), answers from 1,672 current users of e-cigarettes were obtained. Across sample subgroups, responses to dependence- and abuse liability–relevant questions differed by how respondents rated the strength of the throat hit ("very weak," "rather weak," "average," "rather strong," and "very strong"). The "throat hit" is the specific sensation felt in the back of the throat by users when they inhale e-cigarette aerosol that is also reported with combustible tobacco cigarettes and is believed to be a pleasant sensation of slight irritation of the airways. Unadjusted comparisons indicated that the time of the first e-cigarette tended to be shorter among users who reported a stronger throat hit (indicating more severe dependence), and the median time across the groups ranged from 15 to 30 minutes, indicating medium levels of dependence. High prevalence estimates for survey questions assessing rewarding effects and euphoria, indicative of product abuse liability, were found overall, including "like the taste of the vapor" (range 75–90 percent across groups differentiated by strength of throat hit), "like sensation of vapor when inhaling" (60–92 percent), and "feels so good to vape" (59–91 percent). For each of these questions, the prevalence tended to be higher among e-cigarette users reporting stronger throat hit in unadjusted comparisons. Overall, this study provides additional suggestive evidence that dependence symptoms and experiences indicative of abuse liability are of moderate to high prevalence and severity and may be higher in those who obtain a stronger throat hit from their product.

In sum, the collective papers across these three studies provide suggestive evidence that e-cigarette dependence symptoms and subjective effects of vaping indicative of abuse liability are of appreciable prevalence and severity in samples of users and may be associated with nicotine concentration and user characteristics.

Additional Descriptive Data on E-Cigarette Dependence Symptoms

In four small laboratory studies of current e-cigarette users (Dawkins et al., 2016 [n = 11]; Goldensen et al., 2016 [n = 20]; Hobkirk et al., 2017 [n = 9]; Nichols et al., 2016 [n = 7]), mean dependence symptom reports were incidentally reported to provide descriptive data on the sample. For the three studies that reported PSECDI composite scores the range was 6.0 to 8.4, indicating low to moderate levels of nicotine dependence. Using a modified FTCD for e-cigarettes, Dawkins and colleagues (2016) reported a mean score of 4.73 and a mean self-rated addiction to e-cigarettes on a 1–5 scale of 3.18 (1.17) in their sample, indicating moderate nicotine dependence (Dawkins et al., 2016). These data provide additional suggestive confirmatory data to reports in the epidemiological data reviewed above that e-cigarette dependence symptoms are non-negligible in various samples of users.

HUMAN LABORATORY STUDIES

The search resulted in 9 articles that reported original data from 12 separate studies that matched the requirements above (see Table 8-2 for a summary of these studies). Review of the articles revealed that five of the studies compared the effects of e-cigarette products varying in e-liquid flavoring on abuse liability outcomes. Three of these five studies as well as three additional studies also addressed the effect of varying e-cigarette nicotine concentration on abuse liability. Four studies compared the effects of e-cigarette administration with combustible tobacco cigarette administration among smokers.

Studies Testing the Effects of Flavor

Goldenson and colleagues (2016) conducted a double-blind, crossover design study among young adults who reported using e-cigarettes in the past 30 days (n = 20, ages 19–34, 80 percent current smokers). Participants used e-cigarette devices with Joyetech "Delta 23 Atomizer" tanks connected to a Joyetech "eVic Supreme" battery (recent-generation device) filled with e-cigarette solutions (Dekang Biotechnology Co., Ltd., 50/50 propylene glycol [PG]/glycerol) in 10 flavors (6 sweet: peach, watermelon, blackberry, cotton candy, cola, and sweet lemon tea; 3 non-sweet: mint, tobacco, and menthol; and 1 flavorless). The participants self-administered 20 standardized 2-puff doses of aerosolized e-cigarette solutions in 3 flavors (sweet versus non-sweet versus flavorless), either with nicotine (6 mg/ml) or without (0 mg/ml [placebo]). After each administration, participants rated three abuse liability indicators (liking, willingness to use again, and perceived monetary value), perceived sweetness, and throat hit strength. Each flavor was presented twice (once in 6 mg/ml and once in placebo) resulting in 20 total administrations all occurring on a single visit. Before testing, participants were trained on how to follow the standardized puffing procedure that was used for each trial to equalize the "dose" of product administered for each condition, which involved a 10-second preparation, 4-second inhalation, 1-second hold, and 2-second exhale—approximating typical vaping topography.

Results showed that sweet-flavored solutions produced significantly greater abuse liability rating for each index compared with non-sweet and flavorless ($p < 0.0001$). Throat hit ratings were greater for nicotine than placebo, but did not significantly increase abuse liability or interact with flavor effects on abuse liability outcomes. Controlling for flavor and nicotine, perceived sweetness was positively associated with each abuse liability outcome. To account for the influence of preexisting flavor preferences, the authors examined results in a subsample of participants who reported regularly using non-sweet flavors ($n = 9$). Consistent with results in the overall sample, all outcomes were positively associated with sweetness ratings ($p < 0.0001$). As in the overall sample, results among the subsample showed higher mean abuse liability ratings for sweet flavored solutions compared with non-sweet and flavorless solutions. However, for each appeal rating, the main effects for flavors (p = 0.09–0.17) and pairwise contrasts of sweet-flavored to non-sweet or flavorless solutions (p = 0.06–0.23) did not reach statistical significance. Additional tests of whether participants could correctly guess the characterizing flavor of each liquid administered after each administration indicated that participants' accuracy was not significantly better than chance guessing, suggesting upholding of the study blind to participants regarding the flavor they received.

The study strengths include the use of three to five different flavors per flavor category and analyses correlating sweetness ratings with abuse liability outcomes, suggesting a more generalized phenomenon across multiple different types of products that e-liquids with flavors that produce perceptions of sweetness also were of higher abuse liability. The standardized puffing procedure to equate the dose of administration was also a strength of the study, because it can prevent confounding of flavor or nicotine condition with the duration of puff taken. The null nicotine finding should be interpreted with the caveat that the study design was not well suited to detect and isolate nicotine's pharmacological effects, given that participants were rapidly exposed to multiple products with and without nicotine in a short time frame and that participants were not required to be deprived of nicotine to participate in the test session. Therefore, the participants likely had to base their ratings on the acute sensory response rather than a more generalized pharmacological effect that may take several minutes to generate. In addition, outcomes were limited to self-reporting, which reflects one aspect of abuse liability that may or may not be parallel to other indicators (e.g., willingness to work for vaping). In sum, this study provides fairly strong evidence that sweet flavorings enhance subjective abuse liability indexes in young adults and provides limited evidence regarding the impact of nicotine on abuse liability.

Using a within-subjects design, Audrain-McGovern and colleagues (2016) conducted three human laboratory sessions among young adult daily smokers who had previously tried e-cigarettes at least once, but used e-cigarettes less often than daily ($n = 32$). Participants used an "e-GO" tank-style e-cigarette with a single 2.2- to 2.4-Ω resistance coil that could not be adjusted, 650-mAh rechargeable lithium ion battery, and a 2.4-ml refillable e-liquid tank. The first session asked participants to rate unflavored and sweet (green apple and chocolate)-flavored e-cigarettes with nicotine on how satisfying and good they tasted to evaluate the rewarding value of flavoring. The sweet flavor that produced the higher reward rating for each respective participant was selected as the "flavored" product to use over the next two sessions for comparison with the unflavored e-cigarette. To assess the relative reinforcing value of a sweet-flavored e-cigarette compared with an unflavored e-cigarette, the second session applied a choice task that evaluated the willingness to "work" in the form of moving a computer mouse to hit targets on one of two computer screens, to earn points toward flavored or unflavored e-cigarette puffs. Session 3 measured the absolute reinforcing value of sweet-flavored versus unflavored e-cigarettes via a 90-minute ad lib e-cigarette use session where puffs from each e-cigarette product (sweet-flavored versus unflavored) were counted.

Results of the study were clear and consistent. Rating on a 1–7 scale, the average subjective rewarding value rating was significantly higher for the chocolate-flavored (mean [SD] = 3.69 [1.78]), and green apple–flavored (mean [SD] = 4.22 [1.55]) product than the unflavored (mean [SD] = 3.11 [1.55]) product. Participants worked harder for flavored e-cigarette puffs than for unflavored e-cigarette puffs ($p < 0.0001$). Total work was 596.31 responses (mouse clicks on targets) for the flavored e-cigarette (SD = 520.25; range 0–1,375) and 126.66 for the unflavored e-cigarette). During ad lib use over a 90-minute period, participants took twice as many flavored puffs than unflavored e-cigarette puffs (40 versus 23 puffs; incidence rate ratio [IRR] = 2.028; 95% CI = 1.183–3.475; $p = 0.01$).

The study strengths include the use of three different abuse liability outcomes, each of which provides unique information about abuse liability (i.e., one addressing the subjective experience, one addressing the motivation to obtain the product, one addressing self-administration under unconstrained conditions) and each yielding convergent results. A limitation was e-cigarette exposure eligibility criteria in the sample—all were ever users who had not progressed to become daily users—which may restrict generalizability to users who may be most prone to dependence (i.e., those who have already become daily e-cigarette users). At the same time, because all had experience using e-cigarettes, the likelihood that inability to use e-cigarettes properly had an impact on findings is low. In addition, the subjective reward finding should be interpreted with the caveat that one of the two items in the subjective reward index was "tasted good," which would be expected to be highly dependent on flavor. A more ideal subjective reward outcome would involve the inclusion of multiple elements indicative of self-reported reward value (e.g., product liking, mood elevation, desire to use again) to parse whether the result depended entirely on the fact that the sweet-flavored products tasted better than the unflavored product. Because all products contained nicotine, whether the effects of flavor on abuse liability would generalize across different nicotine concentrations (including no nicotine) is unknown. Overall, the study provides clear and consistent evidence across three different types of abuse liability outcomes indicating that sweet-flavored products produced higher abuse liability than unflavored products in young adult smokers.

Rosbrook and Green (2016) conducted two experiments testing the effects of e-cigarette administration varying in menthol and nicotine concentration on subjective abuse liability ratings and sensory effects. Each experiment involved 32 adult smokers age 18–45 (6 subjects participated in both experiments). In both experiments, the majority of subjects were self-reported menthol cigarette smokers (25 in experiment 1 and 26 in experiment 2). Five subjects in experiment 1 and 12 subjects in experiment 2 reported using e-cigarettes regularly. Both studies used the V2 Standard E-Cigarette device (79 mm; VMR Products, LLC) and V2 blank cartridges. In the first experiment, cartridges were filled with 15 different e-liquids (Pace Engineering Concepts, LLC) with 5 different concentrations of nicotine (0, 6, 12, 18, or 24 mg/ml) and 3 different concentrations of menthol (0.0 percent, 0.5 percent, or 3.5 percent l-menthol) in a 70/30 PG/glycerol base. In the second experiment, the cartridges were filled with six different e-liquids, each at 0 or 24 mg/ml nicotine: two menthol and two menthol–mint commercial flavors (70/30 PG/glycerol; AmericaneLiquidStore) and two unflavored e-liquids (PG/glycerol base only; Pace Engineering Concepts, LLC). Participants were trained in the puffing and rating procedure prior to the testing, which involved taking two "priming puffs" into the mouth only, then to fully inhale the third puff as they normally would when smoking a combustible tobacco cigarette and to exhale through the mouth. After exhalation the subject was prompted to rate liking or disliking the flavor on a scale with 11 semantic labels, ranging from "most dislike imaginable" to "most like imaginable" with "neutral" in the middle and other intermediate descriptors. Participants also rated three other sensory effects. Testing occurred on a single day for both experiments, and participants were required to be deprived of tobacco overnight. The study was double blind.

For both experiments, the e-liquids were only "slightly liked" on average. For the first experiment, the degree of liking did not vary significantly across nicotine or menthol concentrations. For the second experiment, the main effect of flavor showed higher ratings for liking of the commercial menthol and menthol–mint flavors over the unflavored e-liquid ($p < 0.001$). Nicotine and nicotine–flavor interactions were not significant. Sensory effect ratings of nicotine and menthol were reported, suggesting independent and interactive effects of nicotine and menthol in an expected direction on outcomes like coolness and harshness/irritation. The sensory effect results were consistent with the known effects of these substances from the combustible tobacco cigarette literature and validate the robustness of the menthol and nicotine manipulations.

The results of these experiments should be interpreted within the following caveats. All participants were combustible tobacco cigarette smokers, most of whom did not report frequent use of e-cigarettes. Hence, most participants may have been unfamiliar with e-cigarettes and how to use them, which could impact sensitivity to manipulations in flavor and nicotine. Also, such individuals would be expected to be less likely to be prone to dependence on e-cigarettes given that most were not (yet) users. The use of a relatively low-powered device that likely delivers less nicotine and flavor constituents than do more powerful devices leaves unclear whether these results would generalize to other popular products. Critically, all e-liquids for the first experiment and the unflavored liquid for the second experiment were created by a private engineering company and were merely PG, glycerol, and l-menthol. E-liquids available in the marketplace generally contain numerous other additives to enhance the sweetness and remove aversive tastes and sensory qualities (see Chapter 5 for discussion of flavorings). Hence, the absence of effects of menthol flavoring on liking in the first experiment may bear modest relevance to the mentholated e-liquids used in the population. Indeed, in the second experiment when commercial menthol and menthol-mint flavorings were used, the liking ratings were significantly higher relative to the unflavored solution containing only PG and glycerol. Finally, the use of a single item rating of liking is a very narrow indicator of abuse liability. In sum, this study provides moderately strong controlled evidence that commercially available menthol and menthol-mint flavors produce greater subjective product liking than unflavored e-liquids among smokers.

In a study by St.Helen and colleagues (2017), 11 men and 3 women participated in a 3-day inpatient crossover study with strawberry, tobacco, and their usual flavor e-liquid on subjective product liking ratings indicative of abuse liability and other outcomes. Exclusive e-cigarette users or dual users of fewer than five combustible tobacco cigarettes per day, who used second- and/or third-generation e-cigarettes at least 25 days per month for the past 3 months or more and had saliva cotinine levels at least 30 ng/ml were eligible. Commercially available strawberry and tobacco test e-liquids (Bulkejuice.com) with 60/40 and 56/44 PG/glycerol and with 19–20 mg/ml nicotine were used in the two test e-liquid conditions, The participant's own e-liquid was used for the comparison condition, each of which had sweet characterizing flavor names (with the exception of one participant who used a flavor that was "tobacco/vanilla"), with a range from 1.6 mg/ml to 186.7 mg/ml across participants (mean [SD] = 7.4 [5.3]) and a mean (SD) PG/glycerol ratio of 63/37 (18/18). For each session from 4:00 to 10:00 pm, subjects could use e-cigarettes ad lib to become acclimatized to the assigned flavor for the next day. Participants were abstinent overnight until the morning standardized session of 15 puffs, which was followed by 4 hours of abstinence, and then a 90-minute ad lib use session followed by subjective measures. For the standardized puffing procedure, participants took 15 puffs, one puff every 30 seconds, from the e-cigarette. Puff duration was not controlled by the study. Multiple blood draws were taken, and subjective questionnaires were administered 5 to 15 minutes post-puffing.

Results showed that for the standardized session, the tobacco and strawberry test e-liquids were not significantly different for mood enhancement or any subjective satisfaction or reward rating. While statistical tests for comparisons to the usual brand e-liquid were not reported, positive mood change mean (SD) scores from pre- to post-administration were 2.8 (1.6) for usual brand compared with 0.2 (1.1) and 0.4 (1.6) for strawberry and tobacco, respectively, which are suggestive of greater mood enhancement for usual brand than the test e-liquids. A similar pattern was found for mean (SD) satisfaction ratings (usual brand = 17.1 [0.9], strawberry = 12.4 [1.2], tobacco = 13.2 [1.5]).

After the ad lib session, mean ± SEM for the "taste good" ratings of the strawberry, tobacco, and usual e-liquids were 3.4 ± 0.4, 3.1 ± 0.5, and 5.9 ± 0.3, respectively (maximum possible score of this item is 7). The usual flavor was rated significantly higher than the strawberry and tobacco e-liquids ($p < 0.001$), while the strawberry and tobacco e-liquids were not significantly different for this outcome. For average satisfaction, subjects reported ratings with the strawberry ($p = 0.002$) and tobacco ($p < 0.001$) e-liquids compared with the usual brand e-liquids. Ratings of enjoyment of sensations in chest and throat were lower for both the strawberry ($p = 0.022$) and tobacco ($p = 0.019$) e-liquids compared with the usual brand e-liquids.

The findings of the study should be interpreted with the caveat that the primary goal was to determine effects of flavorings on nicotine pharmacokinetics, and subjective measures were secondary outcomes. Hence, the study sample size, although appropriate for studying effects on nicotine blood yield, was underpowered to detect meaningful effects for subjective abuse liability–relevant outcomes. Nonetheless, the controlled design, inclusion of both standardized and ad lib testing conditions, and inclusion of regular e-cigarette users with experimentally controlled tobacco product deprivation enhances the internal validity of the study, particularly for the standardized session test results. The ad lib session subjective ratings are subject to between-condition variations in the "dose" of product self-selected by the participants. Because the e-liquids self-selected by the user varied widely in nicotine concentration, PG/glycerol, and characterizing flavor, the particular product characteristics driving differences between usual brand and test e-liquids cannot be determined. At the same time, there is ecological validity to be gained by the using the participants' own e-liquids given their ability to self-select the product likely to be highly rewarding to their own preferences. In sum, the study provides tentative evidence that self-selected e-liquids produce greater satisfaction and potential other indicators of abuse liability than experimenter-provided e-liquids in experienced e-cigarette users.

Studies Testing the Effects of Nicotine Concentration

Using a double-blind within-participants design, counterbalanced design with two conditions (low and high nicotine), Dawkins and colleagues (2016) conducted a study of experienced e-cigarette users who completed 60 minutes of ad lib use in two separate sessions. The participants were 11 experienced male e-cigarette users (reported using e-cigarettes daily for more than 3 months) who currently used a second- or third-generation e-cigarette, and used 24 mg/ml at least once in the past 6 months. Participants abstained from nicotine use (including from e-cigarettes) for 12 hours prior to study commencement and were tested individually. In the laboratory, the investigators provided the participants with the study device—a Joyetech "eVic™ supreme" e-cigarette with a "Nautilus Aspire" tank, 3.9 V (8.5 W, 1.8-Ω resistance), adjusted to the largest airflow and filled with Halo Smokers' Angels brand e-liquid (50/50 PG/glycerol, 6 mg/ml [low] or 24 mg/ml [high] labeled nicotine). The researchers asked study participants to use e-cigarettes ad lib for 60 minutes, after which they completed a visual analogue scale rating assessing positive effects indicative of abuse liability (e.g., hit and satisfaction) and other effects for the preceding product self-administered.

Hit and satisfaction levels (mean percentage [SD]) were higher in the high nicotine condition (hit = 61.86 [31.50], satisfaction = 60.70 [17.30]) than in the low nicotine condition (hit = 44.73 [23.00], satisfaction = 46.89 [16.93]), but these differences did not reach statistical significance. Given that the sample size was small ($n = 11$), it is likely that the study was underpowered to detect effects, which raises the possibility that the non-significant differences may be type-II errors. Liquid consumption, puff number, and puff duration were significantly higher in the low nicotine condition compared with the high nicotine condition (all $p < 0.01$), which the authors interpreted engaging in compensatory puffing behavior in order to increase nicotine yield toward titration to achieve equal nicotine exposure in the two conditions. Approximately twice the overall puff consumption was recorded from the 6-mg/ml versus the 24-mg/ml conditions.

Despite the fact that the amount of product consumed was clearly more in low versus high nicotine condition, the evidence trended toward greater subjective abuse liability indicators addressing a pharmacological drug effect (i.e., "hit" rating) and subjective satisfaction in the higher nicotine condition. Thus, even though the study design allowing consumption to be uncontrolled was likely biased toward larger effects for low nicotine due to more consumption in this condition, the results tended to show the opposite. Strengths include the inclusion of experienced users and experimentally controlled deprivation from nicotine prior to the test session, which is a strong design for detecting abuse liability effects due to the pharmacological effects of nicotine exposure. Limitations include very small sample limited to men only. Taken together, these findings provide tentative evidence that nicotine may enhance some subjective effects indicative of abuse liability; however, no firm conclusion can be drawn due to the absence of statistically significant results ($p = 0.09$ to 0.11).

In a fully within-subjects design involving adult DSM-IV diagnosed nicotine-dependent smokers ($n = 28$), Perkins and colleagues (2015) examined the effect of controlled administration of e-cigarettes with 36 mg/ml nicotine concentration compared with a placebo on subjective abuse liability ratings and other measures. None of the participants reported using e-cigarettes weekly either currently or in the past, and none had used within the prior 2 weeks of participating, suggesting relatively little e-cigarette use experience. In two counterbalanced laboratory sessions, each following overnight abstinence, participants self-administered e-cigarettes from PrimeVapor LLC, with prefilled cartridges containing a glycerol-based e-liquid (labeled nicotine concentration 36 mg/ml or 0 mg/ml) in either the rawhide red (tobacco) non-menthol flavor and Freeport (menthol) flavor. A KR808D-1 type automatic e-cigarette battery was used. The procedure involved self-administration of 10 four-second puffs over 5 minutes. To control the "dose" of exposure, the researchers employed computer-presented instructions to guide and standardize the precise timing and duration of each puff inhalation. After the first set of 10 puffs, subjects indicated on a 0–100 visual analog scale (anchored by "not at all" and "extremely") several ratings relevant to abuse liability (e.g., "liking").

Results showed that participants provided significantly higher ratings on an indicator of strength of drug effect (e.g., "how much nicotine") and on two indicators of subjective reward (i.e., "liking" and "satisfied") for the nicotine e-cigarette than the placebo product (see Figure 8-3). Other outcomes were studied that are not considered within the scope of the review.

The highly controlled tight design with an adequately sized sample

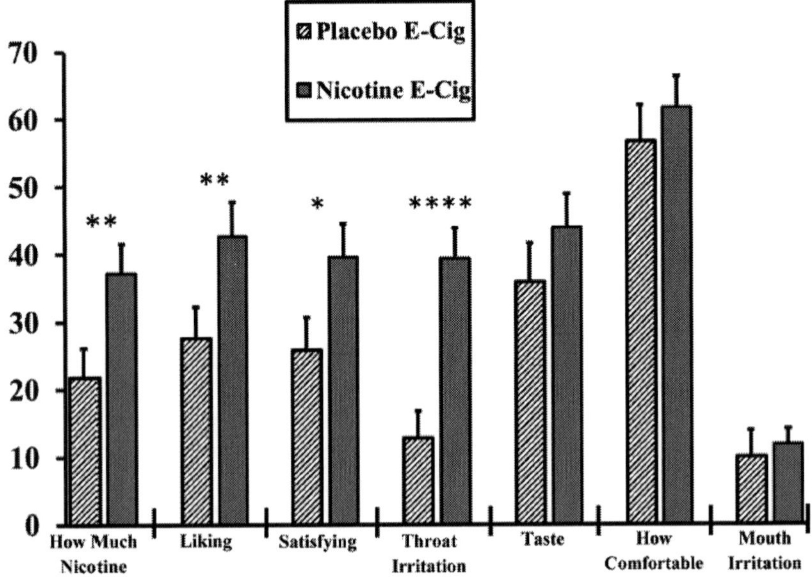

FIGURE 8-3 Subjective reward responses for the nicotine e-cigarette and the placebo (non-nicotine) e-cigarette.
NOTE: *p < 0.05 between e-cigarettes; **p = < 0.01 between e-cigarettes; ****p = < 0.001 between e-cigarettes.
SOURCE: Adapted from Perkins et al., 2015.

for a within-subject laboratory study makes this study highly rigorous. Because subjective abuse liability reports were not a primary outcome, the data collected were fairly cursory and do not address multiple manifestations of abuse liability. Outside of this factor and the use of what would be considered a less powerful device, the methods were very strong. In sum, this study provides rigorous evidence that e-cigarettes with a high dose of nicotine versus placebo increase abuse liability ratings among combustible tobacco cigarette-dependent smokers.

A study conducted by Baldassarri and colleagues (2017) included four daily e-cigarette users who had been using e-cigarettes for 1 month or longer and three smokers who had consumed more than 10 combustible tobacco cigarettes per day for the past year. The goal was to study nicotine receptor occupancy using a positron emission tomography neuroimaging protocol examining responses to an e-cigarette or combustible tobacco cigarette challenge. Self-reported product liking ratings were collected. However, inspection of the study showed that four e-cigarette users participated in two scans each (8-mg/ml and 36-mg/ml e-cigarette), and only two of the users underwent a third scan with a placebo (0-mg/ml e-cigarette). Hence, the sample was too small to permit meaningful within-person comparisons across e-cigarette nicotine doses. The three healthy smokers participated in one scan with the combustible tobacco cigarette challenge, but did not participate in the e-cigarette challenge, making cross-product comparisons confounded by between-subject group differences. Thus, this study could not be used to make any conclusions regarding the evidence.

As reviewed above in the section on studies testing the flavor effects, Goldenson and colleagues (2016) and Rosbrook and Green (2016) each examined the effects of varying nicotine concentrations on study outcomes and found no significant effect of nicotine variation on abuse liability–relevant measures. However, both studies used a multicondition exposure paradigm in which conditions of varying nicotine levels were administered within a short time frame and in small doses (e.g., either a single puff or two puffs). These designs are aimed to address the sensory effects of manipulations and are poorly suited for isolating the effect of a single pharmacologically active dose of nicotine, which requires a sufficient dosage amount (e.g., likely at least 10 puffs), following a period of nicotine deprivation. Hence, the nicotine effect findings from these studies are considered to provide little weight to the evidence determinations regarding whether nicotine concentration alters the abuse liability of e-cigarettes.

Comparisons of E-Cigarettes to Combustible Tobacco Cigarettes and Other Products

In 28 e-cigarette–naïve current smokers, Strasser and colleagues (2016) compared the effects of own-brand combustible tobacco cigarette smoking on abuse liability outcomes versus an e-cigarette product as a within-subject design factor. As an additional between-subject factor, when the participants were challenged with an e-cigarette, subjects were randomized to receive one of five brands of e-cigarette cigalike brands to determine whether brand variation within the e-cigarette class affected study outcomes: (1) NJOY = 18 mg nicotine; (2) V2 = 18 mg nicotine; (3) Green Smoke = 18.9–20.7 mg nicotine; (4) blu = 20–24 mg nicotine; and (5) White Cloud = 23–24 mg nicotine. On day 1, participants were allowed to smoke their own regular brand of combustible tobacco cigarette for a 10-minute period and then provided subjective rewarding effects of the combustible tobacco cigarette (e.g., satisfying, calming, pleasant, smoke another right now). Participants were then provided with their supply of e-cigarettes based on randomization and instructed to refrain from any tobacco/nicotine use aside from the e-cigarette provided for the remaining 9 study days. Participants were instructed to use their assigned e-cigarette as much as desired. Participants returned to lab on days 5 and 10 for two identical testing sessions that followed the exact procedures as described for day 1, except that participants used the e-cigarette ad lib during a 10-minute vaping period, and ratings were based on the e-cigarette challenge.

The main finding of the study in regard to the abuse liability outcome was that when comparing the relative self-reported liking assessed at day 1 (mean [SE] = 627.0 [43.0]; in reference to their own combustible tobacco cigarette), and later, reports of liking of the e-cigarette were significantly lower at day 5 (mean [SE] = 340.4 [31.2]) and day 10 (mean [SE] = 343.6 [39.6]). There was no main effect for e-cigarette brand or an interaction effect for e-cigarette liking ($p > 0.05$). The study result should be interpreted with the caveat of having a very small sample size for brand versus brand between-group comparisons ($n = 6$ per group). All participants were current daily combustible tobacco cigarette smokers who had no or minimal prior e-cigarette use experience and who were willing to switch to e-cigarettes for 10 days, making this particular group perhaps not generalizable to certain segments of the population at risk for e-cigarette dependence. As noted by the author, the study used an older cigalike model and results may not extend to newer-generation devices. The use of only tobacco flavor also tempered the authors' conclusions. Hence, the test might have been biased toward detecting lower product liking for e-cigarettes relative to the standard brand. In addition, the ad lib uncontrolled puff administration resulted in the participants using their own combustible tobacco cigarette for a longer period of time during the 10-minute self-administration interval than the duration of use of the e-cigarette products in the 10-minute interval. In sum, this study provides fairly weak evidence regarding lower abuse liability of first-generation e-cigarette devices relative to own-brand combustible tobacco cigarettes among e-cigarette–naïve smokers and inconclusive evidence whether or not product variation within the e-cigarette product class affects abuse liability.

Stiles and colleagues (2017) evaluated the abuse liability of three e-cigarettes (Vuse Solo brand, labeled nicotine concentrations of 14, 29, or 36 mg per e-liquid cartridge; solvent, flavoring additives, or characterizing labels and device properties not reported) relative to "high- and low-abuse liability" comparator products (usual brand combustible tobacco cigarettes and nicotine gum, respectively) among 45 e-cigarette–naïve smokers. For inclusion in the study, subjects were required to be adults age 21–60, smoke 10 or more non-menthol 83-mm (king size) to 100-mm combustible tobacco cigarettes per day for at least 6 months, and typically smoke their first combustible tobacco cigarette of the day within 30 minutes of waking. Products used as comparators were any combustible, filtered, non-menthol brand style, 83 mm (king size) to 100 mm in length for the high-abuse liability comparator and Nicorette® White Ice Mint nicotine polacrilex gum, 4 mg (GlaxoSmithKline Consumer Healthcare, L.P.) for the low-abuse liability product. Subjects participated in a 7-day ambulatory home use trial of each product before each of five test visits to allow subjects to become accustomed to using the new products. Subjects were required to abstain from smoking for 12 hours prior to reporting to the clinic on the morning of each test visit. The testing consisted of up to 10 minutes use of Vuse Solo or smoking of one combustible tobacco cigarette, or up to 30 minutes using nicotine gum according to the package instructions. Five questionnaires were administered to assess subjective endpoints: Product Liking, Intent to Use Product Again, Product Effects, Urge to Smoke, and Urge for Product measured at multiple time points out to 2 hours following use.

Results showed that product liking was lower for the three Vuse Solo e-cigarettes (least square [LS] mean peak scores ranging from 4.13 to 4.57) compared with combustible tobacco cigarettes (LS mean peak score value = 9.06, $p < 0.001$ for all), and higher than nicotine gum (LS mean peak score value = 3.21, $p < 0.05$ for all). Ratings of Intent to Use Again followed a similar pattern. Whether the three different doses of nicotine were different from one another on abuse liability outcomes was not reported, though inspection of mean scores across the conditions suggests the differences are smaller among the different e-cigarette products than relative difference from combustible tobacco cigarette and gum conditions (see Table 8-4).

Subjects used the greatest e-liquid in the Vuse Solo 14-mg device (0.061 g), followed by Vuse Solo 29-mg (0.048 g), and Vuse Solo 36-mg (0.026 g) based on the average difference in the weights of the e-liquid cartridges.

Strengths of the study include use of multiple doses of nicotine to elucidate pharmacological dose–response effects and inclusion of both combustible tobacco cigarette and nicotine gum as active comparator conditions. However, the failure to control the amount of product administered across visits due to the ad lib design for the test session as well as uncontrolled exposure during the 7-day ambulatory period leaves the confounding effects of exposure on study outcomes unclear. Furthermore, the study did not provide data on the flavoring additives, vehicle compound, and device parameters (e.g., voltage, resistance) used. Hence, the generalizability beyond the product to other e-cigarettes that vary in nicotine concentration is unclear. In sum, this study provides suggestive evidence that an e-cigarette product may have intermediate abuse liability relative to nicotine gum (low abuse liability) and combustible tobacco cigarettes (higher abuse liability) among e-cigarette–naïve smokers.

TABLE 8-4 Product Liking for Vuse Solo E-Cigarettes with Different Nicotine Concentrations Compared with Usual Brand Combustible Tobacco Cigarette and Nicotine Gum

Parameter	LS Mean				
	Vuse Solo 14 mg	Vuse Solo 29 mg	Vuse Solo 36 mg	Usual Brand Cigarette	Nicotine Gum
Product Liking ($AUEC_{15–360}$)	1,396.68[a,b]	1,430.66 [a,b]	1,190.01 [a,b]	3,116.52	799.38
E_{max}	4.36 [a,b]	4.57 [a,b]	4.13 [a,b]	9.06	3.21
Intent to Use Again ($AUEC_{15–360}$)	1,619.43 [a,b]	1,635.82 [a,b]	1,400.99 [a,b]	2,369.30	1,091.84
E_{max}	4.71 [a,b]	4.75 [a,b]	4.07 [a,b]	6.81	3.29
Liking of Positive Effects ($AUEC_{15–360}$)	727.42	800.57 [a]	673.67	889.74	444.17
E_{max}	6.71 [a,b]	6.51 [a,b]	5.99 [a]	8.31	5.47
Disliking of Negative Effects ($AUEC_{15–360}$)	502.66	827.42	740.85	423.38	422.14
E_{max}	6.03	6.41	6.67	5.80	6.28

NOTE: AUEC = area under the effect curve; LS = least square.
[a] = Significantly different from usual brand cigarette, $p < 0.05$.
[b] = Significantly different from nicotine gum, $p < 0.05$.
SOURCE: Stiles et al., 2017.

Vansickel and colleagues (2012) conducted a study of e-cigarette–naïve current smokers. Participants completed a behavioral choice abuse liability task evaluating the relative reinforcing value of e-cigarette and usual brand combustible tobacco cigarettes versus money; subjective abuse liability ratings were also collected. Participants were given a "Vapor King" (KR808 model) e-cigarette with a rechargeable 3.7-V battery and airflow sensor with a lighted display end and disposable cartomizer to use. WOW cowboy or WOW cowboy menthol tobacco–flavored cartomizers (18 mg/ml nicotine; commonly used nicotine strength; Vapor4Life) were matched to participants' combustible tobacco cigarette flavor preference (i.e., non-menthol or menthol). The first of four, within-subject sessions was an e-cigarette administration session that involved six, 10-puff bouts (30-second interpuff interval) with each bout separated by 30 minutes. In the remaining three sessions, participants made choices among 10 e-cigarette puffs and varying amounts of money, 10 own-brand puffs and varying amounts of money, and 10 e-cigarette puffs and a varying number of own-brand combustible tobacco cigarette puffs, respectively, using a standardized multiple-choice procedure. The primary outcome for three choice sessions was the "crossover value," the point at which participants chose to receive (1) money over 10 puffs from the e-cigarette; (2) money over 10 puffs of their own-brand combustible tobacco cigarette; or (3) own-brand puffs over 10 puffs from the e-cigarette, for each respective session.

Results showed that after the first administration session, e-cigarette administration increased ratings on these measures with each successive sampling session, for ratings of "pleasant" ($F_{6,114} = 21.1$, $p < 0.0001$), "satisfying" ($F_{6,114} = 19.5$, $p < 0.0001$), "taste good" ($F_{6,114} = 20.2$, $p = 0.0001$), and "use another right now." For the choice procedure sessions, crossover values were greater in the own-brand combustible tobacco cigarettes versus money choice condition relative to the crossover or the e-cigarette versus money condition. Collapsed across time, the average crossover value was $1.06 (SD = $0.16) for choosing money versus e-cigarette, but was $1.50 (SD = $0.26) for choosing money over own-brand combustible tobacco cigarette, indicating greater reinforcing effects of smoking. For the task of pitting choices of e-cigarette and own-brand combustible tobacco cigarette puffs, the average crossover value, collapsed across time, was 3 own-brand puffs (SD = 0.4 puffs), indicating that 10 e-cigarette puffs were equivalent to 3 own-brand puffs. It can be concluded that the e-cigarette carried some abuse liability (albeit lower than combustible tobacco cigarettes) because probability of choosing vaping systematically increased as monetary values decreased, suggesting there was a significant reward value ascribed to e-cigarettes, and participants were willing to forgo a meaningful amount of money for e-cigarette puffs.

The use of multiple operationalizations of abuse liability and a rigorous behavioral choice procedure to ascribe a relative value of e-cigarettes versus both money and combustible tobacco cigarettes are key strengths. The study also showed that the e-cigarette administration significantly increased plasma nicotine, verifying that the manipulation was robust. However, the nicotine boost was lower than what is typically observed via a standard combustible tobacco cigarette. Hence, the abuse liability estimates could reflect conditions and products that may underestimate what regular smokers may choose to use. In sum, this study provides strong evidence that e-cigarettes possess abuse liability in regular smokers and suggestive evidence that the relative abuse liability is lower than the smoker's usual combustible tobacco cigarette brand used.

In a study by Vansickel and colleagues (2010), 32 e-cigarette–naïve smokers took 10 standardized puffs from one of four conditions in a within-subject crossover design: own brand combustible tobacco cigarette, "NPRO" e-cigarettes (NPRO, NJOY; 18-mg cartridge), "Hydro" e-cigarettes (Hydro, Crown 7; 16-mg cartridge), or sham (unlit combustible tobacco cigarette) conditions. Participants were daily smokers of 15 or more cigarettes per day and e-cigarette–naïve. Flavor (tobacco or menthol) of the product was matched to the preferred flavor of participants' own combustible tobacco cigarette brand. Participants responded to the subjective effect questionnaires 5, 15, 30, and 45 minutes after the 10 puffs of the respective product (including puffs of the unlit "sham" combustible tobacco cigarette). This cycle was repeated twice for each study visit/product condition.

The authors found significant condition-by-time interactions for ratings of "satisfying," "pleasant," and "taste good." In particular, ratings of "satisfying" and "pleasant" increased significantly at all time points with use of the Hydro e-cigarette, NPRO e-cigarette, and own-brand combustible tobacco cigarette. Ratings of "satisfying" and "pleasant" increased significantly higher for own-brand combustible cigarettes than those for Hydro e-cigarette or NPRO e-cigarette (see Figure 8-4).

This study had strengths in that a detailed four-condition comparison was made, including two separate products with a strong inactive control condition (i.e., sham) and an active comparison condition (i.e., usual brand combustible tobacco cigarette). The multi-time-point detailed assessment strategy increased statistical power. One strength was the assessment of biomarkers and physiological outcomes sensitive to nicotine. These results indicated that, within the first 5 minutes of administration, smoking own-brand combustible tobacco cigarettes significantly increased plasma nicotine and heart rate, but use of the NPRO e-cigarette, Hydro e-cigarette, and sham smoking did not. Thus, the first-generation products used in this study were likely ineffective at delivering nicotine and thus reflect an insensitive test of abuse liability relative to the prod-

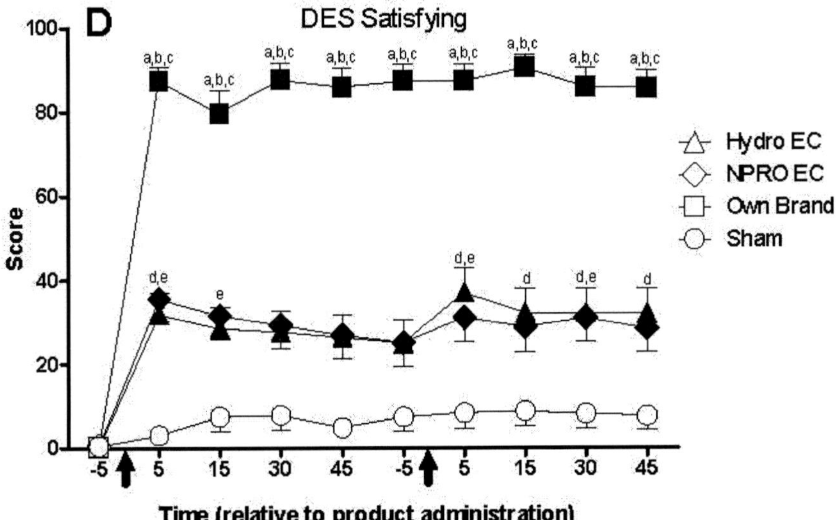

FIGURE 8-4 Interactions between time and condition (Hydro e-cigarette, NPRO e-cigarette, own-brand combustible tobacco cigarette, and sham [unlit combustible tobacco cigarette]) for subjective effects.
NOTES: An "a," "b," or "c" indicates that own brand was significantly different from sham, Hydro EC, or NPRO EC at that time point. A "d" indicates that Hydro EC was significantly different from sham at that time point. An "e" indicates that NPRO EC was significantly different from sham at that time point (Tukey's HSD, $p < 0.05$). Unidirectional error bars, one standard error. DES = direct effects of smoking; EC = e-cigarette.
SOURCE: Vansickel et al., 2010.

ucts available in the marketplace today. Furthermore, the e-cigarette–naïve participants were likely not well versed in proper use of e-cigarettes for obtaining efficient nicotine yield. Nonetheless, there were still some differences between these products and the sham condition. In sum, this study provides additional suggestive evidence that e-cigarette products may carry some abuse liability, but not at levels as high as combustible tobacco cigarettes.

Clinical Trials

The search revealed two clinical trials in which smokers were provided products to use at their own leisure. This section describes secondary outcomes, which involved ratings of e-cigarette and other comparison products based on recall of use experiences.

In a crossover trial, 38 current smokers (age 18 and older) used e-cigarettes or nicotine oral inhalers each for 3 days, in random order, with a washout period in between (Steinberg et al., 2014). The researchers provided the participants with three e-cigarettes (disposable, regular-flavor blu e-cigarettes with 20–24 mg/ml nicotine) and nicotine inhalers (plastic, pen-shaped containers with cartridges containing 10 mg nicotine and that deliver up to 2 mg nicotine each; Pfizer). Participants were instructed on how to use each device. As recommended by the blu instruction manual, the researchers instructed the participants to puff the device as they would their usual combustible tobacco cigarettes; participants were also instructed to use a new device each day. As described in the package insert for the inhalers, participants were instructed to inhale deeply into back of throat or puff in short breaths, trying to use 80 inhalations over 20 minutes. Participants were instructed to use the first product assigned as they wished for a 3-day period, which provided sufficient time for participants to learn how to use the devices. After the first product-use period, subjects participated in a post-use visit during which researchers collected product ratings. This was followed by a 3-day washout period, during which participants were instructed to smoke their usual combustible tobacco cigarettes as they wished before using the next product. To gain insight into craving and satisfaction during the product use periods, subjects were instructed to use the e-cigarettes and nicotine inhalers as combustible tobacco cigarette substitutes, but were told that cigarette smoking was permissible if absolutely necessary. The researchers collected retrospective ratings at three time points: baseline, after the 3-day e-cigarette use period, and after the 3-day inhaler use period. The e-cigarette had a higher total satisfaction score (13.9 versus 6.8 [$p < 0.001$], range for responses = 3–21) and higher reward score (15.8 versus 8.7 [$p < 0.001$], range for responses = 5–35) than the inhaler. Ratings of combustible tobacco cigarettes and e-cigarette did not differ significantly.

In a study, Meier and colleagues (2017) used a double-blind randomized crossover design, smokers (n = 24, 75 percent male; mean age = 48.5 years) smoked as usual for 1 week, followed by 2 counterbalanced weeks of ad lib use of first-generation e-cigarettes (blu) with up to seven prefilled cartridges containing either 16 mg or 0 mg nicotine (regular tobacco flavor or menthol flavor available only). Participants were instructed "this e-cig may or may not contain nicotine; we ask that you try it at least once, but use it however you like; smoke regular cigarettes as you wish." At the end of each visit, participants reported no differences between the active and placebo e-cigarettes in satisfaction (nicotine mean [SD] = 3.49 [0.3] versus placebo mean [SD] = 3.18 [0.3]) or rewarding effects (mean [SD] = 2.38 [0.2] versus placebo mean [SD] = 2.36 [0.2]).

Collectively these findings provide little additional weight to conclusions given the uncontrolled nature of e-cigarette exposure and use of early-generation products.

CONCLUSIONS

*Conclusion 8-1. There is **substantial evidence** that e-cigarette use results in symptoms of dependence on e-cigarettes.*

Finding: There are several supportive findings from good-quality observational studies with very few or no credible opposing findings that (1) dependence symptoms are of appreciable prevalence or severity or higher in epidemiological studies of users; and (2) greater frequency or chronicity of use is associated with greater likelihood or severity of dependence symptoms. These are supported by well-designed abuse liability studies that e-cigarette use increases abuse liability, with less credible studies also providing supportive evidence. A firm conclusion can be made, but minor limitations, including chance, bias, and confounding factors, cannot be ruled out with reasonable confidence.

*Conclusion 8-2. There is **moderate evidence** that risk and severity of dependence are lower for e-cigarettes than combustible tobacco cigarettes.*

Finding: There are several supportive findings from fair-quality studies with very few or no credible opposing findings. A general conclusion can be made, but limitations, including chance, bias, and confounding factors, cannot be ruled out with reasonable confidence.

*Conclusion 8-3. There is **moderate evidence** that variability in e-cigarette product characteristics (nicotine concentration, flavoring, device type, and brand) is an important determinant of risk and severity of e-cigarette dependence.*

Finding: Some findings support that nicotine concentration, flavoring, device generation, and brand are associated with outcomes indicative of level of dependence risk, with very few or no credible opposing findings. A general conclusion can be made, but limitations, including chance, bias, and confounding factors, cannot be ruled out with reasonable confidence.

REFERENCES

ADAMHA (Alcohol, Drug Abuse, and Mental Health Administration). 1989. *Testing for abuse liability of drugs in humans*. https://archives.drugabuse.gov/sites/default/files/monograph92.pdf (accessed October 9, 2017).

APA (American Psychiatric Association). 2013. *Diagnostic and statistical manual of mental disorders*, 5th edition. Washington, DC: American Psychiatric Association.

Audrain-McGovern, J., A. A. Strasser, and E. P. Wileyto. 2016. The impact of flavoring on the rewarding and reinforcing value of e-cigarettes with nicotine among young adult smokers. *Drug and Alcohol Dependence* 166:263–267.

Baldassarri, S. R., A. T. Hillmer, J. M. Anderson, P. Jatlow, N. Nabulsi, D. Labaree, K. P. Cosgrove, S. S. O'Malley, T. Eissenberg, S. Krishnan-Sarin, and I. Esterlis. 2017. Use of electronic cigarettes leads to significant beta2-nicotinic acetylcholine receptor occupancy: Evidence from a PET imaging study. *Nicotine & Tobacco Research* 20(4):425–433.

Benowitz, N. L. 2008. Neurobiology of nicotine addiction: Implications for smoking cessation treatment. *American Journal of Medicine* 121(4 Supplement 1):S3–S10.

Breland, A., E. Soule, A. Lopez, C. Ramoa, A. El-Hellani, and T. Eissenberg. 2017. Electronic cigarettes: What are they and what do they do? *Annals of the New York Academy of Sciences* 1394(1):5–30.

Caggiula, A. R., E. C. Donny, M. I. Palmatier, X. Liu, N. Chaudhri, and A. F. Sved. 2009. The role of nicotine in smoking: A dual-reinforcement model. *Nebraska Symposium on Motivation* 55:91–109.

Carter, L. P., M. L. Stitzer, J. E. Henningfield, R. J. O'Connor, K. M. Cummings, and D. K. Hatsukami. 2009. Abuse liability assessment of tobacco products including potential reduced exposure products (PREPs). *Cancer Epidemiology, Biomarkers and Prevention* 18(12):3241–3262.

CDC (Centers for Disease Control and Prevention). 2016. Quickstats: Cigarette smoking status among current adult e-cigarette users, age group—National Health Interview Survey, United States, 2015. *Morbidity and Mortality Weekly Report* 65(42):1177.

Chou, S. P., R. B. Goldstein, S. M. Smith, B. Huang, W. J. Ruan, H. Zhang, J. Jung, T. D. Saha, R. P. Pickering, and B. F. Grant. 2016. The epidemiology of DSM–5 nicotine use disorder: Results from the National Epidemiologic Survey on Alcohol and Related Conditions—III. *Journal of Clinical Psychiatry* 77(10):1404–1412.

Dawkins, L., and O. Corcoran. 2014. Acute electronic cigarette use: Nicotine delivery and subjective effects in regular users. *Psychopharmacology (Berl)* 231(2):401–407.

Dawkins, L., J. Turner, A. Roberts, and K. Soar. 2013. "Vaping" profiles and preferences: An online survey of electronic cigarette users. *Addiction* 108(6):1115–1125.

Dawkins, L. E., C. F. Kimber, M. Doig, C. Feyerabend, and O. Corcoran. 2016. Self-titration by experienced e-cigarette users: Blood nicotine delivery and subjective effects. *Psychopharmacology (Berl)* 233(15–16):2933–2941.

DiFranza, J. R., J. A. Savageau, K. Fletcher, J. K. Ockene, N. A. Rigotti, A. D. McNeill, M. Coleman, and C. Wood. 2002. Measuring the loss of autonomy over nicotine use in adolescents: The DANDY (Development and Assessment of Nicotine Dependence in Youths) study. *Archives of Pediatrics & Adolescent Medicine* 156(4):397–403.

Domino, E. F., L. Ni, J. S. Domino, W. Yang, C. Evans, S. Guthrie, H. Wang, R. A. Koeppe, and J. K. Zubieta. 2013. Denicotinized versus average nicotine tobacco cigarette smoking differentially releases striatal dopamine. *Nicotine & Tobacco Research* 15(1):11–21.

Donny, E. C., E. Houtsmuller, and M. L. Stitzer. 2007. Smoking in the absence of nicotine: Behavioral, subjective and physiological effects over 11 days. *Addiction* 102(2):324–334.

Donny, E. C., R. L. Denlinger, J. W. Tidey, J. S. Koopmeiners, N. L. Benowitz, R. G. Vandrey, M. al'Absi, S. G. Carmella, P. M. Cinciripini, S. S. Dermody, D. J. Drobes, S. S. Hecht, J. Jensen, T. Lane, C. T. Le, F. J. McClernon, I. D. Montoya, S. E. Murphy, J. D. Robinson, M. L. Stitzer, A. A. Strasser, H. Tindle, and D. K. Hatsukami. 2015. Randomized trial of reduced-nicotine standards for cigarettes. *New England Journal of Medicine* 373(14): 1340–1349.

Etter, J. F. 2015. Explaining the effects of electronic cigarettes on craving for tobacco in recent quitters. *Drug and Alcohol Dependence* 148:102–108.

Etter, J. F. 2016. Throat hit in users of the electronic cigarette: An exploratory study. *Psychology of Addictive Behaviors* 30(1):93–100.

Etter, J. F., and C. Bullen. 2014. A longitudinal study of electronic cigarette users. *Addictive Behaviors* 39(2):491–494.

Etter, J. F., and T. Eissenberg. 2015. Dependence levels in users of electronic cigarettes, nicotine gums and tobacco cigarettes. *Drug and Alcohol Dependence* 147:68–75.

Fagerström, K. 2012. Determinants of tobacco use and renaming the FTND to the Fagerström Test for Cigarette Dependence. *Nicotine & Tobacco Research* 14(1):75–78.

Farsalinos, K. E., D. Tsiapras, S. Kyrzopoulos, M. Savvopoulou, and V. Voudris. 2014. Acute effects of using an electronic nicotine-delivery device (electronic cigarette) on myocardial function: Comparison with the effects of regular cigarettes. *BMC Cardiovascular Disorders* 14:78. https://doi.org/10.1186/1471-2261-14-78 (accessed February 5, 2018).

Fiore, M. C., C. R. Jaen, and T. B. Baker. 2008. *Treating tobacco use and dependence: 2008 update, Clinical practice guideline*. Rockville, MD: U.S. Department of Health and Human Services, Public Health Service. https://bphc.hrsa.gov/buckets/treatingtobacco.pdf (accessed February 5, 2018).

Foulds, J., S. Veldheer, J. Yingst, S. Hrabovsky, S. J. Wilson, T. T. Nichols, and T. Eissenberg. 2015. Development of a questionnaire for assessing dependence on electronic cigarettes among a large sample of ex-smoking e-cigarette users. *Nicotine & Tobacco Research* 17(2):186–192.

Goldenson, N. I., M. G. Kirkpatrick, J. L. Barrington-Trimis, R. D. Pang, J. F. McBeth, M. A. Pentz, J. M. Samet, and A. M. Leventhal. 2016. Effects of sweet flavorings and nicotine on the appeal and sensory properties of e-cigarettes among young adult vapers: Application of a novel methodology. *Drug and Alcohol Dependence* 168:176–180.

Gonzalez-Roz, A., R. Secades Villa, and S. Weidberg. 2017. Evaluating nicotine dependence levels in e-cigarette users. *Adicciones* 29(2):136–138.

Griffiths, R. R., and B. Wolf. 1990. Relative abuse liability of different benzodiazepines in drug abusers. *Journal of Clinical Psychopharmacology* 10(4):237–243.

Heatherton, T. F., L. T. Kozlowski, R. C. Frecker, and K. O. Fagerström. 1991. The Fagerström Test for Nicotine Dependence: A revision of the Fagerström Tolerance Questionnaire. *British Journal of Addiction* 86(9):1119–1127.

Henningfield, J. E., D. K. Hatsukami, M. Zeller, and E. Peters. 2011. Conference on abuse liability and appeal of tobacco products: Conclusions and recommendations. *Drug and Alcohol Dependence* 116(1–3):1–7.

Hobkirk, A. L., T. T. Nichols, J. Foulds, J. M. Yingst, S. Veldheer, S. Hrabovsky, J. Richie, T. Eissenberg, and S. J. Wilson. 2017. Changes in resting state functional brain connectivity and withdrawal symptoms are associated with acute electronic cigarette use. *Brain Research Bulletin*. https://doi.org/10.1016/j.brainresbull.2017.05.010 (accessed February 5, 2018).

Hughes, J. R. 2006. Clinical significance of tobacco withdrawal. *Nicotine & Tobacco Research* 8(2):153–156.

Jamal, A., A. Gentzke, S. Hu, K. A. Cullen, B. J. Apelberg, D. M. Homa, and B. A. King. 2017. Tobacco use among middle and high school students—United States, 2011–2016. *Morbidity and Mortality Weekly Report* 66(23):597–603.

Japuntich, S. J., M. E. Piper, T. R. Schlam, D. M. Bolt, and T. B. Baker. 2009. Do smokers know what we're talking about? The construct validity of nicotine dependence questionnaire measures. *Psychological Assessment* 21(4):595–607.

Johnson, J. M., J. L. Muilenburg, S. L. Rathbun, X. Yu, L. P. Naeher, and J.-S. Wang. 2017. Elevated nicotine dependence scores among electronic cigarette users at an electronic cigarette convention. *Journal of Community Health*. 43:164–174.

Kasza, K. A., B. K. Ambrose, K. P. Conway, N. Borek, K. Taylor, M. L. Goniewicz, K. M. Cummings, E. Sharma, J. L. Pearson, V. R. Green, A. R. Kaufman, M. Bansal-Travers, M. J. Travers, J. Kwan, C. Tworek, Y. C. Cheng, L. Yang, N. Pharris-Ciurej, D. M. van Bemmel, C. L. Backinger, W. M. Compton, and A. J. Hyland. 2017. Tobacco-product use by adults and youths in the United States in 2013 and 2014. *New England Journal of Medicine* 376(4):342–353.

Kollins, S. H. 2003. Comparing the abuse potential of methylphenidate versus other stimulants: A review of available evidence and relevance to the ADHD patient. *Journal of Clinical Psychiatry* 64(Supplement 11):14–18.

Liu, G., E. Wasserman, L. Kong, and J. Foulds. 2017. A comparison of nicotine dependence among exclusive e-cigarette and cigarette users in the PATH study. *Preventive Medicine* 104:86–91.

Markou, A. 2008. Review. Neurobiology of nicotine dependence. *Philosophical Transactions of the Royal Society B: Biological Sciences* 363(1507):3159–3168.

Meier, E., A. E. Wahlquist, B. W. Heckman, K. M. Cummings, B. Froeliger, and M. J. Carpenter. 2017. A pilot randomized crossover trial of electronic cigarette sampling among smokers. *Nicotine & Tobacco Research* 19(2):176–182.

Nichols, T. T., J. Foulds, J. M. Yingst, S. Veldheer, S. Hrabovsky, J. Richie, T. Eissenberg, and S. J. Wilson. 2016. Cue-reactivity in experienced electronic cigarette users: Novel stimulus videos and a pilot FMRI study. *Brain Research Bulletin* 123:23–32.

Perkins, K. A., J. L. Karelitz, and V. C. Michael. 2015. Reinforcement enhancing effects of acute nicotine via electronic cigarettes. *Drug and Alcohol Dependence* 153:104–108.

Piper, M. E., T. M. Piasecki, E. B. Federman, D. M. Bolt, S. S. Smith, M. C. Fiore, and T. B. Baker. 2004. A multiple motives approach to tobacco dependence: The Wisconsin Inventory of Smoking Dependence Motives (WISDM-68). *Journal of Consulting and Clinical Psychology* 72(2):139–154.

Quester, S., and N. Romanczuk-Seiferth. 2015. Brain imaging in gambling disorder. *Current Addiction Reports* 2(3):220–229.

Reyes–Guzman, C. M., R. M. Pfeiffer, J. Lubin, N. D. Freedman, S. D. Cleary, P. H. Levine, and N. E. Caporaso. 2017. Determinants of light and intermittent smoking in the United States: Results from three pooled national health surveys. *Cancer Epidemiology, Biomarkers & Prevention* 26(2):228-239.

Rosbrook, K., and B. G. Green. 2016. Sensory effects of menthol and nicotine in an e-cigarette. *Nicotine & Tobacco Research* 18(7):1588–1595.

Rose, J. E. 2006. Nicotine and nonnicotine factors in cigarette addiction. *Psychopharmacology* 184(3):274–285.

Rostron, B. L., M. J. Schroeder, and B. K. Ambrose. 2016. Dependence symptoms and cessation intentions among US adult daily cigarette, cigar, and e-cigarette users, 2012–2013. *BMC Public Health* 16(1):814.

Schoenborn, C. A., and R. M. Gindi. 2015. Electronic cigarette use among adults: United States, 2014. *NCHS Data Brief* (217):1–8.

Shiffman, S., A. J. Waters, and M. Hickcox. 2004. The Nicotine Dependence Syndrome Scale: A multidimensional measure of nicotine dependence. *Nicotine & Tobacco Research* 6(2):327–348.

Shihadeh, A., and T. Eissenberg. 2015. Electronic cigarette effectiveness and abuse liability: Predicting and regulating nicotine flux. *Nicotine & Tobacco Research* 17(2):158–162.

Soneji, S., J. L. Barrington-Trimis, T. A. Wills, A. M. Leventhal, J. B. Unger, L. A. Gibson, J. Yang, B. A. Primack, J. A. Andrews, R. A. Miech, T. R. Spindle, D. M. Dick, T. Eissenberg, R. C. Hornik, R. Dang, and J. D. Sargent. 2017. Association between initial use of e-cigarettes and subsequent cigarette smoking among adolescents and young adults: A systematic review and meta-analysis. *JAMA Pediatrics* 171(8):788–797.

St.Helen, G., D. A. Dempsey, C. M. Havel, P. Jacob, 3rd, and N. L. Benowitz. 2017. Impact of e-liquid flavors on nicotine intake and pharmacology of e-cigarettes. *Drug and Alcohol Dependence* 178:391–398.

Steinberg, M. B., M. H. Zimmermann, C. D. Delnevo, M. J. Lewis, P. Shukla, E. J. Coups, and J. Foulds. 2014. E-cigarette versus nicotine inhaler: Comparing the perceptions and experiences of inhaled nicotine devices. *Journal of General Internal Medicine* 29(11):1444–1450.

Stiles, M. F., L. R. Campbell, D. W. Graff, B. A. Jones, R. V. Fant, and J. E. Henningfield. 2017. Pharmacodynamic and pharmacokinetic assessment of electronic cigarettes, combustible cigarettes, and nicotine gum: Implications for abuse liability. *Psychopharmacology (Berl)* 234(17):2643–2655.

Strasser, A. A., V. Souprountchouk, A. Kaufmann, S. Blazekovic, F. Leone, N. L. Benowitz, and R. A. Schnoll. 2016. Nicotine replacement, topography, and smoking phenotypes of e-cigarettes. *Tobacco Regulatory Science* 2(4):352–362.

Strong, D. R., J. Pearson, S. Ehlke, T. Kirchner, D. Abrams, K. Taylor, W. M. Compton, K. P. Conway, E. Lambert, V. R. Green, L. C. Hull, S. E. Evans, K. M. Cummings, M. Goniewicz, A. Hyland, and R. Niaura. 2017. Indicators of dependence for different types of tobacco product users: Descriptive findings from Wave 1 (2013–2014) of the Population Assessment of Tobacco and Health (PATH) study. *Drug and Alcohol Dependence* 178:257–266.

Vansickel, A. R., and T. Eissenberg. 2013. Electronic cigarettes: Effective nicotine delivery after acute administration. *Nicotine & Tobacco Research* 15(1):267–270.

Vansickel, A. R., C. O. Cobb, M. F. Weaver, and T. E. Eissenberg. 2010. A clinical laboratory model for evaluating the acute effects of electronic "cigarettes:" Nicotine delivery profile and cardiovascular and subjective effects. *Cancer Epidemiology, Biomarkers & Prevention* 19(8):1945–1953.

Vansickel, A. R., M. F. Weaver, and T. Eissenberg. 2012. Clinical laboratory assessment of the abuse liability of an electronic cigarette. *Addiction* 107(8):1493–1500.

Volkow, N. D., G. F. Koob, and A. T. McLellan. 2016. Neurobiologic advances from the brain disease model of addiction. *New England Journal of Medicine* 374(4):363–371.

Wagner, F. A., and J. C. Anthony. 2002. From first drug use to drug dependence; developmental periods of risk for dependence upon marijuana, cocaine, and alcohol. *Neuropsychopharmacology* 26(4):479–488.

Yingst, J. M., S. Veldheer, S. Hrabovsky, T. T. Nichols, S. J. Wilson, and J. Foulds. 2015. Factors associated with electronic cigarette users' device preferences and transition from first generation to advanced generation devices. *Nicotine & Tobacco Research* 17(10): 1242–1246.

9

Cardiovascular Disease

Active smoking of combustible tobacco cigarettes and exposure to secondhand tobacco smoke are established causes of clinical cardiovascular disease. Prior Surgeon General reports concluded that the evidence is sufficient to infer that active combustible tobacco cigarette smoking causes coronary heart disease, stroke, atherosclerotic peripheral artery disease, and aortic aneurysm and early abdominal aortic atherosclerosis, and that for secondhand tobacco smoke, the evidence is sufficient to infer that it causes coronary heart disease and stroke (HHS, 2014). Evidence on the cardiovascular effects of active smoking and cardiovascular disease is derived from multiple epidemiological and experimental studies, from studies showing the relatively short-term benefits on the cardiovascular system of quitting smoking, and from the reduction in cardiovascular hospitalizations following the implementation of smoke-free legislation in multiple countries and communities around the world.

When evaluating the potential cardiovascular effects of e-cigarette use, it is important to consider what is known about the dose–response or the exposure–response relationship between exposure to airborne fine particulate matter and cardiovascular disease (Pope et al., 2009). Data combined from multiple studies to estimate adjusted relative risks of cardiovascular mortality plotted against the estimated average daily dose of fine particulate matter from combustible tobacco cigarette smoke, secondhand tobacco smoke, and ambient air pollution showed that the exposure–response relationship between fine particulate matter and cardiovascular disease mortality is relatively steep at low levels of exposure and it plateaus at higher levels. Because the particle characteristics and composition of e-cigarettes differ from those emitted by combustible tobacco cigarettes (see Chapter 3), it is not possible to extrapolate at this time whether the ultrafine particles and liquid particles emitted by e-cigarettes are toxic to the cardiovascular system. The possibility that they could be toxic, however, makes research in this area very important.

In addition to the particles, some toxicants in combustible tobacco cigarette smoke have been specifically related to cardiovascular disease risk, in particular metals, such as lead, nickel, and cadmium (Cosselman et al., 2015; Nigra et al., 2016). Because increasing evidence supports that e-cigarettes, particularly the heating coil, are a source of metals (see Chapter 5), the cardiotoxicity of e-cigarettes that use metallic coils to heat the e-liquid should be evaluated. Nicotine, moreover, as it has been reviewed in Chapter 4, stimulates the sympathetic nervous system, which results in short-term increases in heart rate, blood pressure, and myocardial contractility (see Figure 9-1). These nicotine mechanisms have been involved in the short-term effects of tobacco as a trigger for myocardial ischemia and myocardial infarction (HHS, 2014), although currently there is no consensus about the health effects of nicotine. While some investigators

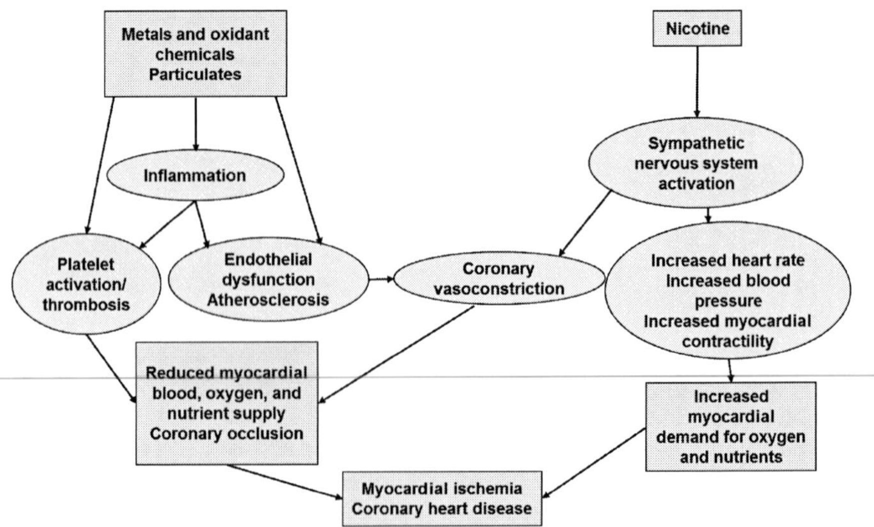

FIGURE 9-1 Conceptual framework of plausible pathways, including mechanisms and intermediate outcomes, by which exposure to e-cigarettes influences cardiovascular disease.
SOURCE: Adapted from HHS, 2014.

have minimized potential effects on cardiovascular disease (Benowitz and Fraiman, 2017), others see greater risk (Bhatnagar, 2016). Possible mechanistic pathways for particulates, metals, and other toxic chemicals, which are also found in e-cigarette aerosols and could thus be by which exposure to e-cigarettes influences cardiovascular disease related to atherosclerosis and coronary heart disease, are summarized in Figure 9-1. This figure is inspired from the well-established evidence of the toxicity of combustible tobacco products on the cardiovascular system, as summarized in the Surgeon General's report (HHS, 2014). A major difference among the potentially cardiotoxic substances that are found in combustible tobacco cigarettes, but not in e-cigarettes, is the lack of combustion chemicals such as polycyclic aromatic hydrocarbons and carbon monoxide (see Chapter 5). The possibility that e-cigarettes may increase the risk of cardiovascular disease must be evaluated carefully given the high burden of cardiovascular disease worldwide and the importance of the burden of disease in the estimation of attributable risk.

CHARACTERIZATION OF DISEASE ENDPOINTS AND INTERMEDIATE OUTCOMES

Relatively few studies have investigated the cardiovascular effects of e-cigarette products. In particular, there are no epidemiological studies evaluating clinical outcomes such as coronary heart disease, stroke, or atherosclerotic peripheral artery disease, or established subclinical outcomes of underlying atherosclerosis such as carotid intima-media thickness or coronary artery calcification. Clinical outcomes such as coronary heart disease (including myocardial infarction and sudden cardiac death), stroke, and peripheral artery disease have been the cornerstone of prospective epidemiological studies evaluating the vascular effects of combustible tobacco cigarettes. Subclinical measures of atherosclerosis, such as carotid intima-media thickness or coronary artery calcification, are also considered excellent measures of cardiovascular risk that can inform on relevant mechanistic pathways (see Figure 9-1). Importantly, these can be measured in cross-sectional designs, allowing for some early assessment as compared with the long-term follow-up needed for clinical cardiovascular outcomes. None of the studies on e-cigarettes and cardiovascular disease conducted so far and summarized below, however, have measured either clinical cardiovascular outcomes or subclinical atherosclerotic outcomes. This lack of data on e-cigarettes and clinical and subclinical atherosclerotic outcomes represents a major research need.

*Conclusion 9-1. There is **no available evidence** whether or not e-cigarette use is associated with clinical cardiovascular outcomes (coro-*

nary heart disease, stroke, and peripheral artery disease) and subclinical atherosclerosis (carotid intima-media thickness and coronary artery calcification).

The evidence available on the possible cardiovascular effects of e-cigarettes can be classified as studies conducted in vitro, evaluating the cytotoxicity of e-cigarette aerosols and other alterations in myocardial cells and human vascular cells; studies conducted in vivo, evaluating relevant mechanistic pathways for cardiovascular toxicity in mice; and clinical experiments, generally crossover experiments that have assessed short-term cardiovascular effects, such as changes in heart rate, blood pressure, and arterial stiffness, of e-cigarettes as compared with combustible tobacco cigarettes and to not smoking. A few studies have evaluated the associations between e-cigarette use and heart rate, heart rate variability, blood pressure levels, and markers of oxidative stress over longer periods, including a cohort study of patients with hypertension who were using e-cigarettes (Polosa et al., 2016), a randomized clinical trial evaluating the effect of switching from smoking to e-cigarette use analyzed also as a cohort study (Farsalinos et al., 2016), and a cross-sectional study comparing heart rate variability and oxidative stress measures in e-cigarette users versus non-users (Moheimani et al., 2017).

Heart rate, controlled by the autonomic nervous system, is a powerful measure of cardiovascular function (Koskela et al., 2013; Poirier, 2014). Slower average resting heart rate is related to higher cardiovascular health and longer life span. Endurance physical exercise can reduce resting heart rate and promote cardiovascular health. The increase in cardiovascular risk associated with high resting heart rate maybe due to elevated blood pressure or sympathetic overactivity (Koskela et al., 2013). Elevated brachial blood pressure is one of the best established contributors to clinical cardiovascular disease and mortality, including myocardial infarction, stroke, and renal failure, when not detected early and treated appropriately (James et al., 2014). Hypertension diagnosis, treatment, and control are critical for cardiovascular disease prevention and control. Hypertension can be defined when either systolic or diastolic blood pressure (SBP or DBP) is elevated. While there are blood pressure cutoffs that are used clinically, the increase in cardiovascular risk is continuous along blood pressure levels. The short-term effects of combustible tobacco cigarettes on both heart rate and blood pressure levels are well established, resulting in short-term elevations that could be related to the effects of nicotine. Long term, however, the effect of combustible tobacco cigarettes on both heart rate and brachial blood pressure levels are less clear, although chronic smoking has been associated with elevated central systolic blood pressure in smokers (Mahmud and Feely, 2003). The short-term effects of smoking in heart rate and brachial blood pressure could also play a role in triggering acute events. Arterial elasticity is essential for blood flow, and the hardening or stiffening of the arteries plays an important role in the development of cardiovascular disease. Arterial stiffness, which can be also defined as arteriosclerosis, or the hardening of the artery wall, can be assessed non-invasively measuring the pulse wave velocity, which measures the speed of the blood pressure wave along the arterial system. Pulse wave velocity can be measured at the carotid, aortic, or brachial levels and it is a strong predictor of clinical cardiovascular events (Mattace-Raso et al., 2006; Willum Hansen et al., 2006). Combustible tobacco cigarette smoking has been associated with arterial stiffness both in short-term experiments and in studies evaluating chronic effects (Levenson et al., 1987; Mahmud and Feely, 2003). In healthy individuals without established cardiovascular disease or major cardiovascular risk factors, endothelial function is also related to increased arterial stiffness. Because endothelial function is an early marker of atherosclerosis (narrowing of the arteries because of the presence of plaque) and clinical cardiovascular disease characterized by a reduced bioavailability of endothelium-derived nitric oxide (NO), it shows the close interrelatedness between these well-established markers of cardiovascular disease (McEniery et al., 2006).

In the sections below, the committee reviews the clinical experiments evaluating the short-term cardiovascular effects of e-cigarettes as well as the few studies that have evaluated the effects of e-cigarettes on the cardiovascular system over longer periods of time or in a cross-sectional setting. The primary focus of this chapter is understanding the cardiovascular effects of e-cigarettes compared with no use, although we also report on findings compared with combustible tobacco cigarettes when those are available in the studies evaluated. A more detailed comparison of the cardiovascular effects of e-cigarettes versus combustible tobacco cigarettes is found in Chapter 18 on harm reduction. In the absence of clinical or subclinical studies on the long-term cardiovascular effects of e-cigarettes, evaluating the potential harm reduction of e-cigarettes is preliminary.

EVIDENCE FROM HUMAN STUDIES OF CARDIOVASCULAR EFFECTS

A total of 13 clinical intervention studies published between 2010 and 2017 have evaluated acute cardiovascular effects of e-cigarette use, such as changes in blood pressure levels, heart rate, arterial stiffness and endothelial function, cardiac geometry and function, and oxidative stress measured in minutes to hours following the intervention (see Table 9-1). Among them, 11 studies were crossover studies in which all participants

TABLE 9-1 Clinical Studies of Short-Term Effects of E-Cigarette Use on Cardiovascular Endpoints

Reference	Study Design	Population	Mean Age % Men % C-Smoker % F-Smoker % Naïve E-Cigarette	E-Cigarette Device Characteristics and E-Liquid
St.Helen et al., 2017	Not blinded, 3-arm randomized crossover trial over 3 consecutive days (in-patient)	Healthy sole and dual e-cigarette user (≤5 cigarettes per day) from colleges campuses in San Francisco, CA	32.3 years 79% 14.3% 71.4% 0%	KangerTech Mini ProTank 3 clearomizer (1.5 Ω) connected to a KangerTech 3.7-V, 1,000-mAh battery; 3 flavors: Bulk e-liquid strawberry (pH 8.29) Bulk e-liquid tobacco (pH 9.10) Own flavor (mean pH 6.80) with 50/50 PG/glycerol and 18 mg/ml nicotine (for strawberry and tobacco)
Spindle et al., 2017	Not blinded, 2-arm ordered crossover trial with a minimum of 48-hour washout period	Healthy sole and dual e-cigarette users (≤5 combustible tobacco cigarettes per day) from Richmond, VA, using e-cigarettes for at least 3 months	29.6 years 76% 7% NR 0%	Own e-cigarette device and e-liquid (≥12 mg/ml nicotine)

Intervention Pattern and Cotinine Levels	Comparison Groups	n[a]	Study Endpoints	Results
Ad libitum (ad lib) acclimatization from 4 to 10 pm, abstinent overnight, 15 puffs/session (1 every 30 seconds) followed by 4 hours of abstinence, and then 90 minutes ad lib. Mean max nicotine concentration (SEM) was 12.1 (2.0), 9.5 (1.2) and 6.2 (1.0) ng/ml for strawberry, tobacco, and own flavor, respectively.	Before and at 5, 10, 15, 20, and 30 minutes after the final puff of: Strawberry Tobacco Own flavor	14	HR (bpm)	Mean max change (SEM) in HR after 15 puffs versus baseline was: 17.2 (2.5) (strawberry), 12.3 (2.3) (tobacco), 9.4 (2.4) (own flavor). Mean maximum increase (95% CI) was 4.6 (0.8, 8.5) bpm higher for strawberry e-liquid than for tobacco e-liquid. Mean (SEM) of HR area under the curve (AUC) after 15 puffs was 245 (37) (strawberry), 210 (45) (tobacco), 169 (53) (own flavor). Mean difference (95% CI) in HR AUC: 34 (–43, 111) comparing strawberry to tobacco. No difference in HR by pH of the e-liquid, mean (SEM) 183 (85) versus 154 (69) for usual acidic and usual basic pH ($p = 0.85$). HR not reported for the ad lib session.
10 puffs, 30-second interpuff interval, and 90-minute ad lib bout. Plasma nicotine increased up to 4.6 ng/ml during ad lib.	Before and continually every 20 seconds for 2.5 hours comparing same device and e-liquid with or without a mouthpiece	29	HR (bpm)	Mean (SEM) HR increased to 73.3 (1.3) bpm after the directed bout and to 73.9 (1.5), 73.6 (1.6), and 74.4 (1.7) at 30, 60, and 90 minutes, respectively, after the onset of the ad lib but compared with baseline of 66.3 (1.3) bpm.

continued

TABLE 9-1 Continued

Reference	Study Design	Population	Mean Age % Men % C-Smoker % F-Smoker % Naïve E-Cigarette	E-Cigarette Device Characteristics and E-Liquid
St.Helen et al., 2016	1-arm trial	Healthy sole and dual e-cigarette users (≤5 cigarettes per day)	38.4 years 54% 23% NR 0%	Usual brand of device and e-liquid
Carnevale et al., 2016	Single blinded 2-arm ordered crossover trial with 1-week washout	Healthy smoking and never smoking participants from Rome, Italy (recruitment dates NR)	28.0 years 47.5% 50% 0% NR	NR leading brand charged; 16-mg nicotine cartridge (~250 puffs)

Intervention Pattern and Cotinine Levels	Comparison Groups	n[a]	Study Endpoints	Results
15 puffs/session, 30-second interpuff interval, followed by 4 hours of abstinence, and then 90 minutes ad lib. Mean plasma nicotine after 15 puffs was 8.4 ng/ml.	Before and 5, 10, 15, 20, and 30 minutes after the final puff	13	HR (bpm)	Compared with baseline HR increased a mean of 8.0 ($p < 0.001$) and 5.2 ($p = 0.04$) bpm after 5 and 10 minutes, respectively, and was not significantly different after 15 minutes.
1 cigarette, 9 puffs (equivalent to 0.6 mg of nicotine). Cotinine NR.	Just before and 30 minutes after - 1 combustible tobacco cigarette - 9 e-cigarette puffs	40	Serum sNOX2-dp (pg/ml), 8-*iso*-PGF2α (pmol/L), Serum NO (µM), Serum vitamin E (µmol/mmol), Brachial artery FMD (%)	Mean (SD) before and after combustible tobacco cigarette/e-cigarette 23.6 (7.8) 38.2 (9.9)/21.6 (6.8) 30.2 (6.2) 135 (56) 203 (81)/133 (54) 187 (62) 35.3 (12.0) 19.5 (9.9)/35.5 (12.5) 25.9 (12.1) 4.6 (1.8) 3.1 (1.9)/3.8 (1.6) 2.8 (1.2) 6.7 (4.3) 3.4 (3.9)/6.7 (3.6) 4.3 (2.2) Stratified results for smokers and non-smokers similar with worse profile for smokers.

continued

TABLE 9-1 Continued

Reference	Study Design	Population	Mean Age % Men % C-Smoker % F-Smoker % Naïve E-Cigarette	E-Cigarette Device Characteristics and E-Liquid
Antoniewicz et al., 2016	Single blinded 2-arm randomized crossover trial with 1-week washout	Healthy sporadic smokers from Stockholm, Sweden, not smoking in the last 7 days (recruitment dates NR)	28 years 64.3% 100% 0% 100%	eGo XL (2nd-generation), 1,100-mAh, 3.7-V, dual-coil CE5 atomizer. E-liquid with nicotine 12 mg/ml, 44.4/49.4% PG/glycerol without flavors (Valeo laboratories GmbH).

Intervention Pattern and Cotinine Levels	Comparison Groups	n[a]	Study Endpoints	Results
10 puffs in 10 minutes in semisupine position. Median (IQR) plasma cotinine after 4 hours was 4.1 (3.5, 4.7) ng/ml.	Before and 1, 4, and 24 hours after: - E-Cigarette - Control (resting)	16	EPC (leukocytes, events) Microvesicles (number) all and by origin (endothelial, platelet or leukocytes) and inflammation markers (HMGB1, P-selectin, CD40, and E-selectin [CD62E]) FeNO (only pre and 24 hours)	EPCs increased after e-cigarette use at 1 hour (p = 0.003) and 4 hours (p = 0.036) and returned to normal at 24 hours. No changes were observed for control periods. Median (IQR) pre, 1, 4, 24 hours e-cigarette/control 1,725 (731, 4,012), 2,600 (1,264, 7,668), 5,102 (2,164, 7,858), 5,731 (1,402, 7,176)/ 1,557 (1,020, 4,997), 3,277 (2,038, 4,987), 3,700 (2,545, 4,494), 2,724 (2,012, 4,858) p = 0.683. NS associations for MVs by origin and inflammation markers except for E-selectin: 8 (2, 17), 14 (8, 43), 28 (17, 65), 20 (15, 40)/ 9 (4, 22), 19 (12, 40), 23 (14, 42), 23 (11, 37) (p = 0.038). Median (IQR) pre, 24 hours e-cigarette/controls 10 (7, 15), 11 (8, 14)/ 10 (7, 15), 11 (8, 14), p = 0.88.

continued

TABLE 9-1 Continued

Reference	Study Design	Population	Mean Age % Men % C-Smoker % F-Smoker % Naïve E-Cigarette	E-Cigarette Device Characteristics and E-Liquid
Fogt et al., 2016	Double blinded, 2-arm ordered crossover trial with 1-week washout	Healthy participants from San Antonio, TX (recruitment dates NR)	23.1 (±2.5) years 50% 0% NR 100%	GreenSmartLiving e-cigarette (details not described). E-liquid with 0 and 18 mg/ml nicotine.
Cooke et al., 2015	Double blinded, randomized, 2-arm crossover trial with 1-week washout	Healthy non-smoking participants from San Antonio, TX (recruitment dates NR)	23 (±1) years 50% 0% NR 100%	GreenSmartLiving e-cigarette (details not described). E-liquid with 0 and 18 mg/ml nicotine.

Intervention Pattern and Cotinine Levels	Comparison Groups	n[a]	Study Endpoints	Results
20 puffs in 10 minutes inhaling as deeply as possible. Urine cotinine 0–10 and 30–100 ng/ml for 18 and 0 mg/ml e-cigarette, respectively.	40 minutes post-exposure: - E-cigarette 0 mg/ml - E-cigarette 18 mg/ml Exercise test starts 55 minutes post–e-cigarette exposure	20	Resting: SBP (mmHg) DBP (mmHg) HR (bpm) RMR (kcal/min) VO_2 (L/min) RQ (energy exp.) Exercise test: SBP_{peak} (mmHg) DBP_{peak} (mmHg) $(VO_2)_{peak}$ (L/min) Power $(W)_{peak}$	Mean (SD) 0/18 mg/ml e-cigarette 115.8 (8.0)/112.1 (6.8), p = 0.04 73.6 (8.3)/76.6 (6.0), p = 0.04 61 (10)/61 (10), p = 0.47 1.19 (0.2)/1.18 (0.2), p = 0.39 0.25 (0.1)/0.25 (0.2), p = 0.5 0.79 (0.01)/0.78 (0.1), p = 0.15 Numbers NR, p = 0.14 74.9 (8.3)/79.4 (7.6), p = 0.02 2.3 (0.7)/2.3 (0.8), p = 0.77 204.8 (57.8)/201.0 (53.8), p = 0.29
20 puffs in 10 minutes. Urine cotinine 0–10 and 30–100 ng/ml for 18 and 0 mg/ml e-cigarette, respectively.	Before and 10–20 (seated), 20–25 (supine), 25–30 (70° head-up tilt), and 30–35 (supine) minutes post-exposure: - E-cigarette 0 mg/ml - E-cigarette 18 mg/ml 1-week washout period	20	Seated: SBP (mmHg) DBP (mmHg) HR (pbm) Supine, tilt, and recovery positions (5 minutes each): SBP (mmHg) DBP (mmHg) Autonomic control: R-R RRISD	Change pre-post 0/18 mg/ml[b] −2/2 (p ≤ 0.03) −2/4 (p = 0.001) −4/1.2 (p ≤ 0.03) Mean BP in each position 0/18 mg/ml[b] 109/117 p = NR, 99/108 (p = 0.03), 110/118 (p = NR) 62/69 (p = 0.02), 61/67 (p = 0.02), 64/71 (p = 0.04). R-R and RRISD decreased with tilt (p ≤ 0.01), but reductions were similar by treatment group.

continued

TABLE 9-1 Continued

Reference	Study Design	Population	Mean Age % Men % C-Smoker % F-Smoker % Naïve E-Cigarette	E-Cigarette Device Characteristics and E-Liquid
Yan and D'Ruiz, 2015	Single blinded, randomized 6-arm crossover trial with 36-hour washout period	Healthy participants smoking in past 12 months from Lincoln, NE, and after a lead-in period for 7 days to get accustomed to using e-cigarette products and abstaining from nicotine for 36 hours	38.7 years 48% 100% 0% 0%	blu e-cigarettes with the following e-liquid formulations: A: classic e-cigarette 2.4% nicotine 75% glycerol B: classic e-cigarette 2.4% nicotine 50/20% glycerol/PG C: menthol e-cigarette, 2.4% nicotine 75% glycerol D: classic e-cigarette 1.6% nicotine 75% glycerol E: classic e-cigarette 1.6% nicotine 50/20% glycerol/PG
Szołtysek-Bołdys et al., 2014	Single blinded, 2-arm ordered cross-over trial with 1-day washout period	Healthy students of University of Silesia, Poland, smoking >5 cigarettes per day for 2 years and used e-cigarettes at least 10 times	23 (±2) years 0% 100% 0% 0%	Ego-3 (clearomizer Crystal 2 with coil, 2.4-Ω voltage battery 900-mAh, 3.4-V) nicotine 24 mg/ml

Intervention Pattern and Cotinine Levels	Comparison Groups	n[a]	Study Endpoints	Results
E-cigarette: 50 5-second puffs at 30-second intervals. Combustible tobacco cigarette: usual puff duration at 30-second intervals. E-cigarette and combustible tobacco cigarette: 1 hour ad lib use. Plasma nicotine (ng/ml) ranged from 2.0 (D) to 3.0 (B) at 5 minutes, from 10.0 (D) to 17.1 (B) at 30 minutes and from 13.7 (D) to 22.4 (B) after 1 extra hour ad lib. For cigarettes, it was 14.4, 7.9, and 29.2 at the same times.	30 minutes pre and 20 minutes following the end of the ad lib period of e-cigarette A, B, C, D, E, and F (Marlboro cigarette)	23	SBP (mmHg) DBP (mmHg) HR (bpm)	Change (SD) post versus pretreatment: A: 1.1 (11.1), $p = 0.63$/ B: 2.8 (11.3), $p = 0.24$/ C: 4.0 (10.0), $p = 0.07$/ D: 5.8 (10.0), $p = 0.02$/ E: 3.8 (10.7), $p = 0.10$/ F: 5.7 (12.4), $p = 0.04$. A: 6.8 (6.7), $p < 0.001$/ B: 6.8 (6.5), $p < 0.001$/ C: 3.2 (7.3), $p = 0.05$/ D: 6.8 (3.8), $p < 0.001$/ E: 4.4 (4.7), $p < 0.001$/ F: 6.8 (7.1), $p < 0.001$. A: 2.3 (5.5), $p = 0.06$/ B: 3.6 (6.0), $p = 0.008$/ C: 4.1 (5.7), $p = 0.002$/ D: 1.9 (7.4), $p = 0.24$/ E: 2.2 (5.9), $p = 0.08$/ F: 4.3 (5.4), $p = 0.001$. Plasma nicotine positively correlated with HR change with a mean increase of 0.16 bpm for 1 ng/ml increase in plasma nicotine (R^2: 0.64).
1-hour sessions: Combustible tobacco cigarette 10–12 puffs (personal brand) E-Cigarette 15 puffs Cotinine NR	10 minutes after: - Combustible tobacco cigarette - E-Cigarette	15	Arterial stiffness: SI (m/s) RI (%) SBP (mmHg) DBP (mmHg) HR (bpm)	Mean (95% CI) before and after cigarette/e-cigarette SI: 6.75 (6.66, 6.85), 6.56 (6.46, 6.65), $p = 0.006$/ 6.73 (6.62, 6.84), 6.75 (6.66, 6.83) p = NS. RI: 54.0 (51.5, 56.7), 49.6 (47.5, 51.8), $p = 0.01$/ 52.0 (49.3, 54.7), 50.8 (48.2, 53.3), p = NS. Both cigarettes and e-cigarette showed a small increase in SBP, DBP, and HR, but it was not significant (only figure) and was hard to see.

continued

TABLE 9-1 Continued

Reference	Study Design	Population	Mean Age % Men % C-Smoker % F-Smoker % Naïve E-Cigarette	E-Cigarette Device Characteristics and E-Liquid
Farsalinos et al., 2014	Not blinded, 2-arm ordered trial with no smoking or nicotine use in the 4 hours before the intervention	Healthy consecutive smokers at Onassis Cardiac Surgery Center, Greece (>14 cigarettes per day for ≥5 years) and e-cigarette users who quit smoking and used 9–12 mg/ml nicotine e-liquid for ≥1 month (mean 6 months). Smokers and e-cigarette users similar at baseline except e-cigarette users formerly smoked 10 combustible tobacco cigarettes per day more when they smoked than current smokers	35 (±5) years 90% 47% 53% NA	eGO-T battery (Nobacco, Greece) with an eGo-C atomizer (2nd generation) 650-mAh rechargeable lithium battery, 3.5 V, manually activated 11 mg/ml nicotine PG >60%, linalool <5%, tobacco essence <5%, methyl vanillin <1%.

Intervention Pattern and Cotinine Levels	Comparison Groups	n[a]	Study Endpoints	Results
Combustible tobacco cigarette smoked ad lib. E-cigarette ad lib for 7 minutes. Cotinine NR. Experiments for e-cigarette and combustible tobacco cigarettes were done in different rooms.	Before and after the experiments - Combustible tobacco cigarette smokers - E-cigarette users	36 40	SBP (mmHg) DBP (mmHg) HR (bpm) Echocardiography E (cm/s) A (cm/s) E/A DT (ms) IVRT (ms) IVRTc (ms) MPI Sm (cm/s) Em (cm/s) Am (cm/s) Em/Am E/Em MPIt GS (%) SRs (s-1) SRe (s-1) SRa (s-1)	Mean (SD) change before after cigarette/e-cigarette Before: 6.6 (5.2) p < 0.001/0.7 (4.6) p = 0.37 After: 4.4 (3.3) p < 0.001/3.0 (3.6) p < 0.001 5.9 (4.7) p < 0.001/0.4 (4.8) p = 0.649 −0.6 (6.1) p = 0.57/1.2 (5.0) p = 0.13 2.9 (5.7) p = 0.007/1.6 (5.6) p = 0.08 −0.10 (0.16) p = 0.001/−0.03 (0.14) p = 0.17 3 (10) p = 0.09/1 (8) p = 0.58 5.6 (9.2) p < 0.001/−1.0 (5.7) p = 0.28 10.4 (10.1) p < 0.001/−1.2 (6.9) p = 0.29 0.03 (0.04) p = 0.002/−0.01 (0.04) p = 0.330 −0.8 (1.1) p = 0.57/0.2 (0.7) p = 0.17 −0.7 (1.4) p < 0.001/0.2 (0.7) p = 0.10 0.1 (0.6) p = 0.80/0.2 (0.8) p = 0.12 −0.08 (0.13) p = 0.004/−0.01 (0.13) p = 0.54 0.29 (0.74) p = 0.02/0.01 (0.47) p = 0.87 0.03 (0.05) p = 0.004/−0.01 (0.04) p = 0.08 0.2 (1.7) p = 0.441/−0.4 (1.2) p = 0.06 −0.2 (0.1) p = 0.15/−0.01 (0.07) p = 0.36 −0.08 (0.12) p < 0.001/0.01 (0.08) p = 0.35 0.03 (0.09) p = 0.11/0.01 (0.08) p = 0.462 *(continues on p. 357)*

continued

TABLE 9-1 Continued

Reference	Study Design	Population	Mean Age % Men % C-Smoker % F-Smoker % Naïve E-Cigarette	E-Cigarette Device Characteristics and E-Liquid
Czogała et al., 2012	Not blinded, 2-arm ordered crossover study with 1-week washout	Healthy daily cigarette smokers (≥5 cigarettes per day) from Sosnowiec, Poland	34.9 (15.3) years 50% 100% 0% 100%	MILD M2001 (1st generation); 14 mg/ml nicotine L&M blu label PM cigarette
Eissenberg, 2010	Not blinded, 4-arm ordered trial with washout period of 48 hours	Healthy smokers from Richmond, VA, with 12 hours of tobacco/nicotine abstinence confirmed with CO <10 ppm	29.8 years 69% 100% 0% 100%	NPRO (NJOY) and Hydro (Crown Seven) 16-mg nicotine cartridge menthol or non-menthol (choice of participant)

Intervention Pattern and Cotinine Levels	Comparison Groups	n[a]	Study Endpoints	Results
				(continued from p. 355) Also run analysis for the effect of combustible tobacco cigarette versus e-cigarette on changes of echocardiographic measures after adjustment for changes in SPB and HR (IVRT, IVRTc, MPI, Em, MPIt, SRe remained significantly associated).
Ad lib e-cigarette use (minimum amount of puffs NR)	- Combustible tobacco cigarette - E-cigarette	42	SBP (mmHg) DBP (mmHg) HR (bpm)	Mean (SD) before and after combustible tobacco cigarette/e-cigarette SBP: 127.1 (15.4) to 131.4 (NS)/122.6 (11.4) to 122.5 (12.6) (NS) DBP: 78.8 (11.0) to 84.1 (10.4) ($p = 0.02$)/76.7 (9.5) to 78.6 (10.8) (NS) HR: 78.5 (12.0) to 90.9 (15.4) ($p < 0.001$)/77.9 (79.4) to 79.4 (13.6) (NS)
Instructed to puff and then puffed ad lib 10 times (30-second intervals) for each product, cycle was repeated 60 minutes later. Plasma nicotine (ng/ml) for own cigarette, NPRO, and Hydro, respectively, were 16.8, 3.5, and 2.5 at 5 minutes and 8.7, 2.6, and 2.2 at 30 minutes	Before and up to 30 minutes after 1st puff: Cigarette (own) Sham puffing NPRO Hydro	16	HR (bpm)	HR increased only after own cigarette ($p < 0.05$). Numbers are not shown in the paper for either combustible tobacco cigarette or e-cigarette.

continued

TABLE 9-1 Continued

Reference	Study Design	Population	Mean Age % Men % C-Smoker % F-Smoker % Naïve E-Cigarette	E-Cigarette Device Characteristics and E-Liquid
Vansickel et al., 2010	Not blinded, randomized 4-arm trial with washout period of ≥48 hours	Healthy smokers from Richmond, VA, with 12 hours of tobacco/nicotine abstinence confirmed with CO < ppm	33.6 years 59% 100% 0% 100%	NPRO (18 mg, NJOY) Hydro (16 mg)

[a] Final sample size used in the analyses. For Antoniewicz and colleagues (2016), 2 participants were excluded from the 16 initially recruited because cotinine levels were compatible with recent smoking. For Yan and D'Ruiz (2015), initially 38 participants were recruited but only 23 participants completed the study.

[b] Numbers approximated because abstracted from a figure.

NOTES: 8-*iso*-PGF2α = 8-*iso*-prostaglandin F2α; EPC = endothelial progenitor cells; FMD = flow-mediated dilation; HR = heart rate; LA = left atrial; LV = left ventricle; MSNA = efferent

received 2 or more interventions (in 6 of them the order of the intervention was randomized) (Antoniewicz et al., 2016; Cooke et al., 2015; Fogt et al., 2016; St.Helen et al., 2017; Vansickel et al., 2010; Yan and D'Ruiz, 2015), and in the other 5, the order was preassigned and the same for everybody (Carnevale et al., 2016; Czogała et al., 2014; Eissenberg, 2010; Spindle et al., 2017; Szołtysek-Bołdys et al., 2014). The remaining studies were a two-arm design to evaluate the short-term effect of smoking a cigarette and of vaping an e-cigarette in smokers and previous users of e-cigarettes, respectively (Farsalinos et al., 2014) and a single-arm before/after trial (St.Helen et al., 2016).

Intervention Pattern and Cotinine Levels	Comparison Groups	n[a]	Study Endpoints	Results
Instructed to puff 10 times with 30-second intervals at 2 separate times during the session (1 hour between them). Plasma nicotine increased for own brand but not for NPRO, Hydro, and sham experiments.	Before and up to 1 hour after: - Combustible tobacco cigarette (own) - Sham puffing - NPRO - Hydro	32	HR (bpm)	HR increased from 66 ppm before the experiment to 80, 75, and 70 ppm 5, 15, and 30 minutes, respectively, after the first experiment and to 74, 73, and 70 ppm after the second experiment with the own-brand cigarette. For NPRO and Hydro, only small changes not statistically significant were observed (from 66 ppm before to a maximum of 69 ppm at 5 minutes after the first experiment and 67 ppm at 5 minutes after the second experiment with NPRO; and even smaller changes with Hydro).

muscle sympathetic nerve activity from the right peroneal nerve; NA = not applicable; nic. = nicotine, NO = nitric oxide; NR = not reported; NS = not significant; Ox = oxidative; PG/VG = propylene glycol/glycerol; RI = reflection index; RMR = resting metabolic rate; R-R = intervals to assess vagal-cardiac control in the time domain; RRISD = R-R interval standard deviations to assess respiratory sinus arrhythmia, SI = stiffness index; sNOX2-dp = soluble NOX2-derived peptide, a marker of nicotinamide adenine dinucleotide phosphate (reduced form) oxidase activation.

The literature search also identified 3 studies evaluating cardiovascular-related outcomes over a longer period than the 13 acute clinical studies (see Table 9-2), including a cross-sectional study of e-cigarette users compared with non-users conducted in Los Angeles, California (n = 34) (Moheimani et al., 2017); a cohort of smokers not intending to quit from Catania, Italy, who were randomized to one of three types of e-cigarette use (0 percent nicotine, 2.4 percent nicotine for 12 weeks, and 2.4 percent nicotine for 6 weeks plus 1.8 percent nicotine for 6 weeks) (n = 183 with complete follow-up) and also analyzed as a cohort study comparing sole e-cigarette users (called quitters in the original publication), dual users (called reducers), and smokers (called failures) according to their continuation of combustible tobacco smoking (n = 145 for participants with continuous e-cigarette/smoking status over time) (Farsalinos et al., 2016); and a cohort of hypertensive patients who were e-cigarette users compared with hypertensive patients who smoked cigarettes (n = 89) also in Catania, Italy (Polosa et al., 2016).

The sample size across the 15 studies ranged from 13 (St.Helen et al., 2016) to 183 (Farsalinos et al., 2016) participants, for a total of 662 participants across the 15 studies (356 in the short-term clinical studies and 306 in the epidemiological studies). Study participants were recruited from Catania (Italy), Khallithea (Greece), Los Angeles (California), Lincoln (Nebraska), Richmond (Virginia), Rome (Italy), San Antonio (Texas), San Francisco (California), Silesia (Poland), Sosnowiec (Poland), and Stockholm (Sweden). In the short-term clinical studies, participants were relatively young (mean age ranged from 23 to 39 years old), required to be healthy (including no hypertension or diabetes risk factors in most studies), and included a balanced number of men and women, except in one study restricted to women (Szołtysek-Bołdys et al., 2014) and another study that included 90 percent men (Farsalinos et al., 2014). Mean age of the participants in the epidemiological studies ranged from 33 to 54 years. In one study, all participants had hypertension at baseline. In a total of seven studies, all participants were current smokers (Antoniewicz et al., 2016; Czogała et al., 2014; Eissenberg, 2010; Farsalinos et al., 2016; Szołtysek-Bołdys et al., 2014; Vansickel et al., 2010; Yan and D'Ruiz, 2015), ranging from sporadic smokers to heavy smokers; five studies included some current smokers; and the remaining were former smokers (Farsalinos et al., 2014; St.Helen et al., 2017) or it was not specified if they were former or never smokers (Polosa et al., 2016; Spindle et al., 2017; St.Helen et al., 2016); one study included half of the participants being current smokers and half never smokers (Carnevale et al., 2016); one study included 65 percent never smokers and 35 percent former smokers; and in two studies the participants were not current smokers, although it is unclear if former smokers were included (Cooke et al., 2015; Fogt et al., 2016). Among the short-term clinical studies, in six studies the participants were e-cigarette–naïve users (Antoniewicz et al., 2016; Cooke et al., 2015; Czogała et al., 2012; Eissenberg, 2010; Fogt et al., 2016; Vansickel et al., 2010); in one study participants were trained to use e-cigarettes during a 7-day period (Yan and D'Ruiz, 2015); in five studies participants were experienced e-cigarette users (Farsalinos et al., 2014; Szołtysek-Bołdys et al., 2014); and one study did not report whether participants were naïve e-cigarette users (Carnevale et al., 2016).

The e-cigarette device used in the experiments included a tank-style device in one study (St.Helen et al., 2017); second-generation devices in three studies (different eGO models) (Antoniewicz et al., 2016; Farsalinos et al., 2014; Szołtysek-Bołdys et al., 2014); cigalikes in six studies (GreenSmartLiving in two studies [Cooke et al., 2015; Fogt et al., 2016]; blu in one study [Yan and D'Ruiz, 2015]; Mild in one study [Czogała et al., 2012]; NJOY NPRO and Hydro in two studies [Eissenberg, 2010; Vansickel et al., 2010]); one leading brand of an unspecified device in one study (Carnevale et al., 2016); and the personal devices of the study participants in two studies (Spindle et al., 2017; St.Helen et al., 2016). Nicotine or cotinine biomarkers were reported in 10 studies and were generally lower than those that would be reached with combustible tobacco cigarettes (Antoniewicz et al., 2016; Cooke et al., 2015; Eissenberg, 2010; Fogt et al., 2016; Yan and D'Ruiz, 2015), except maybe for studies using tank-style devices and the personal e-cigarettes of the participants (Spindle et al., 2017; St.Helen et al., 2016, 2017). Few studies provided details on actual wattage and resistance (Antoniewicz et al., 2016; Farsalinos et al., 2014; St.Helen et al., 2017; Szołtysek-Bołdys et al., 2014) and no studies provided details on the coils. The e-liquid concentration of nicotine ranged from 0 mg/ml (Cooke et al., 2015; Fogt et al., 2016) to 24 mg/ml (Szołtysek-Bołdys et al., 2014), although some studies reported the total amount of nicotine in the cartridge, but not the actual concentration (Carnevale et al., 2016; Eissenberg, 2010). Only one study tested multiple propylene glycol (PG)/glycerol concentrations (Yan and D'Ruiz, 2015), and only two other studies actually reported the concentrations of other constituents beyond nicotine (Antoniewicz et al., 2016; Farsalinos et al., 2014). Regarding flavors, only one study used a vanillin flavor (Farsalinos et al., 2014); two studies mentioned menthol, one allowing the choice of a menthol flavoring (Eissenberg, 2010), and another study specifically tested menthol (Yan and D'Ruiz, 2015); and one study compared strawberry flavor, tobacco flavor, and the personal flavor used by the participant (St.Helen et al., 2017).

The interventions tested were substantially different across the short-term clinical studies. Seven studies compared the short-term effects of one or more e-cigarettes versus combustible tobacco cigarettes (Carnevale et al., 2016; Czogała et al., 2012; Eissenberg, 2010; Farsalinos et al., 2014; Szołtysek-Bołdys et al., 2014; Vansickel et al., 2010; Yan and D'Ruiz, 2015) (one of those also included one arm with sham puffing [Eissenberg et al., 2010]). One study compared e-cigarettes to a resting period in the same conditions as the e-cigarette use period (Antoniewicz et al., 2016). Two studies compared the same e-cigarette with e-liquids with and without nicotine (Cooke et al., 2015; Fogt et al., 2016) and with different flavors. One study compared the same e-cigarette and e-liquid with and without a mouthpiece (Spindle et al., 2017). The washout periods ranged from less than 24 hours (St.Helen et al., 2017) to 1 week in crossover studies (Antoniewicz et al., 2016; Carnevale et al., 2016; Cooke et al., 2015;

TABLE 9-2 Epidemiological Studies on Chronic E-Cigarette Use and Cardiovascular Endpoints

Reference	Study Design	Population	Age Range % Men % C-Smoker % F-Smoker	E-Cigarette Device Characteristics	E-Cigarette Pattern of Use and Cotinine Levels
Moheimani et al., 2017	XS	Los Angeles, CA, recruited in 2015–2016 (source or recruitment methods NR)	21–45 years 59% 0% 35%	NR	Mean = 241 minutes per day Mean = 1.6 years Plasma cotinine range = 2.6–27.3 mg/L

Comparison Groups	n[a]	Study Endpoints	Results	Adjustment[b]
- E-cigarette users - Non-users E-cigarette users asked not to use the e-cigarette the day of the study	16/18 12/18	SBP (mmHg) DBP (mmHg) MAP (mmHg) HR (bpm) HRV: HF (non-user) - LF (non-user) - LF/HF HRV-controlled breathing oxLDL (user) paraxonase-1 (nmol) HDLantiox. index (user) Fibrinogen (mg/dl) CRP (number abnormal)	Mean user/non-user 115.8/109.0 (p = 0.07) 73.5/70.0 (p = 0.27) 87.6/83.0 (p = 0.15) 64.0/63.0 (p = 0.73) 46.5/57.8 (p = 0.04) 52.7/39.9 (p = 0.03) 1.37/0.85 (p = 0.05) NS (no. not shown) 3,801/2,413 (p = 0.01) 649.9/892.8 (p = 0.17) 0.42/0.38 (p = 0.55) 270.9/251.9 (p = 0.24) 3/1 (p = 0.15) Correlations of plasma cotinine with: HF (−0.34, p = 0.04) LF (0.35, p = 0.03) LF/HF (0.36, p = 0.03) oxLDL (0.35, p = 0.05) other biomarkers (NS)	None (e-cigarette users more likely to be men and former smokers)

continued

TABLE 9-2 Continued

Reference	Study Design	Population	Age Range % Men % C-Smoker % F-Smoker	E-Cigarette Device Characteristics	E-Cigarette Pattern of Use and Cotinine Levels
Farsalinos et al., 2016	RCT also analyzed as a CO	Smokers not attempting to quit from Catania, Italy, followed for 52 weeks, recruited in 2010–2011 through a smoking cessation clinic and offered to use e-cigarettes	44.0 years (mean) 63% 100% 0%	"Categoria" e-cigarette model 401, Arbi Group Srl (disposable cartridge and 3.7-V, 90mAh lithium ion battery). E-liquid nicotine: - 2.4% 12 weeks - 2.4% 6 weeks + 1.8% 6 weeks - 0% 12 weeks	NR
Polosa et al., 2016	CO	Regular smokers on treatment for hypertension at an outpatient clinic in Catania, Italy (period of recruitment NR)	53.9 years (mean) 56% 48% (some dual users) 52%	NR	Daily use from 10 to 14 months (83.7% more than 12 months)

Comparison Groups	n[a]	Study Endpoints	Results	Adjustment[b]
RCT arms: - 0% nicotine - 1.8% - 2.4% CO groups: - Smokers - Dual users - Sole users (called failures, reducers, and quitters in the paper)	63/ 66/ 61 93/ 34/ 18	SBP (mmHg) DBP (mmHg) HR (bpm) at baseline and at 8 follow-up visits over 52 weeks	RCT: mean (SD) SBP decreased from 128 (15) at baseline to 123 (14) mmHg at 52 weeks ($p = 0.004$) with no difference by treatment group. CO: adjusted mean change (95% CI) in SBP over time compared with smokers: Dual users: −6.76 (−13.39, −0.13) mmHg e-cigarette users: −14.25 (−23.70, −4.81) mmHg Stratified analysis by baseline BP:[c] Elevated (n = 66): mean (SD) change in SBP (mmHg) over time was 6.0 (12.5) ($p = 0.002$), 10.8 (10.1) ($p < 0.001$), and 16.3 (11.3) ($p = 0.005$) for smokers, dual users, and sole users, respectively. Normal (n = 79): No difference by group. No differences over time were observed for HR or for DBP by RCT treatment and CO group overall or stratified by baseline BP (elevated or normal).	Some analyses adjusted for sex, age, and weight change
- Smokers - Dual users - Single users	46/ 23/ 20	SBP (mmHg) DBP (mmHg) HR (bpm) Measured at baseline, 6 and 12 months % HT control smokers/ e-cigarette users	Median (IQR) 145 (137, 152)/137 (132, 144)/ 134 (130, 142) 87 (85, 90)/83 (80, 92)/81 (74, 84) 78 (72, 85)/77 (70, 83)/80 (75, 86) 145 (136, 150)/130 (121, 140)/ 130 (123, 138) 85 (85, 90)/80 (71, 90)/80 (75, 87) 79 (72, 84)/76 (71, 92)/80 (76, 90) p-value comparing e-cigarette users versus smokers from baseline to 12 months < 0.001 for SBP and DBP and 0.71 for HR 20/37 at 6 months and 22/49 at 12 months	Sex, age, weight, changes in SBP between pre-baseline and baseline <10 mmHg

continued

TABLE 9-2 Continued

NOTES: C-smoker = current smoker; CO = crossover; DBP = diastolic blood pressure; F-smoker = former smoker; HF = high frequency; HR = heart rate; HRV = heart rate variability; HT = hypertension; LF = low frequency; MAP = mean arterial pressure; NR = not reported; NS = not significant; RCT = randomized controlled trial; SBP = systolic blood pressure; XS = cross-sectional.

[a] Final sample size used in the analyses. For Moheimani and colleagues (2017), the sample size was initially larger, but 1 participant among non-users of e-cigarettes was excluded because of active smoking, and 2 and 5 e-cigarette users were excluded because of active smoking or because of e-cigarette use the day of the study, respectively. Also, only 12 e-cigarette users had sufficient bio-specimens available to measure biomarkers. For Farsalinos and colleagues (2016), 300 (100 in each group) were initially recruited for the RCT, but 183 completed the study at 52 weeks (61 percent response rate with no difference by treatment group, so the estimated sample size is 61 participants in each treatment group available for the statistical analysis).

[b] Adjustment for potential confounding through regression modeling, matching, stratification, or other strategy.

[c] Elevated BP defined as SBP/DBP greater than or equal to 130/85 mmHg.

Czogała et al., 2012; Fogt et al., 2016). The two-arm separate comparison groups study (Farsalinos et al., 2014) and the one-arm before/after study (St.Helen et al., 2016) required no smoking or e-cigarette use several hours prior to the interventions.

In the 13 short-term clinical studies, outcomes were measured before and after the interventions. These studies contribute to assessing the short-term effect of using an e-cigarette regardless of the comparison group. In the remaining studies, the outcomes were measured cross-sectionally with the assessment of e-cigarette exposure in one study, and over 1 year in two studies. The following study outcomes were measured:

- heart rate in 14 studies (Cooke et al., 2015; Czogała et al., 2012; Eissenberg, 2010; Farsalinos et al., 2014, 2016; Fogt et al., 2016; Moheimani et al., 2017; Polosa et al., 2016; Spindle et al., 2017; St.Helen et al., 2016, 2017; Szołtysek-Bołdys et al., 2014; Vansickel et al., 2010; Yan and D'Ruiz, 2015);
- blood pressure in 9 studies (Cooke et al., 2015; Czogała et al., 2012; Farsalinos et al., 2014, 2016; Fogt et al., 2016; Moheimani et al., 2017; Polosa et al., 2016; Szołtysek-Bołdys et al., 2014; Yan and D'Ruiz, 2015);
- hypertension control in 1 study (Polosa et al., 2016);
- biomarkers of oxidative stress in 2 studies (Carnevale et al., 2016; Moheimani et al., 2017);
- biomarkers of inflammation in 1 study (Moheimani et al., 2017);

- endothelial function based on brachial artery flow–mediated dilation in 1 study (Carnevale et al., 2016);
- arterial stiffness in 1 study (Szołtysek-Bołdys et al., 2014);
- endothelial progenitor cells and microvesicles in 1 study (Antoniewicz et al., 2016);
- autonomic control and heart rate variability in 2 studies (Cooke et al., 2015; Moheimani et al., 2017); and
- cardiac geometry and function in 1 study (Farsalinos et al., 2014).

The summary of the main results for these outcomes is presented below.

Heart Rate

Among the 11 studies that have evaluated short-term changes in heart rate, 10 studies measured heart rate before and after the intervention and 1 study measured heart rate only at the end of the intervention (Fogt et al., 2016). Five studies found higher heart rate levels after versus before e-cigarette use (Cooke et al., 2015; Spindle et al., 2017; St.Helen et al., 2016, 2017; Yan and D'Ruiz, 2015), all of them published between 2015 and 2017, while five studies published between 2010 and 2014 found no difference in heart rate after versus before e-cigarette use (Czogała et al., 2012; Eissenberg, 2010; Farsalinos et al., 2014; Szołtysek-Bołdys et al., 2014; Vansickel et al., 2010). The study by Fogt and colleagues (2016) also found similar heart rate levels after using an e-cigarette with 0 versus 18 mg/ml nicotine. The studies that found increases in heart rate were characterized by using tank-style devices, own devices, and/or confirmed that nicotine or cotinine biomarkers had increases following e-cigarette use. In those studies, the change in heart rate after versus before e-cigarette use ranged from an increase in 1.2 beats per minute (bpm) in a study of a GreenSmartLiving e-cigarette with nicotine 18 mg/ml (Cooke et al., 2015) to 17.2 bpm in a study of a tank-style e-cigarette device with strawberry flavoring with nicotine 18 mg/ml that closely evaluated the maximum change, which occurred at 5 minutes after completing a 15-puff session (St.Helen et al., 2017). Studies that found no changes generally used first- and second-generation e-cigarette devices and had no or small changes in nicotine-related biomarkers. Studies that compared changes in heart rate levels before and after smoking a combustible tobacco cigarette found marked increases in heart rate, generally larger than those found with e-cigarettes. However, most of the studies comparing e-cigarettes with combustible tobacco cigarettes have been done using first- and second-generation devices that did not markedly increase nicotine or cotinine levels in plasma. In the Yan and D'Ruiz (2015) study comparing a blu e-cigarette to a Marlboro cigarette (plasma nicotine levels ranged from 13.7 ng/ml to 22.5 ng/ml plasma nicotine after 1 hour of ad lib e-cigarette use depending on the e-liquid formulation compared with 29.5 ng/ml after 1 hour of ad lib use of Marlboro cigarettes), the change in heart rate after versus before e-cigarette ranged from a mean (SD) of 1.9 (7.4) bpm ($p = 0.24$) for a blu e-cigarette with classic e-liquid with 1.6 percent nicotine and 75 percent glycerol to 4.1 (5.7) bpm ($p = 0.002$) for a blu e-cigarette with menthol e-liquid, 2.4 percent nicotine and 75 percent glycerol, which compared with a change of 4.3 (5.4) bpm ($p = 0.001$) following a Marlboro cigarette. These results indicate that in some instances the changes in heart rate induced by e-cigarettes are similar to those induced by combustible tobacco cigarettes.

Short-term effects of e-cigarette use on heart rate do not necessarily mean that chronic e-cigarette use increases resting heart rate, which is an established predictor of poor clinical cardiovascular health. In a cross-sectional study of daily e-cigarette users from Los Angeles, resting heart rate was similar among e-cigarette users compared with non-users (Moheimani et al., 2017) (see Table 9-2). An important limitation of this study is the lack of adjustment for sociodemographic characteristics and cardiovascular disease risk factors between e-cigarette users and non-users. Resting heart rate was also similar over a 52-week period comparing e-cigarettes "Categoria model 401" with different levels of nicotine (0 percent, 2.4 percent + 1.8 percent, and 2.4 percent) randomly assigned to smokers in a cessation clinic (Farsalinos et al., 2016), as well as in a group of hypertensives using e-cigarettes as single or dual use compared with smoking.

Synthesis

Recent intervention studies using tank-style devices and devices owned by e-cigarette users and with confirmation of nicotine intake have consistently found increases in heart rate shortly after e-cigarette use. Earlier studies, using first- and second-generation devices, found no changes in heart rate following e-cigarette use. However, those studies were characterized by small or no increase in nicotine or cotinine biomarker levels. The crossover design, including randomization of the intervention order in several studies, is an ideal experimental design to evaluate short-term effects minimizing interindividual sources of variability in heart rate. The effect estimates, although generally smaller than those observed for tobacco cigarettes, get closer in value for some types of e-cigarettes, generally related to higher nicotine intake. It is well known that nicotine increases heart rate, which provides biological plausibility to these findings. For studies evaluating the association between e-cigarette use and heart rate over longer-term periods, the three studies available found no association, although the studies did not adjust for sociodemographic variables and the type of e-cigarettes was not well characterized.

Blood Pressure

A total of six clinical studies measured short-term changes in SBP/DBP following e-cigarette use, five of them including measures before and after the experiments (Cooke et al., 2015; Czogała et al., 2012; Farsalinos et al., 2014; Szołtysek-Bołdys et al., 2014; Yan and D'Ruiz, 2015). All the studies indicated that they had recruited healthy participants without hypertension. Some studies had confirmed that SBP/DBP were less than or equal to 140/90 mmHg or even lower. In a crossover study assessing GreenSmartLiving e-cigarettes (Cooke et al., 2015), the mean (SD) change in SBP before and 10 minutes after the intervention was approximately –2.0 (3.0) and 2.0 (3.0) mmHg for 0 and 18 mg/ml nicotine concentrations, respectively, and the differences between those two groups were significant ($p \leq 0.03$). The corresponding changes for DBP were –2.0 (3.0) and 4.0 (6.0) mmHg ($p = 0.001$). SBP and DBP in that experiment were also higher with nicotine compared with no nicotine during supine, tilt, and recovery experiments in addition to the rest measures. In the cross-over trial using blu e-cigarettes with five different e-liquids (Yan and D'Ruiz, 2015), the increase in mean (SD) SBP measured before and after the intervention (which included an ad lib period) ranged from 1.1 (11.1) mmHg ($p = 0.63$) for Classic Tobacco with 2.4 percent nicotine and 75 percent glycerol to 5.8 (10.0) mmHg ($p = 0.02$) for Classic Tobacco with 1.6 percent nicotine and 75 percent glycerol. The corresponding increase after smoking a Marlboro cigarette was 5.7 (12.4) mmHg ($p \leq 0.04$). The corresponding changes for DBP ranged from 3.2 (7.3) mmHg ($p = 0.05$) for blu with menthol and 2.4 percent nicotine and 75 percent glycerol to 6.8 mmHg for three other types of blu cigarettes with different compositions ($p < 0.001$). The increase in DBP for a Marlboro cigarette was also 6.8 (7.1) mmHg ($p < 0.001$). Consistent with these findings, in the study by Farsalinos and colleagues (2014), DBP increased both after exposure to a cigarette (mean change [SD] = 4.4 [3.3], $p < 0.001$) and to an e-cigarette (3.0 [3.6], $p < 0.001$), while SBP increased after a cigarette (6.6 [5.2], $p < 0.001$) but not after an e-cigarette (0.7 [4.6], $p = 0.37$). In the study that compared blood pressure levels before and 10 minutes after a personal cigarette or an e-cigarette (Ego-3) in female students from Silesia, Poland (Szołtysek-Bołdys et al., 2014), the investigators reported small, statistically insignificant increases in SBP and DBP after both e-cigarettes and cigarettes, but the numbers are not shown. In another study in Poland, a first-generation e-cigarette was not associated with short-term changes in SBP/DBP, while a combustible tobacco cigarette was associated with increases in DBP. In the study that reported blood pressure levels only at the end of the experiments (and thus does not allow assessment of the effect of using the e-cigarette compared with baseline) (Fogt et al., 2016), mean (SD) SBP was lower for the e-cigarette with 18 versus 0 mg/ml, 112.1 (6.8) versus 115.8 (8.0), $p = 0.04$, while mean (SD) DBP was higher at 76.6 (6.0) versus 73.6 (8.3), $p = 0.04$. During the exercise test, peak SBP was similar for both levels of nicotine, while peak DBP was higher for those with nicotine.

Short-term effects of e-cigarette use on SBP/DBP do not necessarily mean that chronic e-cigarette use increases resting blood pressure levels. In a cross-sectional study of daily e-cigarette users from Los Angeles, mean SBP was borderline significantly higher in e-cigarette users versus non-users (115.8 versus 109.0 mmHg, $p = 0.07$), while DBP was similar (Moheimani et al., 2017) (see Table 9-2), although the study did not adjust for sociodemographic characteristics and cardiovascular disease risk factors between e-cigarette users and non-users. In the studies from Catania, Italy, SBP and DBP decreased over time in participants who switched from tobacco cigarettes to e-cigarettes, especially those who achieved sole use (Farsalinos et al., 2016; Polosa et al., 2016). In the group of hypertensives, there was an improvement in hypertension control at 6 months and 12 months (Polosa et al., 2016). The study without hypertensives is limited by

- a relatively large loss of study participants during follow-up;
- lack of detailed reporting for the initial study design based on three treatment groups; and
- the observational design comparing sole and dual e-cigarette user to smokers in the secondary analyses, although the three groups were comparable at baseline by sex, age, pack-years, and blood pressure levels.

The study among hypertensives is limited by

- small sample size;
- unclear description of how many participants with hypertension were available initially and if they were selected using a random sampling strategy;
- lack of details on the e-cigarette devices and the e-liquid used by the participants; and
- the retrospective data collection based on clinical records.

The study matched for age, sex, and lack of fluctuation in SBP comparing a pre-baseline visit occurring 6–13 months prior with the baseline visit. It is unclear how the authors ensured recruitment of participants who have not had changes in their blood pressure levels of more than 10 mmHg for 6–12 months, but studied the change in the following year. It is possible that the study has been done completely retrospectively.

Synthesis

Overall, for SBP, there are some inconsistent findings, with the majority of studies finding weak positive increases or no changes with the use of e-cigarettes, while experiments with combustible tobacco cigarettes found consistent increases. From studies with different levels of nicotine, it seems that lower nicotine concentrations resulted in weaker increases in SBP or even lower SBP levels than no nicotine. For DBP, on the other hand, the studies consistently show short-term increases in DBP following the use of an e-cigarette that delivers nicotine with a magnitude of the effect similar to the increase observed when smoking a cigarette. The crossover design, including randomization of the intervention order in several studies, is an ideal experimental design to evaluate short-term effects minimizing interindividual sources of variability in SBP/DBP. These findings are consistent with other studies in humans supporting short-term effects of e-cigarette use on markers of endothelial function and arterial stiffness (see below). The short-term effect of nicotine from e-cigarettes on SBP and DBP is consistent with findings from other nicotine delivery products including tobacco cigarettes and even nicotine replacement products. Regarding chronic health effects on blood pressure levels, the evidence is very limited as there is only one study comparing e-cigarette use to non-use, and two studies comparing e-cigarette use to smoking, one including patients with hypertension.

Oxidative Stress, Inflammation, Endothelial Function, and Arterial Stiffness (Arteriosclerosis)

Two studies have measured biomarkers of oxidative stress, one evaluating short-term changes in a study of 20 current smokers and 20 never smokers exposed to a cigarette or an e-cigarette in a non-randomized crossover design (all participants exposed first to the cigarette and 1 week later to the e-cigarette) (Carnevale et al., 2016), and the other a cross-sectional study of e-cigarette users compared with non-users from Los Angeles (Moheimani et al., 2017). In the crossover study, the following biomarkers of oxidative stress were measured in serum before and 30 minutes after exposure to a cigarette or an e-cigarette: soluble NOX2-derived peptide (sNOX2-dp), a marker of nicotinamide adenine dinucleotide phosphate (reduced form) oxidase activation, nitric oxide bioavailability, a signaling molecule with a major role in the regulation of vasodilation and endothelial function, and 8-*iso*-prostaglandin F2α (8-*iso*-PGF2α). The study reported the mean (SD) before and after the cigarettes and the e-cigarettes. The mean change in serum before and after cigarette and e-cigarette exposure was 14.6 ($p < 0.001$) and 8.6 ($p < 0.001$) pg/ml for sNOX2-dp, 68 ($p < 0.001$) and 54 ($p < 0.001$) pmol/L for 8-*iso*-PGF2α, −15.8 ($p < 0.001$) and −9.6 ($p < 0.001$) μM for NO bioavailability, and −1.5 ($p < 0.001$) and −1.0 ($p < 0.001$) μmol/mmol for vitamin E, respectively. Although the magnitude of the effect was weaker compared with the changes induced by a combustible tobacco cigarette, these experiments suggest that e-cigarettes can also increase levels of oxidative stress and reduce the levels of antioxidants. A major limitation of this study is the lack of information on the type of e-cigarette device and e-liquid used. Additional research would be needed to confirm these short-term effects and for which types of devices, as well as to evaluate the long-term effects of e-cigarette use on biomarkers of oxidative stress. These findings are consistent with in vitro and in vivo studies that are discussed in more detail in Chapter 7. In summary, several studies in vitro have shown that human vascular endothelial cells show increased reactive oxygen species with e-cigarette extract compared with controls (Anderson et al., 2016). Mice exposed to e-cigarette aerosol for several weeks showed increased levels of oxidative stress, macrophage-mediated inflammation, and inflammatory cytokines including interleukin-6 (Lerner et al., 2015).

In the cross-sectional study from Los Angeles (see Table 9-2), oxidized LDL was higher in e-cigarette users versus non-users, while there were no differences in other biomarkers of oxidative stress or inflammation, although the sample size was small (Moheimani et al., 2017). The same crossover study that measured oxidative stress biomarkers also assessed endothelial function by measuring flow-mediated dilation (FMD) (Carnevale et al., 2016), a marker of vascular reactivity in large arteries that measures the change in arterial diameter following reactive hyperemia. FMD was measured based on ultrasound assessment of basal brachial diameter and endothelial-dependent FMD of the brachial artery following established guidelines. FMD is expressed as a change in post-stimulus diameter evaluated as a percentage of the baseline diameter, with a lower percentage reflecting worse endothelial function. Mean (SD) brachial artery FMD changed from 6.7 (4.3) percent to 3.4 (3.9) percent ($p < 0.001$) and from 6.7 (3.6) percent to 4.3 (2.2) percent ($p = 0.001$) before and after, respectively, a cigarette and an e-cigarette. Although the change was larger after a cigarette (−3.3 percent change) than an e-cigarette (−2.4 percent change), both were statistically significant. The study did not provide detailed information on changes in pulse-wave velocity. The implications of these findings for long-term endothelial function in long-term e-cigarette users need to be evaluated.

The short-term effect of e-cigarettes on endothelial function has also been evaluated based on changes in endothelial progenitor cells (EPCs) measured with flow cytometry and reported as EPC events (Antoniewicz et al., 2016). EPCs are stem cells mainly derived from the bone marrow that have been proposed as a biomarker of endothelial function as they play a critical role in the maintenance, differentiation, and regeneration of endothelial cells following vascular injury or neogenesis (Lekakis et al., 2011). In experiments comparing EPC levels before and 1 hour, 4 hours, and 24 hours after exposure to an eGoXL e-cigarette with nicotine 12 mg/ml and 49.4 percent/44.4 percent PG/glycerol without flavors, EPC events increased at 1 hour and 4 hours and returned to normal at 24 hours (see Figure 9-2). No changes were observed for control periods conducted with 1-week washout in a randomized crossover manner and in the same conditions as the e-cigarette experiment. These short-term effects of e-cigarettes on EPCs could be related to nicotine, as nicotine has been shown to increase short-term increases of EPCs. In addition to EPCs, the same experiment also measured microvesicles (MVs) from the cell membrane. The MVs consist of a lipid bilayer that can be released from all cell types in the circulation, such as leukocytes, erythrocytes, endothelial cells, and platelets. No differences were found in MVs overall, by cell origin (endothelial, platelet, or leukocyte) or by markers of inflammation (high-mobility group protein B1 [HMGB1], P-selectin, CD40 ligand), but a statistically significant difference was found for endothelial MVs with E-selectin (CD144 + CD62E), with higher levels at 4 hours after the experiment (median = 28 [IQR = 17, 65] versus 23 [14, 42]) that returned to normal at 24 hours (20 [15, 40] versus 23 [11, 37]), $p = 0.038$.[1] More research is needed to understand the short-term effects of e-cigarettes on endothelial function and the long-term implications of these findings. Indeed, a short-term increase in EPCs does not necessarily translate to acute endothelial injury. In epidemiological studies, lower rather than higher EPC levels are associated with higher risk of coronary heart disease. The use of novel, relatively easy-to-obtain biomarkers such as EPCs and MVs could be useful to assess both the short-term and the long-term effects of e-cigarettes on cardiovascular disease.

Arterial elasticity is essential for blood flow. The hardening or stiffening of the arteries, which is also called arteriosclerosis, plays an important role in the development of cardiovascular disease. The term arterial

[1] Chapter 7 also includes this study in its review and presents effects of e-cigarette exposure on overall MVs. The committee finds no conflict between the evidence presented in this chapter and the evidence presented in Chapter 7.

stiffness is commonly used when arteriosclerosis is measured based on the pulse wave graph using photoplethysmography. One study has measured arterial stiffness at the height of the phalanges artery before and 10 minutes after a personal cigarette or an e-cigarette (Ego-3) exposure in female students from Silesia, Poland (Szołtysek-Bołdys et al., 2014). The main study outcomes are the stiffness index (SI) measured in meters per second and the reflection index (RI) measured in percentage. SI is the ratio of the patient height in meters and the time between peaks of the systolic and diastolic components in the pulse wave graph. The RI is the ratio of diastolic and systolic component heights, expressed as percentage. In those experiments, in which SI and RI were measured before and 10 minutes after smoking a cigarette, and 1 week later after using an e-cigarette (Ego-3) with nicotine 24 mg/ml, SI was reduced from 6.75 to 6.56 ($p = 0.006$) after the cigarette but remained similar (6.73 and 6.75, changes not statistically significant) after an e-cigarette. RI was reduced (54.0 to 49.6 percent, $p = 0.01$) after a cigarette. The reduction after an e-cigarette (52.0 percent to 50.8 percent) was not statistically significant, although the exact p-value was not reported. The findings of this experiment would indicate that e-cigarettes would not induce short-term changes in arterial stiffness, contrary to combustible tobacco cigarettes. Given the findings

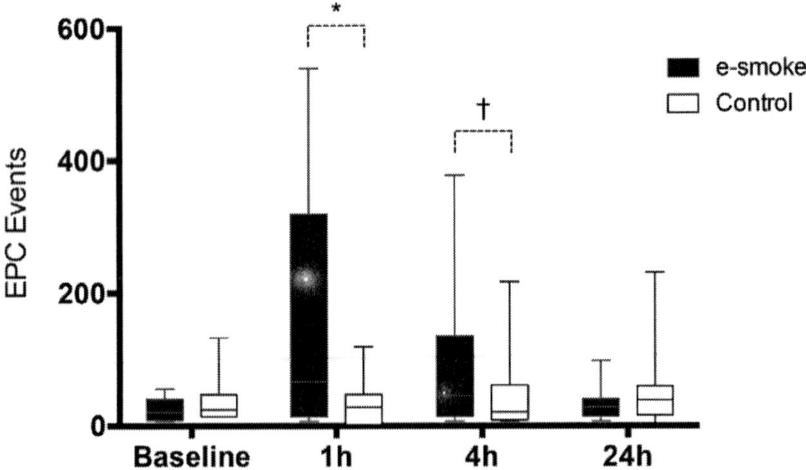

FIGURE 9-2 Endothelial progenitor cells (EPCs) during e-cigarette inhalation and control.
NOTES: Two-way, multiple measures ANOVA were significant for the interaction of exposure and time ($p = 0.002$). Separate time-point analysis was significant for 1 hour versus baseline, $^{*}p = 0.003$; and 4 hours versus baseline, $^{\dagger}p = 0.036$.
SOURCE: Antoniewicz et al., 2016.

for DBP as well as some of the findings reported for endothelial dysfunction, it is important to further evaluate the short- and long-term effects of e-cigarette smoking on arterial stiffness in larger studies.

Synthesis

Although the number of studies evaluating the effects of e-cigarettes on measures of oxidative stress, endothelial dysfunction, and arterial stiffness is small, these outcomes are interrelated and are considered in the underlying pathophysiological pathway toward clinical cardiovascular disease, including coronary heart disease, stroke, and peripheral artery disease. A major limitation is that these outcomes were evaluated short term rather than long term and it is unknown if these short-term findings have long-term consequences for the cardiovascular system. Research further evaluating these subclinical measures of cardiovascular disease is needed.

Cardiac Geometry and Function

The two-arm intervention study comparing the short-term effects of combustible tobacco cigarettes in smokers and e-cigarettes in e-cigarette users conducted measures of echocardiography before and 5 minutes after smoking a cigarette or using an e-cigarette (Farsalinos et al., 2014). During the echocardiography measures of flow diastolic velocities (E, A), their ratio (E/A), deceleration time (DT), isovolumetric time (IVRT), and corrected-to-heart rate IVRT (IVRTc) were measured. Mitral annulus systolic (Sm) and diastolic (Em, Am) velocities were estimated. Myocardial performance index was calculated from Doppler flow (MPI) and tissue Doppler (MPIt). Longitudinal deformation measurements of global strain (GS), systolic (SRs) and diastolic (SRe, SRa) strain rate were also performed. While the study focused its presentation of the findings comparing the effects of smoking a cigarette in smokers to vaping an e-cigarette among e-cigarette users, the comparability of those two groups is unclear. A better study design would be to evaluate the changes that occur before and after within each group. For e-cigarette users, none of the changes in the echocardiograph measures were statistically significant. However, some were borderline. For example, there was a mean (SD) change of 1.6 (5.6) cm/second in A flow diastolic velocity ($p = 0.08$), which was in the same direction as that observed for combustible tobacco cigarette smokers. The change in Em of 0.2 (0.7) cm/second MPIt (−0.01 [0.04], $p = 0.08$) was in the opposite direction from that among smokers. For GS the change (SD) was −0.4 (1.2) and almost statistically significant ($p = 0.06$), although also in the opposite direction from that among smokers. Overall, the implications of this study are unclear. First, because the study is not using a crossover design, the interventions were not randomized, and the comparability of smokers and e-cigarette users is unclear. Second, the usefulness of echocardiographic measures to assess short-term changes is unclear. Cardiac function and echocardiographic measures can be difficult to obtain and it is unclear if changes in those measures can be observed so quickly. These measures, moreover, are user dependent and if the examiner is aware of the intervention and the before and after status of the participant, the results may be influenced. Finally, this study used an early-generation e-cigarette device, so the relevance for currently used e-cigarettes is also unknown.

Autonomic Control

One study measured short-term effects of e-cigarette use on autonomic cardiovascular control under conditions of orthostatic stress (Cooke et al., 2015). No differences were observed by treatment group. In the cross-sectional study of e-cigarette users from Los Angeles compared with non-users, heart rate variability was measured with an echocardiogram (ECG) obtained during 5 minutes of quiet rest and during 5 minutes of controlled breathing at 12 breaths per minute (stimulus for the vagal tone). Three main spectral components were distinguished: high frequency (HF = 0.15–0.4 Hz, indicator of vagal activity), low frequency (LF = 0.04–0.15 Hz, a mixture of both vagal and sympathetic activity), and the ratio of LF to HF, reflecting cardiac sympathetic balance. Time-domain analysis was not applied because the ECG recording was too short.

In a second study, Moheimani and colleagues (2017) found the HF component decreased significantly in e-cigarette users compared with non-users (mean 46.5 versus 57.8, $p = 0.04$) while the LF and the LF/HF ratio increased significantly (52.7 versus 39.9, $p = 0.03$ and 1.37 versus 0.85, $p = 0.05$). No differences were observed between e-cigarette users and non-users in the changes of HF, LF, and LF/HF ratio during the controlled breathing maneuver. Study limitations include the small sample size, unclear description of the sources and forms of recruitment and response rate, the lack of adjustment or matching for sociodemographic and lifestyle risk factors (in particular given the imbalance by sex, former smoking status, and pack-years), and the lack of details on the e-cigarette devices and the e-liquid used by the participant. Outcome assessment was conducted using high-quality protocols and is described in detail.

CONCLUSIONS

The level of evidence regarding the association between e-cigarette use and biomarkers of cardiovascular disease risks varies:

> *Conclusion 9-2. There is **substantial evidence** that heart rate increases shortly after nicotine intake from e-cigarettes.*

> *Conclusion 9-3. There is **moderate evidence** that diastolic blood pressure increases shortly after nicotine intake from e-cigarettes.*

> *Conclusion 9-4. There is **limited evidence** that e-cigarette use is associated with a short-term increase in systolic blood pressure, changes in biomarkers of oxidative stress, increased endothelial dysfunction and arterial stiffness, and autonomic control.*

> *Conclusion 9-5. There is **insufficient evidence** that e-cigarette use is associated with long-term changes in heart rate, blood pressure, and cardiac geometry and function.*

REFERENCES

Anderson, C., A. Majeste, J. Hanus, and S. Wang. 2016. E-cigarette aerosol exposure induces reactive oxygen species, DNA damage, and cell death in vascular endothelial cells. *Toxicological Sciences* 154(2):332–340.

Antoniewicz, L., J. A. Bosson, J. Kuhl, S. M. Abdel-Halim, A. Kiessling, F. Mobarrez, and M. Lundback. 2016. Electronic cigarettes increase endothelial progenitor cells in the blood of healthy volunteers. *Atherosclerosis* 255:179–185.

Benowitz, N. L., and J. B. Fraiman. 2017. Cardiovascular effects of electronic cigarettes. *Nature Reviews Cardiology* 14(8):447–456.

Bhatnagar, A. 2016. E-cigarettes and cardiovascular disease risk: Evaluation of evidence, policy implications, and recommendations. *Current Cardiovascular Risk Reports* 10(7):24.

Carnevale, R., S. Sciarretta, F. Violi, C. Nocella, L. Loffredo, L. Perri, M. Peruzzi, A. G. M. Marullo, E. De Falco, I. Chimenti, V. Valenti, G. Biondi-Zoccai, and G. Frati. 2016. Acute impact of tobacco vs. electronic cigarette smoking on oxidative stress and vascular function. *Chest* 150(3):606–612.

Cooke, W. H., A. Pokhrel, C. Dowling, D. L. Fogt, and C. A. Rickards. 2015. Acute inhalation of vaporized nicotine increases arterial pressure in young non-smokers: A pilot study. *Clinical Autonomic Research* 25(4):267–270.

Cosselman, K. E., A. Navas-Acien, and J. D. Kaufman. 2015. Environmental factors in cardiovascular disease. *Nature Reviews Cardiology* 12(11):627–642.

Czogała, J., M. Cholewinski, A. Kutek, and W. Zielinska-Danch. 2012. [Evaluation of changes in hemodynamic parameters after the use of electronic nicotine delivery systems among regular cigarette smokers]. *Przegląd Lekarski* 69(10):841–845.

Czogała, J., M. L. Goniewicz, B. Fidelus, W. Zielinska-Danch, M. J. Travers, and A. Sobczak. 2014. Secondhand exposure to vapors from electronic cigarettes. *Nicotine & Tobacco Research* 16(6):655–662.

Eissenberg, T. 2010. Electronic nicotine delivery devices: Ineffective nicotine delivery and craving suppression after acute administration. *Tobacco Control* 19(1):87–88.

Farsalinos, K. E., D. Tsiapras, S. Kyrzopoulos, M. Savvopoulou, and V. Voudris. 2014. Acute effects of using an electronic nicotine-delivery device (electronic cigarette) on myocardial function: Comparison with the effects of regular cigarettes. *BMC Cardiovascular Disorders* 14:78. https://bmccardiovascdisord.biomedcentral.com/articles/10.1186/1471-2261-14-78 (accessed January 31, 2018).

Farsalinos, K., F. Cibella, P. Caponnetto, D. Campagna, J. B. Morjaria, E. Battaglia, M. Caruso, C. Russo, and R. Polosa. 2016. Effect of continuous smoking reduction and abstinence on blood pressure and heart rate in smokers switching to electronic cigarettes. *Internal and Emergency Medicine* 11(1):85–94.

Fogt, D. L., M. A. Levi, C. A. Rickards, S. P. Stelly, and W. H. Cooke. 2016. Effects of acute vaporized nicotine in non-tobacco users at rest and during exercise. *International Journal of Exercise Science* 9(5):607–615.

HHS (U.S. Department of Health and Human Services). 2014. *The health consequences of smoking—50 years of progress: A report of the Surgeon General.* Atlanta, GA: U.S. Department of Health and Human Services, Centers for Disease Control and Prevention, National Center for Chronic Disease Prevention and Health Promotion, Office on Smoking and Health.

James, P. A., S. Oparil, B. L. Carter, W. C. Cushman, C. Dennison-Himmelfarb, J. Handler, D. T. Lackland, M. L. LeFevre, T. D. MacKenzie, O. Ogedegbe, S. C. Smith, L. P. Svetkey, S. J. Taler, R. R. Townsend, J. T. Wright, A. S. Narva, and E. Ortiz. 2014. 2014 Evidence-based guideline for the management of high blood pressure in adults: Report from the panel members appointed to the eighth Joint National Committee (JNC 8). *Journal of the American Medical Association* 311(5):507–520.

Koskela, J. K., A. Tahvanainen, A. Haring, A. J. Tikkakoski, E. Ilveskoski, J. Viitala, M. H. Leskinen, T. Lehtimaki, M. A. Kahonen, T. Koobi, O. Niemela, J. T. Mustonen, and I. H. Porsti. 2013. Association of resting heart rate with cardiovascular function: A cross-sectional study in 522 Finnish subjects. *BMC Cardiovascular Disorders* 13:102.

Lekakis, J., P. Abraham, A. Balbarini, A. Blann, C. M. Boulanger, J. Cockcroft, F. Cosentino, J. Deanfield, A. Gallino, I. Ikonomidis, D. Kremastinos, U. Landmesser, A. Protogerou, C. Stefanadis, D. Tousoulis, G. Vassalli, H. Vink, N. Werner, I. Wilkinson, and C. Vlachopoulos. 2011. Methods for evaluating endothelial function: A position statement from the European Society of Cardiology Working Group on Peripheral Circulation. *European Journal of Cardiovascular Prevention and Rehabilitation* 18(6):775–789.

Lerner, C. A., I. K. Sundar, H. Yao, J. Gerloff, D. J. Ossip, S. McIntosh, R. Robinson, and I. Rahman. 2015. Vapors produced by electronic cigarettes and e-juices with flavorings induce toxicity, oxidative stress, and inflammatory response in lung epithelial cells and in mouse lung. *PLoS ONE* 10(2):e0116732. https://doi.org/10.1371/journal.pone.0116732 (accessed February 8, 2018).

Levenson, J., A. C. Simon, F. A. Cambien, and C. Beretti. 1987. Cigarette smoking and hypertension. Factors independently associated with blood hyperviscosity and arterial rigidity. *Arteriosclerosis, Thrombosis, and Vascular Biology* 7(6):572.

Mahmud, A., and J. Feely. 2003. Effect of smoking on arterial stiffness and pulse pressure amplification. *Hypertension* 41(1):183.

Mattace-Raso, F. U. S., T. J. M. van der Cammen, A. Hofman, N. M. van Popele, M. L. Bos, M. A. D. H. Schalekamp, R. Asmar, R. S. Reneman, A. P. G. Hoeks, M. M. B. Breteler, and J. C. M. Witteman. 2006. Arterial stiffness and risk of coronary heart disease and stroke. *Circulation* 113(5):657.

McEniery, C. M., S. Wallace, I. S. Mackenzie, B. McDonnell, Yasmin, D. E. Newby, J. R. Cockcroft, and I. B. Wilkinson. 2006. Endothelial function is associated with pulse pressure, pulse wave velocity, and augmentation index in healthy humans. *Hypertension* 48(4):602.

Moheimani, R. S., M. Bhetraratana, F. Yin, K. M. Peters, J. Gornbein, J. A. Araujo, and H. R. Middlekauff. 2017. Increased cardiac sympathetic activity and oxidative stress in habitual electronic cigarette users: Implications for cardiovascular risk. *JAMA Cardiology* 2(3):278–284.

Nigra, A. E., A. Ruiz-Hernandez, J. Redon, A. Navas-Acien, and M. Tellez-Plaza. 2016. Environmental metals and cardiovascular disease in adults: A systematic review beyond lead and cadmium. *Current Environmental Health Reports* 3(4):416–433.

Poirier, P. 2014. Exercise, heart rate variability, and longevity: The cocoon mystery? *Circulation* 129(21):2085–2087.

Polosa, R., J. B. Morjaria, P. Caponnetto, E. Battaglia, C. Russo, C. Ciampi, G. Adams, and C. M. Bruno. 2016. Blood pressure control in smokers with arterial hypertension who switched to electronic cigarettes. *International Journal of Environmental Research and Public Health* 13(11):E1123.

Pope, C. A., 3rd, R. T. Burnett, D. Krewski, M. Jerrett, Y. Shi, E. E. Calle, and M. J. Thun. 2009. Cardiovascular mortality and exposure to airborne fine particulate matter and cigarette smoke: Shape of the exposure–response relationship. *Circulation* 120(11):941–948.

Spindle, T. R., M. M. Hiler, A. B. Breland, N. V. Karaoghlanian, A. L. Shihadeh, and T. Eissenberg. 2017. The influence of a mouthpiece-based topography measurement device on electronic cigarette user's plasma nicotine concentration, heart rate, and subjective effects under directed and ad libitum use conditions. *Nicotine & Tobacco Research* 19(4):469–476.

St.Helen, G., K. C. Ross, D. A. Dempsey, C. M. Havel, P. Jacob, 3rd, and N. L. Benowitz. 2016. Nicotine delivery and vaping behavior during ad libitum e-cigarette access. *Tobacco Regulatory Science* 2(4):363–376.

St.Helen, G., D. A. Dempsey, C. M. Havel, P. Jacob, 3rd, and N. L. Benowitz. 2017. Impact of e-liquid flavors on nicotine intake and pharmacology of e-cigarettes. *Drug and Alcohol Dependence* 178:391–398.

Szołtysek-Bołdys, I., A. Sobczak, W. Zielińska-Danch, A. Bartoń, B. Koszowski, and L. Kośmider. 2014. Influence of inhaled nicotine source on arterial stiffness. *Przegląd Lekarski* 71(11):572–575.

Vansickel, A. R., C. O. Cobb, M. F. Weaver, and T. E. Eissenberg. 2010. A clinical laboratory model for evaluating the acute effects of electronic "cigarettes": Nicotine delivery profile and cardiovascular and subjective effects. *Cancer Epidemiology, Biomarkers & Prevention* 19(8):1945–1953.

Willum Hansen, T., J. A. Staessen, C. Torp-Pedersen, S. Rasmussen, L. Thijs, H. Ibsen, and J. Jeppesen. 2006. Prognostic value of aortic pulse wave velocity as index of arterial stiffness in the general population. *Circulation* 113(5):664.

Yan, X. S., and C. D'Ruiz. 2015. Effects of using electronic cigarettes on nicotine delivery and cardiovascular function in comparison with regular cigarettes. *Regulatory Toxicology and Pharmacology* 71(1):24–34.

10

Cancers

In prior Surgeon General reports, active smoking of combustible tobacco cigarettes has been determined to be causally associated with increased risk of 13 different malignancies (HHS, 2014). The biological mechanisms driving combustible tobacco cigarette smoking as a cause of such a diverse spectrum of cancers is due in large part to the wide array of carcinogens present in combustible tobacco cigarette smoke, many of which are generated by the combustion of the tobacco. There are more than 7,000 chemicals in combustible tobacco cigarette smoke, and more than 70 are established human carcinogens (HHS, 2010; IARC, 2012). In addition to combustible tobacco cigarette smoking, pipe and cigar smoking are established causes of lung cancer (HHS, 2014). Furthermore, even exposure to secondhand tobacco smoke, which results in much lower levels of smoke exposure than active smoking, is causally associated with lung cancer (HHS, 2006).

The cancer risk associated with the use of electronic cigarettes hypothetically would be expected to be less than combustible tobacco cigarettes based on the rationale that e-cigarettes include nicotine from tobacco—but not all the other tobacco constituents—and would therefore result in a reduced burden of carcinogens delivered to the user. Additionally, the nicotine present in e-cigarette aerosols does not contain appreciable amounts of tobacco-specific nitrosamines, nor are other pyrolysis products from nicotine formed. Moreover, compared with combustible tobacco smoke, potentially carcinogenic components of e-cigarette aerosols may be orders of magnitude less "carcinogenic" compared with those present in tobacco smoke (Chen et al., 2017; Stephens, 2018). (Comparisons of combustible tobacco smoke and e-cigarette aerosols are described in more detail in Chapter 18 on Harm Reduction.) By contrast, there is uncertainty about the potential mutagenicity and carcinogenicity of other e-cigarette substances, such as flavorants and humectants, present in the aerosol emitted from e-cigarettes that result from the heating and aerosolization of the liquid in these products. Furthermore, as described in Chapter 5, carcinogens such as formaldehyde and arsenic have been detected in electronic cigarette aerosol.

CHARACTERIZATION OF DISEASE ENDPOINTS AND INTERMEDIATE OUTCOMES

As shown in Figure 10-1, the etiology of cancers induced by environmental exposures is a complex, multistep process that generally takes years to develop. There are several biologically plausible pathways for

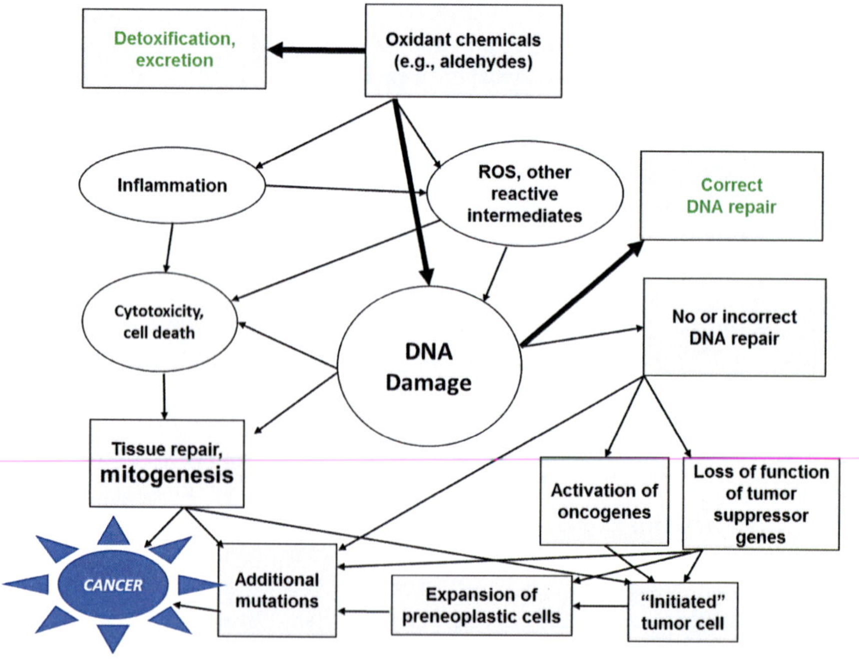

FIGURE 10-1 Conceptual framework of plausible pathways, including mechanisms and intermediate outcomes, by which exposure to e-cigarettes influences cancer outcomes.
NOTE: ROS = reactive oxygen species.

which components of e-cigarette aerosols could conceptually influence cancer development. As discussed in Chapter 5, numerous compounds identified in e-cigarette aerosols can form reactive oxygen species (ROS), and/or can be converted to reactive intermediates capable of binding to DNA. Oxidative damage to DNA, and/or the direct adduction of reactive molecules to DNA, such as can occur with formaldehyde, is the most important intermediate outcome of chemical carcinogenesis. As discussed later in this chapter, some studies have identified cytotoxicity of e-cigarette aerosols, potentially contributing to tissue repair and mitogenic response, which is another important pathway in the development of chemically induced cancers. Formaldehyde is perhaps the most prevalent component of e-cigarette aerosols capable of inducing ROS formation. A 2014 National Research Council report on the carcinogenesis of formaldehyde determined that epidemiological evidence was strongest for an association between formaldehyde exposure and cancers of the nasopharyngeal region and sinonasal cavities and myeloid leukemia (NRC, 2014). However, it should be recognized that formaldehyde is highly reactive, and potential DNA damage induced by it is most likely to occur at the site of exposure, the upper airways. It is also formed in small amounts by endogenous processes, so whether toxicologically significant amounts of formaldehyde from exogenous exposures can cause DNA damage in tissues distant from the site of exposure is controversial (Swenberg et al., 2011). Nevertheless, the presence of levels of formaldehyde in e-cigarette aerosols at concentrations that reportedly can exceed occupational exposure limits by an order of magnitude or more (see Chapter 5) are of concern for the potential risk to nasopharyngeal and lung cancer. It should be noted that, as described in earlier chapters, the levels of formaldehyde in e-cigarette aerosols can vary by many orders of magnitude, depending in large part on the device parameters (e.g., power), e-liquid contents (e.g., propylene glycol [PG] and glycerol), and user characteristics (e.g., puff topography). Thus, the presence of formaldehyde and other potentially mutagenic and cytotoxic constituents provides biologically relevant mechanisms whereby long-term use of e-cigarettes could affect cancer risk.

OPTIMAL STUDY DESIGN

The strongest evidence to characterize the potential association between e-cigarette use and the risk of human cancer will be methodologically rigorous epidemiological studies with human cancer as the outcome. Importantly, many e-cigarette users will be current or former combustible tobacco cigarette smokers, especially in the near term, and the effects of current and former smoking will be a challenging confounder to account for in observational studies. The second strongest level of evidence will be studies of intermediate cancer endpoints; for example, a study of e-cigarette use in relation to colorectal adenomas would have direct relevance to colorectal cancer because adenomas are precursor lesions in the colon carcinogenesis pathway. An important result of this comprehensive review is that the published literature is currently devoid of any evidence that includes rigorously designed epidemiological studies that include intermediate cancer endpoints, let alone cancer as an endpoint. Except for a study that included self-reported cancer as an adverse event (Manzoli et al., 2017), the published data have used biomarkers (oxidative stress and inflammation) as study outcomes.

EPIDEMIOLOGY

The literature search identified two studies on e-cigarette products in humans that refer to cancer. One of these was the study by Manzoli and colleagues (2017), which was composed of three groups (total n = 932) with the following sample sizes at the end of the 24-month follow-up: smokers of only combustible tobacco cigarettes throughout follow-up (n = 363), users of only e-cigarettes throughout follow-up (n = 97), and users of both e-cigarettes and combustible tobacco cigarettes throughout follow-up (n = 37). The authors defined e-cigarette users as users of any type of e-cigarette for 6 months or more. The authors report "any cancer" under serious adverse events, with the following results: only combustible tobacco cigarettes 0.8 percent (3/363), only e-cigarettes 2.1 percent (2/97), and dual users, 0 percent (0/37). The risk ratios the committee calculated from these data, using combustible tobacco cigarettes only as the referent category, are 2.49 (95% CI = 0.42–14.72) for e-cigarettes only and 0 (95% CI not estimable) for dual use. The results do not provide any indication for cancer risk reduction from sole use of e-cigarettes. These data are extremely limited by sample size and are of low quality; for example, the cancer data are presumably self-reported and not pathologically confirmed, the sample size is very small to assess the endpoint of any cancer and precludes assessment of specific malignancies, and there is no consideration of complete combustible tobacco cigarette smoking history or potential confounding factors.

In another human study, oral cells were collected by scraping the oral mucosa; the micronucleus assay was then applied to these oral mucosa cells (Franco et al., 2016) as a biomarker of potential genotoxicity and/or chromosomal instability (Luzhna et al., 2013). The Franco and colleagues (2016) study population had a total of 65 participants from three groups: (1) combustible tobacco cigarette smokers (n = 23); (2) e-cigarette users (defined as use of any e-cigarette device and liquid; n = 22); and

(3) non-smokers of combustible tobacco cigarettes and e-cigarettes (n = 20). The results revealed that compared with non-users of e-cigarettes and non-smokers of combustible tobacco cigarettes, the mean number of micronucleated cells/1,000 cells was 21 percent higher in e-cigarette users and 160 percent higher in combustible tobacco cigarette smokers. The results were also presented for the measure of total micronuclei/1,000 cells; compared with non-smokers of combustible tobacco cigarettes and e-cigarettes, e-cigarette users had mean levels that were 133 percent higher and combustible tobacco cigarette smokers had mean levels that were 633 percent greater. The pattern of associations for both micronuclei measures presented were thus consistent in showing that the average micronuclei burden was elevated in e-cigarette users relative to that in never smokers, and was elevated fourfold or more in combustible tobacco cigarette smokers compared with e-cigarette users. The only p-values reported were for the comparison of combustible tobacco cigarette smokers with e-cigarette users; these differences were statistically significant for both mean micronucleated cells/1,000 cells ($p = 0.001$) and total micronuclei/1,000 cells ($p = 0.004$). Weaknesses of this study include not presenting any evidence on the reliability of the micronucleus assay, not presenting all relevant p-values, and the lack of consideration of potential confounding factors even though the e-cigarette user group was on average 10 years older than the other study groups. This latter point is important because other studies have demonstrated age-related associations with micronuclei formation (Bonassi et al., 2011; Fenech et al., 2011).

Also relevant to a consideration of the potential association between electronic cigarettes and cancer are studies of e-cigarette use in relation to oxidative stress and inflammation; both of these biomarkers have been reviewed in detail earlier in this report. For the study of oxidative stress, the detailed results were not presented, but the graphical evidence presented failed to show a clear association between active and passive combustible tobacco smoking or active and passive e-cigarette use on acute measures of oxidative stress in an experimental setting (Poulianiti et al., 2016). A major limitation of the study by Poulianiti and colleagues is that the well-established role of combustible tobacco cigarette smoking in increasing oxidative stress (HHS, 2004, 2010) was not observed, raising major questions about the study's validity. Whether this was due to problems with the research protocol or suboptimal assay quality is unclear.

The study of inflammation (Flouris et al., 2012) was embedded within the exact same study as the aforementioned study of oxidative stress (Poulianiti et al., 2016), in that it was the identical study population except the assay results were presented for markers of inflammation (i.e., same study, two different publications). Once again, the complete results were not presented, but the authors reported that under the experimental conditions, both active tobacco smoking and secondhand exposure to tobacco smoke were significantly associated with increased circulating concentrations of inflammatory markers, including leucocytes, lymphocytes, and granulocytes (Flouris et al., 2012). These associations are consistent with the known effects of tobacco smoke exposure (HHS, 2004, 2010), and thus these findings suggest greater internal validity than for the oxidative stress results from this exact same study. The results did not show similar associations with e-cigarettes, which were not associated with these inflammatory markers.

CASE REPORTS AND OTHER CLINICAL STUDIES

Two case reports were identified that provided evidence relevant to the association between e-cigarette use and cancer. One case reported on a white male combustible tobacco cigarette smoker who had chronically elevated leucocyte and neutrophil counts in the absence of overt clinical disease; this is a clinical scenario consistent with chronic idiopathic neutrophilia (Farsalinos and Romagna, 2013). The patient was followed clinically for 6.5 years, during which he was unable to quit smoking and the symptoms persisted. The patient was then able to successfully quit smoking by using e-cigarettes. Even though the patient still used e-cigarettes after he stopped smoking combustible tobacco cigarettes, 6 months after quitting the latter, all the patient's markers of inflammation were significantly reduced, including leucocytes, lymphocytes, neutrophils, and C-reactive protein (Farsalinos and Romagna, 2013). Case reports provide only a weak form of evidence, but this single patient's experience suggests that e-cigarettes have less detrimental impacts than combustible tobacco cigarettes on inflammation and immune status.

In a case report published by Madsen and colleagues (2016), a 45-year-old female who used e-cigarettes presented after experiencing abdominal pain and fever for 4 months. Radiographic images revealed numerous pulmonary nodules and liver lesions consistent with extensive metastasis, but after a complete clinical workup, no evidence of malignancy was detected. A lung biopsy found an area with multinucleated giant cells. The authors reported that the biopsied lesion was consistent with a foreign-body reaction to lipophilic material. The patient subsequently stopped use of e-cigarettes; shortly thereafter, the lung nodules and liver lesions disappeared. The authors noted that the presence of multinucleated giant cells was consistent with the presence of glycerol-based oils detected in e-cigarette aerosol, and concluded that using e-cigarettes was associated with an inflammatory reaction that produces symptoms that can create the appearance of metastatic cancer.

These two case reports both relate to inflammation/immune status, with the case report of Farsalinos and Romagna (2013) suggesting that e-cigarettes are associated with substantially less inflammation than combustible tobacco cigarettes. However, the case report of Madsen and colleagues (2016) indicated that e-cigarettes are a strong enough source of inflammation to elicit symptoms that could be misdiagnosed as a form of cancer. These case reports raise interesting questions and reinforce the long-term need for carefully designed epidemiological studies of e-cigarette use in relation to cancer risk that include appropriate comparisons based on jointly considering the use of combustible tobacco cigarettes and e-cigarettes.

IN VIVO ANIMAL STUDIES

The literature search identified no in vivo animal studies focused on the potential carcinogenic actions of long-term e-cigarette use (Dodmane et al., 2014; Haussmann and Fariss, 2016; Toth, 1982; Waldum et al., 1996).

In Vitro Mutagenicity by the Ames *Salmonella* Reverse Mutation Assay

Three studies used the Ames mutagenicity assay with and without S9 metabolic activation (Canistro et al., 2017; Misra et al., 2014; Thorne et al., 2016) (see Table 10-1). Canistro and colleagues (2017) evaluated urine from male rats exposed in vivo to e-cigarette aerosols. They used two different *Salmonella* strains: TA100, which detects predominantly base substitution mutations, and YG1024, which detects primarily frame-shift mutations. They found that urine from e-cigarette aerosol-exposed rats was directly mutagenic in TA100, and metabolic activation decreased mutagenicity in this strain. Conversely, they found that urine was not directly mutagenic in YG1024 strain, but addition of the metabolic activation system significantly increased mutagenicity of urine above the background rate in non-exposed rats. Thorne and colleagues (2016) directly tested e-cigarette aerosol collected matter (ACM) from a Vype® ePen e-liquid cartridge containing blended tobacco flavor in TA98 and TA100 strains, with and without metabolic activation at nine different concentrations, up to 2,400 μg/plate. They reported no significant increases in mutagenicity in any of the assays. Misra and colleagues (2014) also assessed two e-liquids for mutagenicity in Ames strains TA98 and TA100, with and without metabolic activation. While extracts from tobacco smoke from standard reference combustible tobacco cigarettes were mutagenic in both strains at higher concentrations (in the presence of S9), there was no increase in mutagenicity in either strain exposed to the e-cigarette aerosol extract at any dose. Thus, of three studies examining mutagenicity of e-liquids, the

TABLE 10-1 In Vitro Mutagenicity/DNA Damage Assessment of E-Cigarette Liquids and Aerosols

Reference	Test Agents	Cells or Tissue Types
Breheny et al., 2017	Vype ePen e-liquid cartridges (blended tobacco flavor) containing 18 mg/ml nicotine; comparison with tobacco smoke total particulate matter (TPM) from reference combustible tobacco cigarette (3R4F).	Bhas 42 mouse fibroblast cells.
Canistro et al., 2017	e-cigarette BandZ S.r.l., (Pisa, Italy). "Essential cloud, red fruit flavor," 20-ml package. Composition per 100 g of product: propylene glycol, glycerol, nicotine (18 mg/ml). Power set at 5.5 V, 15 W.	Blood and urine collected from in vivo animal exposures; male S-D rats exposed via inhalation chamber. Peripheral blood for alkaline comet assay and micronucleus test. DNA extracted from lung. Urine for Ames assay, *Salmonella* strains TA100 and YG1024 with and without S9.
Misra et al., 2014	blu e-cigarettes containing glycerol-based e-liquids, with and without nicotine and two market leader flavors (classic tobacco and magnificent menthol), were used. Combustible tobacco cigarettes (Kentucky reference 3R4F, 1R5F, and Marlboro Gold), were used for comparison.	*Salmonella* strains TA98 and TA100. CHO-K1 cells.

Dose and Time Course	Assay Employed	Results
Aerosol collected material (ACM) from the e-cigarette was produced using a Borgwaldt LM20X linear smoking machine with 3-second duration using a square-wave puff profile, 55-ml puff volume, 30-second frequency, 3-second puff duration. ACM concentrations 3, 6, 12, 24, 48, 60, and 120 µg/ml. Comparison to same concentrations of TPM.	"Promoter activity" via cell transformation assay.	ACM from the e-cigarette was shown to be negative in all three promoter experiments, whereas TPM was positive in all three experiments.
Equivalent to 1 ml/day e-liquid. One cycle of treatment consisted of 17-second puff (6 seconds on, 5 seconds off, 6 seconds on) followed by 20-minute stop. At the end of the cycle, the animals were transferred to a clean chamber to begin the next cycle. Animals were submitted to 11 cycles per day for 5 consecutive days per week, and for 4 consecutive weeks.	Alkaline comet assay on blood. Micronucleus test on smears of peripheral blood. 8-OHdG (oxidative damage to DNA). Ames test on urine extracts.	"Extensive DNA damage in leukocytes measured as tail comet length of the fragmented DNA determined by single- and double-strand breaks." "Increase in the percentage of immature micronucleated reticulocytes (MN-RET) over normal reticulocyte RT." "8-OHdG markedly increased in the lungs." "Urine of e-cig-exposed animals induced a dose-dependent increase in the number of *S. typhimurium* revertants in different strains. The highest sensitivity was shown by the TA100 strain."
Cells were treated for approximately 24 hours with increasing levels of e-liquids. The cellular treatment dose range used for e-cigarettes (e-liquids and pad-collected aerosols) was 0–20 mg/ml and for combustible tobacco cigarettes, 0–0.5 mg/ml.	Ames assay TA98 and TA100 with S9 activation. Micronucleus assay.	No significant induction in the number of revertants over respective controls was observed for all e-liquids. No significant induction in the MN formation over respective controls was observed for all e-liquids.

continued

TABLE 10-1 Continued

Reference	Test Agents	Cells or Tissue Types
Thorne et al., 2016	E-cigarette ACM from Vype® ePen e-liquid cartridges (blended tobacco flavor) contained 18 mg/ml nicotine.	*Salmonella* strains TA98 and TA100.
Thorne et al., 2017	Emissions of three aerosol products. Kentucky reference combustible tobacco cigarettes (3R4F) and 2 e-cigarette formats: (1) a puff-activated closed "cigalike" device (eStick); (2) a "closed modular" system, dual-voltage, button-activated product (ePen).	Human bronchial epithelial cells (BEAS-2Bs).
Welz et al., 2016	E-liquids with the fruit flavors apple and cherry and one tobacco-flavored liquid; base mixture of 80% propylene glycol, 10% glycerol, and 10% water. All liquids had a nicotine concentration of 12 mg/ml.	Fresh tissue samples of healthy human oropharyngeal mucosa assembled into mucosal tissue cultures (spheroidal in vitro model).
Yu et al., 2016	V2 e-cigarette in red American tobacco flavor and VaporFi e-cigarette in classic tobacco flavor; both brands used a mixture of 70% propylene glycol/30% glycerol liquid formulas. Both 1.2% (12 mg/ml) nicotine e-liquid and nicotine-free versions in the same flavors were used for each.	Immortalized human keratinocytes (HaCaT). HNSCC cell lines UMSCC10B and HN30.

Dose and Time Course	Assay Employed	Results
All TPM/ACM experiments were conducted using final concentrations of 0, 50, 100, 150, 200, 250, 300, 500, 1,000 and 2,400 µg/plate.	Ames assay TA98 and TA100 with S9 activation.	Non-mutagenic in the 85-mm plate incorporation assay.
Average Delivered Deposition (µg/cm^2). 3R4F 0 3.1 ± 0.3 5.4 ± 1.8 10.5 ± 1.2 26.9 ± 2.1 eStick 0 35.2 ± 0.9 71.3 ± 2.0 ePen 0 42.5 ± 4.1 85.7 ± 2.7	DNA double strand breaks (γ-H2Ax immunofluorescence).	eStick and ePen were non-genotoxic and non-cytotoxic. Combustible tobacco cigarette smoke aerosols were genotoxic at a 3.1-µg/cm^2 dose and cytotoxic at 26.9 µg/cm^2.
Two different types of incubation: (1) one-time incubation for 24 hours and (2) incubation for 2.5 hours on five sequential days. DNA-damage experiments used one dose, a 15% solution of each e-liquid.	Alkaline elution DNA damage assay (neutral comet assay)	Tobacco liquid and base liquids were negative when treated once for 24 hours or when treated for 5 days. By contrast, apple and cherry liquids induced significant DNA damage in both single and repetitive 5-day treatments.
Single concentration 1% aerosol by volume. HaCaT cells treated for 8 weeks. UMSCC10B and HN30 each treated for 1 week.	Neutral comet assay DNA double strand breaks (γ-H2Ax immunofluorescence).	All four e-cigarette extracts (both nicotine and non-nicotine) were positive, in all three cell types; nicotine response greater.

two that looked directly at the e-liquid extracts did not find any evidence of mutagenicity, although the study that exposed animals (rats) in vivo to e-cigarette aerosols did find an increase in the mutagenicity of urine.

Micronucleus Assay

Both Canistro and colleagues (2017) and Misra and colleagues (2014) used the micronucleus assay to assess potential mutagenicity of e-liquids. The micronucleus assay detects clastogenic and aneugenic DNA damage that results in the disruption or breakage of chromosomes, leading to portions of the chromosome being added, deleted, or rearranged following cell division. Canistro and colleagues (2017) found an increase in the percentage of micronucleated reticulocytes (immature red blood cells) following in vivo exposure to e-liquids. In contrast, Misra and colleagues (2014) found no significant increase in Chinese hamster ovary (CHO) cells exposed to e-liquids for 24 hours, including cells exposed to tobacco smoke extract. Again, although the same endpoint assay was used in each of these studies, the differences in outcomes may be due to substantial differences in experimental design, with the in vivo study of e-cigarette exposure finding a positive effect, whereas the study in a cell line exposed directly to e-liquids had no effect.

Oxidative Damage to DNA (8-OHdG Formation)

Canistro and colleagues (2017) evaluated two measures of oxidative stress following in vivo, whole-body exposure of male Sprague-Dawley rats to the equivalent of 1 ml/day of e-liquid containing 18 mg/ml of nicotine in an inhalation chamber. Levels of 8-hydroxy-2′-deoxyguanosine (8-OHdG) in the lung, and the reducing power of the lung tissue (ferric reducing antioxidant power, or FRAP) were assessed in the animals after 4 consecutive weeks of exposure via a smoking machine (11 17-second puff cycles per day, 5 days per week). The formation of 8-OHdG is a widely used biomarker of oxidative damage to DNA. It has been associated with increased mutagenesis in a number of test systems, and is often considered as an intermediate biomarker of carcinogenic potential (Curtin, 2012; Kasai, 1997). They found a statistically significant, approximately fourfold increase in the levels of 8-OHdG in the lung tissue of exposed rats. There was a strong inverse correlation between the FRAP activity in lung tissue and 8-OHdG levels ($r = 0.845$, $n = 5$), further supporting the conclusion that e-cigarette aerosols increase oxidative stress in the lung. The authors also measured the levels of antioxidant enzymes, including catalase, NQO1, superoxide dismutase, and glutathione *S*-transferase, and found a 25–35 percent decrease in activities in all four enzymes. Because the expression of these enzymes is driven in large part by the levels of antioxidant "stress" through the Keap1-Nrf2/antioxidant response element, an increase in oxidative stress would normally be expected to increase, rather than decrease, the levels of expression of these enzymes' pathway (Ma, 2013). It is not clear why the levels of these enzymes would be decreased, rather than increased, following exposures to e-cigarette aerosols that appear to be inducing oxidative stress in the lung.

Although oxidative damage to DNA is widely regarded as a potentially significant contributor to carcinogenesis, the vast majority of oxidative damage to DNA occurs via endogenous processes. The extent to which exogenous factors that induce oxidative stress and thus the formation of 8-OHdG contribute to actual tumor development is uncertain, and thus the utility of 8-OHdG to serve as a predictive biomarker of carcinogenesis is very limited.

Cell Transformation (Promoter Activity)

Although most in vitro assays focused on evaluating carcinogenic potential of xenobiotics use mutagenesis and/or oxidative free radical production, a few in vitro tests can assess the potential for a substance to act as a promoter of carcinogenesis. Breheny and colleagues (2017) used a cell transformation assay to assess the potential promoter activity of e-cigarette–generated ACM, and compared it to the promoter activity from tobacco smoke total particulate matter (TPM) collected from a reference combustible tobacco cigarette (3R4F). ACM was collected from a Vype ePen with an e-liquid cartridge containing blended tobacco flavor and 18 mg/ml of nicotine, using a linear smoking machine. Seven different ACM concentrations, ranging from 3 to 120 μg ACM/ml, were used in exposures to Bhas 42 mouse fibroblasts. They found that TPM was positive in all of three experiments, whereas ACM was negative in all three experiments (see Table 10-1).

Relevance of DNA-Damage/Mutagenicity Studies and the Presence of DNA-Reactive Chemicals in E-Cigarette Aerosols to Potential Human Cancer Risk from E-Cigarette Use

As discussed above, some of the in vitro studies have found evidence that chemical constituents of e-cigarette aerosols are capable of reacting with DNA and in some instances inducing mutations in vitro and following in vivo exposure (Canistro et al., 2017). Some of the chemical constituents found in e-cigarette aerosols, including especially the reactive aldehydes formaldehyde and acrolein, are DNA-reactive, and formaldehyde has been shown to cause nasopharyngeal cancers in animals exposed via inhalation, and is considered by the Environmental Protection Agency and the International Agency for Research on Cancer to be a "known human carcinogen." Although highly reactive with both protein and DNA, acrolein to date has not been shown to be carcinogenic in laboratory animals following long-term exposure via ingestion. However, no long-term inhalation studies in laboratory animals have been completed. As discussed in Chapter 5, formaldehyde and acrolein are present in e-cigarette aerosols. It should be noted that both of these reactive aldehydes are formed endogenously at low levels, and are present in many food items and may "off-gas" from commercial products, leading to frequent and widespread, but low-level, exposures to these compounds. It should also be noted that both acrolein and formaldehyde are highly reactive, and adverse health effects, including potentially cancer, are most likely to occur at the site of exposure (e.g., in the oral cavity and tracheobronchial tree). Cancer risk from environmental exposures to potentially DNA-reactive/mutagenic chemicals is a function of dose of the chemical at the target site. Using formaldehyde as an example, it is informative to put the levels of formaldehyde in e-cigarette vapors in perspective with other sources of exposure. As discussed in Chapter 18 (Harm Reduction), Goniewicz (2014) measured the levels of formaldehyde and other carbonyl compounds in e-cigarettes and compared them with the levels present in combustible tobacco cigarettes. When adjusted to "cigarette equivalents" (amount emitted in one combustible tobacco cigarette, and amount present in 15 "typical" puffs of an e-cigarette), the predicted exposures to both formaldehyde and acrolein were about 10- and 50-fold lower from e-cigarettes in most circumstances (see Table 10-2).

Gillman and colleagues (2016) did a similar comparison, using five different devices, each at four different "power" levels. Two of these devices generated remarkably high levels of both formaldehyde and acrolein—levels well above those found in cigarette smoke, and levels that exceed occupational standards for both of these substances (see Table 10-3). They noted that these two devices likely suffered from poor "wicking" of e-liquid to the heating element, which would generate much higher temperatures, facilitating decomposition of the humectant (PG) to carbonyls. They also noted that device 1 was not widely used, likely because of the frequency with which it would generate highly irritating aerosol (so-called "dry puff"). The other three devices generated levels of both formaldehyde and acrolein that were similar to those reported by Goniewicz and colleagues (2014).

Furthermore, it should be recognized that the contributions of formaldehyde, acrolein, and other reactive carbonyls present in cigarette smoke are likely relatively insignificant contributors to the known cancer risks

TABLE 10-2 Comparison of Formaldehyde and Acrolein Levels in Smoke from One Combustible Tobacco Cigarette and in Aerosol from 15 Puffs of an E-Cigarette

	Tobacco Smoke, 1 Cigarette (Roemer et al., 2004)		E-Cigarette Aerosols per 15 Puffs (Goniewicz et al., 2014)	
	Formaldehyde	Acrolein	Formaldehyde	Acrolein
Mean	25.39	53.88	2.83	1.15
SD	21.80	31.81	1.82	1.35
Min	3.70	15.50	0.32	0.01
Max	75.50	98.20	5.61	4.19
Ratio cigarette/ e-cigarette mean			8.97	46.98

NOTE: SD = standard deviation.
SOURCES: Adapted from Roemer et al., 2004, and Goniewicz et al., 2014.

from combustible tobacco products. Thus, although there is substantial evidence that these DNA-reactive and potentially mutagenic compounds are formed and present in e-cigarette aerosols, the relatively low levels of exposure, coupled with the relatively low carcinogenic potential of these compounds, suggest that cancer risk from long-term use of e-cigarettes, if any, is likely to be very low, when compared with that from combustible tobacco cigarettes.

STUDIES OF EFFECTS OF MAJOR COMPONENTS OF E-CIGARETTES ON CANCER OUTCOMES

As described earlier regarding optimal study design, given the relatively recent introduction of e-cigarettes, there is a paucity of evidence on the long-term effects of e-cigarettes on cancer outcomes. Consequently, the committee drew on existing evidence of major components of e-cigarettes—namely, nicotine and the humectants PG and glycerol—with an emphasis on cancer outcomes. The committee discusses findings from epidemiological and in vivo animal studies in this section, from which the committee could draw inferences about the potential carcinogenic effects of e-cigarettes, but the discussion does not represent results of a systematic review.

TABLE 10-3 Formaldehyde and Acrolein Levels Generated from Five E-Cigarette Devices at Different Power Levels

	Units Adjusted to µg/15 Puffs									
	Device 1		Device 2		Device 3		Device 4		Device 5	
Power Level	Form.	Acro.	Form.	Acro.	Form.	Acro.	Form.	Acro.	Form.	Acro.
P1	128	104	4	0.9	1.1	0.6	2.0	0.8	2.0	1.2
P2	315	255	23	5.0	1.1	0.9	4.2	0.9	3.2	2.4
P3	480	375	120	39.0	0.8	0.5	2.1	0.8	4.7	2.3
P4	765	615	255	124.5	8.9	8.0	3.2	0.9	5.1	2.4
Mean	422	337	100	42.3	2.9	2.5	2.9	0.8	3.7	2.1
SD	270	216	115	57.4	4.0	3.7	1.0	0.1	1.4	0.6
Min	128	104	4	0.9	0.8	0.5	2.0	0.8	2.0	1.2
Max	765	615	255	124.5	8.9	8.0	4.2	0.9	5.1	2.4
Ratio	0.1	0.2	0.3	1.3	8.7	21.8	8.9	65.3	6.8	26.1

NOTE: Acro. = acrolein; Form. = formaldehyde; SD = standard deviation.
SOURCE: Adapted from Gillman et al., 2016.

Epidemiological Studies

As reviewed below and elsewhere (Grando, 2014; HHS, 2014; IARC, 2000; Shields, 2011), the potential carcinogenicity of nicotine has been studied extensively in the in vitro and in vivo settings. However, there is a paucity of epidemiological evidence assessing the potential association between nicotine per se and the risk of cancer in humans. This is largely because studying the potential association between nicotine exposure and human cancer poses methodological challenges that severely compromise the generation of meaningful data. This is because prior to the advent of e-cigarettes, in recent decades the "purest" form of nicotine exposure has been via nicotine replacement therapies (NRTs). Given that these are smoking cessation medications, teasing an isolated contribution of NRTs in relation to cancer risk in the context of extensive prior/current combustible tobacco cigarette smoking histories is complex. For example, among smokers the overall contribution of nicotine exposure from NRT can only be expected to be a very small fraction of a smoker's overall nicotine exposure because it will be greatly outweighed by the nicotine exposure from years of smoking combustible tobacco cigarettes. Continued greater use of NRT usually occurs in more addicted smokers who have a more difficult time quitting (Alberg et al., 2005), introducing the potential for strong confounding.

With these inherent challenges, the Lung Health Study provides the highest quality evidence on this topic to date (Murray et al., 2009). The advantages of the Lung Health Study are that it was a smoking cessation trial that tested an NRT (nicotine gum) and thus had detailed NRT use and combustible tobacco cigarette smoking data in the intervention group for a period of 5 years. In this study 3,320 participants from this intervention group were followed up for an additional 7.5 years to ascertain cancer outcomes, thus providing evidence on this topic from a prospective cohort study that emanated from the original randomized trial. Despite these strengths, in addition to the generic limitations noted above are limitations introduced by the fact that the cohort size and duration of follow-up are limited for yielding adequate statistical precision, the nicotine doses from nicotine gum are small, and the NRT exposure use and assessment occurred so near in time to the follow-up for cancer outcomes that the study could only be expected to detect contributions that occur in the latter stages of carcinogenesis. Thus, the inferences from the study results that indicated no statistically significant or clinically meaningful increased risk of lung cancer, gastrointestinal cancer, or all cancers are twofold: (1) it is unlikely there is a strong association between NRT use and cancer risk in the short term, and (2) the evidence provided by this null finding does not rule out the possibility of a weaker association between nicotine and cancer in the short term.

No epidemiological studies have addressed the long-term health consequences, including cancer, of propylene glycol and glycerol. Despite the fact that propylene glycol has been widely used in theatrical settings and in a few other occupations (see Chapter 5), the absence of evidence on cancer related to this topic is demonstrated by the fact that the Department of Health and Human Services, the International Agency for Research on Cancer, and the Environmental Protection Agency have yet to classify the carcinogenicity of propylene glycol in humans.

In Vivo Animal Studies

Typically, rodent bioassays for carcinogenesis involve 2 years of continuous exposures, and no studies of this nature have been identified in rats, mice, or other laboratory animals. However, *N'*-nitrosonornicotine (NNN) and 4-(methylnitrosamino)-1-(3-pyridyl)-1-butanone (NNK), derived from the tobacco leaves, formed during the tobacco curing process, and reported in e-liquids and aerosol, may contribute to the overall carcinogenic activity of tobacco products. As noted previously, however, because the nicotine in e-cigarette liquids is not extracted from cured tobacco leaves, where NNN and NNK are formed, the levels of these potent mutagens in e-cigarette aerosols are extremely low compared with tobacco smoke. Nicotine itself, as used in nicotine replacement therapies, is challenging to study in relation to cancer risk in epidemiological studies; the one high-quality study to evaluate the potential carcinogenicity of nicotine in NRT, the Lung Health Study, yielded null findings (see Murray et al., 2009, above).

Several studies have evaluated the consequences of long-term exposure to nicotine in animal models (Haussmann and Fariss, 2016). Two lifetime (2-year) bioassays evaluating the carcinogenicity of nicotine have been completed. Waldum and colleagues (1996) conducted a 2-year inhalation exposure study of nicotine using young adult female rats exposed to a constant concentration (501 ± 151 μg/m^3) of nicotine. Although more animals had tumors in the nicotine-exposed group (21/59; 36 percent) than the controls (6/25; 24 percent) (see Table 10-4), the types of tumors found in the exposed group were common in this strain of rat. The authors concluded that there were no "tumorigenic effects of nicotine on any organ in the body" (Waldum et al., 1996, p. 1345), although they did note that tumors in the pituitary gland (adenoma) were seen only in the nicotine-treated animals, and noted that nicotine has been shown to have "neuroendocrine actions" (Waldum et al., 1996, p. 1345).

Toth (1982) evaluated the potential carcinogenic effects of lifetime exposure of 0.5 or 0.7 mg/ml of nicotine, administered in drinking water for 24 months to groups of male and female Swiss mice. These concentrations translate to an average nicotine dose of approximately 150

TABLE 10-4 Occurrence of Tumors in Female Sprague-Dawley Rats Exposed to Nicotine for Up to 24 Months and Controls

Tumors (Site and Type)	Nicotine Exposed (%)	Controls (%)
Mammary gland		
Fibroadenoma	15	24
Adenocarcinoma	2	0
Pituitary gland		
Adenoma	7	0
Atypical adenoma	2	0
Ovary		
Granulosa-theca cell tumor	2	0
Adenocarcinoma	3	0
Skin		
Histiocytoma	2	0
Metastasis (origin unknown)		
Liver	2	0
Abdominal cavity	2	0
Total percentage of rats with tumors	36 (21/59)	24 (6/25)

NOTE: Percentages may not add up to 100 percent due to varied reporting, rounding, and missing data from source.
SOURCE: Adapted from Waldum et al., 1996.

mg/kg per day assuming a body weight of 25 g. Due to higher water consumption in the low-dose group, the daily dose per mouse at the 0.5 mg/ml concentration was only slightly smaller than in the 0.7 mg/ml group. Although this was generally a well-designed study with a reasonably large sample size, it could be argued that the highest dose was not sufficiently high, as there were no indications of toxicity, and no impact on body weight development or survival, so it would not be defined as a "maximal tolerated dose," which is often an expectation in carcinogenicity bioassays. A thorough histopathological examination was completed. The authors reported no increase in tumor incidence in either nicotine-exposed group. The author of the study concluded that nicotine was "not carcinogenic under the experimental conditions" (Haussmann and Fariss, 2016, p. 712; Toth, 1982, p. 72).

Murphy and colleagues (2011) evaluated whether nicotine administration could enhance the development of NNK-initiated lung tumors in A/J mice. They found that nicotine alone, administered at a daily dose of 0.15 mg/mouse for 46 weeks did not increase lung tumor multiplicity. NNK-treated mice had much higher lung tumor multiplicity compared with controls, but administration of nicotine for 46 weeks had no significant effect on the multiplicity of lung tumors in mice.

Another recent in vivo study in rats investigated whether oral nicotine exposure could cause early histopathological changes in urinary bladder epithelium that might be consistent with early-stage bladder carcinogenesis. Dodmane and colleagues (2014) administered nicotine hydrogen tartrate to rats and mice at doses of 52 and 514 ppm, respectively, for 4 weeks in drinking water. They then did a detailed histological evaluation of the urothelial lining. They found histopathological changes (hyperplasia) in 70 percent of the rats and 40 percent of the mice, compared with none in control animals. They also found that rats had a non-significant increase in the mean BrdU labeling index relative to controls, although there was no evidence of cytotoxicity via scanning electron microscopy. The authors concluded that "these findings suggest that oral nicotine administration induced urothelial hyperplasia (increased cell proliferation), possibly due to a mitogenic effect of nicotine and/or its metabolites" (Dodmane et al., 2014, p. 49). They further hypothesized that such nicotine-induced urothelial cell proliferation could possibly "act synergistically with DNA adduct-forming aromatic amines to increase the incidence of tumor formation in the urinary bladder in tobacco users" (Dodmane et al., 2014, p. 53).

VULNERABLE/SUSCEPTIBLE POPULATIONS

Population characteristics that identify subgroups that bear a disproportionate burden of cancer in the United States are race/ethnicity, sex, and socioeconomic status. Among these, the groups with the highest cancer burden are African Americans, males, and those of lower socioeconomic status. When looking across these characteristics, African American males are a particularly high-risk group. Among African Americans, the use of NRT products has historically been very low (Fu et al., 2005, 2008; Trinidad et al., 2011), and the emerging surveillance data on e-cigarette use also indicate low prevalence of use by African Americans. The results of the literature search revealed that the few relevant human studies were largely or entirely carried out in predominantly white populations outside the United States. Future research that includes diverse U.S. populations will be essential.

Children and adolescents are also vulnerable populations. For lung cancer, the younger the age of initiation of combustible tobacco cigarette smoking, the greater the risk of developing lung cancer in adulthood even after adjusting for lifetime combustible tobacco cigarette smoke exposure dose (HHS, 2014). This enhanced lung cancer risk associated with smoking at younger ages is hypothesized to be due to increased susceptibility of the developing lung to carcinogens due to more rapidly dividing cells compared with mature lungs.

SYNTHESIS

A systematic review of the current body of evidence relevant to the potential association between electronic cigarette use and cancer leads to the clear conclusion that the present body of evidence is simply too sparse to permit meaningful inferences to be drawn about either cancer or intermediate cancer endpoints. Furthermore, the human studies published on cancer-related lines of inquiry to date are not only few in number, but have not had an optimal level of methodological rigor to permit drawing even preliminary inferences. The sparseness of the current evidence and the low quality of the human evidence on this topic preclude making any evidence-based conclusions about the potential association between e-cigarette use and risk of cancer in human populations.

> **Finding:** There are no available epidemiological studies on the potential association between e-cigarette use and cancer in humans to make any conclusions. This holds true for comparisons of e-cigarette use compared with combustible tobacco cigarettes and e-cigarette use compared with no use of tobacco products.

> *Conclusion 10-1. There is* ***no available evidence*** *whether or not e-cigarette use is associated with intermediate cancer endpoints in humans. This holds true for e-cigarette use compared with use of combustible tobacco cigarettes and e-cigarette use compared with no use of tobacco products.*

> *Conclusion 10-2. There is* ***limited evidence*** *from in vivo animal studies using intermediate biomarkers of cancer to support the hypothesis that long-term e-cigarette use could increase the risk of cancer; there is* ***no available evidence*** *from adequate long-term animal bioassays of e-cigarette aerosol exposures to inform cancer risk.*

> *Conclusion 10-3. There is* ***limited evidence*** *that e-cigarette aerosol can be mutagenic or cause DNA damage in humans, animal models, and human cells in culture.*

> *Conclusion 10-4. There is* ***substantial evidence*** *that some chemicals present in e-cigarette aerosols (e.g., formaldehyde, acrolein) are capable of causing DNA damage and mutagenesis. This supports the biological plausibility that long-term exposure to e-cigarette aerosols could*

increase risk of cancer and adverse reproductive outcomes. Whether or not the levels of exposure are high enough to contribute to human carcinogenesis remains to be determined.

While evidence in humans for associations between e-cigarette use and cancer is extremely sparse, more abundant data have been generated in the in vitro and in vivo settings, including some positive studies and some negative studies on mutagenesis of e-cigarette components. Due to the mixed results across different experimental conditions and for different outcomes, clear, consistent signals have yet to be observed.

REFERENCES

Alberg, A. J., J. L. Patnaik, J. W. May, S. C. Hoffman, J. Gitchell, G. W. Comstock, and K. J. Helzlsouer. 2005. Nicotine replacement therapy use among a cohort of smokers. *Journal of Addictive Diseases* 24(1):101–113.

Bonassi, S., R. El-Zein, C. Bolognesi, and M. Fenech. 2011. Micronuclei frequency in peripheral blood lymphocytes and cancer risk: Evidence from human studies. *Mutagenesis* 26(1):93–100.

Breheny, D., O. Oke, K. Pant, and M. Gaça. 2017. Comparative tumor promotion assessment of e-cigarette and cigarettes using the in vitro Bhas 42 cell transformation assay. *Environmental and Molecular Mutagenesis* 58(4):190–198.

Canistro, D., F. Vivarelli, S. Cirillo, C. Babot Marquillas, A. Buschini, M. Lazzaretti, L. Marchi, V. Cardenia, M. T. Rodriguez-Estrada, M. Lodovici, C. Cipriani, A. Lorenzini, E. Croco, S. Marchionni, P. Franchi, M. Lucarini, V. Longo, C. M. Della Croce, A. Vornoli, A. Colacci, M. Vaccari, A. Sapone, and M. Paolini. 2017. E-cigarettes induce toxicological effects that can raise the cancer risk. *Scientific Reports* 7(1):2028.

Chen, J., C. Bullen, and K. Dirks. 2017. A comparative health risk assessment of electronic cigarettes and conventional cigarettes. *International Journal of Environmental Research and Public Health* 14(4):382.

Curtin, N. J. 2012. DNA repair dysregulation from cancer driver to therapeutic target. *Nature Reviews Cancer* 12(12):801–817.

Dodmane, P. R., L. L. Arnold, K. L. Pennington, and S. M. Cohen. 2014. Orally administered nicotine induces urothelial hyperplasia in rats and mice. *Toxicology* 315:49–54.

Farsalinos, K. E., and G. Romagna. 2013. Chronic idiopathic neutrophilia in a smoker, relieved after smoking cessation with the use of electronic cigarette: A case report. *Clinical Medicine Insights: Case Reports* 6:15–21.

Fenech, M., N. Holland, E. Zeiger, W. P. Chang, S. Burgaz, P. Thomas, C. Bolognesi, S. Knasmueller, M. Kirsch-Volders, and S. Bonassi. 2011. The HUMN and HUMNxL international collaboration projects on human micronucleus assays in lymphocytes and buccal cells—Past, present and future. *Mutagenesis* 26(1):239–245.

Flouris, A. D., K. P. Poulianiti, M. S. Chorti, A. Z. Jamurtas, D. Kouretas, E. O. Owolabi, M. N. Tzatzarakis, A. M. Tsatsakis, and Y. Koutedakis. 2012. Acute effects of electronic and tobacco cigarette smoking on complete blood count. *Food and Chemical Toxicology* 50(10):3600–3603.

Franco, T., S. Trapasso, L. Puzzo, and E. Allegra. 2016. Electronic cigarette: Role in the primary prevention of oral cavity cancer. *Clinical Medicine Insights: Ear, Nose and Throat* 9:7–12.

Fu, S. S., S. E. Sherman, E. M. Yano, M. van Ryn, A. B. Lanto, and A. M. Joseph. 2005. Ethnic disparities in the use of nicotine replacement therapy for smoking cessation in an equal access health care system. *American Journal of Health Promotion* 20(2):108–116.

Fu, S. S., M. M. Kodl, A. M. Joseph, D. K. Hatsukami, E. O. Johnson, N. Breslau, B. Wu, and L. Bierut. 2008. Racial/ethnic disparities in the use of nicotine replacement therapy and quit ratios in lifetime smokers aged 25–44. *Cancer Epidemiology, Biomarkers & Prevention* 17(7):1640–1647.

Gillman, I. G., K. A. Kistler, E. W. Stewart, and A. R. Paolantonio. 2016. Effect of variable power levels on the yield of total aerosol mass and formation of aldehydes in e-cigarette aerosols. *Regulatory Toxicology and Pharmacology* 75:58–65.

Goniewicz, M. L., J. Knysak, M. Gawron, L. Kosmider, A. Sobczak, J. Kurek, A. Prokopowicz, M. Jablonska-Czapla, C. Rosik-Dulewska, C. Havel, P. Jacob, and N. Benowitz. 2014. Levels of selected carcinogens and toxicants in vapour from electronic cigarettes. *Tobacco Control* 23(2):133–139.

Grando, S. A. 2014. Connections of nicotine to cancer. *Nature Reviews Cancer* 14(6):419–429.

Haussmann, H. J., and M. W. Fariss. 2016. Comprehensive review of epidemiological and animal studies on the potential carcinogenic effects of nicotine per se. *Critical Reviews in Toxicology* 46(8):701–734.

HHS (U.S. Department of Health and Human Services). 2004. *The 2004 Surgeon General's report on bone health and osteoporosis: What it means to you*. Rockville, MD: Department of Health and Human Services, U.S. Public Health Service.

HHS. 2006. *The health consequences of involuntary exposure to tobacco smoke: A report of the Surgeon General*. Atlanta, GA: U.S. Department of Health and Human Services, Centers for Disease Control and Prevention, National Center for Chronic Disease Prevention and Health Promotion, Office on Smoking and Health.

HHS. 2010. *A report of the Surgeon General: How tobacco smoke causes disease: What it means to you*. Atlanta, GA: U.S. Department of Health and Human Services, Centers for Disease Control and Prevention, National Center for Chronic Disease Prevention and Health Promotion, Office on Smoking and Health.

HHS. 2014. *The health consequences of smoking—50 years of progress: A report of the Surgeon General*. Atlanta, GA: U.S. Department of Health and Human Services, Centers for Disease Control and Prevention, National Center for Chronic Disease Prevention and Health Promotion, Office on Smoking and Health.

IARC (International Agency for Research on Cancer). 2000. *IARC monographs on the evaluation of carcinogenic risks to humans, Volume 77: Some industrial chemicals*. http://publications.iarc.fr/Book-And-Report-Series/Iarc-Monographs-On-The-Evaluation-Of-Carcinogenic-Risks-To-Humans/Some-Industrial-Chemicals-2000 (accessed October 19, 2017).

IARC. 2012. *Monographs: Tobacco smoking*. http://monographs.iarc.fr/ENG/Monographs/vol100E/mono100E-6.pdf (accessed December 19, 2017).

Kasai, H. 1997. Analysis of a form of oxidative DNA damage, 8-hydroxy-2'-deoxyguanosine, as a marker of cellular oxidative stress during carcinogenesis. *Mutation Research* 387(3):147–163.

Luzhna, L., P. Kathiria, and O. Kovalchuk. 2013. Micronuclei in genotoxicity assessment: From genetics to epigenetics and beyond. *Frontiers in Genetics* 4:131.

Ma, Q. 2013. Role of Nrf2 in oxidative stress and toxicity. *Annual Review of Pharmacology and Toxicology* 53:401–426.

Madsen, L. R., N. H. V. Krarup, T. K. Bergmann, S. Brentzen, S. Neghabat, L. Duval, and S. T. Knudsen. 2016. A cancer that went up in smoke: Pulmonary reaction to e-cigarettes imitating metastatic cancer. *Chest* 149(3):e65–e67.

Manzoli, L., M. E. Flacco, M. Ferrante, C. La Vecchia, R. Siliquini, W. Ricciardi, C. Marzuillo, P. Villari, and M. Fiore. 2017. Cohort study of electronic cigarette use: Effectiveness and safety at 24 months. *Tobacco Control* 26(3):284–292.

Misra, M., R. D. Leverette, B. T. Cooper, M. B. Bennett, and S. E. Brown. 2014. Comparative in vitro toxicity profile of electronic and tobacco cigarettes, smokeless tobacco and nicotine replacement therapy products: E-liquids, extracts and collected aerosols. *International Journal of Environmental Research & Public Health* 11(11):11325–11347.

Murphy, S. E., L. B. von Weymarn, M. M. Schutten, F. Kassie, and J. F. Modiano. 2011. Chronic nicotine consumption does not influence 4-(methylnitrosamino)-1-(3-pyridyl)-1-butanone induced lung tumorigenesis. *Cancer Prevention Research* 4(11):1752–1760.

Murray, R. P., J. E. Connett, and L. M. Zapawa. 2009. Does nicotine replacement therapy cause cancer? Evidence from the Lung Health Study. *Nicotine & Tobacco Research* 11(9):1076–1082.

NRC (National Research Council). 2014. *Review of the formaldehyde assessment in the National Toxicology Program 12th report on carcinogens*. Washington, DC: The National Academies Press.

Poulianiti, K., C. Karatzaferi, A. D. Flouris, I. G. Fatouros, Y. Koutedakis, and A. Z. Jamurtas. 2016. Antioxidant responses following active and passive smoking of tobacco and electronic cigarettes. *Toxicology Mechanisms and Methods* 26(6):455–461.

Roemer, E., R. Stabbert, K. Rustemeier, D. J. Veltel, T. J. Meisgen, W. Reininghaus, R. A. Carchman, C. L. Gaworski, and K. F. Podraza. 2004. Chemical composition, cytotoxicity and mutagenicity of smoke from US commercial and reference cigarettes smoked under two sets of machine smoking conditions. *Toxicology* 195(1):31–52.

Shields, P. G. 2011. Long-term nicotine replacement therapy: Cancer risk in context. *Cancer Prevention Research* 4(11):1719–1723.

Stephens, W. E. 2018. Comparing the cancer potencies of emissions from vapourised nicotine products including e-cigarettes with those of tobacco smoke. *Tobacco Control* 27(1):10.

Swenberg, J. A., K. Lu, B. C. Moeller, L. Gao, P. B. Upton, J. Nakamura, and T. B. Starr. 2011. Endogenous versus exogenous DNA adducts: Their role in carcinogenesis, epidemiology, and risk assessment. *Toxicological Sciences* 120(Supplement 1):S130–S145.

Thorne, D., I. Crooks, M. Hollings, A. Seymour, C. Meredith, and M. Gaça. 2016. The mutagenic assessment of an electronic-cigarette and reference cigarette smoke using the Ames assay in strains TA98 and TA100. *Mutation Research/Genetic Toxicology and Environmental Mutagenesis* 812:29–38.

Thorne, D., S. Larard, A. Baxter, C. Meredith, and M. Gaça. 2017. The comparative *in vitro* assessment of e-cigarette and cigarette smoke aerosols using the γH2AX assay and applied dose measurements. *Toxicology Letters* 265:170–178.

Toth, B. 1982. Effects of long term administration of nicotine hydrochloride and nicotinic acid in mice. *Anticancer Research* 2(1–2):71–73.

Trinidad, D. R., E. J. Pérez-Stable, M. M. White, S. L. Emery, and K. Messer. 2011. A nationwide analysis of US racial/ethnic disparities in smoking behaviors, smoking cessation, and cessation-related factors. *American Journal of Public Health* 101(4):699–706.

Waldum, H. L., O. G. Nilsen, T. Nilsen, H. Rorvik, V. Syversen, A. K. Sanvik, O. A. Haugen, S. H. Torp, and E. Brenna. 1996. Long-term effects of inhaled nicotine. *Life Sciences* 58(16):1339–1346.

Welz, C., M. Canis, S. Schwenk-Zieger, S. Becker, V. Stucke, F. Ihler, and P. Baumeister. 2016. Cytotoxic and genotoxic effects of electronic cigarette liquids on human mucosal tissue cultures of the oropharynx. *Journal of Environmental Pathology, Toxicology and Oncology* 35(4):343–354.

Yu, V., M. Rahimy, A. Korrapati, Y. Xuan, A. E. Zou, A. R. Krishnan, T. Tsui, J. A. Aguilera, S. Advani, L. E. Crotty Alexander, K. T. Brumund, J. Wang-Rodriguez, and W. M. Ongkeko. 2016. Electronic cigarettes induce DNA strand breaks and cell death independently of nicotine in cell lines. *Oral Oncology* 52:58–65.

11

Respiratory Diseases

Smoking of combustible tobacco products is the number one cause of chronic obstructive pulmonary disease (COPD) worldwide. Although the proportion of smokers has decreased over the past 25 years, approximately 1.1 billion people continue to smoke as of 2015 (Rabe and Watz, 2017). COPD leads to more than 3 million deaths per year worldwide, with only ischemic heart disease and cerebrovascular disease causing more deaths. Individuals who smoke also have an increased risk of sleep apnea and asthma exacerbations (Jayes et al., 2016). Respiratory complications from smoking can be further confounded by the increase in cardiovascular disease in individuals who smoke (Rabe and Watz, 2017).

In addition to the adverse respiratory health effects caused by smoking combustible tobacco products, secondhand smoke exposure has been reported to be associated with significant respiratory morbidities in non-users (Jayes et al., 2016). Tobacco smoke exposure has been shown to increase the severity of asthma exacerbations in children exposed to secondhand smoke (Merianos et al., 2016). Exposure to tobacco smoke in utero has been associated with abnormalities in lung development and small airway dysfunction in school-age children, manifested by reductions in forced expiratory volume in 1 second (FEV1) and forced expiratory flow 25–75 percent (FEF25–75 percent) (den Dekker et al., 2015; Duijts et al., 2012; Hayatbakhsh et al., 2009). A study in China found that school-age children exposed to secondhand smoke had increased cough and decreased lung function compared with children not exposed to secondhand smoke (He et al., 2011), and a study from Finland found that children of mothers who smoked combustible tobacco cigarettes during pregnancy were more likely to have increased airway resistance than children of mothers who did not smoke (Kalliola et al., 2013). Postnatal exposure to tobacco smoke also has been associated with an increased risk of wheeze and upper and lower respiratory tract illnesses in exposed children compared with unexposed children (Jayes et al., 2016).

Currently there is a lack of information regarding the short- and long-term effects of e-cigarettes on the respiratory system. This is due in part to the relative newness of the delivery system, the vast assortment of devices being used, and the variety of nicotine concentrations and flavorings that are currently available. Nevertheless, exposure of the lungs to various components of the e-cigarette aerosol could potentially damage the respiratory system or worsen preexisting lung disease through a variety of mechanisms (see Figure 11-1). For example,

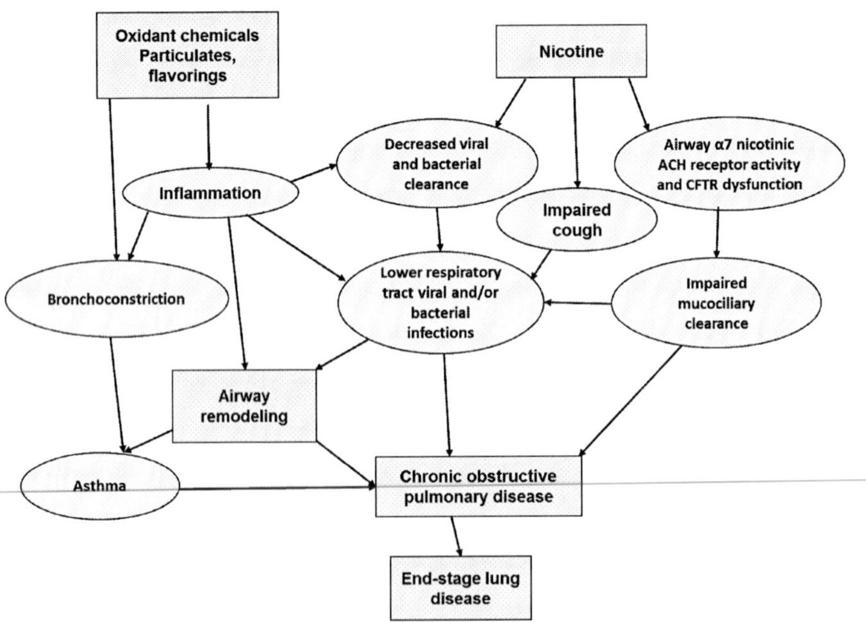

FIGURE 11-1 Conceptual framework of plausible pathways, including mechanisms and intermediate outcomes, by which exposure to e-cigarettes influences respiratory disease.
NOTE: ACH = acetylcholine receptors; CFTR = cystic fibrosis transmembrane conductance regulator.

nicotine-containing e-cigarette aerosols have the potential to adversely impact several host defense mechanisms in the lungs. In a murine model, α7 nicotinic acetylcholine receptors (α7 nAChRs) were shown to regulate cystic fibrosis transmembrane conductance regulator (CFTR) activity in the airways. Exposure to nicotine downregulated α7 nAChR activity, which in turn impaired CFTR function, causing impaired mucociliary clearance (MCC) (Maouche et al., 2013). In humans, CFTR dysfunction has been shown to be associated with the development of COPD and asthma hyperresponsiveness (Saint-Criq and Gray, 2017). Exposure to nicotine in tobacco smoke and e-cigarette aerosols also has been reported to impair cough (Dicpinigaitis, 2017; Dicpinigaitis et al., 2006; Sitkauskiene and Dicpinigaitis, 2010). Furthermore, nicotine has been shown to downregulate Th1 immune responses to lipopolysaccharide (Yanagita et al., 2012), consistent with an immunomodulatory effect of nicotine on viral and bacterial clearance.

Independent of nicotine, exposure to particulates and flavorings in e-cigarette aerosols could also potentially impair lung function. The presence of ultrafine particles has been measured in the aerosols of e-cigarettes (Laube et al., 2017), and particulates in the submicron range have the potential to damage airways and lung parenchyma. As noted in Chapter 3, the health risks from exposure to particles will depend on their nature, not simply their size. Nevertheless, certain ultrafine particles, which encompass particle sizes less than 100 nm, can cause DNA damage, induce pro-inflammatory cytokine expression, and adversely affect the immune system through the production of free oxygen radicals (Li et al., 2016). In addition, inhalation of ultrafine particles has been reported to increase the rate of asthma exacerbations (Li et al., 2016). Flavorings in e-cigarettes may also alter cellular redox balances in the airways by increasing pro-inflammatory cytokines (Lerner et al., 2015), and high temperatures generated by e-cigarette devices may cause formation of formaldehyde, leading to toxic effects on the lungs (Geiss et al., 2015).

In established smokers who are trying to quit or reduce combustible tobacco use, e-cigarettes may be less deleterious to the respiratory system when compared with exposure to combustible tobacco smoke (see Chapter 18). However, initiation of e-cigarette use by a person who has never smoked may cause harm to the respiratory system compared with never using e-cigarettes, particularly if initiation of e-cigarettes occurs at a young age. Therefore, understanding the health effects of e-cigarettes is dependent on the context of age, current and prior use of combustible tobacco products, and whether the user has preexisting lung conditions such as asthma and COPD. In addition, there is a need to examine the short- and long-term effects of secondhand and thirdhand e-cigarette aerosols on the respiratory health of non-users, who may inhale or come in contact with exhaled mainstream aerosol, which can settle on hard surfaces. Infants and preschool children who live with e-cigarette users may be at higher risk for secondary exposures because this age group spends much of their time in the residence of the e-cigarette user. Finally, exposure of the dual user to both combustible tobacco products and e-cigarette aerosols may cause unique health risks to the respiratory system.

CHARACTERIZATION OF DISEASE ENDPOINTS AND INTERMEDIATE OUTCOMES

In studying the effects of e-cigarette use on respiratory disease endpoints, an important question is whether or not e-cigarette use by itself can lead to the development of chronic respiratory conditions such as asthma and COPD or if e-cigarette use can worsen preexisting lung conditions compared with people who do not smoke. Additionally, researchers should determine if substitution of e-cigarettes for combustible tobacco use lessens the development of chronic respiratory conditions or lessens progression of preexisting lung conditions compared with people who continue to smoke. Because these respiratory disease endpoints may take years or even decades to realize, it becomes necessary to measure intermediate outcomes that may predict a disease state. The intermediate outcomes most relevant to the clinician include measurements of lung function and lung structure. The most common measurements of lung function include forced vital capacity (FVC), FEV1, FEV1/FVC ratio, and FEF25–75 percent, with the latter three the most useful in detecting presence and progression of obstructive lung diseases, such as asthma and COPD. These measurements are easily obtainable using spirometry. Body plethysmography can be used to detect an increase in residual volume, which can correlate with worsening airflow obstruction. In addition, impulse oscillometry can be used to detect changes in large and small airway resistance, and may be more sensitive than spirometry in detecting reversibility of airway obstruction in people with COPD (Saadeh et al., 2015). Structural changes in the lung such as the development of emphysematous changes or mucus plugging can be determined using computed tomography (CT) of the chest. Ultra-low-dose CT (Messerli et al., 2017), and more recently, MRI of the chest, has been shown to be an alternative modality to conventional chest CT in assessing COPD changes (Saadeh et al., 2015; Washko et al., 2012). Finally, standardized respiratory questionnaires can be helpful in evaluating outcomes; however, instrument responsiveness may differ among questionnaires (Puhan et al., 2006). Research on other intermediate outcomes in respiratory health should include the effect of e-cigarette aerosols, with and without nicotine, on cough reflex sensitivity, urge to cough, and nasal MCC because cough and MCC are integral defense mechanisms that help clear pathogens and environmental pollutants from the lungs and sinuses (Chatwin et al., 2003; Lee et al., 2017; Tarrant et al., 2017).

Quantification of inflammatory cell numbers from bronchoalveolar lavage (BAL) (Levanen et al., 2016; Siew et al., 2017) and measurement of pro-inflammatory cytokines from bronchial biopsies (Shields et al., 2017) could be used as intermediate respiratory endpoints to assess inflammation in the lower respiratory tract inflammation caused by e-cigarette use. In addition, combustible tobacco smoke has been shown to alter microbiome diversity; therefore, examination of sputum, nasal, and pharyngeal microbiome diversity may also help predict the impact of e-cigarette use on respiratory health (Diao et al., 2017). Other intermediate outcomes that could be used as markers of respiratory health include self-reported wheeze, bronchitis, shortness of breath, mucus production, other respiratory symptoms, and quality of life measurements.

OPTIMAL STUDY DESIGN

Since the potential health effects of e-cigarettes on the respiratory system are not completely understood, randomized controlled trials (RCTs) would not be appropriate at this time. Alternatively, prospective cohort studies that assess respiratory health outcomes in e-cigarettes users compared with combustible tobacco users and dual users could help determine the risks and benefits of using e-cigarettes. In addition, RCTs testing the efficacy of e-cigarette substitution as a method of smoking cessation in smokers unable to quit using nicotine replacement therapy (NRT) could concurrently measure lung function, lung structure, lung symptoms, and quality of life in individuals substituting e-cigarettes for combustible tobacco products. These additional studies could provide valuable information regarding the respiratory health effects of e-cigarette substitution on established smokers and help determine if switching completely or partly to e-cigarettes from combustible tobacco products in people with preexisting lung disease can alter progression or stability of lung disease.

Prospective cohort studies in adolescents and young adult e-cigarette users without a history of combustible tobacco product use should be performed to determine the likelihood of e-cigarette use leading to the development of chronic respiratory symptoms or decline in lung function. Furthermore, since asthma is a common respiratory disease of childhood, it is also important to determine if adolescents and young adults with asthma are at increased risk for asthma exacerbations and a more rapid decline in lung function when using e-cigarettes. Potential confounding factors, such as dual tobacco or cannabinoid use, exposure to secondhand smoke, and prior history of tobacco use, could introduce bias into the comparisons across exposure groups and need to be considered. Rigorous, objective assessment of the spectrum of endpoints, including lung function, respiratory symptoms, and cardiovascular and other comorbidities would also be essential to these studies.

QUESTIONS ADDRESSED BY THE LITERATURE

Due to the relatively recent widespread acceptance of e-cigarettes, there is a lack of understanding regarding the positive and negative effects of e-cigarettes on respiratory health. This is due in part to the paucity of long-term observational studies of adolescent/young adult never smokers who initiate e-cigarette use and observational studies and RCTs of adult smokers who switch to e-cigarettes for smoking cessation. Human studies are also needed that examine how exhaled mainstream aerosols affect the respiratory system of non-users when inhaled. As previously noted, exposure to these aerosols may disproportionately impact infants and children in the homes of indoor e-cigarette users because the very young often spend the majority of their time in this environment. However, since e-cigarettes, unlike combustible tobacco products, lack substantial sidestream emissions, it is unclear how detrimental exposure to secondhand e-cigarette emissions is to the non-user.

Further investigations into the effects of e-cigarette aerosols on the lung defense mechanisms such as cough, MCC, and the innate and adaptive immune system are needed. In addition, a better understanding of the impact of particle size on the development of DNA damage in respiratory cells is needed as is the relationship between flavorings and development of reactive oxygen species.

CLINICAL AND EPIDEMIOLOGICAL STUDIES IN HUMANS

Effects on Users of Combustible Tobacco Products

The literature search identified 17 studies that examined respiratory or pulmonary outcomes in people using e-cigarettes (see Table 11-1). Subjects in these studies include adult users of combustible products who switch to e-cigarettes completely or become dual users and include subjects with or without preexisting respiratory disease. Outcomes in the studies include standard measures of function ranging from self-reported symptoms of cough to asthma to exhaled carbon monoxide or nitric oxide. Six of these studies were from the same study group (Campagna et al., 2016; Cibella et al., 2016; Polosa et al., 2014a,b, 2016a,b). Three of these studies were observational studies in which the subject population included smokers not intending to quit. These subjects were invited to switch to first-generation e-cigarettes (Campagna et al., 2016; Cibella et al., 2016; Polosa et al., 2014b). Cibella and colleagues (2016) reported significant improvement in self-reported respiratory symptoms of cough/phlegm at 52 weeks in smokers who switched completely to e-cigarettes (18 of 130 subjects) and a significant increase in FEF25–75 percent, but not in FEV1 or FVC. No difference in lung function was found in dual users at 52 weeks (Cibella et al., 2016). In a similar study population of smokers not intending to quit, Campagna and colleagues (2016) found significant decreases in the fractional concentration of carbon monoxide in exhaled breath (FeCO) in smokers who switched completely to e-cigarettes (18 of 134 subjects) and significant increases in the fractional concentration of nitric oxide in exhaled breath (FeNO) at 52 weeks. Polosa and colleagues (2014b) reported on 40 smokers not intending to quit, 17 of whom were lost to follow-up, and found that when invited to use e-cigarettes, 5 of the 40 switched completely to e-cigarettes at 24 months.

In two studies from Polosa and colleagues (2014a, 2016a), they identified retrospectively 18 mild to moderate asthmatic smokers who switched to e-cigarettes (either single or dual users). They reported an improvement in FEV1, performance in the methacholine challenge test, and asthma control questionnaire but no change in asthma exacerbations when these subjects were followed prospectively over a 12-month period (Polosa et al., 2014a, 2016a). In a similar study design, Polosa and colleagues (2016b) identified patients with COPD from medical records who switched to e-cigarettes (single or dual users) and reported that they had significantly fewer COPD exacerbations. D'Ruiz and colleagues (2017) reported on pulmonary function tests in smokers who were switched to e-cigarettes for 5 days and found no significant difference in lung function between the groups.

These studies suggest that smokers with preexisting lung conditions such as asthma and COPD may experience some benefits from switching to e-cigarettes. As reported in the Polosa and colleagues (2016a,b) studies, such benefits may include an increase in FEV1, improved performance in a methacholine challenge test and in asthma control, and a decrease in COPD exacerbations. However, a limitation of these studies is that they were performed in a small number of subjects selected retrospectively. In addition, a reasonably high-quality RCT was negative: Cravo and colleagues (2016), in a clinical study that recruited subjects from two centers in the United Kingdom, reported no difference in lung function in subjects who switched to e-cigarettes. Their study had two cohorts. In both cohorts, smokers were randomized to either change to e-cigarettes containing 2 percent nicotine (with or without menthol flavoring) or to continue smoking. The authors reported no significant changes in pulmonary function tests after 12 weeks between the two groups. In this study,

TABLE 11-1 Clinical and Epidemiological Studies in Humans

Reference	Sample Size	Study Design	E-Cigarette Product	Control Conditions	Operationally Defined Outcomes
Effects in Users of Combustible Tobacco Products					
Campagna et al., 2016	n = 134	3-arm, double-blind, controlled, randomized, clinical trial; longitudinal. Return Rate 75% at week 12, 70.3% at week 24, and 61% at week 52. No difference in characteristics between those who remained or dropped out, except gender (71% of those lost to follow-up were male). No difference in dropout rate among the three experimental groups.	"Categoria" e-cigarette (model "401"). E-cigarette kit with either "original" (2.4% nicotine—Group A), or "Categoria" (1.8% nicotine—Group B), or "original" without nicotine ("sweet tobacco" aroma—Group C) cartridges	Those participants receiving e-cigarettes with 0% nicotine	(1) FeNO in ppb from 10-second exhalation; (2) eCO in ppm from a single expiratory breath; (3) adverse event symptom score for 8 different symptoms

Confounders or Factors Adjusted for	Results
Demographic characteristics, smoking reduction, and quit rates were not significantly different among study groups	(1) FeNO showed significant changes over the time: at baseline (BL), FeNO ppb (medians and interquartile range) were 6.6 (4.3–8.4), 5.9 (5.0–7.8), and 5.5 (4.5–6.9) for failures, reducers, and quitters (as per continuous classification at week 52), respectively. At week 52, it was 7.0 (5.5–9.9), 7.9 (6.0–10.8) and 17.7 (13.3–18.9) ppb, respectively. Repeated-measures ANOVA showed that effect of smoking phenotype was significant ($p < 0.0001$). No significant difference in FeNO changes from baseline was observed in quitters who stopped using e-cigarettes [+11.8 (7.4–13.4) ppb] compared with quitters who were still using e-cigarettes [+14.3 (9.9–15.3) ppb] at any study time points; (2) Significant within-subject effect (i.e., time, $p < 0.0001$) was found for changes in eCO. Exhaled CO ppm (medians and interquartile range) were 21 (14–29), 20 (15–26), and 17 (12–20) at BL for failures, reducers, and quitters (as per continuous classification at week 52), respectively. The same figures at week 52 were 20 (14–30), 13 (6–19), and 3 (1–4) ppm. Repeated-measures ANOVA showed a significant between-subject effect (i.e., smoking phenotype, $p < 0.0001$). Linear regression analysis showed that changes in FeNO were significantly correlated ($p < 0.0001$) with those in eCO at all time points; (3) High prevalence of respiratory symptoms was reported at baseline and virtually disappeared very quickly in both quitters and reducers. Among failures and reducers, the slopes were flat or not significant. Significant and steeper slopes (positive for eCO and negative for FeNO) were found among quitters. Differences among slopes were significant for both eCO and FeNO ($p < 0.0001$, ANCOVA).

continued

TABLE 11-1 Continued

Reference	Sample Size	Study Design	E-Cigarette Product	Control Conditions	Operationally Defined Outcomes
Polosa et al., 2016a	n = 16	Review of longitudinal medical records	Varied	N/A	(1) Juniper's ACQ score, spirometry for FEV1, FVC, and FEF25–75%, bronchial provocation tests assessing AHR for methacholine PC20. (2) Number of exacerbations from previous visit. (3) eCO monitoring and self-reported cigarette consumption. (4) E-cigarette smoking patterns.

Confounders or Factors Adjusted for	Results
Not stated; missing measurements were not included in the analyses	(1) At follow-up 1, there were significant improvements in ACQ scores; at follow-up 2 and follow-up 3, significant improvements were observed on ACQ scores, and all lung function parameters including methacholine PC20. Improvements at 12 months were still present at 24 months. Similar improvements were also observed in the dual users. At follow-up 1, there were significant improvements in ACQ scores and FEF25–75%. At follow-up 2, and follow-up 3, significant improvements from baseline (except for FVC at follow-up 3) were observed on ACQ scores, lung function parameters, and methacholine PC20. Deterioration in objective and subjective asthma outcomes noted in the two patients who relapsed to exclusive tobacco smoking. The normal FEV1/FVC of 79.5% at 12 months (follow-up 2) decreased to 71.0% at 24 months (follow-up 3). Their methacholine PC20 was reduced threefold from 2.95 mg/ml to 1.05 mg/ml and their ACQ score increased substantially from 1.45 to 2.3. (2) No significant differences in number of respiratory exacerbations throughout the study. Average number of exacerbations at baseline of 1.13 were not significantly different from 0.93 exacerbations at follow-up 1, 0.87 exacerbations at follow-up 2, and 0.81 exacerbations at follow-up 3. Of note, exacerbation rate increased from 0 at 12 months (follow-up 2) to 2 at 24 months (follow-up 3) in the two patients who relapsed to exclusive tobacco smoking. (3) Marked reduction in combustible tobacco cigarette use among e-cigarette users, the mean cigarette/day consumption of 21.9 at baseline decreasing to 2.3 at follow-up 1, 1.9 at follow-up 2, and 1.5 at follow-up 3. Substantial reduction in combustible tobacco cigarette use also observed in dual users; their mean cigarette/day consumption at baseline decreasing from 20.7 to 5.3 at follow-up 1, 3.7 at follow-up 2, and 3.5 at follow-up 3. Out of 16 asthmatics, 10 were still exclusively using e-cigarettes at 24 months and not smoking combustible tobacco cigarettes throughout the study (single users). (4) Duration of regular e-cigarette use ranged from 20 to 26 months, with 10 patients using them for at least 2 years. All participants were using standard refillable e-cigarettes by the end the study. The preferred nicotine strength of their e-liquid was 9 mg/ml and 18 mg/ml, which was consumed by 62.5% and 18.8% of e-cigarette users respectively. Most of the participants preferred tobacco flavors over other flavors.

continued

TABLE 11-1 Continued

Reference	Sample Size	Study Design	E-Cigarette Product	Control Conditions	Operationally Defined Outcomes
Cibella et al., 2016	Varied, depending on outcome (generally 103+)	3-arm, double-blind, controlled, randomized, clinical trial; longitudinal. Return rate 75% at week 12, 70.3% at week 24, and 61% at week 52. No difference in characteristics between those who remained or dropped out, except gender (71% of those lost to follow-up were male). No difference in dropout rate between three experimental groups.	"Categoria" e-cigarette (model "401"). E-cigarette kit with either "original" (2.4% nicotine—Group A), or "Categoria" (1.8% nicotine—Group B), or "original" without nicotine ("sweet tobacco" aroma—Group C) cartridges	Participants receiving e-cigarette with 0% nicotine (n varied depending on outcome)	(1) Subjective respiratory problems (frequency of cough/phlegm, wheezing, shortness of breath, or difficulty breathing). (2) Spirometry metrics (FEV1, FVC, FEF25–75%, and FEV1/FVC ratio).
Cravo et al., 2016	n = 419	Randomized, parallel group clinical study; combustible tobacco cigarette smokers switched to e-cigarettes for 12 weeks	E-cigarette with rechargeable battery, atomizer, capsule with e-liquid; 2% nicotine; subjects in combustible tobacco cigarette arm smoked own usual brand	Combustible tobacco cigarette smokers	Primary outcomes: AEs, vital signs, 12-lead ECG, lung function tests, hematology, clinical biochemistry, urinalysis

Confounders or Factors Adjusted for	Results
Demographic characteristics, smoking reduction, and quit rates were not significantly different among study groups.	(1) Cough/phlegm was significantly more frequent at BL among those resulting quitters (64%) with respect to reducers (55%) and failures (36%). No reported wheezing or chest tightness. High prevalence of cough/phlegm and shortness of breath (SoB) reported at BL: frequency of cough/phlegm decreased at each follow-up visit with respect to BL regardless of subjects' smoking phenotypes classification. SoB showed a similar frequency. Symptoms of cough/phlegm and SoB disappeared completely in quitters during the study. Significant effect of smoking phenotype on the reduction in cough/phlegm and SoB with time. Of note, changes in respiratory symptoms from BL were greater for both reducers and quitters with respect to failures ($p < 0.0001$). The presence/absence of respiratory symptoms at all time points (BL, week 12, week 24, and week 52) was not associated with significant differences in any of evaluated spirometric variables. (2) Significant within-subject effect was found for changes in FEV1, FVC, and FEF25–75% over the time (at BL, and at week 12, week 24, and week 52, $p < 0.0001$). No effect of smoking phenotype classification was evident for FEV1, FVC, and FEV1/FVC. Effect of smoking phenotype classification was evident on FEF25–75% that significantly ($p = 0.034$) increased over time among quitters. FEF25–75% was (mean ± SD) 80.6 ± 18.2, 78.3 ± 19.3, and 85.7 ± 15.6 at BL for failures, reducers, and quitters (as per continuous classification at week 52), respectively. The same figures at week 52 were 83.1 ± 18.4, 87.0 ± 20.0, and 100.8 ± 14.6 ($p < 0.0001$).
Not stated.	No clinically significant findings in vital signs, electrocardiogram, lung function tests and standard clinical laboratory parameters. AEs reported: more frequent during the first week and then reduced; 1,515 reported AEs, 495 related to nicotine withdrawal symptoms. Most frequent were headache, sore throat, desire to smoke, and cough; 6% judged as probably or definitely related to the e-cigarette. Additional observations: up to 33.8% decrease in level of urine nicotine equivalents, and decreases in the level of benzene, acrolein, and 4-(methylnitrosamino)-1-(3-pyridyl)-1-butanone.

continued

TABLE 11-1 Continued

Reference	Sample Size	Study Design	E-Cigarette Product	Control Conditions	Operationally Defined Outcomes
D'Ruiz et al., 2017	n = 105	Randomized, open-label, forced-switch parallel-arm study (exclusive e-cigarette use group, dual-use group, cessation group)	3 closed-system blu™ E-cigarette products: Rechargeable tobacco flavor, rechargeable cherry flavor, and disposable cherry flavor; all contained 24 mg/mL (2.4%) nicotine	Complete tobacco and nicotine product cessation	Pulmonary function (FVC, FEV1, and exhaled CO and NO); safety and tolerability
Polosa et al., 2014a	n = 18	Review of longitudinal medical records	Varied	N/A	(1) FEF25–75%, BHR, and ACQ scores; (2) Combustible tobacco cigarette use; (3) Exacerbations; (4) Safety and tolerability

Confounders or Factors Adjusted for	Results
Not stated.	Use of the e-cigarettes for 5 days did not lead to negative respiratory health outcomes or serious AEs. Pulmonary function tests: small but not significant improvements in FVC and FEV1 measurements in most use groups. Statistically significant benefits associated with smoking reduction were also noted in exhaled CO and NO levels.
Not stated; Missing measurements were not included in the analyses.	No significant differences in the parameters of lung function, BHR, or ACQ scores between the pre-baseline and baseline visits (except for a small change in FEF25–75%). (1) Compared with baseline, at 6 months, there were significant improvements in FEF25–75% and ACQ scores; at 12 months significant improvements were observed on all asthma outcomes measures. At 12 months both dual and single users had considerable improvements compared with baseline in all parameters (except for FVC in single users). (2) There was a reduction in combustible tobacco cigarette use amongst all e-cigarette users from a mean combustible tobacco cigarette/day use of 21.9 at baseline decreasing to 1.7 at follow-up visit 2 ($p < 0.001$). Similar reduction in combustible tobacco cigarette smoking was observed in dual users as well (22.4 at baseline to 3.9 at follow-up visit 2; $p < 0.001$). Importantly, 10 asthmatics gave up combustible tobacco cigarette use in favor of the e-cigarette (single users). (3) Prior to e-cigarette use in the 18 patients the average number of exacerbations was 1.06 (at pre-baseline) and 1.17 (at baseline). Over the period of observation none of the subjects in the cohort reviewed had a hospital or intensive care unit admission. (4) No severe adverse reactions or acute exacerbation of asthma symptoms were reported during the period of observation with e-cigarette use.

continued

TABLE 11-1 Continued

Reference	Sample Size	Study Design	E-Cigarette Product	Control Conditions	Operationally Defined Outcomes
Polosa et al., 2014b	n = 40	Observational prospective study following a cohort of smokers in a naturalistic setting after a 24-week intervention phase during which participants were issued Categoria e-cigarettes. Used a "Categoria" e-cigarette 6 months and followed prospectively for 2 years. After an initial 6-month intervention phase using the e-cigarette, participants attended two follow-up visits, at 18 and 24 months.	Categoria e-cigarette, "original" flavor, 7.4-mg nicotine cartridges (no more than 4 cartridges per day)	None	(1) >50% reduction in number of cigarettes from baseline and corresponding eCO level (reducers). (2) >80% reduction in number of cigarettes from baseline, with corresponding eCO (heavy reducers). (3) Abstinence from smoking with corresponding eCO (quitters). Failure to meet any of those benchmarks was defined as smoking cessation failure. (4) Product usage. (5) Adverse smoking-related events or symptoms.

Confounders or Factors Adjusted for	Results
Not stated.	(1) Sustained 50% reduction in the number of cigarettes per day at 24 months was shown in 11/40 subjects, with a median of 24 cigarettes per day decreasing significantly to 4 cigarettes per day ($p = 0.003$). (2) Of these 11 combustible tobacco cigarette reducers, 6 could be classified as sustained heavy reducers at 24 months. They had a median consumption of 27.5 cigarettes per day at baseline, decreasing significantly to 4 cigarettes per day by 24 months ($p = 0.012$). (3) There were 5/40 quitters by the end of the study. (4) Mean of 1.82 (±1.44) cartridges/day was used at 6 months. At 24 months, some e-cigarette users were not using the product (and stayed quitters), some relapsed back to tobacco smoking, and four upgraded their entry-level e-cigarette to better performing intermediate products using e-liquid nicotine from refill bottles (all categorized as heavy reducers). (5) At 6 months, mouth irritation, throat irritation, and dry cough were reported, respectively, by 14.8%, 7.4%, and 11.1% of the participants. Dry mouth, dizziness, headache, and nausea were infrequent. Overall, these symptoms remained stable during the whole duration of the observation phase, with the exception of dizziness and nausea, which disappeared by 24-month study visit.

continued

TABLE 11-1 Continued

Reference	Sample Size	Study Design	E-Cigarette Product	Control Conditions	Operationally Defined Outcomes
Polosa et al., 2016b	n = 48	Reviewed clinical notes of COPD patients attending clinics; 2 follow-up visits (12, 24 months after baseline). Analyses include data from the 3 visits.	Not stated; varied	Age- and sex-matched COPD patients who smoked combustible tobacco cigarettes but not e-cigarettes	(1) Changes in smoking behavior and e-cigarette use. (2) COPD exacerbations. (3) Lung function assessments and COPD staging. (4) CAT scores and 6-MWD.

Confounders or Factors Adjusted for	Results
Not stated; no significant differences in baseline characteristics between e-cigarette and control groups.	(1) Significant reduction in combustible tobacco cigarette consumption in COPD e-cigarette users. Complete abstinence from tobacco smoking in 13/24 (54.2%) of COPD e-cigarette users. Dual usage was reported by 11/24 (45.8%) COPD e-cigarette users. Significant reduction in combustible tobacco cigarette consumption in dual users. More than 75% reduction from baseline in cigarettes per day consumption reported by all COPD e-cigarette dual users at both follow-up visits. (2) Significant reduction in annual COPD exacerbations within the COPD e-cigarette user group but not in control group. Significant reduction in COPD exacerbations observed in dual users, but only at 24 months. In the single users there was significant reduction in exacerbations at both follow-ups. (3) Compared with baseline there were no significant differences in the post-bronchodilator FEV1, FVC, and % FEV1/FVC between study groups. Significant difference in the rate of FEV1 decline at the 24-month follow-up visit in COPD e-cigarette users than in the control group. A few COPD patients in the e-cigarette study group downstaged from GOLD Stage 4 to GOLD Stage 3 and 2. (4) COPD symptoms, as assessed using the CAT, at both follow-up visits decreased statistically and clinically significantly in the e-cigarette group, but no change in control group. Over the 24-month observation period, the median 6-MWD improved more than 60 minutes in the e-cigarette user group compared with just over a median of 3 minutes in the control group.

continued

TABLE 11-1 Continued

Reference	Sample Size	Study Design	E-Cigarette Product	Control Conditions	Operationally Defined Outcomes
Acute Exposures					
Ferrari et al., 2015	n = 20	Laboratory-based, randomized crossover design.	The NF e-cigarette used in this study: elips-C Series (steel shell, microprocessor powered by a battery, a filter, and a removable cartridge); nicotine-free liquid with hazelnut flavor ("Natur Smoke aroma Nocciola Antistress 0 mg/ml nicotina"). The commercial combustible tobacco cigarette (Marlboro® Red) contained 0.8 mg nicotine.	Crossover design (both smokers and non-smokers were randomized to smoke both the NF e-cigarette and a commercial combustible tobacco cigarette ad lib for 5 minutes in 2 different sessions)	(1) FeNO (2) FeCO (3) FVC (4) FEV1 (5) FEF (6) PEF

Confounders or Factors Adjusted for	Results
Not stated (except that smoking habit and crossover design were considered as factors in the ANOVA).	(1) No significant changes of FeNO were observed in the two groups. (2) Baseline FeCO values were significantly higher in smokers than in non-smokers. The combustible tobacco cigarette significantly increased FeCO values; this effect was significant in both groups of subjects. The e-cigarette did not have any significant effects on FeCO. The increase of FeCO values observed after smoking the combustible tobacco cigarette was significantly different from the effect of the e-cigarette. (3) Smoking a combustible tobacco cigarette significantly decreased the FEV1/FVC in non-smokers. (4) Both types of cigarettes significantly decreased FEV1 values in smokers while the decreases in non-smokers were not significant; thus FEV1 decreased significantly in the overall population after smoking a combustible tobacco cigarette while the effect of the e-cigarette did not reach a statistically significant level. (5) The combustible tobacco cigarette significantly decreased FEF25, FEF50, and FEF75 in the overall population, particularly due to the significant reductions of FEF25 in smokers and FEF75 in non-smokers while the reduction of FEF50 did not reach the significant levels in either smokers or non-smokers. The only significant effect of the e-cigarette was a reduction of FEF25 in smokers. Comparing the effects of combustible tobacco and e-cigarette smoking, only a significantly greater reduction of FEF50 was found after combustible tobacco cigarette smoking in non-smokers. Higher values of FEF75 were found after smoking an e-cigarette than after smoking a combustible tobacco cigarette, whereas the inverse was the case in smokers. (6) The combustible tobacco cigarette significantly decreased PEF values in the overall population due to effect in the smokers. The changes in FEV1, FVC, FEV1/FVC, and PEF between the two types of cigarettes were not significantly different in either smokers or non-smokers or in the overall population.

continued

TABLE 11-1 Continued

Reference	Sample Size	Study Design	E-Cigarette Product	Control Conditions	Operationally Defined Outcomes
Vardavas et al., 2012	n = 30	Laboratory-based, intervention design. Two groups: experimental group (n = 30) and control group (n = 10). Control group randomly selected from experimental group to participate in an extra session at a separate time. The role of using an e-cigarette was assessed through: (1) comparing the changes noted among control group participants with changes noted among experimental group participants after the intervention (intragroup comparison); and (2) comparing pre- versus post-respiratory function among experimental group participants (intergroup comparison).	NOBACCO e-cigarettes, black line. Medium cartridge, 11 mg nicotine. The subjects in the experimental group were instructed to use the e-cigarette ad lib for 5 minutes as they would usually smoke.	Control group subjects were asked to use the e-cigarette ad lib for 5 minutes, but without the e-cigarette cartridge included (not blinded).	(1) FeNO, ppb. (2) Dynamic lung volumes. (3) Total respiratory resistance.

Confounders or Factors Adjusted for	Results
Adjustments for the group (control versus experimental) and the relative baseline measurement (pre versus post). After controlling for baseline responses in linear regression, results are strengthened compared with the simple bivariate associations.	(1) FeNO in the experimental group decreased by 16% after the use of an e-cigarette, but not in control group. (2) Pulmonary function assessed via spirometry did not change in either group. (3) Airway impedance at 5 Hz increased in the experimental group by 0.033 kPa/(L/s), whereas no differences were noted among control group participants. Lung resistance in the experimental group also increased at 5 Hz, 10 Hz, and 20 Hz by an average of 0.031 kPa/(L/s), 0.029 kPa/(L/s), and 0.030 kPa/(L/s), respectively. Peripheral pulmonary resistance also increased significantly from 0.22 kPa/(L/s) to 0.25 kPa/(L/s).

continued

TABLE 11-1 Continued

Reference	Sample Size	Study Design	E-Cigarette Product	Control Conditions	Operationally Defined Outcomes
Cough and Mucociliary Clearance					
Dicpinigaitis et al., 2016a	n = 30	Pre-post cough test (before e-cigarette exposure, and after)	30 puffs from a disposable e-cigarette (blu, classic tobacco flavor; approximately 1.5–1.8 mg nicotine)	No control group (instead, pre-post analysis)	(1) C5, measured by the number of coughs following a capsaicin challenge. (2) Secondary analysis with non-nicotine e-cigarette in 8 subjects who demonstrated large degrees of inhibition of cough reflex sensitivity.
Dicpinigaitis et al., 2016b	n = 17	Pre-post cough test (before e-cigarette exposure, and after)	30 puffs from a disposable e-cigarette (blu, classic tobacco flavor; approximately 1.5–1.8 mg nicotine)	No control group (instead, pre-post analysis)	(1) C5, measured by the number of coughs following a capsaicin challenge. (2) Cu.

Confounders or Factors Adjusted for	Results
Not stated.	(1) After e-cigarette exposure, cough reflex sensitivity was significantly diminished compared with baseline. This effect was transient. Mean log C_5 at baseline was 0.50 ± 0.09 (SEM); 15 minutes after e-cigarette exposure it was 0.79 ± 0.11; and 24 hours subsequently it was 0.55 ± 0.10. Difference between log C_5 at baseline and post–e-cigarette exposure was significant as was the difference between post–e-cigarette use and 24 hours later. Twenty-three of 30 subjects demonstrated an inhibition of cough reflex sensitivity after e-cigarette exposure; 5 subjects had no change, and 2 subjects had a one-doubling concentration decrease in C_5. Twenty-six of the 30 subjects coughed to some degree. The median number of coughs for the study group was 15.5 (range 0–114) coughs. No correlation was found between the number of coughs induced by e-cigarette inhalation and subsequent change in cough reflex sensitivity. (2) No inhibition of cough reflex sensitivity was observed after exposure to the non-nicotine–containing e-cigarette, by contrast to the change in C_5 after use of the nicotine-containing e-cigarette. Significantly less coughing was observed after 30 puffs of the non-nicotine–containing e-cigarette compared with the nicotine-containing product.
Not stated.	Seventeen subjects had a demonstrable Cu and formed the subject population: (1) after e-cigarette exposure, C_5, and (2) the Cu was significantly diminished compared with baseline. Mean log C_5 at baseline was 0.60 ± 0.11 (SEM) and 0.92 ± 0.16, 15 minutes after e-cigarette exposure. Mean log Cu was –0.035 ± 0.08 at baseline and 0.21 ± 0.12 at 15 minutes after e-cigarette exposure. The difference between log C_5 at baseline and 15 minutes post–e-cigarette exposure was significant as was the difference in log Cu. This effect was transient. Fourteen of the 17 subjects coughed to some degree in response to inhalation. The median total number of coughs for the study group was 9 with a range of 0–30 coughs.

continued

TABLE 11-1 Continued

Reference	Sample Size	Study Design	E-Cigarette Product	Control Conditions	Operationally Defined Outcomes
Kumral et al., 2016	n = 98	Prospective randomized single-blind clinical trial.	Participants selected brand of device and flavor of the cartridge; 11–12 mg/ml e-liquid for all e-cigarettes.	Non–e-cigarette users (n = 40) were the smokers who quit smoking without the aid of medical therapy or a device, although they were provided cognitive behavioral treatment.	(1) SNOT-22 for subjective symptoms. (2) Saccharin transit test to evaluate nasal MCC function.

Confounders or Factors Adjusted for	Results
Not stated.	(1) SNOT-22 scores were insignificant between groups before the cessation of cigarette smoking; there was a significant difference between the groups at the third-month measurements. Comparison of SNOT-22 results of groups at the beginning of the study and after 3 months revealed statistically significantly lower scores after the 3 months. (2) MCC measurements were insignificant between groups before the cessation of cigarette smoking; there was a significant difference between the groups at the third-month measurements. Comparison of MCC results of group 2 at the beginning of the study and after 3 months revealed statistically significantly lower scores after the 3 months. Group 1 did not show any significant difference after 3 months.

continued

TABLE 11-1 Continued

Reference	Sample Size	Study Design	E-Cigarette Product	Control Conditions	Operationally Defined Outcomes
Respiratory Symptoms in Adolescents					
Cho and Paik, 2016	n = 35,904	Cross-sectional survey study	E-cigarette use assessed by "Have you ever used an e-cigarette in your life?" (yes/no). Answering no: "never user." Answering yes: asked a follow-up question "Have you used e-cigarettes in the past 30 days?" (yes/no). Answering yes: "current user" and answering no: "former user." Cigarette smoking assessed by question "Have you ever smoked, even one puff in your life?" (yes/no). Answering no: "never smoker." Answering yes: asked a follow-up question "In the past 30 days, how many days did you smoke?" Answering "one or more days": "current smoker," answering "none:" "former smoker."	"Current e-cigarette users" are compared with "former e-cigarette users" and "never e-cigarette users" as well as those who had used combustible tobacco cigarettes.	(1) Asthma based on student's self-reported doctor's diagnosis of asthma. (2) Severe asthma based on days of missing school due to symptoms.

Confounders or Factors Adjusted for	Results
Seven variables were included in the model: gender, city size, multicultural family status, overweight status, secondhand smoking at home, atopic dermatitis history, allergic rhinitis history. A variable for combustible tobacco cigarette smoking was added. Multiple logistic regression analyses performed for each potential confounder.	(1) Prevalence rates of asthmatics in "current e-cigarette users," "former e-cigarette users," and "never e-cigarette users," were 3.9%, 2.2%, and 1.7%, respectively. Comparing "current e-cigarette" users with "never e-cigarette" users, the unadjusted OR for asthma was 2.36. Comparing "current e-cigarette" users with "never e-cigarette" users, the adjusted OR for gender only was 2.09, and the adjusted OR for combustible tobacco cigarette smokers only was 1.73. The combustible tobacco cigarette smoking was the highest factor that affected the effect of e-cigarettes on asthma. Gender was the second factor. For all other factors, the changes in estimate of the effect of e-cigarettes on asthma were comparable to that of the unadjusted model. (2) Within the "never combustible tobacco cigarette" group, the OR for "more than 4 day absence from school due to asthma symptoms" was 18.59 in Model A, 13.21 in Model B, and 15.42 in Model C. Differences were not significant for the "former combustible tobacco cigarette" group and "current combustible tobacco cigarette" group. Within the "never combustible tobacco cigarette" group, the OR for "1–3 day absence from school due to asthma symptoms" was 6.81 in Model A, 5.67 in Model B, and 5.04 in Model C. Within the "current combustible tobacco cigarette" group, the OR for "1–3 day absence from school due to asthma symptoms" was 2.48 in Model A, 2.46 in Model B, and 2.23 in Model C. Differences were not significant for the "former combustible tobacco cigarette" group.

continued

TABLE 11-1 Continued

Reference	Sample Size	Study Design	E-Cigarette Product	Control Conditions	Operationally Defined Outcomes
Choi and Bernat, 2016	n = 36,085	Cross-sectional survey	E-cigarettes described to students as "battery-operated devices that look, feel, and taste like a [combustible] tobacco cigarette." Students were asked about e-cigarette use (asked if had ever tried using e-cigarettes [yes/no] and if had used e-cigarettes in past 30 days [yes/no]).	N/A	(1) Asthma status (determined by asking if currently had asthma [never diagnosed, currently has asthma, does not currently have asthma, unsure] and if had an asthma attack in last 12 months [yes/no]). (2) E-cigarette use. (3) Susceptibility to combustible tobacco cigarette smoking (asked about number of days smoked in past 30 days; if said never tried, assessed for susceptibility to combustible tobacco cigarette smoking).

Confounders or Factors Adjusted for	Results
Analyses were weighted to account for cluster sampling and were stratified by county-level metropolitan status. Additional associations adjusted for demographic variables, living with combustible tobacco cigarette smokers, days smoked in the past 30 days, positive social norms toward smoking, and exposure to secondhand combustible tobacco cigarette smoking.	The weighted prevalence of ever e-cigarette use was 8.2% (8.0% among students in metropolitan counties and 11.0% in non-metropolitan/rural counties). Students in metropolitan counties who reported currently having asthma were significantly more likely to have ever used e-cigarettes compared with those never diagnosed with asthma. The prevalence of ever e-cigarette use in students with current asthma was significantly higher among students in non-metropolitan/rural counties (18.2%) compared with those students with current asthma in metropolitan areas (9.9%). The weighted prevalence of past 30-day e-cigarette use was 3.3% (3.2% in students in metropolitan counties and 4.8% in students in non-metropolitan/rural counties). The prevalence of past 30-day e-cigarette use in students with current asthma was significantly higher among students in non-metropolitan/rural counties (9.5%) compared with those students with current asthma in metropolitan areas (5.1%). Among students with current asthma who had never smoked combustible tobacco cigarettes, ever e-cigarette use was associated with higher odds of being susceptible to combustible tobacco cigarette smoking (AOR = 3.96) compared with those who never used e-cigarettes. Past 30-day use of e-cigarettes was associated with an asthma attack in the last 12 months (AOR = 1.78) among those with current asthma.

continued

TABLE 11-1 Continued

Reference	Sample Size	Study Design	E-Cigarette Product	Control Conditions	Operationally Defined Outcomes
McConnell et al., 2017	n = 2086	Cross-sectional survey with past data included. Logistic regression used to evaluate the association of bronchitic symptoms and current wheeze with e-cigarette use. Dummy variables were created to assess effects of past and current use, compared with never use, and of frequency of use among current users. The linear trend in effects of frequency of current e-cigarette use assessed across 3 categories of use (never users, 1–2, and 3 or more days in the previous 30 days).	Students were asked the age at which they first tried cigarettes or e-cigarettes and number of days they used the product in the past 30 days. Participants who had "never tried" a product were classified as "never users." Those who had used a product, but not in the last 30 days, were classified as "past users." Participants who had used a product on at least 1 of the past 30 days were classified as "current users" of that product. Frequency of current e-cigarette use was categorized as 1–2 days or 3 or more days. Students reported number of cigarettes smoked in the previous month and the lifetime number of cigarettes smoked. Lifetime number of cigarettes smoked was categorized as 0 (never smokers), >0–10, 11–99, and >99 cigarettes.	N/A	(1) Chronic bronchitis symptoms (daily cough for 3 months, congestion or phlegm other than when accompanied by a cold, or bronchitis in the previous 12 months). (2) Wheeze assessed based on a report of wheezing or whistling in the chest during the previous 12 months. Analysis based on subjects with complete information on e-cigarette use.

Confounders or Factors Adjusted for	Results
Asthma was based on student's self-report of ever having had asthma. Parent-completed questionnaire assessed sociodemographic characteristics. Confounding assessed by including covariates in model. Models were adjusted for lifetime number of cigarettes. In sensitivity analyses, associations of e-cigarettes with bronchitic symptoms and wheeze were adjusted for these same conditions in 2010 and were restricted to children without symptoms in 2010. Twenty-three interaction terms of e-cigarette use with a dog or cat at home were examined for this outcome. For each outcome, the interactions of gender, ethnicity (Hispanic and non-Hispanic white) and asthma (in separate models) with e-cigarette use were also evaluated by calculating a likelihood ratio test for models with and without the interaction across categories of e-cigarette use. In all models, missing data were assumed to occur at random.	(1) Survey included 502 participants (24.0%) who had ever used e-cigarettes; 301 (14.4%) were past and 201 (9.6%) current users. Among current users, 107 (53.3%) used e-cigarettes on 1–2 days monthly and 94 (46.8%) on 3 or more days. Among past and current e-cigarette users, 132 (44.2%) and 81 (40.5%), respectively, were never cigarette users). Compared with Hispanic participants, non-Hispanic white youth were more likely to have bronchitic symptoms or wheeze. Parental education greater than high school was associated with greater risk of both outcomes. Secondhand smoke exposure in the home was associated with increased risk of bronchitic symptoms but not of wheeze. Current and non-current use of cigarettes was associated with greater risk of each outcome. Bronchitic symptoms were associated with both past (OR = 1.85) and current use of e-cigarettes (OR = 2.02). They were attenuated by additional adjustment for lifetime number of cigarettes smoked and secondhand smoke exposure in the home (OR = 1.71, for past and 1.41 for current use). There were no statistically significant interactions of e-cigarette use with gender, ethnicity (Hispanic and non-Hispanic white), asthma, and presence of a dog or cat in the home. The risk of bronchitic symptoms increased with number of days used in the previous 30 days (OR = 1.66 for 1–2 days and OR = 2.52 for 3 or more days) compared with e-cigarette–never users. This association with e-cigarette use frequency was not confounded by demographic characteristics, but was attenuated by additional adjustment for secondhand smoke exposure and lifetime number of cigarettes smoked (OR = 1.37 for 1–2 days and OR = 1.64 for 3 or more days of use) and the trend was no longer significant. (2) Wheeze was associated with current (OR = 1.86) but not with past use of e-cigarettes (OR = 1.02). The effect of current e-cigarette use was not confounded by sociodemographic characteristics but was markedly attenuated by adjustment for secondhand smoke exposure and lifetime number of cigarettes smoked (OR = 1.24), and after adjustment the association of past use of e-cigarettes with wheeze became negative (OR = 0.70). The magnitude of effect estimates for e-cigarette exposure in analyses restricted to never smokers were similar to those found in the entire population after adjustment for sociodemographic characteristics, smoking history, and secondhand smoke exposure.

continued

TABLE 11-1 Continued

Reference	Sample Size	Study Design	E-Cigarette Product	Control Conditions	Operationally Defined Outcomes
Wang et al., 2016	n = 45,128	Cross-sectional survey (current and past smoking status, e-cigarette use status, respiratory symptoms, demographic characteristics, secondhand smoke exposure)	Not stated; varied	N/A	(1) E-cigarette use. (2) Respiratory symptoms.

NOTES: 6-MWD = 6-minute walk distance; ACQ = asthma control questionnaire; AE = adverse event; AHR = airway hyperresponsiveness; ANCOVA = analysis of covariance; ANOVA = analysis of variance; AOR = adjusted odds ratios; BHR = bronchial hyperresponsiveness; BL = baseline; C_5 = cough reflex sensitivity; CAT = COPD Assessment Test; CO = carbon monoxide; COPD = chronic obstructive pulmonary disease; Cu = urge to cough; eCO = exhaled carbon monoxide; ECG = echocardiogram; FeCO = fractional concentration

smokers with respiratory conditions were excluded from the study and subjects in the e-cigarette randomized arm, although encouraged not to use combustible tobacco cigarettes, did often report dual use (Cravo et al., 2016).

Taken together the majority of studies in the literature examining respiratory outcomes of e-cigarette use and their benefit on respiratory function in current smokers come from the same region of Italy, which limits generalizability of their results. In addition, with the exception of the study by Cravo and colleagues (2016), the sample sizes were generally small and subjects were selected retrospectively.

Acute Exposures

Two studies focused on the short-term effects of e-cigarettes on exhaled breath measurements (FeCO and FeNO) and pulmonary function tests. The first study examined the effects of nicotine-free e-cigarettes on lung function and exhaled breath measurements. Ferrari and col-

Confounders or Factors Adjusted for	Results
AORs of respiratory symptoms due to e-cigarette use calculated using logistic regression for all students and by smoking status, adjusting for sociodemographic characteristics, SHS exposure, school clustering effects, and smoking status.	(1) Only 1.1% of all students, 0.1% of never smokers, 5.8% of ever smokers, 2.0% of experimenters, 9.6% of ex-smokers, and 9.6% of current smokers had used e-cigarettes in the past 30 days. (2) Respiratory symptoms were reported by 18.8% of all students, 17.7% of never smokers, 25.8% of ever smokers, 21.7% of experimenters, 27.2% of ex-smokers, and 34.3% of current smokers. E-cigarette use was significantly associated with respiratory symptoms (AOR = 1.28). The corresponding AORs were 2.06 in never smokers, 1.39 in ever smokers, and 1.40 in ex-smokers. Positive but non-significant associations were observed in experimenters and current smokers.

of carbon monoxide; FeNO = fractional concentration of nitric oxide; FEF25–75% = forced expiratory flow at 25–75 percent of the pulmonary volume; FEV1 = forced expiratory volume; FVC = forced vital capacity; GOLD Stages 1–4 = Global Initiative for Chronic Obstructive Lung Disease Stages of COPD (1 = mild, 2 = moderate; 3 = severe; 4 = very severe); MCC = mucociliary clearance; NF = nicotine free; NO = nitric oxide; PEF = peak expiratory flow; SHS = secondhand smoke; SNOT-22 = Sino-Nasal Outcome Test; SoB = shortness of breath.

leagues (2015) recruited 10 smokers and 10 non-smokers and found no significant decline in lung function after 5 minutes in the subjects using nicotine-free e-cigarettes by contrast to subjects who smoked combustible tobacco cigarettes. Vardavas and colleagues (2012) recruited healthy smokers and found that after 5 minutes of using a nicotine-containing e-cigarette, airway flow resistance increased and FeNO decreased from baseline. Although the mechanisms underlying the lower FeNO in e-cigarette users are unclear, smokers also have been shown to have low FeNO levels compared with non-smokers (Malinovschi et al., 2012; Torén et al., 2006). This suggests that the mechanisms that cause lower FeNO in e-cigarette users are similar to those that cause lower FeNO levels in smokers. Although higher FeNO levels have been demonstrated in people with eosinophilic-induced asthma and are considered a marker of airway inflammation (Malinovschi et al., 2012), studies of subjects with other respiratory conditions including cystic fibrosis (CF) have reported lower FeNO levels, possibly associated with impaired CFTR function (Korten et al., 2018).

Cough and Mucociliary Clearance

Airway exposure to nicotine has also been implemented as a causal factor in inhibiting cough and MCC defenses (Dicpinigaitis et al., 2016a; Laube et al., 2017; Maouche et al., 2013). Specifically, nicotine may modulate perceptual and motor responses to irritant cough stimulants (capsaicin), inhibiting the urge to cough (Davenport et al., 2009). Four studies reported on the effects of e-cigarettes on cough and nasal MCC (Dicpinigaitis, 2017; Dicpinigaitis et al., 2016a,b; Kumral et al., 2016). In a randomized single-blind clinical trial, Kumral and colleagues (2016) used Sino-Nasal Outcome Test (SNOT-22) scores and measured nasal MCC of subjects recruited from a smoking cessation clinic in which they were assigned to either e-cigarettes or non-e-cigarette cessation therapy. At 3 months, subjects assigned to the e-cigarette group had significantly worse sino-nasal symptoms and nasal MCC than subjects assigned to the non–e-cigarette group (Kumral et al., 2016). Two studies from Dicpinigaitis and colleagues (2016a,b) recruited healthy adult nonsmokers. Subjects were challenged with capsaicin at baseline and then at 15 minutes and 24 hours after a short exposure to nicotine-containing or non–nicotine-containing e-cigarettes. They found that urge to cough as measured by capsaicin challenge was depressed at 15 minutes following nicotine-containing e-cigarettes, but not nicotine-free e-cigarettes. At 24 hours after nicotine-containing e-cigarette use, cough reflex sensitivity returned to baseline (Dicpinigaitis et al., 2016b). Dicpinigaitis and colleagues (2016a) also reported that nicotine-containing e-cigarettes caused a decrease in cough reflex sensitivity (C_5), analyzed using mixed-effects modeling, at 15 minutes after nicotine-containing e-cigarette use but not after nicotine-free e-cigarette use. Dicpinigaitis (2017) again highlighted the role of nicotine causing centrally mediated suppression of cough in a study in which he reported suppression of cough at 15 minutes after capsaicin challenge in both combustible tobacco cigarette users and users of nicotine-containing e-cigarettes. Following cessation of combustible tobacco cigarette smoking, this centrally mediated cough reflex returned (Dicpinigaitis, 2017).

Respiratory Symptoms in Adolescents

Four studies examined respiratory symptoms in adolescents using or who have used e-cigarettes. Using self-reported questionnaires from participants in the Southern California Children's Health Study, McConnell and colleagues (2017) found a significant association between increased rates of chronic bronchitis symptoms among past, but not current, e-cigarette users over the previous 12 months. Cho and Paik (2016), using a Web-based questionnaire in a population of high school students from

South Korea, found that students who used e-cigarettes were more likely to have a self-reported clinical diagnosis of asthma and were more likely to have been absent from school due to severe asthma symptoms. Using an anonymous questionnaire with Chinese adolescents in Hong Kong, Wang and colleagues (2016) reported a higher rate of respiratory symptoms in those who used e-cigarettes regardless of previous or current history of smoking and observed that adolescents who used e-cigarettes had more days absent from school because of asthma. Choi and Bernat (2016) examined the prevalence of ever and past 30-day use of e-cigarettes by adolescents, using the 2012 Florida Youth Tobacco Survey. They reported an association between past 30-day e-cigarette use and having an asthma exacerbation in adolescents with asthma. Interestingly, adolescents with asthma in this study were more likely to have used e-cigarettes ever and in the past 30 days compared with adolescents not diagnosed with asthma.

IN VIVO ANIMAL STUDIES AND IN VITRO MECHANISTIC STUDIES

Animal studies in combination with in vitro studies have provided some unique insights into the potential health effects associated with e-cigarette use. Larcombe and colleagues (2017) exposed 4-week-old female BALB/c mice to 8 weeks of either tobacco smoke or propylene glycol (PG) or glycerol e-cigarette solutions with and without nicotine. They found that mice exposed to tobacco smoke had increased pulmonary inflammation and changes in pulmonary function, including methacholine hyperresponsiveness. Although inflammation was not increased in the e-cigarette–exposed mice, pulmonary function abnormalities were found. A limitation to the study is that they excluded male mice from analysis.

Garcia-Arcos and colleagues (2016) examined the effects of aerosolized nicotine-free and nicotine-containing e-cigarette fluid via inhalation in mice and normal human airway epithelial cells. Exposure in mice was for 1 hour per day for 4 months. Human bronchial epithelial (HBE) cells were cultured at an air–liquid interface with exposure to e-cigarette aerosols or nicotine solutions. Exposure to inhaled nicotine-containing e-cigarette fluids triggered effects normally associated with the development of COPD, including increased airway hyperreactivity, distal airspace enlargement, mucin production, and cytokine and protease expression. Exposure to nicotine-free e-cigarettes did not affect these lung parameters, suggesting effects were nicotine dependent in the mouse lung. These effects were also nicotine dependent in human airway cells in culture, further suggesting that inhaled nicotine contributes to airway and lung disease in addition to its addictive properties. Exposure of HBE cells to nicotine-containing e-cigarette fluids also demonstrated impaired ciliary beat frequency, airway surface liquid volume, cystic fibrosis transmembrane regulator, and ATP-stimulated K^+ ion conductance and decreased expression of *FOXJ1* and *KCNMA1*. The major concerns for this study include the matter of aerosolization and the dose delivered to animals by inhalation compared with human use, as well as the dose delivered to cells in culture versus actual exposure conditions in vivo (Garcia-Arcos et al., 2016).

Acute exposure to e-cigarettes compared with combustible tobacco cigarette smoke has been studied by Husari and colleagues (2016). Mice were exposed for 6 hours per day to air, e-cigarette, or combustible tobacco cigarette smoke for 3 days with higher particulate levels for e-cigarettes compared with combustible tobacco cigarette smoke. Human alveolar cells (A549) in culture were also exposed to various concentrations of e-cigarette aerosol and combustible tobacco cigarette smoke extracts. The authors found a significant increase in interleukin-1β (IL-1β) with exposure to e-cigarette, while combustible tobacco cigarette smoke resulted in significant increases in IL-1β, IL-6, TNF-α expression, and oxidative stress. TUNEL staining demonstrated significant cell death with combustible tobacco cigarette smoke, but not with exposure to e-cigarettes. Concerns about this study include the manner of exposure delivery to animals and the relevance of the A549 cell test results to the assessment of human implications for health (Husari et al., 2016).

Lim and Kim (2014) examined e-cigarette cartridge solution and its potential to aggravate allergen-induced airway inflammation and hyperresponsiveness in BALB/c mice. These investigators used diluted e-cigarette cartridge solution, which was delivered to mice by intratracheal instillation two times a week for 10 weeks. The mice had been previously sensitized to ovalbumin (OVA) by intratracheal, intraperitoneal, and aerosol allergen challenge. E-cigarette exposure increased infiltration of inflammatory cells, including eosinophils, into airways; enhanced the asthmatic AI and airway hyperresponsiveness; and stimulated cytokine production of IL-4, IL-5, and IL-13, as well as OVA-specific IgE production. These data suggest e-cigarette solutions can exacerbate allergy-induced asthma symptoms. This study is limited by its use of intratracheal instillation of dilute e-cigarette solution rather than true delivery of e-cigarette exposure by inhalation.

Hwang and colleagues (2016) examined the effects of e-cigarette inhalation on immune function. Mouse inhalation of e-cigarette aerosols was done 1 hour daily for 4 weeks, leading to alterations in inflammatory markers within the airways and elevation of an acute-phase reactant in serum. Exposure of human epithelial cells at the air–liquid interface to aerosols from an e-cigarette device resulted in dose-dependent cell death; in mice, reduced antimicrobial activity against *Staphylococcus aureus* in epithelial cells, alveolar macrophages, and neutrophils were observed. The authors concluded that inhalation of e-cigarette aerosols alters immunomodulatory cytokines in the airways of mice and increases markers of inflammation in BAL and serum, thus enhancing the virulence of *Staphylococcus aureus*. Although observations of e-cigarette impact are similar in mice and cells in culture, the actual mechanisms based on dose are difficult to ascertain (Hwang et al., 2016).

Additional studies, by Sussan and colleagues (2015), also questioned how e-cigarettes may impair antibacterial and antiviral defenses in mice. They found e-cigarette aerosol exposure for 2 weeks produced a significant increase in oxidative stress and moderate macrophage-mediated inflammation, and significantly impaired pulmonary bacterial clearance, compared with air-exposed mice, following an intranasal infection with *Streptococcus pneumonia*. For mice infected with influenza A virus, e-cigarette exposure was associated with increased lung viral titers and enhanced virus-induced illness and mortality. These findings demonstrate that e-cigarettes may impair the immune response and enhance susceptibility to bacterial and viral infections (Sussan et al., 2015).

Laube and colleagues (2017) exposed 10-week-old male mice to e-cigarette aerosol containing PG alone or PG in combination with nicotine for 20 minutes per day for either 1 or 3 weeks. Following exposure, mice were examined for MCC using technectium-labeled sulfur colloid with clearance of the colloid determined using an X-SPECT gamma camera. The research showed that daily exposure for 3 weeks to PG and nicotine slowed MCC compared with exposure to PG alone. This finding supports the potential biological plausibility of the previous study by Sussan and colleagues (2015), which also used mice and showed impaired bacterial clearance in the lungs of mice. Together, these studies provide evidence that exposure to e-cigarette aerosols during adolescence and early adulthood is not harmless to the lungs and can result in significant impairments in lung function even in the absence of lung inflammation.

Toxicity, oxidative stress, and inflammatory response in mice and human airway epithelial cells were examined by Lerner and colleagues (2015). E-cigarette exposure in C57BL/6J mice increased pro-inflammatory cytokines, while diminishing glutathione levels in the lungs, critical in maintaining a balance of cellular redox in the lungs. E-cigarette aerosol exposure of human airway epithelial cells (H292) in an air–liquid interface system resulted in increased secretion of inflammatory cytokines IL-6 and IL-8. Delivery of unaerosolized e-liquids was also found to be oxidative dependent on flavor additives. They found sweet or fruit flavors to be stronger oxidizers than tobacco flavors. Thus, exposure to e-cigarette aerosols/e-liquids produces measurable oxidative and inflammatory responses in lung cells and tissues that might lead to unrealized health consequences. Concerns about this study are minimal, but include the methods of delivery to cells in culture and the extrapolation of in vitro results to humans.

E-cigarette exposure has been found to have potential implications on the larynx as well. Salturk and colleagues (2015) found that exposure of Wistar albino rats to e-cigarette aerosol for 1 hour per day for 4 weeks caused hyperplasia and metaplasia of the laryngeal mucosa of rats, but this finding was not statistically significant. This study, although interesting, is inconclusive as to the relevance of how possible health effects to the larynx should be considered in e-cigarette use. Laube and colleagues (2017) examined MCC changes in C57BL/6 mice after 3 weeks of daily exposure and found that young adult male mice exposed to PG alone had significantly higher MCC than mice exposed to nicotine/PG aerosol. This study suggested that chronic exposure to nicotine-containing e-cigarette aerosols can impair airway MCC.

A 90-day inhalation study in rats, followed by a 42-day recovery period, was conducted by Werley and colleagues (2016). Exposure was done with low-, mid-, and high-dose levels of aerosols composed of vehicle (glycerol and PG mixture); vehicle and 2.0 percent nicotine; or vehicle, 2.0 percent nicotine, and flavor mixture. Daily targeted aerosol total particulate matter (TPM) doses of 3.2, 9.6, and 32.0 mg/kg/day were achieved by exposure to 1 mg/L aerosol for 16, 48, and 160 minutes, respectively. Treatment-related effects following 90 days of exposure included changes in body weight, food consumption, and respiratory rate. Also observed were dose-related decreases in thymus and spleen weights, and increased BALF lactate dehydrogenase, total protein, alveolar macrophages, neutrophils, and lung weights. This study in rats provides some insight for establishing a threshold level based on body-weight decreases at the mid-dose level for each formulation, equivalent to a daily TPM exposure dose of approximately 9.6 mg/kg/day. Histopathology changes appear to be isolated to the nasal mucosa. Concerns for this study include how to extrapolate these findings to human exposure and the relevance of the e-cigarette device used and non-respiratory parameters used for comparison. Further, lung weights and body weights are crude measures of effect.

One study reported that neonatal exposure to aerosol from nicotine-containing e-cigarettes was associated with diminished alveolar cell proliferation and impairment in postnatal lung growth (McGrath-Morrow et al., 2015).

SYNTHESIS AND CONCLUSIONS

The human observational studies examining the effect of switching to e-cigarettes (single or dual use) provide support for a finding of beneficial health effects relative to continued use of combustible tobacco products, with most favoring that conclusion. These studies were judged to be of fair quality. A major limitation of them, however, is that they are primarily from a single study group. In addition, the one RCT was negative, finding no improvement in lung function after 12 weeks in subjects who switched to e-cigarettes compared with people who continued to smoke combustible tobacco cigarettes (Cravo et al., 2016). Therefore, the committee concludes that there is limited evidence supporting improvements in lung function in smokers who switch to e-cigarettes.

Studies examining the long-term effects of e-cigarettes on the development of chronic respiratory symptoms are completely lacking due to the newness of the product. It is of importance to know whether chronic e-cigarette use by itself can cause COPD and if substitution of e-cigarettes for combustible tobacco products can prevent or slow the development of COPD in smokers who quit or reduced use of combustible tobacco products. At this time, there is a lack of well-designed epidemiological studies examining either question.

Studies examining the short-term effects of e-cigarettes indicate that nicotine-containing e-cigarettes, but not nicotine-free e-cigarettes, can have short-term adverse effects on lung defense mechanisms, including MCC, urge to cough, and cough sensitivity. These studies are of fair quality. They include subjects with and without a history of smoking and there are few-or-no credible opposing findings. These studies provide moderate evidence supporting short-term adverse effects of nicotine-containing e-cigarettes on lung defense mechanisms.

The committee identified four studies examining the effects of e-cigarette use on adolescent respiratory health—all are cross-sectional and use self-reported questionnaires. They include large groups of adolescents from three countries and reach similar results, thus providing moderate evidence of an association between respiratory symptoms in adolescents and e-cigarette use.

In non-users who are exposed to secondhand smoke and in healthy adolescents and young adult users, common respiratory endpoints can include an increase in asthma symptoms and severity and a higher prevalence of upper and greater lower respiratory tract symptoms and infections (Liu et al., 2016; Shargorodsky, 2016; Shargorodsky et al., 2015; Wilson et al., 2013). Currently, there is a lack of rigorously designed epidemiological studies examining the relationship between chronic e-cigarette use in adolescents and young adults and increased prevalence of respiratory symptoms and respiratory illnesses. There are also no epidemiological studies reporting on the respiratory effects of exposure to exhaled mainstream smoke from an e-cigarette user on a non-user.

The animal studies that have examined the effects of e-cigarettes on respiratory outcomes have used different e-cigarette devices, pumps, solutions, and exposures, limiting the ability to compare results among studies. Confounding factors such as aerosol temperature and particle size have not been taken into account. These methodological differences among studies can result in differences in particle deposition in the lungs and differences in systemic absorption of particles, nicotine, and toxins, resulting in different respiratory outcomes. In addition, not all studies evaluating the effects of nicotine aerosols on lung inflammation, MCC, and lung immune responses have included biomarkers of systemic nicotine absorption, which would help to standardize exposures in animal studies. The utility of studies using whole-body exposures in animal models when examining health effects of e-cigarette aerosols is limited because this type of exposure may overestimate or underestimate an exposure in the human condition. Furthermore, in vitro cell studies would be more informative and representative of the human condition if aerosols rather than liquid e-cigarette solutions are used and if primary, instead of immortalized, cell lines are used. Despite these limitations, the animal and in vitro studies described provide additional evidence of adverse effects of e-cigarette exposure on the respiratory system and do not change the committee's conclusions regarding the evidence of human health effects.

There is coherence across studies in humans, animals, and in vitro systems regarding the effect of e-cigarette exposure and respiratory symptoms. This adverse effect on respiratory symptoms is likely associated with an increase in cellular inflammation and oxidative stress and decreased cough reflexes and MCC. The observation that past e-cigarette use was associated with an increase in chronic bronchitic symptoms in adolescents and an increase in school absenteeism from asthma symptoms in current e-cigarette users is potentially concerning since a more rapid decline in lung function in later life has been linked to asthma and chronic bronchitis in early life (Bernal et al., 1989; Vestbo and Lange, 2016). In addition, there is limited evidence to indicate that e-cigarette substitution for tobacco product use in established smokers is associated with a decrease in cellular oxidative stress and improved respiratory symptoms and lung function.

Conclusion 11-1. There is ***no available evidence*** *whether or not e-cigarettes cause respiratory diseases in humans.*

Conclusion 11-2. There is ***limited evidence*** *for improvement in lung function and respiratory symptoms among adult smokers with asthma who switch to e-cigarettes completely or in part (dual use).*

*Conclusion 11-3. There is **limited evidence** for reduction of chronic obstructive pulmonary disease (COPD) exacerbations among adult smokers with COPD who switch to e-cigarettes completely or in part (dual use).*

*Conclusion 11-4. There is **moderate evidence** for increased cough and wheeze in adolescents who use e-cigarettes and an association with e-cigarette use and an increase in asthma exacerbations.*

*Conclusion 11-5. There is **limited evidence** of adverse effects of e-cigarette exposure on the respiratory system from animal and in vitro studies.*

VULNERABLE/SUSCEPTIBLE POPULATIONS

Chronic Obstructive Pulmonary Disease

Despite a number of studies, the results are unclear about whether use of e-cigarettes as a substitute for combustible tobacco use in people with COPD may be beneficial, neutral, or harmful. Harm may occur if e-cigarette use prevents the smoker from quitting entirely and instead prolongs the use of combustible tobacco products through dual use. Harm may also occur in an individual with COPD if single use of an e-cigarette as a substitute for combustible tobacco cigarettes causes additional airway inflammation in already damaged lungs. No studies have examined whether e-cigarette use alone can cause lower respiratory tract (LRT) inflammation in healthy adults or increase or decrease existing LRT inflammation in adults with COPD. If the use of e-cigarettes by a smoker with COPD can reduce use of combustible tobacco products and can decrease lung inflammation secondary to the reduction of exposure to toxicants found in combustible tobacco smoke but not e-cigarettes, this could be beneficial to the patients with COPD. In addition, individuals with COPD who failed or who are resistant to conventional NRT or other cessation strategies may be more willing to use e-cigarettes to quit smoking.

Asthma and Other Respiratory Diseases of Childhood

Asthma is one of the most common chronic respiratory diseases in the United States and is prevalent in young children and adolescents. In recent years since the introduction of e-cigarettes in the United States, substantial numbers of adolescents have tried and have used e-cigarettes (Backinger, 2017; HHS, 2016; Jamal et al., 2017; Kann et al., 2016; Miech et al., 2017).

Recent longitudinal studies have shown that children with asthma may have an accelerated decline in lung function as they age (Martinez, 2016). Smoking and other environmental exposures, including air pollution, can increase severity of asthma symptoms and these exposures have been associated with a more rapid decline in lung function in children (Gautier and Charpin, 2017; Schultz et al., 2017; Vanker et al., 2017). An area that remains unclear is if e-cigarette use can cause neutrophilic inflammation, similar to that which can be found in the asthmatic smoker and the smoker with COPD (Andelid et al., 2015; Siew et al., 2017). If so, then e-cigarette use by people with asthma may further exacerbate lower airway inflammation regardless of whether their asthma phenotype is predominately allergic or neutrophilic in origin. As discussed above, adolescents with asthma—a disease characterized by reversible airway obstruction—who use e-cigarettes may be more likely to have an increase in respiratory symptoms and exacerbations compared with adolescent non-users, as indicated by one cross-sectional study (Cho and Paik, 2016).

Cystic Fibrosis

Children and adolescents with other respiratory diseases who use e-cigarettes may also be at increased risk for worsening of respiratory symptoms. CF and primary ciliary dyskinesia (PCD) are respiratory diseases also characterized by lower respiratory tract neutrophilic inflammation. In the United States, the carrier frequency of CF mutations is 1/36, with whites having a carrier rate of 1/27 and African Americans with a carrier rate of 1/79 (Zvereff et al., 2014). It is unclear whether adolescents with CF or PCD would be more likely to try e-cigarettes if they perceive them to be less harmful than combustible tobacco cigarettes.

Nicotine alone has been shown to cause dysregulation of the CFTR chloride channel in the airways in animal studies, causing impaired airway MCC (Maouche et al., 2013). Another study found an association between secondhand smoke exposure in children with CF and lower FEV1 and weight percentile (Ong et al., 2017). Nicotine exposure from e-cigarette use could potentially cause a higher rate of respiratory symptoms in CF carriers if nicotine causes dysregulation of CFTR in the airways.

Preterm Infants

Exposure to nicotine in utero may have long-lasting negative effects on lung function in vulnerable populations such as preterm infants. Recently, maternal smoking during pregnancy has been associated with the development of bronchopulmonary dysplasia and later respiratory morbidities in preterm infants (Morrow et al., 2017). No studies have examined the respiratory health effects of e-cigarettes on the preterm infants of mothers who used e-cigarettes during pregnancy.

REFERENCES

Andelid, K., A. Andersson, S. Yoshihara, C. Ahren, P. Jirholt, A. Ekberg-Jansson, and A. Linden. 2015. Systemic signs of neutrophil mobilization during clinically stable periods and during exacerbations in smokers with obstructive pulmonary disease. *International Journal of Chronic Obstructive Pulmonary Disease* 10:1253–1263.

Backinger, C. L. 2017. *Youth use of electronic cigarettes.* http://c.ymcdn.com/sites/www.srnt.org/resource/resmgr/conferences/2017_annual_meeting/FDA_PreCon_Slides/Backinger_youth_e-cig_SRNT20.pdf (accessed September 18, 2017).

Bernal, J. E., P. Sarmiento, I. Briceno, and S. S. Papiha. 1989. Polymorphism of serum proteins (C3, BF, HP and TF) of six populations in Colombia. *Human Hereditary* 39(2):94–98.

Campagna, D., F. Cibella, P. Caponnetto, M. D. Amaradio, M. Caruso, J. B. Morjaria, M. Malerba, and R. Polosa. 2016. Changes in breathomics from a 1-year randomized smoking cessation trial of electronic cigarettes. *European Journal of Clinical Investigation* 46(8):698–706.

Chatwin, M., E. Ross, N. Hart, A. H. Nickol, M. I. Polkey, and A. K. Simonds. 2003. Cough augmentation with mechanical insufflation/exsufflation in patients with neuromuscular weakness. *European Respiratory Journal* 21(3):502–508.

Cho, J. H., and S. Y. Paik. 2016. Association between electronic cigarette use and asthma among high school students in South Korea. *PLoS ONE* 11(3):e0151022. http://journals.plos.org/plosone/article?id=10.1371/journal.pone.0151022 (accessed January 31, 2018).

Choi, K., and D. Bernat. 2016. E-cigarette use among Florida youth with and without asthma. *American Journal of Preventive Medicine* 51(4):446–453.

Cibella, F., D. Campagna, P. Caponnetto, M. D. Amaradio, M. Caruso, C. Russo, D. W. Cockcroft, and R. Polosa. 2016. Lung function and respiratory symptoms in a randomized smoking cessation trial of electronic cigarettes. *Clinical Science* 130(21):1929–1937.

Cravo, A. S., J. Bush, G. Sharma, R. Savioz, C. Martin, S. Craige, and T. Walele. 2016. A randomised, parallel group study to evaluate the safety profile of an electronic vapour product over 12 weeks. *Regulatory Toxicology and Pharmacology* 81:S01-S14.

Davenport, P. W., A. Vovk, R. K. Duke, D. C. Bolser, and E. Robertson. 2009. The urge-to-cough and cough motor response modulation by the central effects of nicotine. *Pulmonary Pharmacology and Therapeutics* 22(2):82–89.

den Dekker, H. T., A. Voort, J. C. de Jongste, I. K. Reiss, A. Hofman, V. W. V. Jaddoe, and L. Duijts. 2015. Tobacco smoke exposure, airway resistance, and asthma in school-age children: The Generation R study. *Chest* 148(3):607–617.

Diao, W., N. Shen, Y. Du, K. Qian, and B. He. 2017. Characterization of throat microbial flora in smokers with or without COPD. *International Journal of Chronic Obstructive Pulmonary Disease* 12:1933–1946.

Dicpinigaitis, P. V. 2017. Effect of tobacco and electronic cigarette use on cough reflex sensitivity. *Pulmonary Pharmacology and Therapeutics* 47:45–48.

Dicpinigaitis, P. V., B. Sitkauskiene, K. Stravinskaite, D. W. Appel, A. Negassa, and R. Sakalauskas. 2006. Effect of smoking cessation on cough reflex sensitivity. *European Respiratory Journal* 28(4):786–790.

Dicpinigaitis, P. V., A. L. Chang, A. J. Dicpinigaitis, and A. Negassa. 2016a. Effect of e-cigarette use on cough reflex sensitivity. *Chest* 149(1):161–165.

Dicpinigaitis, P. V., A. L. Chang, A. J. Dicpinigaitis, and A. Negassa. 2016b. Effect of electronic cigarette use on the urge-to-cough sensation. *Nicotine & Tobacco Research* 18(8):1763–1765.

D'Ruiz, C. D., G. O'Connell, D. W. Graff, and X. S. Yan. 2017. Measurement of cardiovascular and pulmonary function endpoints and other physiological effects following partial or complete substitution of cigarettes with electronic cigarettes in adult smokers. *Regulatory Toxicology and Pharmacology* 87:36–53.

Duijts, L., V. W. V. Jaddoe, R. J. P. van der Valk, J. A. Henderson, A. Hofman, H. Raat, E. A. P. Steegers, H. A. Moll, and J. C. de Jongste. 2012. Fetal exposure to maternal and paternal smoking and the risks of wheezing in preschool children: The Generation R study. *Chest* 141(4):876–885.

Ferrari, M., A. Zanasi, E. Nardi, A. M. M. Labate, P. Ceriana, A. Balestrino, L. Pisani, N. Corcione, and S. Nava. 2015. Short-term effects of a nicotine-free e-cigarette compared to a traditional cigarette in smokers and non-smokers. *BMC Pulmonary Medicine* 15(1):120.

Garcia-Arcos, I., P. Geraghty, N. Baumlin, M. Campos, A. J. Dabo, B. Jundi, N. Cummins, E. Eden, A. Grosche, M. Salathe, and R. Foronjy. 2016. Chronic electronic cigarette exposure in mice induces features of COPD in a nicotine-dependent manner. *Thorax* 71(12):1119–1129.

Gautier, C., and D. Charpin. 2017. Environmental triggers and avoidance in the management of asthma. *Journal of Asthma and Allergy* 10:47–56.

Geiss, O., I. Bianchi, F. Barahona, and J. Barrero-Moreno. 2015. Characterisation of mainstream and passive vapours emitted by selected electronic cigarettes. *International Journal of Hygiene and Environmental Health* 218(1):169–180.

Hayatbakhsh, M. R., S. Sadasivam, A. A. Mamun, J. M. Najman, G. M. Williams, and M. J. O'Callaghan. 2009. Maternal smoking during and after pregnancy and lung function in early adulthood: A prospective study. *Thorax* 64(9):810–814.

He, Q. Q., T. W. Wong, L. Du, Z. Q. Jiang, T. S. Yu, H. Qiu, Y. Gao, A. H. Wong, W. J. Liu, and J. G. Wu. 2011. Environmental tobacco smoke exposure and Chinese schoolchildren's respiratory health: A prospective cohort study. *American Journal of Preventive Medicine* 41(5):487–493.

HHS (U.S. Department of Health and Human Services). 2016. *E-cigarette use among youth and young adults: A report of the Surgeon General*. Atlanta, GA: U.S. Department of Health and Human Services, Centers for Disease Control and Prevention, National Center for Chronic Disease Prevention and Health Promotion, Office on Smoking and Health.

Husari, A., A. Shihadeh, S. Talih, Y. Hashem, M. El Sabban, and G. Zaatari. 2016. Acute exposure to electronic and combustible cigarette aerosols: Effects in an animal model and in human alveolar cells. *Nicotine & Tobacco Research* 18(5):613–619.

Hwang, J. H., M. Lyes, K. Sladewski, S. Enany, E. McEachern, D. P. Mathew, S. Das, A. Moshensky, S. Bapat, D. T. Pride, W. M. Ongkeko, and L. E. C. Alexander. 2016. Electronic cigarette inhalation alters innate immunity and airway cytokines while increasing the virulence of colonizing bacteria. *Journal of Molecular Medicine* 94(6):667–679.

Jamal, A., A. Gentzke, S. Hu, K. A. Cullen, B. J. Apelberg, D. M. Homa, and B. A. King. 2017. Tobacco use among middle and high school students—United States, 2011–2016. *Morbidity and Mortality Weekly Report* 66(23):597–603.

Jayes, L., P. L. Haslam, C. G. Gratziou, P. Powell, J. Britton, C. Vardavas, C. Jimenez-Ruiz, J. Leonardi-Bee, and Tobacco Control Committee of the European Respiratory Society. 2016. Smokehaz: Systematic reviews and meta-analyses of the effects of smoking on respiratory health. *Chest* 150(1):164–179.

Kalliola, S., A. S. Pelkonen, L. P. Malmberg, S. Sarna, M. Hamalainen, I. Mononen, and M. J. Makela. 2013. Maternal smoking affects lung function and airway inflammation in young children with multiple-trigger wheeze. *Journal of Allergy and Clinical Immunology* 131(3):730–735.

Kann, L., T. McManus, W. A. Harris, S. L. Shanklin, K. H. Flint, J. Hawkins, B. Queen, R. Lowry, E. O. Olsen, D. Chyen, L. Whittle, J. Thornton, C. Lim, Y. Yamakawa, N. Brener, and S. Zaza. 2016. Youth risk behavior surveillance—United States, 2015. *Morbidity and Mortality Weekly Report* 65(6):1–174.

Korten, I., M. Liechti, F. Singer, G. Hafen, I. Rochat, P. Anagnostopoulou, D. Müller-Suter, J. Usemann, A. Moeller, U. Frey, P. Latzin, and C. Casaulta. 2018. Lower exhaled nitric oxide in infants with cystic fibrosis compared to healthy controls. *Journal of Cystic Fibrosis* 17(1):105–108.

Kumral, T. L., Z. Salturk, G. Yildirim, Y. Uyar, G. Berkiten, Y. Atar, and M. Inan. 2016. How does electronic cigarette smoking affect sinonasal symptoms and nasal mucociliary clearance? *B-ENT* 12(1):17–21.

Larcombe, A. N., M. A. Janka, B. J. Mullins, L. J. Berry, A. Bredin, and P. J. Franklin. 2017. The effects of electronic cigarette aerosol exposure on inflammation and lung function in mice. *American Journal of Physiology—Lung Cellular and Molecular Physiology* 313(1):L67–L79.

Laube, B. L., N. Afshar-Mohajer, K. Koehler, G. Chen, P. Lazarus, J. M. Collaco, and S. A. McGrath-Morrow. 2017. Acute and chronic in vivo effects of exposure to nicotine and propylene glycol from an e-cigarette on mucociliary clearance in a murine model. *Inhalation Toxicology* 29(5):197–205.

Lee, A. L., B. M. Button, and E. L. Tannenbaum. 2017. Airway-clearance techniques in children and adolescents with chronic suppurative lung disease and bronchiectasis. *Frontiers of Pediatrics* 5:2. https://www.frontiersin.org/articles/10.3389/fped.2017.00002/full (accessed January 31, 2018).

Lerner, C. A., I. K. Sundar, H. Yao, J. Gerloff, D. J. Ossip, S. McIntosh, R. Robinson, and I. Rahman. 2015. Vapors produced by electronic cigarettes and e-juices with flavorings induce toxicity, oxidative stress, and inflammatory response in lung epithelial cells and in mouse lung. *PLoS ONE* 10(2):e0116732. http://journals.plos.org/plosone/article?id=10.1371/journal.pone.0116732 (accessed January 31, 2018).

Levanen, B., P. Glader, B. Dahlen, B. Billing, I. Qvarfordt, L. Palmberg, K. Larsson, and A. Linden. 2016. Impact of tobacco smoking on cytokine signaling via interleukin-17A in the peripheral airways. *International Journal of Chronic Obstructive Pulmonary Disease* 11:2109–2116.

Li, N., S. Georas, N. Alexis, P. Fritz, T. Xia, M. A. Williams, E. Horner, and A. Nel. 2016. A work group report on ultrafine particles (American Academy of Allergy, Asthma & Immunology): Why ambient ultrafine and engineered nanoparticles should receive special attention for possible adverse health outcomes in human subjects. *Journal of Allergy and Clinical Immunology* 138(2):386–396.

Lim, H. B., and S. H. Kim. 2014. Inhalation of e-cigarette cartridge solution aggravates allergen-induced airway inflammation and hyper-responsiveness in mice. *Toxicological Research* 30(1):13–18.

Liu, A. H., D. C. Babineau, R. Z. Krouse, E. M. Zoratti, J. A. Pongracic, G. T. O'Connor, R. A. Wood, G. K. Khurana Hershey, C. M. Kercsmar, R. S. Gruchalla, M. Kattan, S. J. Teach, M. Makhija, D. Pillai, C. I. Lamm, J. E. Gern, S. M. Sigelman, P. J. Gergen, A. Togias, C. M. Visness, and W. W. Busse. 2016. Pathways through which asthma risk factors contribute to asthma severity in inner-city children. *Journal of Allergy and Clinical Immunology* 138(4):1042–1050.

Malinovschi, A., V. Backer, H. Harving, and C. Porsbjerg. 2012. The value of exhaled nitric oxide to identify asthma in smoking patients with asthma-like symptoms. *Respiratory Medicine* 106(6):794–801.

Maouche, K., K. Medjber, J. M. Zahm, F. Delavoie, C. Terryn, C. Coraux, S. Pons, I. Cloez-Tayarani, U. Maskos, P. Birembaut, and J. M. Tournier. 2013. Contribution of α7 nicotinic receptor to airway epithelium dysfunction under nicotine exposure. *Proceedings of the National Academy of Sciences of the United States of America* 110(10):4099–4104.

Martinez, F. D. 2016. Early-life origins of chronic obstructive pulmonary disease. *New England Journal of Medicine* 375(9):871–878.

McConnell, R., J. L. Barrington-Trimis, K. Wang, R. Urman, H. Hong, J. Unger, J. Samet, A. Leventhal, and K. Berhane. 2017. Electronic cigarette use and respiratory symptoms in adolescents. *American Journal of Respiratory and Critical Care Medicine* 195(8):1043–1049.

McGrath-Morrow, S. A., M. Hayashi, A. Aherrera, A. Lopez, A. Malinina, J. M. Collaco, E. Neptune, J. D. Klein, J. P. Winickoff, P. Breysse, P. Lazarus, and G. Chen. 2015. The effects of electronic cigarette emissions on systemic cotinine levels, weight and postnatal lung growth in neonatal mice. *PLoS ONE* 10(2):e0118344. http://journals.plos.org/plosone/article?id=10.1371/journal.pone.0118344 (accessed January 31, 2018).

Merianos, A. L., C. A. Dixon, and E. M. Mahabee-Gittens. 2016. Secondhand smoke exposure, illness severity, and resource utilization in pediatric emergency department patients with respiratory illnesses. *Journal of Asthma* 54(8):798–806.

Messerli, M., T. Ottilinger, R. Warschkow, S. Leschka, H. Alkadhi, S. Wildermuth, and R. W. Bauer. 2017. Emphysema quantification and lung volumetry in chest x-ray equivalent ultralow dose CT—intra-individual comparison with standard dose CT. *European Journal of Radiology* 91:1–9.

Miech, R., M. E. Patrick, P. M. O'Malley, and L. D. Johnston. 2017. What are kids vaping? Results from a national survey of U.S. adolescents. *Tobacco Control* 26(4):386–391.

Morrow, L. A., B. D. Wagner, D. A. Ingram, B. B. Poindexter, K. Schibler, C. M. Cotten, J. Dagle, M. K. Sontag, P. M. Mourani, and S. H. Abman. 2017. Antenatal determinants of bronchopulmonary dysplasia and late respiratory disease in preterm infants. *American Journal of Respiratory and Critical Care Medicine* 196(3):364–374.

Ong, T., M. Schechter, J. Yang, L. Peng, J. Emerson, R. L. Gibson, W. Morgan, M. Rosenfeld, and E. S. Group. 2017. Socioeconomic status, smoke exposure, and health outcomes in young children with cystic fibrosis. *Pediatrics* 139(2). http://pediatrics.aappublications.org/content/139/2/e20162730.long (accessed January 31, 2018).

Polosa, R., J. Morjaria, P. Caponnetto, M. Caruso, S. Strano, E. Battaglia, and C. Russo. 2014a. Effect of smoking abstinence and reduction in asthmatic smokers switching to electronic cigarettes: Evidence for harm reversal. *International Journal of Environmental Research and Public Health* 11(5):4965–4977.

Polosa, R., J. B. Morjaria, P. Caponnetto, D. Campagna, C. Russo, A. Alamo, M. D. Amaradio, and A. Fisichella. 2014b. Effectiveness and tolerability of electronic cigarette in real-life: A 24-month prospective observational study. *Internal and Emergency Medicine* 9(5):537–546.

Polosa, R., J. B. Morjaria, P. Caponnetto, M. Caruso, D. Campagna, M. D. Amaradio, G. Ciampi, C. Russo, and A. Fisichella. 2016a. Persisting long term benefits of smoking abstinence and reduction in asthmatic smokers who have switched to electronic cigarettes. *Discovery Medicine* 21(114):99–108.

Polosa, R., J. B. Morjaria, P. Caponnetto, U. Prosperini, C. Russo, A. Pennisi, and C. M. Bruno. 2016b. Evidence for harm reduction in COPD smokers who switch to electronic cigarettes. *Respiratory Research* 17(1):116.

Puhan, M. A., I. Soesilo, G. H. Guyatt, and H. J. Schunemann. 2006. Combining scores from different patient reported outcome measures in meta-analyses: When is it justified? *Health and Quality of Life Outcomes* 4:94. https://hqlo.biomedcentral.com/articles/10.1186/1477-7525-4-94 (accessed January 31, 2018).

Rabe, K. F., and H. Watz. 2017. Chronic obstructive pulmonary disease. *Lancet* 389(10082): 1931–1940.

Saadeh, C., B. Cross, M. Gaylor, and M. Griffith. 2015. Advantage of impulse oscillometry over spirometry to diagnose chronic obstructive pulmonary disease and monitor pulmonary responses to bronchodilators: An observational study. *SAGE Open Medicine* 3:2050312115578957. https://www.ncbi.nlm.nih.gov/pmc/articles/PMC4679284 (accessed January 31, 2018).

Saint-Criq, V., and M. A. Gray. 2017. Role of CFTR in epithelial physiology. *Cellular and Molecular Life Sciences* 74(1):93–115.

Salturk, Z., C. Cakir, G. Sunnetci, Y. Atar, T. L. Kumral, G. Yildirim, G. Berkiten, and Y. Uyar. 2015. Effects of electronic nicotine delivery system on larynx: Experimental study. *Journal of Voice* 29(5):560–563.

Schultz, E. S., A. A. Litonjua, and E. Melen. 2017. Effects of long-term exposure to traffic-related air pollution on lung function in children. *Current Allergy and Asthma Reports* 17(6):41.

Shargorodsky, J. 2016. Secondhand smoke and rhinitis. *Current Opinion in Otolaryngology and Head and Neck Surgery* 24(3):241–244.

Shargorodsky, J., E. Garcia-Esquinas, I. Galan, A. Navas-Acien, and S. Y. Lin. 2015. Allergic sensitization, rhinitis and tobacco smoke exposure in U.S. adults. *PLoS ONE* 10(7):e0131957. http://journals.plos.org/plosone/article?id=10.1371/journal.pone.0131957 (accessed January 31, 2018).

Shields, P. G., M. Berman, T. M. Brasky, J. L. Freudenheim, E. Mathe, J. P. McElroy, M. A. Song, and M. D. Wewers. 2017. A review of pulmonary toxicity of electronic cigarettes in the context of smoking: A focus on inflammation. *Cancer Epidemiology, Biomarkers & Prevention* 26(8):1175–1191.

Siew, L. Q. C., S. Y. Wu, S. Ying, and C. J. Corrigan. 2017. Cigarette smoking increases bronchial mucosal IL-17A expression in asthmatics, which acts in concert with environmental aeroallergens to engender neutrophilic inflammation. *Clinical & Experimental Allergy* 47(6):740–750.

Sitkauskiene, B., and P. V. Dicpinigaitis. 2010. Effect of smoking on cough reflex sensitivity in humans. *Lung* 188(Supplement):S29–S32.

Sussan, T. E., S. Gajghate, R. K. Thimmulappa, J. Ma, J. H. Kim, K. Sudini, N. Consolini, S. A. Cormier, S. Lomnicki, F. Hasan, A. Pekosz, and S. Biswal. 2015. Exposure to electronic cigarettes impairs pulmonary anti-bacterial and anti-viral defenses in a mouse model. *PLoS ONE* 10(2):e0116861. http://dx.plos.org/10.1371/journal.pone.0116861 (accessed January 31, 2018).

Tarrant, B. J., C. Le Maitre, L. Romero, R. Steward, B. M. Button, B. R. Thompson, and A. E. Holland. 2017. Mucoactive agents for chronic, non-cystic fibrosis lung disease: A systematic review and meta-analysis. *Respirology* 22(6):1084–1092.

Torén, K., M. Palmqvist, O. Löwhagen, B. Balder, and A. Tunsäter. 2006. Self-reported asthma was biased in relation to disease severity while reported year of asthma onset was accurate. *Journal of Clinical Epidemiology* 59(1):90–93.

Vanker, A., R. P. Gie, and H. J. Zar. 2017. The association between environmental tobacco smoke exposure and childhood respiratory disease: A review. *Expert Review of Respiratory Medicine* 11(8):661–673.

Vardavas, C. I., N. Anagnostopoulos, M. Kougias, V. Evangelopoulou, G. N. Connolly, and P. K. Behrakis. 2012. Short-term pulmonary effects of using an electronic cigarette: Impact on respiratory flow resistance, impedance, and exhaled nitric oxide. *Chest* 141(6):1400–1406.

Vestbo, J., and P. Lange. 2016. Natural history of COPD: Focusing on change in FEV1. *Respirology* 21(1):34–43.

Wang, M. P., S. Y. Ho, L. T. Leung, and T. H. Lam. 2016. Electronic cigarette use and respiratory symptoms in Chinese adolescents in Hong Kong. *JAMA Pediatrics* 170(1):89–91.

Washko, G. R., G. Parraga, and H. O. Coxson. 2012. Quantitative pulmonary imaging using computed tomography and magnetic resonance imaging. *Respirology* 17(3):432–444.

Werley, M. S., D. J. Kirkpatrick, M. J. Oldham, A. M. Jerome, T. B. Langston, P. D. Lilly, D. C. Smith, and W. J. McKinney. 2016. Toxicological assessment of a prototype e-cigarette device and three flavor formulations: A 90-day inhalation study in rats. *Inhalation Toxicology* 28(1):22–38.

Wilson, K. M., J. C. Pier, S. C. Wesgate, J. M. Cohen, and A. K. Blumkin. 2013. Secondhand tobacco smoke exposure and severity of influenza in hospitalized children. *JAMA Pediatrics* 162(1):16–21.

Yanagita, M., R. Kobayashi, Y. Kojima, K. Mori, and S. Murakami. 2012. Nicotine modulates the immunological function of dendritic cells through peroxisome proliferator-activated receptor-gamma upregulation. *Cellular Immunology* 274(1–2):26–33.

Zvereff, V. V., H. Faruki, M. Edwards, and K. J. Friedman. 2014. Cystic fibrosis carrier screening in a North American population. *Genetics in Medicine* 16(7):539–546.

12

Oral Diseases

Smoking is a significant risk factor for the development of periodontal disease. This is a plaque-induced inflammatory disease of the mouth characterized by the presence of gum recession, loss of periodontal ligaments, bone resorption, and loss of teeth (Gross et al., 2017). The global prevalence of severe periodontitis in 2010 was between 10.1 and 11.6 percent of the world's population, affecting approximately 743 million people worldwide (Kassebaum et al., 2014). Pathogenic bacteria in the mouth contribute to the development and severity of periodontitis (Chahboun et al., 2015).

Tobacco smoke can alter the oral microbiota, leading to more severe periodontal disease in the smoker (Coretti et al., 2017). Souto and colleagues (2014a) reported suppression of immune responses in smokers, leading to more severe periodontal disease. In another study by Souto and colleagues (2014b), higher levels of CCL3 and CXCL8 were found in people with more severe periodontitis. Host characteristics have also been shown to contribute to the aggressiveness of periodontal disease, resulting in subsets of people who are at highest risk for developing a rapid form of progressive periodontal disease (Nibali, 2015). Few studies have examined the impact of e-cigarette use on periodontal disease. Emerging research suggests that switching to e-cigarettes may improve periodontal disease in smokers (Tatullo et al., 2016). Other studies indicate that e-cigarette use may have a detrimental effect on gingival health in smokers who switched to e-cigarettes (Wadia et al., 2016).

CHARACTERIZATION OF DISEASE ENDPOINTS AND INTERMEDIATE OUTCOMES

In studying the effects of e-cigarette use on oral health, development and severity of periodontal disease should be a primary disease endpoint. The presence and status of periodontal disease in people who smoke tobacco should be compared with people who use e-cigarettes to quit or reduce smoking. In addition, the presence and status of periodontal disease in adolescents and adults who use e-cigarettes, but who were never smokers should be compared with age-matched people who never used e-cigarettes or smoked. Intermediate outcomes to assess presence and severity of periodontitis should include indexes that are used to diagnose periodontitis and to determine severity of periodontitis. These include bleeding after probing, plaque index, quantification of gingival crevicular fluid, gum recession, bone resorption, and tooth loss. Measurements of gingival cytokines and subgingival microbiota should be used to determine the impact of e-cigarette aerosols on immune responses that impact oral health.

OPTIMAL STUDY DESIGN

The optimal study design to address potential benefits and harms of e-cigarettes on oral health would be a randomized controlled study. Such studies assess whether e-cigarette substitution can attenuate severity of periodontal disease in smokers unable to quit using standard nicotine replacement therapy. Observational studies also are needed to address the long-term effects on the oral health of adolescents and young adults who initiate e-cigarette use and to determine if e-cigarette aerosol can increase prevalence of periodontal disease in non-smokers. Studies are also needed that investigate the effects of e-cigarette aerosols on the microbiota of the oral cavity, the immune responses of the gingiva, and other markers of inflammation.

QUESTIONS ADDRESSED BY THE LITERATURE

Because e-cigarettes are so new, there is a lack of rigorously designed studies examining the effects of e-cigarettes on oral health.

STUDIES IN HUMANS (CLINICAL AND EPIDEMIOLOGICAL)

A study from Javed and colleagues (2017) examined the dental health of three groups of adult men from Saudi Arabia. These groups consisted of men who smoked combustible tobacco cigarettes (group 1), men who smoked e-cigarettes exclusively (group 2), and men who were non-smokers (group 3). The men who smoked cigarettes had a significantly higher plaque index and probing depth than men in group 2 or group 3. The men in group 1 also reported more gum pain compared with individuals in groups 2 ($p < 0.01$) and 3 ($p < 0.01$). This finding suggested poorer dental health in the men who smoked combustible tobacco cigarettes. However, limitations to the study may confound these comparisons because the men in group 1 smoked for a mean of 5.4 years whereas men in group 2 used e-cigarettes for an average of 2.2 years, and the men in group 1 were exposed to higher daily nicotine levels.

Tatullo and colleagues (2016) conducted a clinical observational pilot study involving 110 smokers who reported that they had switched to e-cigarettes. A small subset of subjects had carbon monoxide (CO) levels measured to assess whether they were smoking during the study. Of the 22 out of 110 subjects tested, most were found to have CO levels consistent with very light combustible tobacco smoking. Smokers were divided into two groups, according to the number of years each group smoked: group 1 (less than 10 years of combustible tobacco cigarette smoking) and group 2 (more than 10 years of combustible tobacco cigarette smoking). Patients were subjected to oral examinations to investigate the following parameters: plaque index, bleeding index, and papillary bleeding index. A questionnaire to self-assess the variations of some parameters of general health and to self-assess the need to smoke combustible tobacco cigarettes was distributed to the subjects involved in the study. At the end of this pilot study, it was noted that the subjects had progressive improvement in the periodontal indexes, as well as in their general health perception. This study suggests a beneficial effect on the oral health of smokers who switch to e-cigarette use.

Reuther and colleagues (2016) performed a pilot study investigating the effect of nicotine and non-nicotine e-cigarette aerosols on blood flow in the buccal mucosa in 10 volunteers after 5 minutes of e-cigarette use. They used a laser Doppler probe at 5-minute intervals after 5 minutes of e-cigarette use and found a small but significant rise ($p = 0.008$) in blood flow in the buccal mucosa. In the volunteers that used the nicotine-containing e-cigarettes, flow fell to the same levels as before within 30 minutes.

Finally, a pilot study by Wadia and colleagues (2016) examined the gingival health in 20 established smokers before and after substituting e-cigarettes for combustible tobacco cigarettes for 2 weeks. The primary outcome measurement of gingival inflammation was bleeding on probing. Levels of selected pro-inflammatory cytokines in gingival crevicular fluid, saliva, and serum samples were also determined. There was a statistically significant increase in gingival inflammation when combustible tobacco smokers switched from smoking to e-cigarette use for 2 weeks.

This study, although a pilot study, suggested that e-cigarette use in smokers who switched caused more gingival inflammation when compared with the gingival inflammation at baseline in smokers.

IN VITRO STUDIES

Ji and colleagues (2016) reported increased cytotoxicity in normal human oral keratinocytes exposed to different nicotine concentrations. They concluded that toxicity in their study was due in part to oxidative stress induced by toxic substances from the nanoparticles and chemicals present in the e-cigarette aerosols. They reported increased oxidative stress in the cells exposed to the e-cigarette aerosols as characterized by a significant decrease in intracellular glutathione levels and adenosine triphosphate (ATP). A decline in intracellular ATP levels has been associated with a decrease in cell proliferation and cell death (Henrich and Buckler, 2008). Rouabhia and colleagues (2016) used primary human gingival epithelial cells retrieved from healthy non-smoking donors. Cells were grown and exposed to nicotine-containing e-cigarette aerosols. The investigators found increased apoptotic/necrotic epithelial cell percentages compared with that observed in the control. Sancilio and colleagues (2016) used gingival fibroblasts exposed to nicotine and non-nicotine e-cigarette aerosols. They found peaked reactive oxygen species production after 24 hours, by measurements of CM-H_2DCFDA oxidation, higher Bax expression at 24 hours, and increased apoptosis after 48 hours post-exposure in both nicotine- and non-nicotine–containing e-cigarette aerosols. Sundar and colleagues (2016) exposed human periodontal ligament fibroblast to nicotine-containing e-cigarette aerosols and non-nicotine, menthol-flavored e-cigarettes and found, using a human 3-D model of EpiGingival tissues, that both nicotine and non-nicotine menthol-flavored e-cigarette aerosols caused increased inflammation and DNA damage. Willershausen and colleagues (2014) examined the effects of nicotine and various flavorings on cell viability and proliferation of human periodontal ligament fibroblasts. They found decreased cell proliferation rates and a decrease in ATP detection in cells incubated with nicotine and with various e-cigarette flavorings when compared with control cells. Menthol e-cigarette solutions also caused a decrease in fibroblast proliferation.

Taken together these in vitro studies suggest a detrimental effect of nicotine and flavorings contained in e-cigarette aerosols on cell viability of epithelial and fibroblast cells in culture. These studies indicate that e-cigarette aerosols may cause harm to cells in the oral cavity, which in turn may contribute to poor oral health. In addition, several of these studies suggest that menthol flavorings can cause additional harm to cells by impairing cell migration and inducing cell inflammation and DNA damage.

SYNTHESIS

Taken together, human studies and in vitro studies suggest that e-cigarette aerosols can cause harm to oral health by inducing gingival inflammation in the oral cavity. In vitro studies indicate that e-cigarette aerosols can cause direct cell death and DNA damage to epithelial cells. Other studies comparing and contrasting the dental health of smokers to e-cigarette users suggest that e-cigarette use may be less harmful to oral health than continued smoking of combustible tobacco cigarettes.

Finding: There are no epidemiological studies examining the associations between e-cigarette use and incidence or progression of periodontal disease.

*Conclusion 12-1. There is **limited evidence** suggesting that switching to e-cigarettes will improve periodontal disease in smokers.*

*Conclusion 12-2. There is **limited evidence** suggesting that nicotine- and non-nicotine–containing e-cigarette aerosol can adversely affect cell viability and cause cell damage in oral tissue in non-smokers.*

REFERENCES

Chahboun, H., M. M. Arnau, D. Herrera, M. Sanz, and O. K. Ennibi. 2015. Bacterial profile of aggressive periodontitis in Morocco: A cross-sectional study. *BMC Oral Health* 15:25. https://doi.org/10.1186/s12903-015-0006-x (accessed February 6, 2018).

Coretti, L., M. Cuomo, E. Florio, D. Palumbo, S. Keller, R. Pero, L. Chiariotti, F. Lembo, and C. Cafiero. 2017. Subgingival dysbiosis in smoker and nonsmoker patients with chronic periodontitis. *Molecular Medicine Reports* 15(4):2007–2014.

Gross, A. J., K. T. Paskett, V. J. Cheever, and M. S. Lipsky. 2017. Periodontitis: A global disease and the primary care provider's role. *Postgraduate Medical Journal* 93(1103):560–565.

Henrich, M., and K. J. Buckler. 2008. Effects of anoxia, aglycemia, and acidosis on cytosolic Mg^{2+}, ATP, and pH in rat sensory neurons. *American Journal of Physiology—Cell Physiology* 294(1):C280–C294.

Javed, F., T. Abduljabbar, F. Vohra, H. Malmstrom, I. Rahman, and G. E. Romanos. 2017. Comparison of periodontal parameters and self-perceived oral symptoms among cigarette smokers, individuals vaping electronic cigarettes, and never-smokers. *Journal of Periodontology* 88(10):1059–1065.

Ji, E. H., B. B. Sun, T. K. Zhao, S. Shu, C. H. Chang, D. Messadi, T. Xia, Y. F. Zhu, and S. Hu. 2016. Characterization of electronic cigarette aerosol and its induction of oxidative stress response in oral keratinocytes. *PLoS ONE* 11(5):e0154447. https://doi.org/10.1371/journal.pone.0154447 (accessed February 6, 2018).

Kassebaum, N. J., E. Bernabe, M. Dahiya, B. Bhandari, C. J. Murray, and W. Marcenes. 2014. Global burden of severe periodontitis in 1990–2010: A systematic review and meta-regression. *Journal of Dental Research* 93(11):1045–1053.

Nibali, L. 2015. Aggressive periodontitis: Microbes and host response, who to blame? *Virulence* 6(3):223–228.

Reuther, W. J., B. Hale, J. Matharu, J. N. Blythe, and P. A. Brennan. 2016. Do you mind if I vape? Immediate effects of electronic cigarettes on perfusion in buccal mucosal tissue—A pilot study. *British Journal of Oral and Maxillofacial Surgery* 54(3):338–341.

Rouabhia, M., H. J. Park, A. Semlali, A. Zakrzewski, W. Chmielewski, and J. Chakir. 2016. E-cigarette vapor induces an apoptotic response in human gingival epithelial cells through the caspase-3 pathway. *Journal of Cellular Physiology* 232:1539–1547.

Sancilio, S., M. Gallorini, A. Cataldi, and V. di Giacomo. 2016. Cytotoxicity and apoptosis induction by e-cigarette fluids in human gingival fibroblasts. *Clinical Oral Investigations* 20(3):477–483.

Souto, G. R., C. M. Queiroz-Junior, F. O. Costa, and R. A. Mesquita. 2014a. Smoking effect on chemokines of the human chronic periodontitis. *Immunobiology* 219(8):633–636.

Souto, G. R., C. M. Queiroz-Junior, F. O. Costa, and R. A. Mesquita. 2014b. Relationship between chemokines and dendritic cells in human chronic periodontitis. *Journal of Periodontology* 85(10):1416–1423.

Sundar, I. K., F. Javed, G. E. Romanos, and I. Rahman. 2016. E-cigarettes and flavorings induce inflammatory and pro-senescence responses in oral epithelial cells and periodontal fibroblasts. *Oncotarget* 7(47):77196–77204.

Tatullo, M., S. Gentile, F. Paduano, L. Santacroce, and M. Marrelli. 2016. Crosstalk between oral and general health status in e-smokers. *Medicine (Baltimore)* 95(49):e5589.

Wadia, R., V. Booth, H. F. Yap, and D. L. Moyes. 2016. A pilot study of the gingival response when smokers switch from smoking to vaping. *British Dental Journal* 221(11):722–726.

Willershausen, I., T. Wolf, V. Weyer, R. Sader, S. Ghanaati, and B. Willershausen. 2014. Influence of e-smoking liquids on human periodontal ligament fibroblasts. *Head & Face Medicine* 10:39. https://doi.org/10.1186/1746-160X-10-39 (accessed February 6, 2018).

13

Developmental and Reproductive Effects

Potential effects of e-cigarette use during pregnancy are of great interest for a number of reasons. The increasing prevalence of use among young women in the reproductive age range, combined with the known hazards of combustible tobacco cigarette smoking and the heightened awareness of health issues in relation to pregnancy, naturally raises the question of the nature of how e-cigarettes may affect the pregnancy. Although there is little evidence to draw on in response to that concern, there are a range of opinions regarding its impact, as summarized recently. A review examining perception and use of electronic cigarettes during pregnancy found that the most common perceptions of e-cigarette use during pregnancy were that they posed some risk to maternal and child health, but were safer than combustible tobacco cigarettes for both mother and baby and that they may be used as a tool for smoking cessation (McCubbin et al., 2017).

The physiological challenges of pregnancy make this a time of vulnerability to other stressors, particularly those associated with cardiovascular health, and thus a time of particular concern regarding potential health effects of e-cigarettes. Changes in blood flow, blood pressure, and glucose tolerance associated with normal pregnancy have been noted to constitute a "stress test" that results in a sizable proportion of women becoming temporarily diabetic or hypertensive. In addition, there may be changes in renal function, immunological responses, and other potentially relevant concerns. Short-term effects of e-cigarette use on maternal physiology would be feasible to assess using non-invasive markers, such as Doppler ultrasound to assess blood flow to the fetus.

The fetus undergoes rapid organ development and tissue growth prior to birth. Many toxins, including nicotine, can cross the maternal placental barrier. In addition, gestational age of the fetus greatly influences susceptibility to a particular toxicant. For example, during embryonic life certain chemical exposures can be teratogenic while at a later gestational age, these same toxins can impair tissue and organ growth. Observational studies of offspring born of mothers who used e-cigarettes during pregnancy are needed to examine the impact of in utero e-cigarette exposure on congenital malformations and fetal growth. Additional observational studies are needed to determine the impact of in utero e-cigarette exposure on postnatal lung function and behavior of offspring in later life. Although some potential adverse effects of nicotine on fetal development and growth are known, nothing is known about the effects of aerosols that contain flavorings.

CHARACTERIZATION OF DISEASE ENDPOINTS AND INTERMEDIATE OUTCOMES

The potential for e-cigarettes to affect the course and outcome of pregnancy is plausible, given the range and magnitude of known effects of combustible tobacco cigarette smoking, which includes placental abruption, ectopic pregnancy, preterm birth, fetal growth restriction, stillbirth, infant mortality, sudden infant death syndrome (SIDS), and orofacial clefts (HHS, 2014). While the specific constituents of tobacco smoke responsible for the harm to the mother and fetus are incompletely understood, nicotine is likely to be one of the sources of risk to the fetus, which would be pertinent to potential effects of e-cigarettes. The harm from other tobacco constituents, including carbon monoxide and tobacco-specific nitrosamines, for example, which pose threats to reproductive health, would not be pertinent or would be far less of a concern. It is possible that chemicals unique to e-cigarettes would affect fetal and neonatal development, but there is little or no direct evidence to guide such inferences.

Broadly, there is the potential for nicotine effects on pregnancy complications and fetal development. Pregnancy complications of concern based on tobacco include an increased risk of placental abruption and a potential protective effect for hypertensive disorders. Fetal and neonatal outcomes of concern include stillbirth, reduced growth, and preterm birth, extending into infant mortality, neurodevelopmental deficits, and increased risk for lower respiratory tract infections and asthma development. The most sensitive neonatal response to nicotine exposure might be a reduction in birth weight (Hayes et al., 2016), which is markedly affected by tobacco use. The most severe, though non-specific, neonatal outcome associated with tobacco use is infant mortality. In a study from Sweden, infant mortality was decreased in subsequent pregnancies in mothers who quit smoking (Johansson et al., 2009). No epidemiological studies or biological studies have yet been performed to examine potential links between maternal e-cigarette use during pregnancy and reduction in birth weight or increased infant mortality. In utero and early postnatal nicotine exposure through e-cigarette use may adversely affect the immune system and lung function of exposed infants. A study from South Africa found that infants had a fivefold greater risk of acquiring bacterial pneumonia if they had a primary caregiver who smoked (Verani et al., 2016). Other studies reported that young children exposed to tobacco smoke in utero were more likely to have impaired lung function (Dezateux et al., 2001; Gray et al., 2017).

The most directly relevant analogy to e-cigarettes would be nicotine replacement therapy (NRT), which is another form of nicotine delivery through means other than inhalation (i.e., ingestion or dermal absorption). However, the epidemiological evidence on NRT and pregnancy is quite limited. An evaluation of the use of NRT versus placebo among pregnant combustible tobacco cigarette smokers resulted in more favorable birthweights for the NRT group despite similar cotinine levels (presumably reflecting similar levels of nicotine intake) in one study (Wisborg et al., 2000). This suggests that constituents of tobacco other than nicotine are the source of harm, though a more recent trial showed no benefit (Coleman et al., 2012), which would be consistent with nicotine being responsible for tobacco's effects. The advisability of using NRT during pregnancy remains unresolved (Osadchy et al., 2009). Nonetheless, the use of NRT and possibly the use of e-cigarettes as a substitute for tobacco would likely reduce the potential for harm given the absence of carbon monoxide and other toxicants present in tobacco smoke.

Despite the lack of direct evidence, e-cigarettes are generally perceived to be less harmful than combustible tobacco by pregnant women who smoke combustible tobacco cigarettes (Baeza-Loya et al., 2014; Mark et al., 2015). Perspectives of clinical experts vary widely, including arguments that e-cigarettes are likely to be just as harmful as combustible tobacco cigarettes during pregnancy (Farquhar et al., 2015) and others advocating for a role for e-cigarettes in harm reduction for pregnant women (Bryce and Robson, 2015). Obstetricians who were surveyed indicated that 13.5 percent judged e-cigarettes to be free of harm, 29.0 percent believed e-cigarettes had adverse effects but were less harmful than combustible tobacco cigarettes, 13.5 percent indicated that e-cigarettes and combustible tobacco cigarettes were equally harmful, and 36.5 percent indicated that they did not know (England et al., 2016).

OPTIMAL STUDY DESIGN

The optimal study design would be a randomized trial in which pregnant women are assigned to smoke combustible tobacco cigarettes or e-cigarettes, or not use either product, which is ethically unacceptable and infeasible to implement. Approximating that, calls for observational designs that attempt to isolate the impact of e-cigarettes on the course and outcome of pregnancy and subsequent neonatal development are warranted. This would require accurate assessment of e-cigarette use throughout the course of pregnancy, recognition of different potential impacts depending on timing during gestation, thorough consideration of potential confounding factors that could introduce bias into the comparisons across exposure groups, and rigorous, objective assessment of the spectrum of endpoints from pregnancy complications through birth outcomes and infant health and development. As is the case for other health endpoints, there is a need to compare e-cigarette users with (1) non-users of any nicotine-containing products and (2) specifically combustible tobacco cigarette users, with careful control for correlated behaviors such as alcohol and marijuana use given their association with smoking (Agrawal et al., 2012; Metz and Stickrath, 2015). This is especially relevant to pregnancy because women are often motivated to take measures to improve the health of their pregnancy and may be more motivated to stop smoking combustible tobacco cigarettes than at other times of their life. It would be important to recognize the potential for effects on the fetus to become manifest over the course of early life and perhaps beyond, given the growing evidence that the prenatal environment influences health outcomes such as neurobehavioral development, cardiovascular and pulmonary disease risks, and mental health through the life course.

QUESTIONS ADDRESSED BY THE LITERATURE

Other than public and clinical perceptions of the relative safety or harm from e-cigarettes, there is almost no directly relevant research in humans to inform an assessment. Laboratory research on toxicity of e-cigarettes in pregnancy has begun, as described below, but there are no clinical or epidemiological studies thus far.

EPIDEMIOLOGY

No studies are currently available that directly assess the impact of e-cigarette use on the health of pregnancy. Not only have clinical endpoints not been examined, but to the committee's knowledge, there are no studies of markers of maternal or child health related to exposure during pregnancy.

CASE REPORTS AND OTHER CLINICAL STUDIES

No case reports or other clinical studies of e-cigarettes in relation to pregnancy were identified.

IN VIVO ANIMAL AND IN VITRO/MECHANISTIC STUDIES

A study by Parker and Rayburn (2017) examined the effects of regular, menthol, and electronic cigarette butt (ECB) leachates on *Xeonopus laevis* embryos and found that all leachates were teratogenic, but the ECB were less toxic and teratogenic than the other two in their model. Another study by Palpant and colleagues (2015), using zebrafish and human embryonic stem cells, found negative health effects on heart development from both combustible tobacco cigarette and e-cigarette exposure of similar nicotine levels, but that combustible tobacco cigarette smoke exposure was more toxic.

STUDIES ON COMBUSTIBLE TOBACCO AND NICOTINE

The scarcity of studies examining the impact of e-cigarettes on fetal and postnatal development and reproductive health during pregnancy presents a significant limitation in predicting health effects of e-cigarette emissions on the fetus and pregnant mother. Consequently, the committee considered research on the effects of combustible tobacco cigarettes and NRT on developmental and reproductive outcomes, which may or may not reflect the real risk of e-cigarette aerosols to fetal and reproductive health, but which the committee could draw on in their assessment of the health risk of e-cigarettes to these outcomes. For example, although there are currently no studies in humans evaluating the effects of nicotine-containing or non-nicotine e-cigarettes on fetal and childhood development and reproductive health, because e-cigarettes often contain nicotine, data examining the effects of nicotine exposure on the fetus and young child may estimate risk of nicotine exposure.

Epidemiological Studies

Nicotinic acetylcholine receptors (nACHRs) are present in the fetal brain and lungs of humans, and nicotine is a nACHR agonist (Smith et al., 2010; Wang et al., 2001). Exposure of the fetus to nicotine through maternal e-cigarette use or combustible tobacco cigarette smoking has the potential to activate nACHRs in the brain and lung prematurely, causing disruption of normal development.

Children of mothers who smoked combustible tobacco cigarettes during pregnancy have been reported to have an increased likelihood of developing behavioral difficulties including attention-deficit/hyperactivity disorder (e.g., Abbott and Winzer-Serhan, 2012), possibly caused by prenatal exposure to constituents of combustible tobacco cigarette smoke. Maternal combustible tobacco cigarette smoking during pregnancy also has been associated with a significant increase in wheezing during childhood in several studies (Gilliland et al., 2001, 2003; Moritsugu, 2007). Whether children exposed to e-cigarette aerosols when in utero are also at increased risk for similar adverse outcomes remains unknown.

Very high nicotine levels have been detected in dried blood spots of neonates of mothers who smoked combustible tobacco cigarettes during pregnancy, indicating the ease with which nicotine can cross the placental barrier (Murphy et al., 2013; Spector et al., 2014). In addition, because drug metabolism of nicotine has been reported to be slower in the fetus and infant compared with the adult (Dempsey et al., 2000), greater cumulative exposure to nicotine may occur in the fetus and infant exposed to nicotine. The consequences of slower drug metabolism could result in greater toxicity to the fetus and neonate when compared with similar nicotine exposure in more mature children and adults.

The observation that combustible tobacco cigarette smoke exposure is causally related to an increased risk of SIDS has been noted (Moritsugu, 2007). Reduction in the number of SIDS cases in European countries in which combustible tobacco cigarette smoking rates declined over a period of years further suggests an association (Boldo et al., 2010). The role of nicotine in SIDS is unclear; however, Lavezzi and colleagues (2014) found that among subjects who died of sudden intrauterine unexpected death syndrome or of SIDS, those whose mothers smoked combustible tobacco cigarettes during pregnancy were more likely to have greater α7 nACHR immunostaining in lung epithelial cells and lung vessel walls compared with those whose mothers did not smoke combustible tobacco cigarettes.

In a study examining the risk of major congenital abnormalities in children of mothers who smoked combustible tobacco cigarettes or used NRT, there were no differences between the two groups with the exception (OR = 4.65; 99% CI = 1.76–12.25) that children of NRT users had an increased risk of respiratory anomalies (Dhalwani et al., 2015).

The adverse effect of nicotine on in utero lung development has been suggested to be caused by an increase in oxidative stress (Maritz and van Wyk, 1997). If nicotine is the primary component in combustible tobacco cigarette smoke that alters lung and brain development in the children of mothers who smoke those cigarettes during pregnancy, then exposure to the nicotine from e-cigarette aerosols may also present an increased health risk to the fetus and neonate, though not necessarily equal to that of combustible tobacco cigarettes.

Animal Studies

Animal studies in rodents and non-human primates have demonstrated an adverse effect of nicotine on fetal airway development and lung histology. When nicotine pumps were implanted in pregnant rhesus monkeys, offspring were found to have a reduced total body weight and alveolar hypoplasia with upregulation of α7 receptors in the airway cartilage and vessels of fetal lungs (Sekhon et al., 1999).

Exposure to nicotine during fetal and early postnatal life also has been shown to transiently disrupt vascularization of the lung and alter lung development, but not lung function in a rodent model. Mean linear intercepts of lungs in mice exposed to prenatal and postnatal nicotine was increased and vascular endothelial growth receptor 2 was decreased in lungs at 3 weeks but not 12 weeks of age (Petre et al., 2011).

Other studies have shown that prenatal nicotine exposure can stimulate lung branching through α7 nicotinic receptors in murine lung explants, possibly contributing to dysanaptic lung growth (Wongtrakool et al., 2007). Supporting this finding was an additional study that demonstrated that offspring of mice exposed to prenatal nicotine had decreased forced expiratory flows and decreased airway diameters (Wongtrakool et al., 2012). Exposure to prenatal combustible tobacco cigarette smoke also has been shown to promote Th2 polarization in mice (Singh et al., 2011).

One study examined the effects of whole-body exposure of pregnant mice and their offspring to nicotine-containing e-cigarette aerosols from late prenatal to early postnatal life, approximating the duration of cortical brain development in the mouse. They reported alterations in risk-taking behaviors in adult mice previously exposed to nicotine-containing e-cigarettes during fetal and early life compared with mice exposed to e-cigarettes without nicotine (Smith et al., 2015). In another study, neonatal mice exposed to nicotine-containing e-cigarettes were found to have impaired alveolar growth and decreased lung cell proliferation compared with controls (McGrath-Morrow et al., 2015).

Taken together, although several animal studies have demonstrated an adverse effect of in utero nicotine on lung development and postnatal lung function and behavior, no dose–response studies were performed. In addition, studies of the effects of nicotine on fetal and early prenatal development in animal models have used nicotine pumps, systemic nicotine injections, and whole-body e-cigarette exposures, which may not replicate the human exposure. In addition, it is unknown whether the particle size of emissions or flavoring contained in some e-cigarette emissions can adversely affect fetal development. Further studies are needed before recommendations can be made regarding the risks of e-cigarette use during pregnancy to fetal development and if e-cigarette use as a substitute for combustible tobacco cigarette smoking is a safer alternative compared with NRT.

SYNTHESIS

Given the lack of direct empirical evidence of e-cigarettes' effects on the mother or fetus, from either human or animal studies, little can be said regarding an integrated evaluation. Although the extensive research on tobacco and limited evidence on nicotine in isolation gives some focus to the questions regarding the potential effects of e-cigarettes, the need for direct evaluation is clear.

Conclusion 13-1. There is ***no available evidence*** *whether or not e-cigarettes affect pregnancy outcomes.*

Conclusion 13-2. There is ***insufficient evidence*** *whether or not maternal e-cigarette use affects fetal development.*

REFERENCES

Abbott, L. C., and U. H. Winzer-Serhan. 2012. Smoking during pregnancy: Lessons learned from epidemiological studies and experimental studies using animal models. *Critical Reviews in Toxicology* 42(4):279–303.

Agrawal, A., A. J. Budney, and M. T. Lynskey. 2012. The co-occurring use and misuse of cannabis and tobacco: A review. *Addiction* 107(7):1221–1233.

Baeza-Loya, S., H. Viswanath, A. Carter, D. L. Molfese, K. M. Velasquez, P. R. Baldwin, D. G. Thompson-Lake, C. Sharp, J. C. Fowler, R. De La Garza, 2nd, and R. Salas. 2014. Perceptions about e-cigarette safety may lead to e-smoking during pregnancy. *Bulletin of the Menninger Clinic* 78(3):243–252.

Boldo, E., S. Medina, M. Oberg, V. Puklova, O. Mekel, K. Patja, D. Dalbokova, M. Krzyzanowski, and M. Posada. 2010. Health impact assessment of environmental tobacco smoke in European children: Sudden infant death syndrome and asthma episodes. *Public Health Reports* 125(3):478–487.

Bryce, R., and S. J. Robson. 2015. E-cigarettes and pregnancy. Is a closer look appropriate? *Australian and New Zealand Journal of Obstetrics and Gynaecology* 55(3):218–221.

Coleman, T., S. Cooper, J. G. Thornton, M. J. Grainge, K. Watts, J. Britton, S. Lewis. 2012. A randomized trial of nicotine-replacement therapy patches in pregnancy. *New England Journal of Medicine* 366(9):808–818.

Dempsey, D., P. Jacob, 3rd, and N. L. Benowitz. 2000. Nicotine metabolism and elimination kinetics in newborns. *Clinical Pharmacology & Therapeutics* 67(5):458–465.

Dezateux, C., J. Stocks, A. M. Wade, I. Dundas, and M. E. Fletcher. 2001. Airway function at one year: Association with premorbid airway function, wheezing, and maternal smoking. *Thorax* 56(9):680–686.

Dhalwani, N. N., L. Szatkowski, T. Coleman, L. Fiaschi, and L. J. Tata. 2015. Nicotine replacement therapy in pregnancy and major congenital anomalies in offspring. *Pediatrics* 135(5):859–867.

England, L. J., V. T. Tong, A. Koblitz, J. Kish-Doto, M. M. Lynch, and B. G. Southwell. 2016. Perceptions of emerging tobacco products and nicotine replacement therapy among pregnant women and women planning a pregnancy. *Preventive Medicine Reports* 4:481–485.

Farquhar, B., K. Mark, M. Terplan, and M. S. Chisolm. 2015. Demystifying electronic cigarette use in pregnancy. *Journal of Addiction Medicine* 9(2):157–158.

Gilliland, F. D., Y. F. Li, and J. M. Peters. 2001. Effects of maternal smoking during pregnancy and environmental tobacco smoke on asthma and wheezing in children. *American Journal of Respiratory & Critical Care Medicine* 163(2):429–436.

Gilliland, F. D., K. Berhane, Y. F. Li, E. B. Rappaport, and J. M. Peters. 2003. Effects of early onset asthma and in utero exposure to maternal smoking on childhood lung function. *American Journal of Respiratory & Critical Care Medicine* 167(6):917–924.

Gray, D., L. Willemse, A. Visagie, D. Czovek, P. Nduru, A. Vanker, D. J. Stein, N. Koen, P. D. Sly, Z. Hantos, G. L. Hall, and H. J. Zar. 2017. Determinants of early-life lung function in African infants. *Thorax* 72(5):445–450.

Hayes, C., M. Kearney, H. O'Carroll, L. Zgaga, M. Geary, and C. Kelleher. 2016. Patterns of smoking behaviour in low-income pregnant women: A cohort study of differential effects on infant birth weight. *International Journal of Environmental Research & Public Health* 13(11):1060. https://doi.org/10.3390/ijerph13111060 (accessed February 6, 2018).

HHS (U.S. Department of Health and Human Services). 2014. *The health consequences of smoking—50 years of progress: A report of the Surgeon General*. Atlanta, GA: U.S. Department of Health and Human Services, Centers for Disease Control and Prevention, National Center for Chronic Disease Prevention and Health Promotion, Office on Smoking and Health.

Johansson, A. L., P. W. Dickman, M. S. Kramer, and S. Cnattingius. 2009. Maternal smoking and infant mortality: Does quitting smoking reduce the risk of infant death? *Epidemiology* 20(4):590–597.

Lavezzi, A. M., M. F. Corna, G. Alfonsi, and L. Matturri. 2014. Possible role of the α7 nicotinic receptors in mediating nicotine's effect on developing lung—Implications in unexplained human perinatal death. *BMC Pulmonary Medicine* 14:11. https://doi.org/10.1186/1471-2466-14-11 (accessed February 6, 2018).

Maritz, G. S., and G. van Wyk. 1997. Influence of maternal nicotine exposure on neonatal rat lung structure: Protective effect of ascorbic acid. *Comparative Biochemistry and Physiology Part C: Pharmacology, Toxicology, and Endocrinology* 117(2):159–165.

Mark, K. S., B. Farquhar, M. S. Chisolm, V. H. Coleman-Cowger, and M. Terplan. 2015. Knowledge, attitudes, and practice of electronic cigarette use among pregnant women. *Journal of Addiction Medicine* 9(4):266–272.

McCubbin, A., A. Fallin-Bennett, J. Barnett, and K. Ashford. 2017. Perceptions and use of electronic cigarettes in pregnancy. *Health Education Research* 32(1):22–32.

McGrath-Morrow, S. A., M. Hayashi, A. Aherrera, A. Lopez, A. Malinina, J. M. Collaco, E. Neptune, J. D. Klein, J. P. Winickoff, P. Breysse, P. Lazarus, and G. Chen. 2015. The effects of electronic cigarette emissions on systemic cotinine levels, weight and postnatal lung growth in neonatal mice. *PLoS ONE* 10(2):e0118344. https://doi.org/10.1371/journal.pone.0118344 (accessed February 6, 2018).

Metz, T. D., and E. H. Stickrath. 2015. Marijuana use in pregnancy and lactation: A review of the evidence. *American Journal of Obstetrics and Gynecology* 213(6):761–778.

Moritsugu, K. P. 2007. The 2006 report of the Surgeon General: The health consequences of involuntary exposure to tobacco smoke. *American Journal of Preventive Medicine* 32(6):542–543.

Murphy, S. E., K. M. Wickham, B. R. Lindgren, L. G. Spector, and A. Joseph. 2013. Cotinine and *trans*-3'-hydroxycotinine in dried blood spots as biomarkers of tobacco exposure and nicotine metabolism. *Journal of Exposure Science & Environmental Epidemiology* 23(5):513–518.

Osadchy, A., A. Kazmin, and G. Koren. 2009. Nicotine replacement therapy during pregnancy: Recommended or not recommended? *Journal of Obstetrics and Gynaecology Canada* 31(8):744–747.

Palpant, N. J., P. Hofsteen, L. Pabon, H. Reinecke, and C. E. Murry. 2015. Cardiac development in zebrafish and human embryonic stem cells is inhibited by exposure to tobacco cigarettes and e-cigarettes. *PLoS ONE* 10(5):e0126259. https://doi.org/10/1371/journal.pone.0126259 (accessed February 6, 2018).

Parker, T. T., and J. Rayburn. 2017. A comparison of electronic and traditional cigarette butt leachate on the development of *Xenopus laevis* embryos. *Toxicology Reports* 4:77–82.

Petre, M. A., J. Petrik, R. Ellis, M. D. Inman, A. C. Holloway, and N. R. Labiris. 2011. Fetal and neonatal exposure to nicotine disrupts postnatal lung development in rats: Role of VEGF and its receptors. *International Journal of Toxicology* 30(2):244–252.

Sekhon, H. S., Y. Jia, R. Raab, A. Kuryatov, J. F. Pankow, J. A. Whitsett, J. Lindstrom, and E. R. Spindel. 1999. Prenatal nicotine increases pulmonary α7 nicotinic receptor expression and alters fetal lung development in monkeys. *Journal of Clinical Investigation* 103(5):637–647.

Singh, S. P., S. Gundavarapu, J. C. Pena-Philippides, J. Rir-Sima-ah, N. C. Mishra, J. A. Wilder, R. J. Langley, K. R. Smith, and M. L. Sopori. 2011. Prenatal secondhand cigarette smoke promotes Th2 polarization and impairs goblet cell differentiation and airway mucus formation. *Journal of Immunology* 187(9):4542–4552.

Smith, A. M., L. P. Dwoskin, and J. R. Pauly. 2010. Early exposure to nicotine during critical periods of brain development: Mechanisms and consequences. *Journal of Pediatric Biochemistry* 1(2):125–141.

Smith, D., A. Aherrera, A. Lopez, E. Neptune, J. P. Winickoff, J. D. Klein, G. Chen, P. Lazarus, J. M. Collaco, and S. A. McGrath-Morrow. 2015. Adult behavior in male mice exposed to e-cigarette nicotine vapors during late prenatal and early postnatal life. *PLoS ONE* 10(9):e0137953. https://doi.org/10.1371.journal.pone.0137953 (accessed February 6, 2018).

Spector, L. G., S. E. Murphy, K. M. Wickham, B. Lindgren, and A. M. Joseph. 2014. Prenatal tobacco exposure and cotinine in newborn dried blood spots. *Pediatrics* 133(6):e1632–e1638. https://doi.org/10.1542/peds.2013-3118 (accessed February 6, 2018).

Verani, J. R., M. J. Groome, H. J. Zar, E. R. Zell, C. N. Kapongo, S. A. Nzenze, C. Mulligan, D. P. Moore, C. G. Whitney, and S. A. Madhi. 2016. Risk factors for presumed bacterial pneumonia among HIV-uninfected children hospitalized in Soweto, South Africa. *Pediatric Infectious Disease Journal* 35(11):1169–1174.

Wang, Y., E. F. Pereira, A. D. Maus, N. S. Ostlie, D. Navaneetham, S. Lei, E. X. Albuquerque, and B. M. Conti-Fine. 2001. Human bronchial epithelial and endothelial cells express α7 nicotinic acetylcholine receptors. *Molecular Pharmacology* 60(6):1201–1209.

Wisborg, K., T. B. Henriksen, L. B. Jespersen, and N. J. Secher. 2000. Nicotine patches for pregnant smokers: A randomized controlled study. *Obstetrics & Gynecology* 96(6):967–971.

Wongtrakool, C., S. Roser-Page, H. N. Rivera, and J. Roman. 2007. Nicotine alters lung branching morphogenesis through the α7 nicotinic acetylcholine receptor. *American Journal of Physiology: Lung Cellular and Molecular Physiology* 293(3):L611–L618.

Wongtrakool, C., N. Wang, D. M. Hyde, J. Roman, and E. R. Spindel. 2012. Prenatal nicotine exposure alters lung function and airway geometry through α7 nicotinic receptors. *American Journal of Respiratory Cell and Molecular Biology* 46(5):695–702.

14

Injuries and Poisonings

There is no question that sources of morbidity and mortality from e-cigarettes are the injuries related to malfunctioning of the devices, leading to burns and projectile injuries, and injuries related to intentional or unintentional consumption of e-liquids. There are no epidemiological studies of these events, but the literature does contain numerous case reports, case series, and reports from passive surveillance systems, such as poison control centers. The committee briefly reviews this evidence. The committee notes that in recognition of these injuries, Congress and the Food and Drug Administration (FDA) have taken action. In 2016, Congress directed the Consumer Product Safety Commission to require special packaging (similar to child-resistant packaging) for e-liquid bottles that contain nicotine.[1] FDA's Center for Tobacco Products recently held a public workshop to discuss battery safety (HHS, 2017). Finally, in recognition of the risks, FDA's recently released comprehensive nicotine strategy includes provisions for setting product standards "to protect against known public health risks such as electronic nicotine delivery systems (ENDS) battery issues" and for "concerns about children's exposure to liquid nicotine" (HHS, 2017).

[1] Child Nicotine Poisoning Prevention Act of 2015, Public Law 114-116 § 142, 114th Cong. (September 29, 2017).

BURNS AND EXPLOSIONS

Most of the information regarding the malfunction of e-cigarettes and injuries comes from case reports, case series, and retrospective reviews of burn center reports. No prospective observational studies have been identified. Although these events are infrequent and the true rate is not known, when they do occur they have the potential to cause great harm. Serious burns from exploding e-cigarette batteries have been reported in the literature. Overheating and explosions of lithium ion batteries in e-cigarettes are most frequently the cause of burns in e-cigarette users. The quality of the components and design of the device, including user modifications, may influence the likelihood of malfunction and explosions in e-cigarettes. The committee reviewed 46 case reports published in the literature as solo case reports or case series documenting burns to the face, chest, abdomen, genitalia, and thigh, with burns to the thigh area most frequently reported. The majority (n = 25) of the cases of burns to the thigh are from devices stored in pants pockets (Bauman et al., 2016; Bohr et al., 2016; Colaianni et al., 2016; Herlin et al., 2016; Jiwani et al., 2017; Kumetz et al., 2016; Nicoll et al., 2016; Serror et al., 2017; Sheckter et al., 2016; Treitl et al., 2016; Walsh et al., 2016). Some explosions are documented to occur when the device could have come into content with metals, such as coins and keys, in the pocket.

There have also been reports of injuries caused by projectiles following an e-cigarette explosion. Vaught and colleagues (2017) reported facial trauma from such an explosion. Another case reported that an 18-year-old suffered oral trauma and tooth avulsion following an e-cigarette explosion while using the device (Rogér et al., 2016). Paley and colleagues (2016) reported two cases of severe corneal injuries, in addition to other facial injuries that occurred in an adult and adolescent when their e-cigarettes exploded, resulting in decreased visual acuity.

Several groups have published summaries of reported explosions causing harm, based on reports from general hospitals or burn treatment centers (Arnaout et al., 2017; Brownson et al., 2016; Hassan et al., 2016; Rudy and Durmowicz, 2016). For example, Ramirez and colleagues (2017) found that 29 people were referred between February 2015 and July 2016 to three regional burn treatment centers in California for burn-related injuries from e-cigarettes. In addition, Arnaout and colleagues (2017) reported on 12 people who were treated for e-cigarette injuries in two burn centers in the United Kingdom, between October 2015 and July 2016. In their study, the thigh region was the most common area for a burn. Another study from California found that 25 patients were treated for burns caused by e-cigarettes at a regional burn center, between November 2015 and March 2017 (Toy et al., 2017). The majority of patients were male and most injuries resulted from the e-cigarette device exploding in a pocket, with thigh and genital areas being most commonly affected. Malfunctions of the lithium battery in the e-cigarettes have been blamed for many of these injuries, but Serror and colleagues (2017) reported on a patient who had a full-thickness thigh burn due to overheating of a resistor component of the e-cigarette, in the absence of the device catching fire or exploding.

INTENTIONAL AND UNINTENTIONAL EXPOSURE TO E-LIQUID

Ingestion of nicotine-containing e-cigarette solutions can result in serious health effects, including death, due to nicotine toxicity. Many of the commercially available e-cigarette solutions contain high concentrations of nicotine. The committee identified 19 case reports (documented in 16 publications) in the literature of poisonings from exposure to e-liquid via oral or dermal routes. Twelve of these incidents are reported as intentional (sometimes associated with a suicide note) (Bartschat et al., 2015; Chen et al., 2015; Christensen et al., 2013; Eberlein et al., 2014; Garat et al., 2016; Lam et al., 2016; Schipper et al., 2014; Sommerfeld et al., 2016; Thornton et al., 2014; You et al., 2016), and six as unintentional (Eggleston et al., 2016; Gill et al., 2015; Gupta et al., 2014; Jamison and Lockington, 2016; Noble et al., 2016; Seo et al., 2016). Fatalities have been reported (Eggleston et al., 2016; Thornton et al., 2014; You et al., 2016). The medical consequences of the non-fatal cases include vomiting, lactic acidosis (Garat et al., 2016), and other outcomes. Several of these unintentional cases involved young children who apparently accessed e-liquid vials in the household (Eggleston et al., 2016; Gill et al., 2015; Gupta et al., 2014).

Further evidence of the consequence of ingestion of e-liquid is found in reports from poison control centers and other passive surveillance systems (Anonymous, 2015; Cantrell and Clark, 2014; Chatham-Stephens et al., 2014, 2016; De La Oliva Urieta and Conejo Menor, 2014; Forrester, 2015; Kamboj et al., 2016; Lovecchio and Zoph, 2015; Ordonez et al., 2015; Thomas et al., 2014; Vakkalanka et al., 2014; Valentine et al., 2016; Weiss et al., 2016). For example, between January 2010 and June 2014, poison control centers in Texas received 203 reports of ingestion by children age 5 or younger (Forrester, 2015). Between January 2013 and April 2014, 64 cases of e-liquid exposure were reported to Spain's poison centers, 28 percent of which were in children younger than 2 years of age (De La Oliva Urieta and Conejo Menor, 2014). Between September 2010 and February 2014, poison control centers in the United States recorded 2,405 calls regarding e-cigarette exposures (Chatham-Stephens et al., 2014). Children age 5 and younger accounted for 51 percent of those calls. In the United States, the number of calls to poison centers for e-cigarette exposures increased 1,492.9 percent between January 2012 and April 2015

(Kamboj et al., 2016). E-cigarette exposures were also more likely to result in a health care admission and a more severe outcome than an exposure related to cigarettes.

Although the committee identified no epidemiological studies about injuries and poisonings, the type of evidence that supports other conclusions in this report, the committee viewed the case studies as sufficient basis for several conclusions.

*Conclusion 14-1. There is **conclusive evidence** that e-cigarette devices can explode and cause burns and projectile injuries. Such risk is significantly increased when batteries are of poor quality, stored improperly, or modified by users.*

*Conclusion 14-2. There is **conclusive evidence** that intentional or accidental exposure to e-liquids (from drinking, eye contact, or dermal contact) can result in adverse health effects including but not limited to seizures, anoxic brain injury, vomiting, and lactic acidosis.*

*Conclusion 14-3. There is **conclusive evidence** that intentionally or unintentionally drinking or injecting e-liquids can be fatal.*

REFERENCES

Anonymous. 2015. Electronic cigarettes: Poisoning in children. 2015. *Prescrire International* 24(156):21.

Arnaout, A., F. Dewi, and D. Nguyen. 2017. Re: Burn injuries from exploding electronic cigarette batteries: An emerging public health hazard. *Journal of Plastic, Reconstructive & Aesthetic Surgery* 70(7):981–982.

Bartschat, S., K. Mercer-Chalmers-Bender, J. Beike, M. A. Rothschild, and M. Jubner. 2015. Not only smoking is deadly: Fatal ingestion of e-juice—A case report. *International Journal of Legal Medicine* 129(3):481–486.

Bauman, Z. M., J. Roman, M. Singer, and G. A. Vercruysse. 2016. Canary in the coal mine—Initial reports of thermal injury secondary to electronic cigarettes. *Burns* 43(3):e38–e42.

Bohr, S., F. Almarzouqi, and N. Pallua. 2016. Extensive burn injury caused by fundamental electronic cigarette design flaw. *Annals of Burns and Fire Disasters* 29(3):231–233.

Brownson, E. G., C. M. Thompson, S. Goldsberry, H. J. Chong, J. B. Friedrich, T. N. Pham, S. Arbabi, G. J. Carrougher, and N. S. Gibran. 2016. Explosion injuries from e-cigarettes. *New England Journal of Medicine* 375(14):1400–1402.

Cantrell, F. L., and R. F. Clark. 2014. More on nicotine poisoning in infants. *New England Journal of Medicine* 371(9):880. https://doi.org/10.1056/NEJMc1407921 (accessed February 6, 2018).

Chatham-Stephens, K., R. Law, E. Taylor, P. Melstrom, R. Bunnell, B. Wang, B. Apelberg, and J. G. Schier. 2014. Notes from the field: Calls to poison centers for exposures to electronic cigarettes—United States, September 2010–February 2014. *Morbidity and Mortality Weekly Report* 63(13):292–293.

Chatham-Stephens, K., R. Law, E. Taylor, S. Kieszak, P. Melstrom, R. Bunnell, B. Wang, H. Day, B. Apelberg, L. Cantrell, H. Foster, and J. G. Schier. 2016. Exposure calls to U.S. poison centers involving electronic cigarettes and conventional cigarettes—September 2010–December 2014. *Journal of Medical Toxicology* 12(4):350–357.

Chen, B. C., S. B. Bright, A. R. Trivedi, and M. Valento. 2015. Death following intentional ingestion of e-liquid. *Clinical Toxicology* 53(9):914–916.

Christensen, L. B., T. van't Veen, and J. Bang. 2013. Three cases of attempted suicide by ingestion of nicotine liquid used in e-cigarettes [abstract]. *Clinical Toxicology* 51:290. https://doi.org/10.3345/kip.2016.59.12.490 (acceessed February 6, 2018).

Colaianni, C. A., L. F. Tapias, R. Cauley, R. Sheridan, J. T. Schulz, and J. Goverman. 2016. Injuries caused by explosion of electronic cigarette devices. *Eplasty* 16:ic9.

De La Oliva Urieta, S., and J. L. Conejo Menor. 2014. Exposures to electronic cigarettes: Calls to the poison center in Spain. *Revista Espanola de Medicina Legal* 40(4):146–149.

Eberlein, C. K., H. Frieling, T. Kohnlein, T. Hillemacher, and S. Bleich. 2014. Suicide attempt by poisoning using nicotine liquid for use in electronic cigarettes. *American Journal of Psychiatry* 171(8):891. https://doi.org/10.1176/appi.ajp.2014.14030277 (accessed February 6, 2018).

Eggleston, W., N. Nacca, C. M. Stork, and J. M. Marraffa. 2016. Pediatric death after unintentional exposure to liquid nicotine for an electronic cigarette. *Clinical Toxicology* 54(9):890–891.

Forrester, M. B. 2015. Pediatric exposures to electronic cigarettes reported to Texas poison centers. *Journal of Emergency Medicine* 49(2):136–142.

Garat, A., P. Nisse, M. Kauv, M. Mathieu-Nolf, D. Allorge, and D. Mathieu. 2016. Lactic acidosis due to voluntary e-liquid ingestion. *Toxicologie Analytique et Clinique* 28(4):329–332.

Gill, N., G. Sangha, N. Poonai, and R. Lim. 2015. E-cigarette liquid nicotine ingestion in a child: Case report and discussion. *Canadian Journal of Emergency Medicine* 17(6):699–703.

Gupta, S., A. Gandhi, and R. Manikonda. 2014. Accidental nicotine liquid ingestion: Emerging paediatric problem. *Archives of Disease in Childhood* 99(12):1149. http://doi.org/10.1136/archdischild-2014-306750 (accessed February 6, 2018).

Hassan, S., M. U. Anwar, P. Muthayya, and S. Jivan. 2016. Burn injuries from exploding electronic cigarette batteries: An emerging public health hazard. *Journal of Plastic, Reconstructive & Aesthetic Surgery* 69(12):1716–1718.

Herlin, C., F. Bekara, N. Bertheuil, P. Frobert, R. Carloni, and B. Chaput. 2016. Deep bums caused by electronic vaping devices explosion. *Burns* 42(8):1875–1877.

HHS (U.S. Department of Health and Human Services). 2017. *Battery safety concerns in electronic nicotine delivery systems (ENDS) public workshop—April 2017*. https://www.fda.gov/tobaccoproducts/newsevents/ucm535185.htm (accessed October 4, 2017).

Jamison, A., and D. Lockington. 2016. Ocular chemical injury secondary to electronic cigarette liquid misuse. *JAMA Ophthalmology* 134(12):1443. https://doi.org/10.1001/jamaophthalmol.2016.3651 (accessed February 6, 2018).

Jiwani, A. Z., J. F. Williams, J. A. Rizzo, K. K. Chung, B. T. King, and L. C. Cancio. 2017. Thermal injury patterns associated with electronic cigarettes. *International Journal of Burns and Trauma* (1):1–5.

Kamboj, A., H. A. Spiller, M. J. Casavant, T. Chounthirath, and G. A. Smith. 2016. Pediatric exposure to e-cigarettes, nicotine, and tobacco products in the United States. *Pediatrics* 137(6):e20160041. https://doi.org/10.1542/peds.2016-0041 (accessed February 6, 2018).

Kumetz, E. A., N. D. Hurst, R. J. Cudnik, and S. L. Rudinsky. 2016. Electronic cigarette explosion injuries. *American Journal of Emergency Medicine* 34(11):2252.e1–2252.e3.

Lam, C. N., N. I. Goldenson, E. Burner, and J. B. Unger. 2016. Cultural buffering as a protective factor against electronic cigarette use among Hispanic emergency department patients. *Addictive Behaviors* 63:155–160.

Lovecchio, F., and O. Zoph. 2015. Incidence of electronic cigarette exposures in children skyrockets in Arizona. *American Journal of Emergency Medicine* 33(6):834–835.

Nicoll, K. J., A. M. Rose, M. A. A. Khan, O. Quaba, and A. G. Lowrie. 2016. Thigh burns from exploding e-cigarette lithium ion batteries: First case series. *Burns* 42(4):e42–e46.

Noble, M. J., B. Longstreet, R. G. Hendrickson, and R. Gerona. 2016. Unintentional pediatric ingestion of electronic cigarette nicotine refill liquid necessitating intubation. *Annals of Emergency Medicine* 69(1):94–97.

Ordonez, J. E., K. C. Kleinschmidt, and M. B. Forrester. 2015. Electronic cigarette exposures reported to Texas poison centers. *Nicotine & Tobacco Research* 17(2):209–211.

Paley, G. L., E. Echalier, T. W. Eck, A. R. Hong, A. V. Farooq, D. G. Gregory, and A. J. Lubniewski. 2016. Corneoscleral laceration and ocular burns caused by electronic cigarette explosions. *Cornea* 35(7):1015–1018.

Ramirez, J. I., C. A. Ridgway, J. G. Lee, B. M. Potenza, S. Sen, T. L. Palmieri, D. G. Greenhalgh, and P. Maguina. 2017. The unrecognized epidemic of electronic cigarette burns. *Journal of Burn Care & Research* 38(4):220–224.

Rogér, J. M., M. Abayon, S. Elad, and A. Kolokythas. 2016. Oral trauma and tooth avulsion following explosion of e-cigarette. *Journal of Oral and Maxillofacial Surgery* 74(6):1181–1185.

Rudy, S. F., and E. L. Durmowicz. 2016. Electronic nicotine delivery systems: Overheating, fires and explosions. *Tobacco Control* 26:10–18.

Schipper, E. M., L. C. de Graaff, B. C. Koch, Z. Brkic, E. B. Wilms, J. Alsma, and S. C. Schuit. 2014. A new challenge: Suicide attempt using nicotine fillings for electronic cigarettes. *British Journal of Clinical Pharmacology* 78(6):1469–1471.

Seo, A. D., D. C. Kim, H. J. Yu, and M. J. Kang. 2016. Accidental ingestion of e-cigarette liquid nicotine in a 15-month-old child: An infant mortality case of nicotine intoxication. *Korean Journal of Pediatrics* 59(12):490–493.

Serror, K., M. Chaouat, A. De Runz, M. Mimoun, and D. Boccara. 2017. Thigh deep burns caused by electronic vaping devices (e-cigarettes): A new mechanism. *Burns* 43(5):1133–1135.

Sheckter, C., A. Chattopadhyay, J. Paro, and Y. Karanas. 2016. Burns resulting from spontaneous combustion of electronic cigarettes: A case series. *Burns Trauma* 4:35. https://doi.org/10.1186/s41038-016-0061-9 (accessed February 6, 2018).

Sommerfeld, K., M. Lukasik-Glebocka, M. Kulza, A. Druzdz, P. Panienski, E. Florek, and B. Zielinska-Psuja. 2016. Intravenous and oral suicidal e-liquid poisonings with confirmed nicotine and cotinine concentrations. *Forensic Science International* 262:E15–E20.

Thomas, E., R. A. Spears, G. Alldridge, C. V. Krishna, J. P. Thompson, M. Eddleston, J. A. Vale, and S. H. L. Thomas. 2014. E-cigarette liquid refills—A safe beverage? Analysis of enquiries to the U.K. National Poisons Information Service from 2007 to 2013. *Clinical Toxicology* 52(4):338–339.

Thornton, S. L., L. Oller, and T. Sawyer. 2014. Fatal intravenous injection of electronic nicotine delivery system refilling solution. *Journal of Medical Toxicology* 10(2):202–204.

Toy, J., F. Dong, C. Lee, D. Zappa, T. Le, B. Archambeau, J. T. Culhane, and M. M. Neeki. 2017. Alarming increase in electronic nicotine delivery systems-related burn injuries: A serious unregulated public health issue. *American Journal of Emergency Medicine* 35(11):1781–1782.

Treitl, D., R. Solomon, D. L. Davare, R. Sanchez, and C. Kiffin. 2016. Full and partial thickness burns from spontaneous combustion of e-cigarette lithium-ion batteries with review of literature. *Journal of Emergency Medicine* 53(1):121–125.

Vakkalanka, J. P., L. S. Hardison, Jr., and C. P. Holstege. 2014. Epidemiological trends in electronic cigarette exposures reported to U.S. poison centers. *Clinical Toxicology* 52(5):542–548.

Valentine, N., E. McClelland, J. Bryant, and R. McMillen. 2016. Electronic cigarettes in Mississippi: Issues facing healthcare providers and policy makers. *Journal of the Mississippi State Medical Association* 57(6):181–189.

Vaught, B., J. Spellman, A. Shah, A. Stewart, and D. Mullin. 2017. Facial trauma caused by electronic cigarette explosion. *Ear, Nose and Throat Journal* 96(3):139–142.

Walsh, K., Z. Sheikh, K. Johal, and N. Khwaja. 2016. Rare case of accidental fire and burns caused by e-cigarette batteries. *BMJ Case Reports*. https://doi.org/10.1136/bcr-2015-212868 (accessed February 6, 2018).

Weiss, D., C. D. Tomasallo, J. G. Meiman, P. D. Creswell, P. C. Melstrom, D. D. Gummin, D. J. Patel, N. T. Michaud, H. A. Sebero, and H. A. Anderson. 2016. Electronic cigarette exposure: Calls to Wisconsin poison control centers, 2010-2015. *Wisconsin Medical Journal* 115(6):306–310.

You, G., J. Rhee, Y. Park, and S. Park. 2016. Determination of nicotine, cotinine and *trans*-3'-hydroxycotinine using LC/MC/MS in forensic samples of a nicotine fatal case by oral ingestion of e-cigarette liquid. *Journal of Forensic Sciences* 61(4):1149–1154.

15

Research Needs: Effects of E-Cigarettes on Health

As described in Chapter 6, the committee was tasked to provide a list of research needs to inform the Food and Drug Administration (FDA) and e-cigarette regulation that will be prioritized with respect to

- Research to gather information of most importance for the regulation of e-cigarettes to protect the population health
- Research that should be a priority for federal funding

The committee identified many gaps in the literature during its review and identified dozens of specific research needs important for understanding the health effects of e-cigarettes and for FDA regulatory action, as other research groups have documented (Walton et al., 2015). The committee identified two overarching research needs: addressing gaps in substantive knowledge and improving research methods and quality. Specific items for consideration identified by the committee are noted for each of these and are not listed in any priority order.

ADDRESSING GAPS IN SUBSTANTIVE KNOWLEDGE

Recommendation 15-1: The committee recommends that the Food and Drug Administration and other federal research sponsors and/or device manufacturers prioritize e-cigarette research that addresses key gaps regarding health effects in individuals.

This might include rapid response funding opportunities. Specific items for consideration follow.

Animal Models and In Vitro Mechanistic Studies:

- Mechanistic and in vivo animal studies should be done to determine the potential effects of e-cigarette aerosol on organ development and tissue growth during embryonic and fetal development. Such studies should assess effects of nicotine and flavorings separately, and include both dose–response and time-course effects throughout the period of gestation.
- Long-term (2-year) animal studies should be conducted, using inhalation exposure to e-cigarette aerosol, to better understand disease risks from inhaling reactive carbonyl compounds and other potentially toxic constituents of e-cigarette aerosol, including flavoring chemicals and additives. These studies should include two controls: combustible tobacco smoke–exposed animals and those exposed to ambient air. Endpoints evaluated should include clinical outcomes and biomarkers relevant for, at a minimum, cancers, cardiovascular disease, and respiratory diseases and other relevant clinical outcomes.
- The effect of e-cigarette aerosol on pulmonary inflammation and clearance of viral and bacterial pathogens in the lungs should be studied in appropriate animal models following inhalation exposures.

Short-Term Human Studies with Clinically Relevant Biomarkers

- Particle deposition in the human airways should be evaluated to assess where e-cigarette–derived particles impact the upper versus lower airways and alveoli, and how area of impaction in the lung may influence health effects caused by e-cigarettes. Such studies should also include evaluation of airway epithelium repair.
- Periodontal disease should be evaluated in e-cigarette users who have not been users of combustible tobacco cigarettes, including the effects of e-cigarettes on the subgingival microbiome.
- Short-term biomarker studies in humans are needed that focus on pathways with relevance to cancers, cardiovascular disease, respiratory diseases, and other disease endpoints, including biomarkers of inflammation and immune status, oxidative stress, and gene expression.

- Panel studies should assess the association of changes in e-cigarette use, including device characteristics and patterns of use, with relevant markers of subclinical cardiovascular disease (blood pressure, endothelial dysfunction, arterial stiffness, cardiac geometry and function, and autonomic function) and respiratory diseases (lung function, lung imaging) under real-life conditions.
- Short-term physiological effects of e-cigarettes on the mother and fetus should evaluate the potential for more clinically consequential changes.

Longer-Term Clinical and Epidemiological Studies

- Longitudinal cohort studies should be done to assess the association of long-term use of e-cigarettes with clinical and subclinical cardiovascular, respiratory, and other health outcomes as compared with smoking combustible tobacco cigarettes, dual use of e-cigarettes and combustible tobacco cigarettes, and never smoking or vaping.
- Because prospective studies for clinical disease take very long, cross-sectional studies of e-cigarette use with subclinical measures of cardiovascular disease and respiratory diseases can be very useful. For instance, carotid atherosclerosis and coronary artery calcification can be measured subclinically and inform on clinical cardiovascular risk. Similarly, lung imaging data can provide relevant information on the effects of chronic e-cigarette use before clinical respiratory disease has manifested.
- Studies are needed on the association of secondhand and thirdhand exposures with health outcomes in vulnerable populations, such as pregnant women, infants, young children, the elderly, and patients with cardiovascular and respiratory diseases, compared with secondhand tobacco smoke and the absence of secondhand exposure to either combustible tobacco smoke or to e-cigarettes.
- More research is needed on clinical and epidemiological studies of e-cigarette use during pregnancy, evaluating the association of patterns of use (including sole and dual e-cigarette use) with maternal and infant outcomes, building on known effects of tobacco on pregnancy complications and neonatal health indexes, compared with mothers who continue to smoke during pregnancy and never smokers or never vapers.
- Systematic collection of data is needed on injuries, poisonings, and other harms caused by e-cigarette devices in prospective observational studies of e-cigarettes.

- Identification and evaluation of strategies, including product standards, are needed to minimize the number of accidental burns and injuries caused by e-cigarette malfunctions and explosions.
- Epidemiological studies should be conducted on the "dependence construct" and whether the symptomatic manifestations of e-cigarette dependence are different from those of other tobacco or nicotine-containing products.
- The relationship between smoking history and nicotine pharmacokinetics (PK) should be assessed. Specific areas for examination include how smokers' history and dependence influence nicotine PK and effects when switching to e-cigarettes and how nicotine PK would be predicted to change over time.
- Longitudinal cohort studies are needed of youth and young adults to understand the trajectory of dependence over time in users with little or no combustible tobacco product exposure.
- Effective communication strategies about the relative risk of e-cigarettes compared with combustible tobacco products are needed.

IMPROVING RESEARCH METHODS AND QUALITY

Recommendation 15-2: The committee recommends that the Food and Drug Administration and other federal research sponsors and/or device manufacturers prioritize research that improves the quality of e-cigarette research on health outcomes. This includes protocol and methods validation and development and use of appropriate study design, including the use of the appropriate control groups and relevant biomarkers. Specific examples are given below.

Animal and Mechanistic Studies

- Develop inhalation exposure models for animal studies that are representative of human inhalation exposure to e-cigarette aerosols.
- Include measures of exposure to e-cigarette constituents to assess relevance to human exposure.

Human Clinical and Epidemiological Studies

- Conduct psychometric studies and measurement development research for developing standardized interview and questionnaire-based assessments of dependence, patterns of use, and device characteristics.

- Develop biomarkers of exposure and biomarkers of potential harm in e-cigarette users and compare these to the same biomarkers in the use of various tobacco products.
- Use methods development research to create or adapt existing abuse liability testing for e-cigarettes to better understand the development of dependence on e-cigarettes.
- In clinical and epidemiological studies, use as comparison groups individuals who continue to smoke, those who try to quit with other evidence-based tobacco cessation treatments, and those who are not users of tobacco products, including e-cigarettes.
- Leverage existing population-based epidemiological cohort studies to enhance the quality and quantity of information collected on the use of e-cigarettes and other tobacco-related products and smoking-cessation pharmacotherapies. Some of the existing cohorts for cancers and cardiorespiratory disease would need to recruit additional e-cigarette users, as very few might have been included in the original study population. Specially designed cohorts such as the Population Assessment of Tobacco and Health study will provide the highest-quality data, but additional evidence from existing cohorts could be essential for accelerating the generation of more evidence on cancer and cardiorespiratory diseases and their related endpoints, including intermediate endpoints for these diseases.
- For cohort studies, the age of the study population is important, as the age should be adequate in order to study cancer or cardiorespiratory outcomes, but not so old that it can cause difficulty in distinguishing the health effects of cigarette smoking versus e-cigarettes.
- Develop guidelines for reporting studies on e-cigarette use to standardize the published information and ensure that the studies are useful to understand the health effects of e-cigarette products and to inform product evaluation and regulation. In particular, it is important that studies of the health effects of e-cigarette use in humans provide information on the product characteristics, including the type of device, coil, and e-liquid used, and the patterns of use.

REFERENCE

Walton, K. M., D. B. Abrams, W. C. Bailey, D. Clark, G. N. Connolly, M. V. Djordjevic, T. E. Eissenberg, M. C. Fiore, M. L. Goniewicz, L. Haverkos, S. S. Hecht, J. E. Henningfield, J. R. Hughes, C. A. Oncken, L. Postow, J. E. Rose, K. L. Wanke, L. Yang, and D. K. Hatsukami. 2015. NIH electronic cigarette workshop: Developing a research agenda. *Nicotine & Tobacco Research* 17(2):259–269.

Section III

Public Health Implications of E-Cigarettes

While e-cigarettes might cause youth who use them to transition to use of combustible tobacco products, they could increase adult cessation of combustible tobacco cigarettes if they are used frequently. Across a range of studies and outcomes, e-cigarettes pose less risk to an individual than combustible tobacco cigarettes. With the range of assumptions used, population modeling projects that there would be net public health harm in the short and long term if the products do not increase combustible tobacco cessation in adults. Factors that would maximize potential health benefits associated with these products include determining with more precision whether and under which conditions e-cigarettes could serve as an effective smoking cessation aid, discouraging their use among youth through standard tobacco control strategies such as education and access restrictions, and increasing their safety through data-driven engineering and design.

Understanding the public health implications of e-cigarette use at the population level requires consideration of not only the risks of e-cigarettes on individual health outcomes, as described in the preceding chapters, but also the relation between e-cigarette use and use of other tobacco products—namely, combustible tobacco cigarettes. Given the well-documented and strong influence of combustible tobacco cigarette smoking on health (HHS, 2014) and the emerging evidence that, although not harm free, e-cigarettes likely expose users to lower health risks compared with combustible tobacco cigarettes, any link between e-cigarette use and patterns of combustible tobacco cigarette smoking would have a considerable impact on both individual and population health. Thus, a question relevant to the committee's task is whether and to what extent e-cigarette use affects patterns of combustible tobacco cigarette smoking. The challenge of evaluating the effect of e-cigarette use on combustible tobacco cigarette use is that e-cigarettes could influence combustible tobacco cigarette smoking through a number of pathways, which together could lead to net public health benefit or harm. To understand the potential effects of e-cigarette use on combustible tobacco cigarette smoking, the committee developed a conceptual framework illustrating these plausible pathways, or the possible transitions among e-cigarette use, cigarette smoking, and non-use (see Figure III-1). There are many plausible pathways, and smoking and tobacco use trajectories are often complex. To assess the potential effects of e-cigarette use on combustible tobacco cigarette smoking and corresponding health effects, this section of the report focuses on the influence of e-cigarette use on combustible tobacco cigarette use initiation and cessation, as well as the harm from e-cigarettes relative to that from combustible tobacco cigarettes.

Combustible tobacco cigarette initiation reflects transitions from no smoking to established or regular smoking, and therefore involves multiple steps within the tobacco progression trajectory. Consequently, to study markers along the continuum of smoking initiation, the committee first examined transitions from never smoking combustible tobacco cigarettes to any report of ever using combustible tobacco cigarettes, alone or concurrent with e-cigarettes (dual use). Ever use could reflect either a period

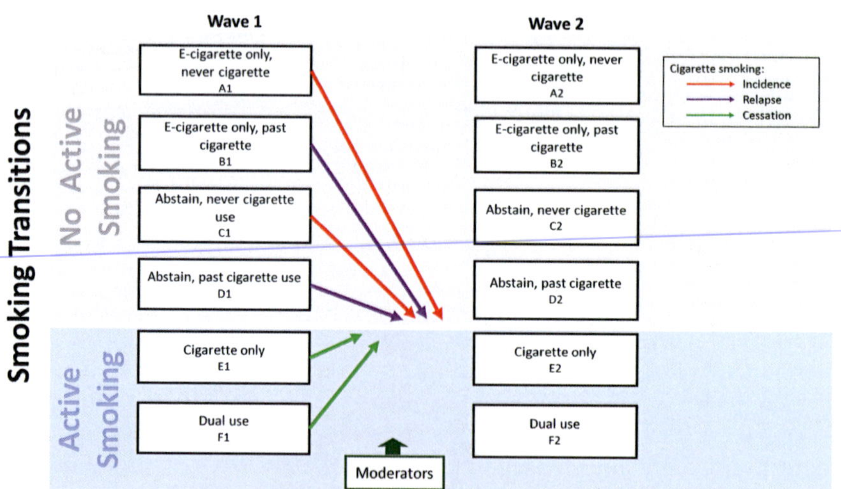

FIGURE III-1 Smoking transitions between e-cigarette use, combustible tobacco cigarette smoking, and non-use.

of temporary experimentation that does not progress to regular smoking or the beginning of a trajectory toward becoming a regular smoker. Thus, the committee then examined the progression to becoming a regular smoker as indicated by increases in the frequency (i.e., number of days used in past 30), intensity (i.e., cigarettes smoked per day on smoking day), and duration (i.e., length of time in which smoking behavior continues versus ceases following initiation) of smoking after becoming an ever smoker. In the framework, cigarette initiation is depicted by the red arrows that denote any transition from non-smoking to smoking. Estimates of e-cigarettes as a risk factor for cigarette initiation most commonly involve a ratio of these red lines, such as the level of combustible tobacco cigarette initiation among e-cigarette users as compared with those who do not use e-cigarettes.

Because nearly all adult combustible tobacco cigarette smokers report first use of cigarettes before age 26 (IOM, 2015), smoking initiation pertains primarily to youth and young adults. E-cigarette use among youth and young adults could influence subsequent combustible tobacco cigarette initiation in several ways. One scenario is that youth and young adults begin using e-cigarettes and subsequently initiate use of combustible tobacco cigarettes, either through switching or in addition to e-cigarettes. In this scenario, e-cigarette use is associated with combustible tobacco cigarette smoking initiation and thus tobacco-related health risks. Another scenario suggests that some portion of youth and young adults who otherwise would have begun smoking combustible tobacco cigarettes would not do so, and would instead begin using e-cigarettes. Here, e-cigarette use would reduce or delay initiation of combustible tobacco cigarette use and could reduce tobacco-related health risks. These potential pathways and corresponding evidence are described further in Chapter 16.

E-cigarette use could affect combustible tobacco use among adult smokers through several pathways, with different implications for public health. For example, it is plausible that e-cigarettes promote cessation of combustible tobacco cigarette smoking. The committee defined cigarette cessation as transitions from any combustible tobacco cigarette smoking to non-smoking. By this definition, cessation may involve the outcome of e-cigarette use alone or non-use of both e-cigarettes and combustible tobacco cigarettes. In other words, smokers could either transition completely from combustible tobacco cigarettes to e-cigarette use only or they could start using e-cigarettes in addition to combustible tobacco cigarettes (dual use) for a limited time, and then completely switch to e-cigarette use alone. Smokers could also subsequently quit both combustible tobacco cigarette and e-cigarette use. As the committee previously concluded, e-cigarettes are likely to expose users to fewer and lower levels of potentially toxic substances compared with exposure from combustible tobacco cigarettes and thus to confer lower health risks. Therefore, complete switching from combustible tobacco cigarettes to e-cigarettes would be expected to reduce tobacco-related health risks. E-cigarette users who subsequently stopped using both e-cigarettes and combustible tobacco cigarettes would incur additional benefits. In the framework, combustible tobacco cigarette cessation is depicted by the green arrows that denote any transition from smoking to non-smoking. Estimates for e-cigarettes as a cessation tool most commonly involve a ratio using at least one of these green lines, such as the level of cigarette cessation among active smokers (E1) compared with smokers who recently quit and use e-cigarettes as a replacement (recent members of B1). In these scenarios, e-cigarettes would benefit public health.

If, on the other hand, e-cigarettes are not effective cessation aids, e-cigarettes could cause relapse, whereby current e-cigarette use by former or non-active combustible tobacco cigarette users leads these users to transition back to combustible tobacco smoking either alone or concurrently with e-cigarettes. This could occur, for example, if a former smoker uses e-cigarettes under the belief that they are safe and will provide many of the same pleasures as combustible tobacco cigarettes, and follow a path that eventually leads back to active cigarette smoking. In the framework, cigarette relapse is depicted by the purple arrows that denote any transition from non-active to active smoking. As with initiation and cessation, estimates of relapse are based primarily on the ratio of the relevant transition probabilities. In this case, cigarette relapse levels among e-cigarette users are compared with relapse levels among former smokers who do not use e-cigarettes. Among e-cigarette users who relapse, the potential reduction in tobacco-related health risks from a period of temporary switching would likely be minimal. The influence of e-cigarettes on relapse would be especially worrying if e-cigarettes cause relapse among those who otherwise would have remained abstinent from combustible tobacco cigarette smoking, as this would increase both individual and overall public health risk. Discussion of the potential influence of e-cigarettes on combustible tobacco cigarette smoking among current and former adult smokers and corresponding evidence can be found in Chapter 17.

Finally, current smokers could start using e-cigarettes in addition to combustible tobacco cigarettes (dual use) and persist in using both products concurrently. If use of both products led to smoking reduction, this could confer health benefits. However, it is also feasible that dual users do not reduce combustible tobacco cigarette use, which could expose them to adverse health effects from the e-cigarettes in addition to those from combustible tobacco use. Discussion and evidence on the influence of concurrent e-cigarette and combustible tobacco cigarette use (dual use) on smoking cessation as well as health outcomes are presented in Chapter 18.

In addition to the tobacco use trajectories, the committee considered whether certain factors (or moderators) might strengthen or weaken the association between e-cigarette use and combustible tobacco cigarette use. Much remains unknown about potential moderators, but potentially important moderators that warrant serious consideration include age, motivation of e-cigarette users to smoke or stop smoking, substance vaped in e-cigarettes (e.g., nicotine concentration or flavorings), and whether e-cigarette use is part of a structured cessation program. Information on these moderators is currently scarce, but noted below when available.

To understand the overall effect of these different hypothesized pathways among e-cigarette use, combustible tobacco cigarette smoking, and non-use on the U.S. population as a whole, the committee used population-dynamic modeling and presents results of a range of scenarios in Chapter 19.

REFERENCES

HHS (U.S. Department of Health and Human Services). 2014. *The health consequences of smoking—50 years of progress: A report of the Surgeon General*. Atlanta, GA: U.S. Department of Health and Human Services, Centers for Disease Control and Prevention, National Center for Disease Prevention and Health Promotion, Office on Smoking and Health.

IOM (Institute of Medicine). 2015. *Public health implications of raising the minimum age of legal access to tobacco products*. Washington, DC: The National Academies Press.

16

Combustible Tobacco Cigarette Smoking Among Youth and Young Adults

The context surrounding e-cigarette use is markedly different in middle-aged and older adults as compared to adolescents and young adults. The proportion of U.S. adults age 25 or older who reported e-cigarette use in the past 30 days is 5.0 percent, much lower than observed among youth (Kasza et al., 2017). Of these adults, nearly all started vaping after having been a regular smoker (CDC, 2016) and most report that quitting smoking and health improvement are major reasons for starting e-cigarette use (Patel et al., 2016; Zhuang et al., 2016). By contrast, use among never smokers is common in adolescents and young adults age 24 or younger. Indeed, past 30-day use of e-cigarettes (use on one or more days in the past 30 days) by U.S. high school students rose from 1.5 percent in 2011 to a high of 16.0 percent in 2015, before declining to 11.3 percent in 2016 (HHS, 2016; Jamal et al., 2016). Among U.S. adults age 18 and older, past 30-day e-cigarette use (any use, even one or two times) is higher among those age 18–24 (12.5 percent) compared to those age 25 and older (5.8 percent) (Kasza et al., 2017). Among U.S. high school student past 30-day e-cigarette users in 2014, 55 percent used an e-cigarette at least 3 days and more than one-quarter (27.4 percent) used an e-cigarette on 10 or more days (Neff et al., 2015). About one-third to one-half of youth and young adult e-cigarette users report no history of regular combustible tobacco product use (CDC, 2016; HHS, 2016). Young populations are more likely to cite enjoyment of flavors and social factors as reasons for vaping, in contrast with adults who typically use e-cigarettes with the intention of reducing or quitting smoking (Ambrose et al., 2015; Bold et al., 2016).

Given the sizable population of adolescents and young adults who initiate e-cigarette use without previously having been a regular user of combustible tobacco cigarettes, it is important to understand the health effects of e-cigarette use, per se, in this population. Apart from any inherent direct effects from exposure to e-cigarette aerosols, the use of e-cigarettes among adolescent and young adult never smokers may affect health by changing combustible tobacco use behavior.

CONCEPTUAL FRAMEWORK: PATTERNS OF USE AMONG YOUTH AND YOUNG ADULTS

Among the population of teens and young adults with no history of smoking, several possible transitions in combustible tobacco use behavior may occur as a result of e-cigarette use. To illustrate this, the overarching tobacco product transitions conceptual model posed in Figure 16-1 has been adapted to address the possible effects of e-cigarette use on combustible tobacco cigarette use among adolescents and young adults with no history of cigarette smoking. The committee recognizes that there are four distinct tobacco product use states (no use, e-cigarette only, combustible tobacco cigarette only, dual use) that each may have unique health consequences. However, the current section amalgamates tobacco product use outcomes into two possible states, as depicted in the adapted model in Figure 16-1: (1) smoking (including combustible tobacco cigarette use only and dual use with e-cigarettes), and (2) no smoking (including e-cigarette use only and no use of either tobacco product). Outcomes were collapsed for this section of the chapter to simplify the conceptual model and because there is a paucity of longitudinal data on adolescents and young adults that distinguishes subtypes of smoking outcomes based on concomitant e-cigarette use.

Concentrating primarily on the population of adolescents and young adults with no substantive history of combustible tobacco cigarette smoking, this section focuses on whether those who become e-cigarette users (Path 1a, Figure 16-1) versus those who do not (Path 1b, Figure 16-1) exhibit different patterns of combustible tobacco cigarette use behavior (Paths 2a, 2b, 3a, and 3b). Two types of combustible tobacco product use outcomes are of interest, which correspond to two key research questions: (1) ever use (i.e., starting any level of cigarette smoking—even merely a few puffs versus sustained abstinence), and (2) progression, defined as increases in smoking frequency (i.e., number of days used in past 30), intensity (i.e., cigarettes smoked per day on smoking day), and duration (i.e., length of time in which smoking behavior continues versus ceases following initiation). Collectively, these two transitions are necessary for the overall initiation process, which involves transition from never

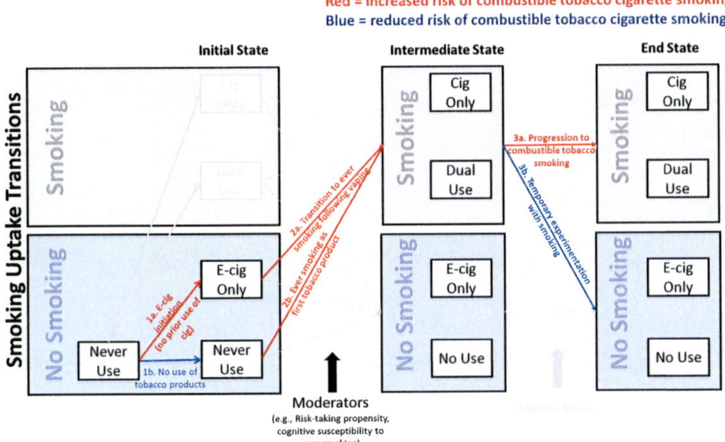

FIGURE 16-1 Conceptual framework for transition from e-cigarette use to combustible tobacco cigarette use initiation and progression.

combustible cigarette smoker to established or regular cigarette use (i.e., not merely temporary experimentation that does not progress to regular smoking).

Transition 1: Among Adolescents and Young Adults with No History of Combustible Tobacco Use, Does E-Cigarette Use Affect Risk of Combustible Tobacco Cigarette Ever Use?

The extent to which factors implicated in ever smoking impact public health is qualified by the fact that a subset of those who become ever users progress to smoke at greater levels of smoking frequency, intensity, or duration (Path 3a, Figure 16-1) and hence become a regular smoker, whereas others may smoke infrequently, smoke very little on each smoking day, and discontinue use shortly following initiation (Path 3b, Figure 16-1) (HHS, 2014). Studying the effect of e-cigarette use on the likelihood of ever smoking is important because ever use is a necessary precursor to progression to regular use. Hence, if e-cigarette use impacts ever smoking, it may have downstream effects on the prevalence of health-damaging courses of smoking. Studying ever use is a particularly useful outcome measure at this time because e-cigarettes have been widely available in the United States only for a short period, leaving the majority of studies lacking sufficient duration of follow-up to study the naturalistic cigarette smoking progression sequence, which can involve a lengthy period between ever use and reaching daily smoking (Chassin et al., 2009; HHS, 2012).

There are three potential ways in which e-cigarette use may impact ever use of combustible tobacco use in young populations. These ways are discussed in the paragraphs below.

Preventive Effect

E-cigarette use could have a preventive effect that deters ever combustible tobacco cigarette use (i.e., probability of transition is lower for Path 2a than 2b, holding all external confounds constant). Some have proposed that for "high-risk" youth with a disposition toward risk-taking behavior (e.g., impulsive personality, novelty-seeking tendency) who are susceptible to smoking initiation, e-cigarettes may provide a diversion that prevents them from experimenting with harmful combustible tobacco products (Etter, 2017; Kozlowski and Warner, 2017). Known sometimes as the "diversion hypothesis," this concept proposes that because some youth possess an elevated drive to engage in exploratory and risk-taking behavior, the availability of e-cigarettes allows such young people to satisfy their curiosity and drive for novelty seeking without needing to resort to combustible tobacco products to satisfy the desire for exploration (Etter, 2017; Kozlowski and Warner, 2017). The diversion hypothesis also proposes that if e-cigarettes were otherwise unavailable, youth prone to risk-taking behavior would be more likely to use combustible tobacco products due to the absence of a suitable non-combustible tobacco substitute (Etter, 2017; Kozlowski and Warner, 2017). In such a case, regulatory policies that reduce e-cigarette use in the population of adolescent and young adult never smokers could indirectly increase the prevalence of smoking and perpetuate the epidemic of tobacco-related illness.

Increased Risk

E-cigarette use could also *increase risk* of ever smoking (i.e., probability of transition is *higher* for Path 2a than 2b, holding all external confounds constant). Sometimes referred to as the "catalyst hypothesis,"[1] this concept proposes a two-step process (Schneider and Diehl, 2016). First,

[1] Some have used the term "gateway" to describe the potential risk-enhancing effect of e-cigarette use on combustible tobacco use initiation (Etter, 2017). Because the term "gateway" has historically been used in colloquial, non-scientific settings and lacks a clear definition, it is not used in this report (Schneider and Diehl, 2016). Instead, this report refers to this potential effect of e-cigarette use on increased smoking initiation as the "catalyst" hypothesis or model as in Schneider and Diehl (2016), which has a clear definition and lends itself to scientifically oriented investigation.

e-cigarettes are suspected to attract "low-risk" teens who would otherwise be deterred from combustible tobacco cigarettes because e-cigarettes possess unique attractive qualities that cigarettes lack, causing e-cigarettes to appeal to a wider segment of the youth population. Relative to combustible tobacco cigarettes, e-cigarettes are perceived to be healthier, be more socially acceptable, be easier to conceal from authority figures, have appealing flavors, have appealing technological features, lack detectable odors, and be easier to access due to inconsistent restriction of sales to youth (Kong et al., 2015; Schneider and Diehl, 2016). Such teens may have a low or moderate risk-taking propensity and may report believing they are not susceptible to trying cigarettes in the future. Second, the exposure to e-cigarettes in this group is suspected to increase proclivity to try combustible tobacco cigarettes (Schneider and Diehl, 2016) for several reasons: (1) the pleasurable sensations caused by nicotine's pharmacological effects or the sensations to the airways and taste may cause adolescent or young adult never smokers to develop more favorable expectations that other tobacco products will also be enjoyable; (2) after successfully engaging in one risky act (i.e., vaping), courage to engage in other risky acts (i.e., smoking) may build; (3) the environments surrounding the procurement of e-cigarettes may increase opportunity to obtain and use combustible tobacco products (e.g., peers who use e-cigarettes may be more likely to smoke and offer cigarettes to their friends; certain e-cigarette retailers may also advertise and sell cigarettes). If e-cigarette use acts as a catalyst for combustible tobacco ever use, regulatory policies that reduce use of e-cigarettes in never smoking adolescents and young adults could ultimately prevent current generations of youth and young adults from developing tobacco-related illness later in life.

No Effect

E-cigarette use could have no effect on combustible tobacco cigarette ever use in adolescents and young adults. That is, if one were to hold constant all possible external confounding influences on the association between e-cigarette use and smoking initiation, there may be an equal probability of transition for Paths 2a and 2b (see Figure 16-1). No effect would be represented by the lack of a statistical association between e-cigarette use and smoking. Alternatively, there could be a statistical association, but the association is entirely due to confounds. For example, often referred to as the "common liability hypothesis" (Etter, 2017; Kozlowski and Warner, 2017), some have proposed that any positive association between e-cigarette use and smoking initiation is due to shared risk factors, such as impulsive and novelty-seeking personality traits or exposure to pro-smoking peers and family members. Under any scenario in which e-cigarette use is deemed not to be associated with smoking combustible tobacco cigarettes (or other substance use and other risky behaviors), the health effects of e-cigarette use on the health of current generations of youth and young adults would be isolated to the direct health effects of exposure to e-cigarette aerosols.

Transition 2: Among Adolescents and Young Adults, Does E-Cigarette Use Affect Risk of Progression to Combustible Tobacco Use Patterns of Greater Frequency, Intensity, or Duration?

Existing evidence on typical smoking trajectories indicate that an appreciable portion of ever users never become frequent smokers, will discontinue, and are temporarily experimenting with smoking (i.e., Path 3b, Figure 16-1) (Dutra et al., 2017; HHS, 2012; Sargent et al., 2017). Other ever users progress to become frequent, heavy, and chronic smokers (i.e., Path 3a, Figure 16-1)—a trajectory that is increasingly more likely the longer someone continues to smoke (Dutra et al., 2017; HHS, 2012; Sargent et al., 2017). A key question is whether adolescents and young adults who become ever smokers after e-cigarette use versus those who become ever smokers with no prior history of e-cigarette use differ in risk of progression in frequency (i.e., days used in the past 30), intensity (i.e., cigarettes per day on smoking day, sometimes termed "heaviness"), or duration of smoking. In Figure 16-1, this question is depicted by whether the probability of progression (versus temporary experimentation) in Path 3a differs as a function if one started smoking through vaping (2a) or not (2b). If e-cigarette use affects post-initiation progression of smoking, the impact of e-cigarette use among never smoking adolescents and young adults on the tobacco-related public health burden will be dependent on e-cigarette effects on both ever use *and* progression to more frequent, heavy, and chronic smoking.

There are three ways in which e-cigarette use may subsequently impact post-initiation adolescent and young adult smoking trajectories.

Preventive Effect

E-cigarette use may reduce risk of smoking progression, such that vapers who become ever smokers may be more likely to be temporarily experimenting with cigarettes, whereas non-vapers who become smokers may be more apt to progress to become more frequent, heavy, and chronic smokers. The "common liability" hypothesis proposes that youth who use e-cigarettes and then transition to combustible tobacco cigarettes are overrepresented by teens with a preference for exploring novel experiences (Etter, 2017; Kozlowski and Warner, 2017). Such youth may be prone to patterns of brief experimentation, wishing to try new activities for the sake of novelty, but they may become bored quickly with tobacco products and move on to other new activities. The common liability hypothesis would predict that young vapers (versus non-vapers) who try cigarettes may be less likely to progress to regular smoking.

Increased Risk

E-cigarette use may increase the risk and speed of progression to more frequent, heavy, and chronic smoking after first trying combustible tobacco cigarettes. For never smokers, the first experience with cigarette smoking can be aversive due to the harsh sensations and bitter taste of cigarette smoke, awkwardness of the smoking self-administration sequence (e.g., puffing, hand-to-mouth movements), and nicotine's aversive pharmacological effects (e.g., nausea, dizziness, airway irritation, bitterness). E-cigarette users may habituate to the aversive pharmacological effects of nicotine and become sensitized to nicotine's addictive effects (e.g., pleasure, anxiolysis) due to nicotine-induced neurobiological changes (Lydon et al., 2014), which would enhance the first few combustible tobacco cigarette smoking experiences. Furthermore, the smoking self-administration ritual may feel more familiar and less awkward to those with previous experience vaping (Wills et al., 2016c). Hence, e-cigarette use could increase the likelihood and speed of progression of the frequency, intensity, and duration of combustible tobacco use.

No Effect

E-cigarette use may have no impact on smoking progression, such that vapers and non-vapers who start smoking show similar likelihood and speed of progression in the frequency, intensity, and duration of smoking. In such a case, youth who start smoking following e-cigarettes may have a risk of tobacco-related illness similar to that of youth who start smoking without a history of e-cigarettes.

EVIDENCE REVIEW: LEVELS OF EVIDENCE AVAILABLE

Because randomized controlled trials to test this research question are not possible and preclinical data testing this question are not entirely relevant, the committee gave extensive consideration to what types of observational data were capable of supporting causal inferences. To this end, the committee applied a framework for determining causality that takes into account multiple streams of evidence to make inferences regarding the causal effect of e-cigarette use on smoking among adolescents and young adults, as in other published work on this topic (Etter, 2017). The framework considered five key criteria in interpreting the principal epidemiological observational evidence as described in greater detail below: (1) strength of the association; (2) consistency across studies, investigators, individuals, research methods, and replications; (3) temporal precedence of e-cigarette use relative to combustible tobacco cigarette smoking; (4) comprehensiveness by which potential confounding effects were addressed and ruled out by covariate adjustment or other methods; and (5) dose responsivity in the association whereby incremental differences in e-cigarette use are associated with proportional differences in smoking initiation and progression outcomes. Supportive evidence addressing the plausibility and concordance with other streams of data were also considered by the committee and are described further below.

Considerations for Observational Data on the Association of E-Cigarette Use with Combustible Tobacco Cigarette Ever Use and Progression

Most evidence addressing this question comes from observational studies of the association between e-cigarette use and ever use and progression of smoking. Although randomized controlled trials are generally considered the strongest study design, randomized studies examining the effects of e-cigarette exposure on never-smoking youth are unethical. A challenge of observational studies is potential confounding, because without randomization, certain factors (confounders) may be systematically and unequally distributed across e-cigarette users and non-users. If these factors are associated with both e-cigarette use and combustible tobacco cigarette smoking initiation and are not in the causal pathway, they could statistically bias the study results and create a spurious effect of e-cigarette use on a combustible tobacco cigarette use outcome. For example, if e-cigarettes attract youth who already have a strong interest in smoking, then e-cigarette use may serve as an indicator of an underlying proclivity to smoke rather than playing a causal role in cigarette initiation. Studies that control for known confounders would be stronger evidence than studies that do not.

In the evidence review of the observational data, studies varied in the breadth of covariates included as confounders for which to statistically control. While residual confounding from unmeasured factors is always possible, the committee considered studies that adjusted for a more comprehensive set of covariates as stronger evidence. These plausible confounders include (1) sociodemographic factors that may address nonspecific shared risk factors; (2) environmental factors that may increase the opportunity, willingness, or interest to use both products (e.g., low monitoring of youth by parents, use of tobacco products by peers or family, permissiveness of tobacco product use by peers or family, exposure to tobacco product advertising); and (3) an endogenous propensity to engage in risk-taking behavior assessed via measures of psychological disposition (e.g., sensation-seeking personality traits, rebelliousness, depression) or risky behaviors (e.g., use of products other than e-cigarettes or combustible tobacco cigarettes, use of non-tobacco drugs of abuse, delinquent behaviors). See Tables 16-1, 16-2, and 16-3 for a listing of the covariates adjusted for in studies that were included in the evidence review.

Among observational study designs, longitudinal studies were considered stronger evidence compared with cross-sectional studies. Given the high plausibility of reverse causality such that combustible tobacco cigarette smoking may also impact e-cigarette use, longitudinal cohort studies that assessed e-cigarette use at baseline and smoking at a future follow-up assessment would provide the strongest evidence to rule out potential reverse causality. Removal of ever smokers at baseline assessment rules out the possibility of reverse causality; however, this approach selects a portion of the population and therefore may not generalize to the entire population of youth and young adults, including those who start smoking at an early age. Alternatively, statistical control of baseline smoking can also address this issue to some extent. The strongest design would follow an entire population of youth beginning at an age at which risk of use of any product is negligible (e.g., 10 years old) and investigate time-varying associations between e-cigarette ever use and later combustible tobacco cigarette use at multiple developmental stages throughout the entire period of risk (e.g., up until age 29), while using multiple methods to establish temporal precedence of vaping relative to smoking. If consistent results are observed across all of the time-varying associations across development through adolescence and young adulthood, a stronger conclusion can be made with confidence in both internal validity and generalizability. Given the brief period in which e-cigarettes have been available, studies with such designs are not available. Hence, the committee considered the body of evidence and whether results were consistent across studies following youth from different regions (e.g., Europe versus North America), youth of different age ranges (e.g., early adolescence versus late adolescence versus emerging adulthood), and those applying different methods (e.g., eliminating baseline smokers versus statistical controls).

Among the longitudinal observational data that are currently available, for the first research question—*Among adolescents and young adults, does e-cigarette use impact risk of ever smoking?*—the committee considered studies that removed ever smokers at baseline from the analytical sample and assessed ever use of smoking at follow-up to reflect the strongest evi-

TABLE 16-1 INITIATION: Summary of Prospective Cohort Studies of the Association Between Ever Use of E-Cigarettes (Versus Never Use) and Subsequent Risk of Ever Smoking of Combustible Tobacco Cigarettes Among Youth/Young Adults Who Were Non-Smokers at Baseline

Reference	Location	Cohort Size	Cohort Age at Baseline	Follow-Up Duration
Barrington-Trimis et al., 2016a	Southern California, USA	298	Median = 17.4 years	Mean = 16 months
Best et al., 2017	Scotland, UK	2,125	11–18 years	12 months
Conner et al., 2017	England, UK	1,726	13–14 years	12 months
Leventhal et al., 2015	Los Angeles, CA, USA	2,530 never users of any combustible tobacco product at baseline	Mean = 14 years	12 months
Loukas et al., 2018	Texas, USA (24 colleges)	2,558	Mean = 19.7 years	18 months
Miech et al., 2017	USA (Monitoring the Future study)	347	High school: 12th grade	Mean = 13.4 months
Primack et al., 2015	USA (Media, Advertising and Health Study)	694	Mean = 20 years	12 months
Primack et al., 2016	USA (nationally representative sample)	915	Mean = 23.5 years	18 months

Measurement Tobacco		OR; 95% CI[c,d]	Adjustments
E-Cigarette[a]	Cigarette[b]		
Ever use	Ever use	5.48; 2.69–11.2	Sex, ethnicity, grade, parental education, and use of hookah, cigar, or pipe at baseline
Ever use	Ever use	2.42; 1.63–3.60	Age, sex, SES, ethnic group, school, smoking susceptibility, peer and family smoking status
Ever use	Ever use	4.06; 2.94–5.60	Age, sex, SES, ethnic group, school, smoking susceptibility, peer and family smoking status
Ever use	Past 6-month use at 6-month and 12-month follow-ups	1.75; 1.10–2.77	Age, sex, ethnicity, parental education, family living situation, peer and family smoking, smoking susceptibility, smoking expectancies, impulsivity, depression, substance use, delinquent behavior
Ever use	Ever use	Overall sample: 1.36; 1.01–1.83. Among baseline never users of any tobacco product: 2.26; CI = 1.35–3.76	Age, sex, race/ethnicity, school, smoking susceptibility, peer smoking, family-of-origin tobacco use, other tobacco use
Ever use	Past 12 months	4.78; 1.91–11.96	Sex, race, baseline marijuana use and binge drinking
Ever use	Ever use	8.3; 1.2–58.6	Age, sex, race/ethnicity, maternal education, peer and parental smoking, sensation-seeking tendency
Ever use	Ever use	6.8; 1.2–58.6	Age, sex, race/ethnicity, relationship status, living situation, education, self-esteem, sensation seeking, rebelliousness

continued

TABLE 16-1 Continued

Reference	Location	Cohort Size	Cohort Age at Baseline	Follow-Up Duration
Spindle et al., 2017	Virginia Commonwealth University	3,757	Mean = 18.5 years	12 months
Wills et al., 2016b	Oahu, Hawaii, USA	1,141	Mean = 14.7 years	12 months

[a] Independent variable.
[b] Dependent variable.
[c] Comparing incidence of combustible tobacco cigarette smoking in baseline users of e-cigarettes compared with the referent category of baseline non-users of e-cigarettes (OR = 1.0).

TABLE 16-2 PROGRESSION: Summary of Prospective Cohort Studies of the Association Between E-Cigarette Use and Subsequent Risk of Recent Smoking/Heavier Smoking of Combustible Tobacco Cigarettes Among Youth/Young Adults

Reference	Location	Cohort Size	Cohort Age at Baseline	Follow-Up Duration
Barrington-Trimis et al., 2016a	Southern California, USA	298 never smokers	Median = 17.4 years	Average = 16 months
Conner et al., 2017	England, UK	318 ever smokers	13–14 years	12 months
Doran et al., 2017	California, USA	391 non-daily smokers	18–24 years	12 months, follow-up every 3 months

Measurement E-Cigarette[a]	Tobacco Cigarette[b]	OR; 95% CI[c,d]	Adjustments
Ever use	Ever use	3.37; 1.91–5.94	Age, sex, race/ethnicity, depression, anxiety, impulsivity, stressful life events, peer deviance, other (non-cigarette) tobacco use
Ever use	Ever use	2.87; 2.03–4.05	Age, sex, race/ethnicity, parental education, family structure, parental support, parental monitoring, rebelliousness

[d] The OR presented for each report is the one adjusted for the largest number of covariates.
NOTE: OR = odds ratio; SES = socioeconomic status.

Measurement E-Cigarette[a]	Tobacco Cigarette[b]	OR, IRR, β; 95% CI[c,d]	Adjustments
Ever use	Past 30-day use	OR = 7.50; 2.41–23.4	Sex, ethnicity, grade, parental education, and use of hookah, cigar, or pipe at baseline
Ever use	Increased use of cigarettes at follow-up among baseline ever users	OR = 1.89; 0.82–4.33	Age, sex, SES, ethnic group, school, smoking susceptibility, peer and family smoking status
Frequency in past 6 months	Total cigarettes smoked	At first follow-up: IRR = 1.13; 1.06–1.21 Interaction with time: IRR = 1.16; 1.09–1.23	A propensity score accounting for sex, race/ethnicity, student status, significant other who smoked, smokers in participant's household, intent to quit

continued

TABLE 16-2 Continued

Reference	Location	Cohort Size	Cohort Age at Baseline	Follow-Up Duration
Hornik et al., 2016	USA (nationally representative sample)	944 baseline non-smokers (total cohort = 1,026)	Mean = 18.3 years	6 months
Leventhal et al., 2016	Los Angeles, CA, USA	2,966	Mean = 15.5 years	6 months
Selya et al., 2017	Chicago, IL, USA	1,007 sample enriched for early adolescent smoking	19–23 years	36 months
Spindle et al., 2017	Virginia Commonwealth University	3,757 never smokers	Mean = 18.5 years	12 months
Unger et al., 2016	Los Angeles, CA, USA	1,056 (all Hispanic) non-smokers	Mean = 22.7 years	12 months

[a] Independent variable.
[b] Dependent variable.
[c] Extent of tobacco cigarette smoking in baseline users of e-cigarettes conditional on e-cigarette use. Odds ratio is reported as estimate of association unless otherwise noted.

Measurement Tobacco		OR, IRR, β; 95% CI[c,d]	Adjustments
E-Cigarette[a]	Cigarette[b]		
Past 30-day use	Past 30-day use	OR = 5.43; 2.59–11.38	Age, sex, race/ethnicity, parental education, ever cigarette use, peer and household smoking, sensation seeking, grades
Four-level use frequency continuum: Never. Prior = ever use, but no use in past 30 days. Infrequent = use 1–2 days in past 30 days. Frequent = used ≥3 days in past 30 days.	Smoking frequency in past 30 days: 0 days, 1–2 days, ≥3 days. Smoking intensity (cigarettes per day on smoking days) in past 30 days: No smoking, <1 cigarette, 1 cigarette, >2 cigarettes.	Frequency proportional odds: OR = 1.37; 1.16–1.31 Intensity proportional odds: OR = 1.26; 1.07–1.48	Age, sex, ethnicity, household structure, parental education, peer and family smoking, smoking susceptibility, smoking expectancies, ever use of alcohol or drugs, ever use of any combustible tobacco product, depression, lack of premeditation, sensation seeking, delinquent behavior
Past 30 day frequency	Past 30 day frequency	β coefficient from a path analysis of prior e-cigarette frequency in relation to later smoking frequency: 0.021 ($p = 0.08$)	Prior-wave e-cigarette frequency, smoking frequency, nicotine dependence
Ever use	Past 30-day use	OR = 3.30; 1.20–9.05	Age, sex, race/ethnicity, depression, anxiety, impulsivity, stressful life events, peer deviance, other (non-cigarette) tobacco use
Past 30 day use status	Past 30-day use	OR = 3.32; 1.55–7.10	Age, sex, past month use of alcohol, hookah, cigars, little cigars, and smokeless tobacco

[d] The estimate of association presented for each report is the one adjusted for the largest number of factors.
NOTE: IRR = incidence rate ratio; OR = odds ratio; SES = socioeconomic status.

TABLE 16-3 DOSE–RESPONSE: Summary of Prospective Cohort Studies of the Association Between E-Cigarette Use Frequency and Subsequent Risk of Smoking of Combustible Tobacco Cigarettes Among Youth/Young Adults

Reference	Location	Cohort Size	Cohort Age at Baseline	Follow-Up Duration
Wills, 2016b	Oahu, Hawaii, USA	1,141 never smokers	Mean = 14.7 years	12 months
Leventhal et al., 2016	Los Angeles, CA, USA	2,966	Mean = 15.5 years	6 months

[a] Independent variable.
[b] Dependent variable.
[c] Comparing incidence of tobacco cigarette smoking in baseline users of e-cigarettes compared with the referent category of baseline non-users of e-cigarettes (OR = 1.0).
[d] The OR presented for each report is the one adjusted for the largest number of factors.

Measurement Tobacco			
E-Cigarette[a]	Cigarette[b]	OR; 95% CI[c,d]	Adjustments
Number of times used at baseline	Ever (versus never) use	Never: 1.0; 95% CI = referent 1–2 times: 2.88; 95% CI = 1.96–4.22 3–4 times: 2.29; 95% CI = 1.35–3.87 Yearly/monthly: 4.17; 95% CI = 2.03–8.57 Weekly/daily: 4.09; 95% CI = 2.43–6.88	Age, sex, race/ethnicity, parental education, parental support, rebelliousness
Frequency: Never. Prior = ever use, but no use in past 30 days. Infrequent = use 1–2 days in past 30 days. Frequent = used ≥3 days in past 30 days.	Smoking frequency in past 30 days: 0 days, 1–2 days, 3 or more days. Smoking intensity (cigarettes per day on smoking days) in past 30 days: No smoking, <1 cigarette, 1 cigarette, >2 cigarettes.	Proportional odds of smoking frequency level versus never use of e-cigarettes: Prior user = 1.51; 95% CI = 0.78–2.93 Infrequent user: 1.94; 95% CI = 0.97–3.91 Frequent user: 2.64; 95% CI = 1.43–4.87 Proportional odds of smoking intensity level versus never use of e-cigarettes: Prior user: 1.44; 95% CI = 0.79–2.64 Infrequent user: 2.02; 95% CI = 1.16–3.53 Frequent user: 1.96; 95% CI = 1.12–3.41	Age, sex, ethnicity, household structure, parental education, peer and family smoking, smoking susceptibility, smoking expectancies, ever use of alcohol or drugs, ever use of any combustible tobacco product, depression, lack of premeditation, sensation seeking, delinquent behavior

NOTES: Additional studies examining associations of e-cigarette use frequency variables with combustible tobacco smoking that did not present pairwise contrasts of varying levels of e-cigarette use are not presented and can be found in Table 16-2. OR = odds ratio.

dence of temporal precedence. For the second research question—*Among adolescents and young adults, does e-cigarette use impact risk of progression in smoking frequency, intensity, and duration?*—the strongest study design for establishing temporal precedence would include at least three time points (see Figure 16-1): a wave 1 in which ever smokers would be eliminated from the sample and e-cigarette use would be assessed as the primary exposure variable. The outcome would address trends in smoking status over time to capture the persistence of use (e.g., smoked since the previous wave of assessment or in the past 30 days leading up to the assessment [yes/no]) as well as trends in frequency (e.g., days smoked in the past 30) or intensity (e.g., cigarettes smoked per day on smoking days). In the case of multiple waves of follow-up data, evidence of a positive baseline e-cigarette use by time interaction term for either smoking status, frequency, or intensity would indicate that e-cigarette use is associated with increased likelihood or speed of progression in the respective outcome, whereas a negative interaction term would indicate that e-cigarette use is associated with reduced likelihood or speed of progression.

Other strategies employed for addressing whether e-cigarette use was associated with progression include two time points, but by contrast with evidence addressing initiation, studies with only two waves would not merely assess ever use at follow-up. Given that youth who ultimately progress to become frequent, heavy, and chronic smokers in adulthood are of greatest public health importance, the weakest evidence of progression to regular use in the two time-point design includes studies that measure recent (e.g., past 30-day) smoking status (yes/no) at follow-up. While past 30-day use typically involves a higher level of smoking than the smoking ever use outcome, the past 30-day outcome is considered a weak indicator of likelihood of progression. Among U.S. high school student past 30-day smokers in 2014, 37.0 percent smoked only 1 or 2 days per month, 22.6 percent smoked every day, and 40.4 percent smoked intermittently (Neff et al., 2015), which underscores the uncertainty of past 30-day use status. Instead, studies that include more detailed measures of smoking frequency that distinguish among monthly, weekly, and daily use and smoking intensity that identify the number of cigarettes smoked per smoking day were considered to provide stronger evidence to address smoking progression. Among studies including only two time points that addressed smoking progression, those that did not eliminate baseline ever smokers and used an alternate strategy for addressing reverse causation (e.g., statistical adjustment of baseline combustible tobacco use, elimination of baseline current combustible tobacco users without eliminating baseline past combustible tobacco users) were considered to provide less robust evidence of temporal precedence of an association of e-cigarette use with smoking progression (Etter, 2017).

Studies in which more frequent or chronic use of e-cigarettes is associated with proportional differences in combustible tobacco use initiation or progression in frequency, intensity, or duration provided further support of causation. Studies using e-cigarette ever use as an assessment of e-cigarette exposure amalgamate youth who may have used e-cigarettes on only one occasion with those who are regular vapers. Such studies were deemed to provide weaker evidence than studies that provide more fine-grained differentiation along a continuum of e-cigarette exposure (e.g., temporary use versus recent use on a monthly basis, recent weekly use versus recent daily use) capable of testing dose–response effects.

Supportive Evidence

While the major emphasis of the evidence review focused on the association of e-cigarette use with smoking initiation and progression in observational data, supplementary lines of evidence were used to provide additional information to address the research questions. Just as studies on the effects of e-cigarettes on health outcomes drew upon in vivo animal and in vitro studies as evidence supporting the biological plausibility of a hypothesized disease pathway, study results that address the specificity of hypothesized biological and psychological mechanisms proposed by the diversion and catalyst hypotheses, respectively, were considered by the committee as supportive lines of evidence of the plausibility that an association identified in the primary review was causal.

Tests of whether the association of e-cigarette use with ever smoking and smoking progression differs by baseline smoking risk status captured by the moderator variables of psychological traits (e.g., rebelliousness) and cognitive susceptibility to smoking (e.g., reported interest and willingness in trying smoking in the future; see Figure 16-1) reflect one line of evidence. That is, evidence of a statistical interaction between e-cigarette use and a moderating variable indicative of a general liability to smoking that is outside of the putative causal pathway from e-cigarette use to changes in smoking was considered. In such research, results consistent with the diversion hypothesis that e-cigarette use prevents ever smoking and smoking progression would demonstrate that there would be a negative association between e-cigarette use and smoking that becomes stronger in higher (versus lower) risk youth in stratified analyses whereby the e-cigarette–combustible tobacco cigarette association is estimated in subgroups differing in level of liability for smoking captured by other moderator variables outside of the causal pathway (e.g., rebelliousness). Results consistent with the catalyst hypothesis would show a positive association between e-cigarette use and smoking initiation that becomes stronger in youth who score lower (versus higher) on such moderator variables.

Also considered were studies examining whether e-cigarette use is associated with changes in intermediate psychosocial mediators that putatively link e-cigarette use with subsequent changes in smoking risk. The mediator variables would include those that are based on concepts proposed in either the diversion or catalyst hypothesis. For instance, evidence that a positive association between baseline e-cigarette use and later combustible tobacco cigarette smoking is mediated by increases in beliefs that smoking is enjoyable would be interpreted as evidence consistent with the catalyst hypothesis and that e-cigarette use increases risk of smoking initiation. Studies demonstrating that e-cigarette use is associated with a subsequent reduction in curiosity or interest in trying cigarettes would support the diversion hypothesis and that e-cigarette use reduces smoking risk. As enjoyment of nicotine's pleasurable effects are hypothesized mechanisms in the catalyst model, studies of whether e-cigarette nicotine concentration is associated with smoking were also considered as relevant to determining plausibility. Qualitative research involving direct testimonials of youth e-cigarette users who explained why they did or did not start smoking were also considered in determining plausibility.

Finally, the committee drew upon additional forms of evidence that provided relevant data to help draw inferences, including ecological studies and studies of other non-cigarette tobacco products. Ecological studies of whether the slope of changes in the prevalence of e-cigarette use and smoking over time are in parallel or opposing directions would cohere with interpretations that e-cigarette use increases or reduces smoking, respectively, and were considered by the committee. As randomized controlled experiments addressing the research questions are unavailable, naturalistic experiments comparing smoking in communities with restrictive e-cigarette use policies for youth (e.g., restrictions against sales to minors) compared with those with permissive youth policies (e.g., no sales restrictions) were considered to provide indirect evidence of the causal effect. Analogous evidence of associations among use of tobacco products popular among youth that are similar to e-cigarettes and cigarette smoking could also provide indirect evidence of causal mechanisms. Like e-cigarettes, hookah and cigarillos are available in characterizing flavors preferred by youth, have not been subject to federal regulation, and have increased in popularity among youth over the past decade. Thus, the committee considered whether analogous associations of relevant, non-cigarette tobacco product use and cigarette smoking initiation existed to interpret the causal effect of e-cigarettes on smoking. Furthermore, the committee reviewed evidence of analogous associations between e-cigarette use and uptake of non-cigarette combustible tobacco products. The committee also reviewed evidence regarding whether e-cigarette use was associated with other risk behavior outcomes (e.g., cannabis use). Among the putative psychosocial and biological mechanisms linking e-cigarette use and changes in smoking proposed by the diversion and catalyst hypotheses are non-specific mechanisms that would also be expected to change risk of other risk behavior outcomes; other mechanisms would be expected to be specific to nicotine and tobacco products. For example, e-cigarette use resulting in satiation of the desire for novelty in the diversion hypothesis and in feeling emboldened to take risks in the catalyst hypothesis are non-specific mechanisms. The enjoyment of the pharmacological effects of nicotine via e-cigarettes in the catalyst hypothesis is a specific mechanism expected to directly increase risk of nicotine and tobacco products more strongly than other risk behaviors. Thus, evidence that the (positive or negative) association between e-cigarette use and subsequent combustible tobacco cigarette use is stronger than the corresponding association of e-cigarette use with another risk behavior, such as cannabis use, would suggest specificity of the association and further strengthen the conclusion from the primary review.

For this supportive evidence, the committee considered study results consistent with the epidemiological data on the association and plausibility as *confirmatory* evidence to strengthen the weight of conclusions. However, because a causal effect can exist in the absence of supporting ecological or analogous evidence due to potential methodological or conceptual limitations that restrict causal inferences from such studies, causal conclusions could be made in the presence of inconsistent evidence across epidemiological studies and these additional forms of evidence.

EVIDENCE REVIEW: METHODS

The primary evidence review was limited to studies of associations between (1) e-cigarette use and (2) ever smoking and progression, including adolescents and young adults age 29 or younger, as risk of smoking onset peaks in adolescence and young adulthood and becomes very low at or after age 30 (HHS, 2012). Because of the difficulty in determining the directionality of associations between e-cigarette and combustible tobacco cigarette use in cross-sectional studies and the presence of a sufficient number of high-quality longitudinal studies, literature review was limited to original primary reports and reviews of studies with a longitudinal design that had a minimum follow-up period of 6 months (i.e., a period in which meaningful changes in youth tobacco use has been demonstrated in prior work). The search strategy is described in Appendix B.

The search identified 5 review papers (4 narrative and commentary papers [Etter, 2017; Kozlowski and Warner, 2017; Phillips, 2015; Schneider and Diehl, 2016] and 1 meta-analysis [Soneji et al., 2017]) and 15 empirical papers that matched these criteria (including those in the review by Soneji and colleagues [Barrington-Trimis et al., 2016a; Best et al., 2017; Conner et al., 2017; Doran et al., 2017; Hornik et al., 2016; Leventhal et al., 2015, 2016; Loukas et al., 2018; Miech et al., 2017; Primack et al., 2015, 2016; Selya et al., 2017; Spindle et al., 2017; Unger et al., 2016; Wills et al., 2016b]).[2] Because the sole review that used meta-analysis (Soneji et al., 2017) was published recently, was deemed to be of high quality based on the ROBIS criteria (Whiting et al., 2016), and included the majority of empirical studies identified (nine studies), the committee reviewed the findings from this meta-analysis. The Soneji and colleagues (2017) paper reviewed and meta-analyzed only the ever and past 30-day use status data at one follow-up from each of the nine studies; the paper does not address dose–response effects and some outcomes indicative of progression in smoking frequency, intensity, or duration. Yet, two of the nine published studies also reported alternative e-cigarette exposure and smoking outcome results of interest, such as smoking or e-cigarette use frequency or multiple follow-up time points, and were reviewed in addition to the overarching results of the Soneji and colleagues (2017) meta-analysis (Leventhal et al., 2015; Wills et al., 2016b). The committee also reviewed the findings from four other studies that fit the criteria for the current evidence review, but were not included in the Soneji and colleagues (2017) meta-analysis because they were published after the publication date (Best et al., 2017; Conner et al., 2017; Doran et al., 2017; Selya et al., 2017). An additional study (Leventhal et al., 2016) that was published prior to, but not included in, the Soneji and colleagues (2017) paper was included in the committee's review. This paper did not meet the Soneji and colleagues inclusion criteria because it included baseline smokers in the sample but was nonetheless relevant to addressing the committee's research question regarding smoking progression.

For the supplemental evidence review, the committee conducted a targeted review of papers based on the premises described in the section above on levels of evidence available. This review included studies of moderators and mediators of the vaping–smoking association that addressed plausibility; ecological evaluations of trends in vaping and smoking over time; effects of age restrictions on e-cigarette sales on smoking that addressed coherence; and studies on the analogous association of non-cigarette tobacco product use with cigarette smoking and e-cigarette use with other tobacco product use.

---

[2] Two studies are abstracts and therefore do not meet the committee's inclusion criteria, but are included here because they were included in the systematic review and meta-analysis by Soneji and colleagues (Hornik et al., 2016; Primack et al., 2016).

EVIDENCE REVIEW: RESULTS

Systematic Review

Method

The Soneji and colleagues (2017) systematic review and meta-analysis included nine studies of U.S. participants age 14 to 26 at baseline based on a search of PubMed, EMBASE, Cochrane Library, Web of Science, the 2016 Society for Research on Nicotine and Tobacco 22nd Annual Meeting abstracts, the 2016 Society of Behavioral Medicine 37th Annual Meeting & Scientific Sessions abstracts, and the 2016 National Institutes of Health Tobacco Regulatory Science Program Conference between February 7 and February 17, 2017. Studies that evaluated the association of ever e-cigarette use among never cigarette smokers at baseline with cigarette ever smoking by follow-up were included. The meta-analysis also included studies that evaluated the association between past 30-day e-cigarette use at baseline with past 30-day smoking at follow-up among baseline non-smokers. Only longitudinal studies were included; cross-sectional studies were excluded. Three independent investigators reviewed the title, abstract, and text of the studies to determine whether the studies met inclusion criteria for the meta-analysis. The interrater agreement among the three reviewers, measured by Fleiss' κ, was 86.1 percent, which is considered to be adequate. The quality of the included studies was evaluated using the Newcastle-Ottawa Scale, which assesses the quality of non-randomized studies and the risk of bias using the Risk of Bias in Non-randomized Studies of Interventions tool, which considers biases from confounding, selection of participants into the studies, missing data, and measurement of outcomes by two independent investigators.

For the meta-analysis, the exposure variables were ever e-cigarette use (yes/no) and past 30-day e-cigarette use status (1 day or more versus 0). The outcome variables were ever smoking status (yes/no) and past 30-day smoking status (1 day or more versus 0). Two parallel sets of associations were analyzed to study the risk of transition from e-cigarette to cigarette use: (1) the relation of baseline ever e-cigarette use with subsequent ever use of combustible tobacco cigarettes at follow-up among baseline never users of combustible cigarettes, and (2) the relation of baseline past 30-day e-cigarette use with subsequent past 30-day use of combustible tobacco cigarettes among those reporting no use of combustible tobacco cigarettes in the past 30 days at baseline. For each outcome, two overall odds ratio (OR) estimates based on a random effects model were reported that combined each study's (1) unadjusted OR and (2) OR after adjusting for covariates in the respective primary literature article. For both analyses, statistical heterogeneity of effect estimates was tested using the I^2 statistic. For the cigarette smoking initiation analysis, the source of heterogeneity between studies was examined by conducting subgroup analyses based on age of the participants, baseline year of study, and whether the sample was a nationally representative sample or regional sample.

Results

Nine studies met inclusion criteria (n = 16,621): seven provided data to address the association with smoking initiation and two addressed the association with past 30-day smoking.

Ever-use analysis The ever-use analysis in Soneji and colleagues (2017) can be used for evaluation of the first research question in this section: Among adolescents and young adults, does e-cigarette use affect risk of ever smoking? Each of the seven ever-use studies eliminated ever smokers of combustible tobacco cigarettes at baseline, providing strong evidence of temporal precedence and eliminating some reverse causation explanations (i.e., past smokers seek out e-cigarette use by baseline and then subsequently return to smoking at follow-up). The combined unadjusted and adjusted ORs for the association of e-cigarette–ever use with ever cigarette use across the seven studies were OR = 3.83 (95% CI = 3.74–3.91) and OR = 3.50 (95% CI = 2.38–5.16), respectively, which reflect strong magnitudes of association. Results are shown in Table 16-4. The seven studies were performed by four independent research groups, included a variety of methodologies (i.e., paper-and-pencil surveys, the Internet, phone), sampling regions and strategies (i.e., three national samples, two from southern California, one from Hawaii, and one from Virginia), and age ranges (mean age at baseline range = 14.1–23.5 years). Given the differences across studies and that each study individually found a statistically significant positive association between e-cigarette ever use and smoking initiation, strong evidence in consistency of the association was determined.

The probability of transition from never use to use of combustible tobacco cigarettes during the follow-up period for baseline–e-cigarette–ever users ranged from a low of 7.9 percent in a sample of 9th-grade students (Leventhal et al., 2015) to 40.4 percent in a sample of 11th- and 12th-grade students (Barrington-Trimis et al., 2016a). These estimates of ever use are high compared to previous results for smoking over 12-month follow-up periods in youth and young adults (HHS, 2014) and the comparison groups of e-cigarette–never users in each study for which use over the follow-up period ranged from 3.0 percent (Leventhal et al., 2015) to 10.6 percent (Spindle et al., 2017) across studies.

TABLE 16-4 Meta-Analysis of Unadjusted and Adjusted Odds of Ever Smoking Combustible Tobacco Cigarettes Among Combustible Tobacco Cigarette–Never Smokers at Baseline and E-Cigarette–Ever Users at Baseline Compared with E-Cigarette–Never Users at Baseline

	Probability of Combustible Tobacco Smoking During Follow-Up Period, %			
Reference	E-Cigarette–Ever Users	E-Cigarette–Never Users	Unadjusted OR; 95% CI	Adjusted OR; 95% CI
Miech et al., 2017	31.1	6.8	6.23; 1.57–24.63	4.78; 1.91–11.96
Spindle et al., 2017	29.4	10.6	3.50; 2.41–5.09	3.37; 1.91–5.94
Primack et al., 2016	37.5	9.0	6.06; 2.15–17.10	6.82; 1.65–28.22
Barrington–Trimis et al., 2016a	40.4	10.5	5.76; 3.12–10.66	6.17; 3.29–11.57
Wills et al., 2016b	19.5	5.4	4.25; 2.74–6.61	2.87; 2.03–4.05
Primack et al., 2015	37.5	9.6	5.66; 1.99–16.07	8.30; 1.19–58.00
Leventhal et al., 2015	8.8	3.1	2.65; 1.73–4.05	1.75; 1.10–2.78
First follow-up	9.7	3.0		
Second follow-up	7.9	3.3		
TOTAL	23.2	7.2	3.83; 3.74–3.91	3.50; 2.38–5.16

NOTES: Heterogeneity: $\tau^2 = 0.13$; $Q_6 = 13.79$; $p = 0.03$; $I^2 = 56\%$. Test for overall effect: $z = 6.34$; $p < 0.001$. The odds ratios (ORs) for the studies are adjusted for a study-specific set of demographic, psychosocial, and behavioral risk factors (see Table 16-1 for covariates).
SOURCE: Adapted from Soneji et al., 2017.

The associations in each of the seven studies were statistically significant and there was heterogeneity in the combined estimate, suggesting variation in effect magnitude across the studies. The authors attempted to explain heterogeneity via subgroup analysis, which found non-significant heterogeneity estimates when the set of studies was limited to the six with young adults only, three studies conducted after 2014, and three nationally representative studies. A limitation of this finding is that a formal interaction test was not conducted to determine whether age, time of publication, or regional versus nationally representative sampling significantly moderated the combined OR estimate across the two groups of studies, perhaps because of the small number of studies precluding formal interaction tests.

This review used a standardized assessment of risk of bias of the individual studies, all of which were deemed as moderate due to potential confounding. There was variability in the types and number of confounding covariates included in the primary articles. Some papers included a more comprehensive set of covariates addressing plausible shared risk factors across demographic, environmental, and intrapersonal/endogenous dispositional domains, providing a more rigorous evaluation of the degree to which an observed association between e-cigarette use and subsequent smoking is direct (i.e., not due to confounding), whereas some included demographic factors and excluded important environmental or intrapersonal factors. The relative difference in ORs between unadjusted and adjusted estimates varied across the seven studies included in the meta-analysis (see Table 16-4). Some studies found larger ORs for unadjusted than adjusted estimates (Leventhal et al., 2015; Miech et al., 2017; Wills et al., 2016b). Others found larger ORs for the adjusted than the unadjusted estimates (Primack et al., 2015, 2016). For two studies, the unadjusted and adjusted ORs did not meaningfully differ (Barrington-Trimis et al., 2016a; Spindle et al., 2017). The net results of this pattern across studies were combined estimates of unadjusted OR = 3.83 (95% CI = 3.74–3.91) and adjusted OR = 3.50 (95% CI = 2.38–5.16) that did not markedly differ from one another as evidenced by highly overlapping confidence intervals for the two estimates. Variation in the disparity in OR estimates between unadjusted and adjusted results across studies could be due to cross-study differences in covariate adjustment. However, inspection of the covariates adjusted for in each study failed to reveal a systematic effect (i.e., the studies with more comprehensive covariate adjustment did not necessarily show reductions in OR estimates from unadjusted to adjusted models). Given this pattern of results, it is difficult to determine the potential influence of residual confounding by unmeasured variables on the associations observed.

An important limitation was the high loss to follow-up in six of the studies (greater than 20 percent). The studies addressed attrition in a number of ways, including (1) comparing associations with complete case analysis to results from analysis using maximum likelihood estimation methods (Wills et al., 2016b), (2) using alternative assumptions that all lost to follow-up are either initiators or non-initiators (Leventhal et al., 2015), and (3) using auxiliary variables to estimate and impute outcome data (Primack et al., 2015). In no cases did the results substantively differ when comparing differing methods for addressing attrition. Because youth and young adults who are lost to follow-up are typically more likely to possess risk factors for cigarette use in previous research (Young et al., 2006) as well as being e-cigarette users at baseline (Barrington-Trimis et al., 2016a; Leventhal et al., 2015; Wills et al., 2016c), the differential loss to follow-up would have resulted in selection bias that most likely would have suppressed the magnitude of the association of the individual articles reviewed for the meta-analysis.

Past 30-day use analysis The combined unadjusted and adjusted ORs for the association of past 30-day e-cigarette use with past 30-day cigarette use were OR = 5.68 (95% CI = 3.49–9.24) and OR = 4.28 (95% CI = 2.52–7.27), respectively (see Figure 16-2). For the past 30-day use analysis, only two primary literature studies were included (Hornik et al., 2016; Unger et al., 2016), raising questions about the generalizability and stability of the combined OR estimate for past 30-day associations. Additionally, youth with a prior history of smoking were permitted in the past 30-day use analysis, which was not adjusted for in one of the studies, allowing for reverse causation. Furthermore, past 30-day use does not address ever use, per se, and provides an imprecise estimate of progression to more frequent, heavy, or chronic smoking. Hence, the past 30-day use analysis in Soneji and colleagues (2017) did not provide rigorous evidence to evaluate either the ever use or progression research questions.

Other Original Studies

Leventhal and colleagues (2015) examined the association between baseline ever use of e-cigarettes with past 6-month smoking status at 6- and 12-month follow-ups among 2,530 baseline never smoker ninth-grade students in Los Angeles. Although this article was reviewed by Soneji and colleagues (2017), they focused on the bivariate association between e-cigarette use and ever-smokers averaged across follow-up, without considering the effects across multiple time points reported in Leventhal and colleagues (2015), which addresses the question of whether e-cigarette use is associated with duration of smoking. Hence,

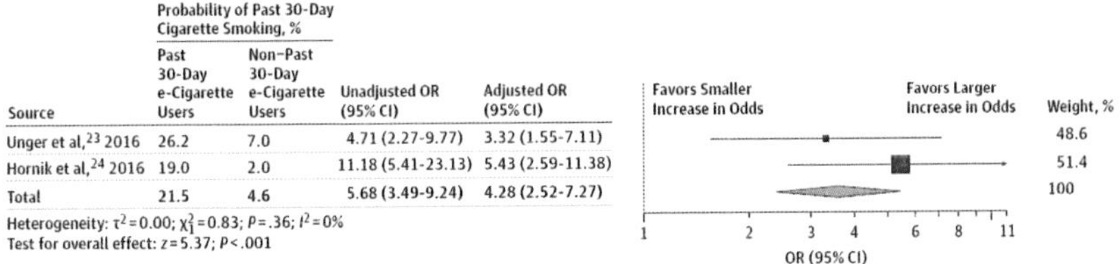

FIGURE 16-2 Meta-analysis of adjusted odds of current (past 30-day) combustible tobacco cigarette smoking at follow-up among non-current combustible tobacco cigarette smokers at baseline and current e-cigarette users at baseline compared with non-current e-cigarette users at baseline.
NOTE: OR = odds ratio.
SOURCE: Soneji et al., 2017.

the multiple-time-point analysis in Leventhal and colleagues (2015) was reviewed by the committee. The exposure variable was ever versus never e-cigarette use at baseline in this study. The outcome was smoking status over the previous 6 months (any smoking versus no smoking). The study found no significant interactions between e-cigarette ever use and time in the prediction of combustible tobacco cigarette smoking (interaction adjusted OR = 0.74; 95% CI = 0.34–1.61, p = 0.44), which suggests that the likelihood of persistence (versus discontinuation) of smoking across the 6- and 12-month follow-ups was non-significantly lower among e-cigarette users. Of baseline e-cigarette–ever users compared to e-cigarette–never users, 9.7 percent versus 3.0 percent smoked in months 1 through 6 of follow-up and 7.9 percent compared to 3.3 percent had smoked in months 7 through 12 of follow-up, respectively. An additional analysis found that baseline e-cigarette–ever users (versus never) were more likely to be sustained users of any combustible tobacco product across both follow-ups (10.0 percent versus 3.6 percent). This study had a high follow-up rate (98 percent), adjusted for a comprehensive set of covariates and potential confounders, and removed baseline smokers to provide temporal precedence. The study was limited because dose–response effects could not be evaluated given the e-cigarette ever use exposure variable. In sum, no conclusive evidence of whether e-cigarette use is associated with duration of smoking among initiators was found in this study.

Wills and colleagues (2016b) reported associations of e-cigarette use with smoking in 9th and 10th graders in Hawaii who were surveyed in 2013 (baseline) and followed up 1 year later. While included in the Soneji meta-analysis, this study was individually reviewed by the committee because it included supplementary analyses of e-cigarette and combustible tobacco cigarette use frequency estimates not addressed in Soneji and colleagues (2017). In analyses of dose–response associations with smoking initiation among 1,070 adolescent never smokers at baseline, the probability of ever smoking at 1-year follow-up was 5 percent among baseline never vapers, which was significantly lower than the probability of ever smoking for youth who had vaped one to two times in their life (14 percent versus 5 percent; adjusted OR = 2.88; 95% CI = 1.96–4.22), three to four times in their life (11 percent versus 5 percent; adjusted OR = 2.29; 95% CI = 1.35–3.87), yearly/monthly (19 percent versus 5 percent; adjusted OR = 4.17; 95% CI = 2.03–8.57), or weekly/daily (19 percent versus 5 percent; adjusted OR = 4.09; 95% CI = 2.43–6.88) at baseline after adjusting for demographic-, environmental-, and psychological/personality-related covariates. Although these estimates suggest a possible threshold effect for association between e-cigarette use frequency and smoking initiation for the two higher versus two lower e-cigarette exposure groups, pairwise comparisons with the Tukey-Kramer adjustment indicated that the four frequency levels of e-cigarette use did not differ significantly from each other in smoking initiation likelihood. Pairwise tests may have been limited in power due to smaller sample sizes for individual group pairs. In the same subsample, analyses examined dose–response associations with probability of initiating and progressing to smoking at least a few times per month or more (versus no initiation or initiating, but not progressing to at least a monthly smoking frequency). The probability of initiating and progressing to monthly smoking was not different between adolescents who vaped one to four times versus never in their life at baseline (0.6 percent versus 1.0 to 1.2 percent, adjusted OR < 1.88), but was higher among those who vaped yearly/monthly (4.2 percent versus 0.6 percent, adjusted OR = 7.13; 95% CI = 1.28–39.73) or weekly/daily (9.7 percent versus 0.6 percent: OR = 17.19; 95% CI = 7.24–40.79) versus never vaped at baseline. These estimates suggest a possible threshold effect whereby at higher frequency levels of vaping, the likelihood of initiating and progressing to more frequent smoking is increased, but at low levels of vaping frequency the likelihood of progression in smoking frequency is not changed. However, the small sample size for the individual groups, and resulting wide confidence intervals of the estimates, tempers conclusive inferences regarding possible threshold effects. In sum, Wills and colleagues (2016b) show suggestive evidence that "dose" of e-cigarette exposure (i.e., use frequency) may differentiate likelihood of smoking initiation and progression in frequency.

Leventhal and colleagues (2016) examined the association between baseline e-cigarette use frequency with progression of combustible tobacco cigarette use frequency and intensity at a 6-month follow-up in 3,084 10th-grade high school students in Los Angeles. This paper included the same cohort as Leventhal and colleagues (2015), but used different time points. This study was not included by Soneji and colleagues (2017) because it was published after their analysis. The e-cigarette use exposure variable was defined as a four-level gradient variable (never versus ever use with no use in past 30 days [prior use] versus 1–2 days in past 30 [current infrequent use] versus ≥3 days in past 30 [current frequent use]). The combustible tobacco cigarette use frequency outcome was a three-level variable based on days used in past 30 (0 versus 1–2 days versus 3 days of use or more). The intensity of combustible cigarette use outcome was characterized with a four-level variable based on the amount of smoking per smoking day (no smoking versus less than one cigarette versus a whole cigarette versus two cigarettes or more). Adjusting for baseline smoking and other covariates, ordinal logistic regression found that each increment higher on the four-level baseline vaping level was associated with proportionally higher odds of smoking at a greater level of frequency (OR = 1.37; 95% CI = 1.16–1.61) and intensity (OR = 1.26; 95%

CI = 1.07–1.48) by follow-up. Adjusting for baseline smoking, pairwise ordinal logistic regression results suggested a dose–response association for smoking frequency, yielding ORs of 4.61 (95% CI = 2.49–8.53) for prior (versus never) baseline vaping, 6.60 (95% CI = 3.48–12.51) for current infrequent (versus never) baseline vaping, and 10.62 (95% CI = 6.46–17.46) for current frequent (versus never) baseline vaping. This study also demonstrated that the positive association between baseline e-cigarette using and follow-up smoking frequency and intensity was stronger among baseline non-smokers than baseline infrequent and frequent smokers in the form of a statistical interaction. In baseline non-smokers, there was evidence of a dose–response association such that smoking frequency at follow-up increased proportionately across baseline vaping frequency, as follows: baseline never users (infrequent smokers = 0.7 percent; frequent smokers = 0.5 percent); prior vapers (infrequent = 3.9 percent; frequent = 2.3 percent); infrequent vapers (7.1 percent, 3.6 percent); and frequent vapers (5.4 percent, 9.7 percent). In baseline smokers, vaping was not significantly associated with smoking frequency at follow-up. Lower strength of vaping–smoking associations in baseline smokers (versus non-smokers) has been reported elsewhere (Conner et al., 2017; Miech et al., 2016; Wills et al., 2016b). As reported in Leventhal and colleagues (2016), this result could suggest that e-cigarette use is more strongly associated with the onset (or return) to smoking as well as the progression to higher levels of cigarette use over the follow-up period, but may have less of an effect among those who are already smokers—many of whom may have started vaping after smoking initiation. In several other studies that report results by baseline smoking status (Conner et al., 2017; Leventhal et al., 2016; Miech et al., 2016; Wills et al., 2016b), the association between vaping and subsequent smoking was null or weakly positive among baseline smokers, which suggests that e-cigarette use is not associated with smoking reduction or cessation in youth and young adults. A strength of the study was the comprehensive adjustment of covariates, which included 15 demographic, environmental, and intrapersonal factors, and high participation (80 percent or more) and retention (99 percent) rates. A limitation was the brief follow-up and the inclusion of youth with a history of smoking, which treated ever smoking as a covariate and baseline current smoking frequency as a moderator rather than eliminating baseline ever-smokers from the analysis to prevent reverse causation. Overall, this study provided fairly strong evidence of dose–response associations between e-cigarette use and progression in smoking frequency and intensity for non-smokers at baseline.

In a sample of 391 non-daily combustible tobacco cigarette smokers age 18 to 24 in California, Doran and colleagues (2017) conducted a longitudinal study that examined whether e-cigarette use frequency was associated with changes in use of combustible tobacco cigarettes over a 12-month follow-up period. This study was published after the Soneji and colleagues (2017) analysis. E-cigarette use frequency was initially assessed via a five-level variable indicative of use over the previous 6 months (never; one to three times; one to two times per month; weekly; two to four times per week; and daily/almost daily). At each follow-up evaluation, the investigators assessed the number of days smoked (i.e., frequency) and total amount of cigarettes smoked (i.e., intensity) over the previous 14 days. Negative binomial regression models adjusting for baseline cigarette use and a propensity score based on a prediction model involving a number of demographic, environmental, and intrapersonal covariates was used. There was a positive association between initial e-cigarette use frequency with cigarette use frequency and intensity at follow-up. For smoking intensity, the incidence rate ratio (IRR) was 1.13 (95% CI = 1.06–1.21), indicating that each one-category increase in initial e-cigarette frequency (e.g., from one to three uses in 6 months to monthly use) was associated with a 13 percent greater number of total cigarettes reported at the second assessment. Analyses of trends in smoking over time across multiple follow-up time points showed a significant interaction for smoking quantity, indicating that this gap widened over time (IRR = 1.16; 95% CI = 1.09–1.23), as illustrated by the higher slope in cigarette intensity across the follow-ups for individuals who used e-cigarettes at a greater frequency at the initial assessment. For smoking frequency outcomes, the interaction between e-cigarette use frequency and time was not significant. A strength of this study was the assessment strategy using frequent follow-ups and short interassessment intervals (i.e., once every 3 months for five total assessments), detailed characterization of exposure and outcome variables to show dose–response relations, and high retention rate (95 percent). In addition, the covariates used to generate a propensity score were comprehensive. Because all participants were smokers at baseline, it is possible that most started smoking before using e-cigarettes, leaving the temporal precedence of the association unclear. It is possible that there is a selection bias whereby those most at risk who are likely to escalate their smoking start using e-cigarettes as a means to help with cravings or because of unsuccessful efforts to quit (rather than a causal effect whereby using e-cigarettes intensifies smoking progression). However, the authors included intention to quit in the propensity score that was adjusted for in the analysis. In sum, this study provides suggestive evidence that e-cigarette use may be associated with increased progression in smoking intensity and in frequency to some degree.

Best and colleagues (2017) examined the association of baseline e-cigarette–ever use (versus never) with cigarette use initiation at 1-year follow-up among 11- to 18-year-old baseline never smokers (n = 2,125) enrolled in four schools in Scotland from 2015 to 2016. This study was published after the Soneji and colleagues (2017) analysis. In an unadjusted model, the OR for ever smokers at follow-up in e-cigarette–ever users versus e-cigarette–never users was 4.62 (95% CI = 3.34–6.38). Adjusting for demographics, susceptibility to smoking, and family/peer smoking, the OR remained significant and was 2.42 (95% CI = 1.63–3.60). A limitation of this study was that other intrapersonal covariates indicative of a propensity toward risk-taking behavior were not included. Also, there was a modest retention rate (70.8 percent), which may reduce the magnitude of the association due to the possibility of dropouts being disproportionately likely to use e-cigarettes at baseline and smoke at follow-up. Finally, e-cigarette exposure level was not reported, precluding investigation of dose–response associations. Strengths are elimination of baseline never smokers from the analytical sample, which permits temporal conclusions about the association that e-cigarette use at baseline was related to an increased probability of transition to becoming an ever smoker at follow-up. In sum, the study methods and results are highly similar to the seven original studies included in the Soneji and colleagues (2017) meta-analysis of initiation and suggests generalization of e-cigarette use–smoking initiation associations to a sample outside the United States.

Conner and colleagues (2017) investigated the association of e-cigarette use at baseline and smoking at a 1-year follow-up among 2,836 adolescents (age 13 to 14 years at baseline) in 20 schools in England from 2014 to 2015. In baseline never smokers (n = 1,726), probability of transitioning from never to ever combustible cigarette use at follow-up was associated with ever (compared to never) use of e-cigarettes at baseline (OR = 5.38; 95% CI = 4.02–7.22), which remained significant when controlling for covariates (OR = 4.06; 95% CI = 2.94–5.60). In adolescents who had tried cigarettes but were not current smokers at baseline (n = 318), ever use was associated with progression in smoking frequency at follow-up (OR = 2.16; 95% CI = 1.01–4.62), which became non-significant when controlling for covariates (OR = 1.89; 95% CI = 0.82–4.33). A unique strength of this study was that smoking was biochemically verified by breath carbon monoxide (CO) readings, and those who had recently smoked or who were defined as having progressed showed significantly higher CO than non-smokers. Due to its half-life, CO is only detected after recent smoking and is thus an insensitive measure for detecting ever use or infrequent smoking. Also, there was a comprehensive set of covariates adjusted for that help to rule out confounding effects. There was a moderate 21 percent attrition rate speculated by the authors to be due to a failure to correctly match anonymous code numbers for students across assessments. Attrition analyses found modest differences between those with and without follow-up data on key variables and no differences in baseline e-cigarette use, suggesting that the impact of attrition on association estimates was small. Adolescents who indicated "I have only tried smoking once" or "I used to smoke sometimes, but I never smoke cigarettes now" at baseline and then selected one of the following, "I sometimes smoke cigarettes now, but I don't smoke as many as one a week," "I usually smoke between one and six cigarettes a week," and "I usually smoke more than six cigarettes a week" at follow-up were classified as having progressed in their smoking. This definition is highly circumscribed and fails to differentiate among low-, moderate-, or high-frequency levels. Also, due to a small number of cases of frequent e-cigarette use, the e-cigarette exposure variables were based on ever use, leaving unclear possible dose–response effects. In sum, this study provides evidence that e-cigarette use is associated with smoking initiation in British youth and weak and inconclusive evidence that e-cigarette use is associated with progression to more frequent smoking.

Selya and colleagues (2017) examined the association between past 30-day e-cigarette and combustible tobacco cigarette use frequency in a young adult sample (age 19–23) originally recruited to be enriched with smokers attending high schools in Chicago, Illinois (81.1 percent had a history of smoking). Participants were surveyed annually four times from 2011 to 2015 and a cross-lagged structural equation model was used to examine the average estimate of association of e-cigarette use with combustible tobacco cigarette use at the subsequent wave for all prospective paths (i.e., Wave 1 → Wave 2, Wave 2 → Wave 3, Wave 3 → Wave 4). The effects of combustible tobacco cigarette dependence severity and use at the previous wave was adjusted for and the lowest possible score on the smoking dependence scale was imputed for never smokers. The results showed that e-cigarette use was not associated significantly with later increases in combustible tobacco cigarette smoking ($\beta = 0.02$, $p = 0.08$). This study was not well positioned to address whether e-cigarette use contributed to ever smoking and subsequent progression of smoking behavior because the sample was recruited to be enriched for smoking in 2006 (prior to the availability of e-cigarettes). Thus, it is likely that the majority of the sample began using combustible tobacco cigarettes prior to using e-cigarettes, including those who sought out e-cigarettes as a cessation aid. The authors acknowledge this limitation and that they did not adjust for any possible confounders of the association. In sum, this study provides negligible evidence that can be used to address the research questions posed in this review.

Loukas and colleagues (2018) administered four semiannual surveys to 2,558 never smoking 18- to 25-year-old (19.71 ± 1.61) students from 24 Texas colleges four times over a 1.5-year follow-up period beginning in 2014–2015 with retention rates ranging from 79 percent to 81 percent across waves. Transition probability from baseline never smoking to ever smoking during the follow-up period was 20.1 percent versus 8.4 percent for baseline e-cigarette–never users (versus ever). Multivariable, multilevel discrete-time hazard models indicated that baseline e-cigarette–ever use was associated with subsequent transition to combustible tobacco cigarette ever smoking (adjusted OR = 1.36; 95% CI = 1.01–1.83) after adjusting for demographics, combustible tobacco cigarette use susceptibility, family-of-origin tobacco use, friend cigarette use, and other tobacco product use. Analyses stratified by other tobacco product use at baseline showed that e-cigarette–ever use was associated with greater odds of combustible tobacco cigarette–ever use during follow-up in baseline never users of cigars, hookah, or smokeless tobacco (OR = 2.26; 95% CI = 1.35–3.76) but not among ever users of other products at baseline (OR = 1.13; 95% CI = 0.81–1.58). The strengths of the study include a longer follow-up period than most prior research (i.e., 18 months here versus 12 months) and comprehensive adjustment of interpersonal risk factors for smoking. The statistical adjustment of use of other tobacco products and the estimation of associations among young adults who had never used any other tobacco products is another strength, which suggests that the associations were not explained entirely by a non-specific constellation of poly-tobacco product use behavior that generalizes to any form of nicotine or tobacco use. Limitations include the application of ever use in operationalizing the e-cigarette exposure, precluding investigation of dose–response associations between level of e-cigarette use and odds of becoming an ever smoker, and the omissions of some covariates that may provide a more comprehensive adjustment for endogenous liability to smoking (e.g., sensation seeking, depression). In sum, this study provides further evidence of an association of e-cigarette use with transition to ever smoking in young adult college students.[3]

[3] Two studies were published after the end of the committee's search dates for their systematic review that otherwise met the committee's inclusion criteria. Hammond and colleagues (2017) surveyed Canadian high school students (n = 17,318) and found that past 30-day e-cigarette use among baseline never smokers was associated with increased likelihood of smoking a whole cigarette by follow-up and that past 30-day e-cigarette use among baseline never daily smokers was associated with increased odds of having smoked daily for at least 7 consecutive days by follow-up after adjusting for covariates. Bold and colleagues (2017) surveyed high school students (n = 808) across three waves (2013, 2014, and 2015) in three public schools in Connecticut. Past-month e-cigarette use was associated with subsequent past month combustible tobacco cigarette use (Wave 1–2, odds ratio [OR] = 7.08, 95% CI = 2.34–21.42; Wave 2–3, OR = 3.87, 95% CI = 1.86–8.06). These studies provide additional evidence consistent with those included in the committee's review, showing an association between e-cigarette use with subsequent ever smoking and past 30-day smoking, and with progression to more frequent (i.e., daily) smoking.

Supporting Evidence

Studies Addressing Conceptually Plausible Mechanisms by Which E-Cigarette Use Affects Smoking

Studies of psychosocial variables expected to moderate or mediate the association of e-cigarette use with smoking based on conceptual models of the e-cigarette use–smoking link were interpreted by the committee as supportive evidence. For possible moderation effects, the catalyst and diversion models lead to distinct predictions regarding the subgroups of youth and young adults for whom the e-cigarette–smoking association may be most salient. The catalyst hypothesis proposes that e-cigarettes increase smoking among low-risk youth who would be unlikely to have started smoking in the absence of e-cigarettes (Schneider and Diehl, 2016). By contrast, the diversion hypothesis proposes that e-cigarettes reduce smoking among high-risk users who would be liable to initiate smoking in the absence of e-cigarettes by providing an alternative to satisfy a propensity to explore novel experiences (Etter, 2017; Warner, 2016). Finally, a common liability hypothesis would propose that e-cigarette use and smoking may be statistically associated due to a shared propensity to experiment with substances (Etter, 2017); thus, a positive association would be present only in youth who possess risk factors indicative of a liability to smoking.

Of longitudinal studies that provide evidence of an association between e-cigarette use and ever smoking among low-risk youth, all six studies have shown that the positive association of e-cigarette use with ever smoking in adolescents and young adults is present in low-risk youth or significantly stronger among lower- (versus higher-) risk youth in the form of a statistical interaction. The e-cigarette–smoking positive association has been shown to be present or significantly amplified for several indicators of lower-risk status, including among youth who report not being susceptible or willing to start smoking (Barrington-Trimis et al., 2016a; Best et al., 2017; Primack et al., 2015; Wills et al., 2016c), have no friends who smoke (Best et al., 2017; Conner et al., 2017), perceive that smoking poses great risk to health (Miech et al., 2017), have high parental support (Wills et al., 2016c), do not perceive themselves as rebellious (Wills et al., 2016c), and have never used other tobacco products (Loukas et al., 2018). Such findings are concordant with the catalyst hypothesis that e-cigarette use increases smoking by changing the likelihood of smoking in low-risk youth who otherwise would not have been liable to become ever smokers.

The catalyst hypothesis also proposes several mediating processes through which e-cigarette use increases smoking (Schneider and Diehl, 2016). Because e-cigarette use may produce positive sensations in the airways and pleasant tastes and lack aversive effects like lung discomfort, the catalyst hypothesis proposes that e-cigarette use may cause adolescent or young adult never smokers to change their perceptions about combustible tobacco cigarettes to be more favorable and increase their willingness to try smoking. Consistent with this notion, longitudinal studies of baseline never smokers have found that e-cigarette use is associated with future increases in positive perceptions about smoking, willingness to smoke, and lower perceptions that smoking is harmful (Miech et al., 2017; Primack et al., 2015; Wills et al., 2016a), which, in turn, mediate increases in probability of becoming an ever smoker (Wills et al., 2016a). Another mediating mechanism proposed by the catalyst model is that youth who enjoy the pharmacological effects of nicotine or develop initial symptoms of nicotine dependence via e-cigarettes may be more inclined to use other tobacco products with nicotine-related pharmacological effects, such as combustible tobacco cigarettes (Schneider and Diehl, 2016). If this mechanism accounted for some of the association of e-cigarette use with increased future smoking, the amount of nicotine used in e-cigarettes should differentiate the future smoking behavior of youth who vape. Concordant with this notion, a dose–response association between the level of nicotine concentration used in e-cigarettes and increases in future smoking frequency and intensity has been reported among adolescent e-cigarette users (Goldenson et al., 2017).

One qualitative focus group study of perceptions about the effect of e-cigarette use on smoking among Swiss youth and young adult (age 16–26) users and non-users and of combustible tobacco cigarettes, e-cigarettes, or both products addresses the plausibility of the catalyst and diversion models (Akre and Suris, 2017). The majority of testimonials were consistent with the catalyst model, and included statements such as

- *"It's maybe a little smoother to start [vaping] … than by directly starting with a normal cigarette"* (Akre and Suris, 2017, p. 450);
- *"The [e-cigarette] can make the gesture a commonplace, one will lose track of the danger of smoking by starting with the [e-cigarette] just for the taste … and after why not pass on to [tobacco cigarettes] which is the following step"* (Akre and Suris, 2017, p. 450);
- *"I think [vaping is] fun for a little while but it lacks the whole aspect of the normal cigarette"* (Akre and Suris, 2017, p. 450); and
- *"I believe [e-cigarettes] could be a trampoline, like me, I started vaping, and finally I started smoking, while maybe I wouldn't have started smoking if I hadn't vaped"* (Akre and Suris, 2017, p. 450).

While the majority of testimonials in this study were consistent with the catalyst model, the authors reported that a minority of dual-user young adults had opinions that vaping could be a diversion for young adolescents with statements such as, *"I think it's not that bad that the tendency goes toward e-cigarettes for the young ones because if it wasn't for the e-cigarettes they would all turn to tobacco"* (Akre and Suris, 2017, p. 452), and *"Youths now discover the e-cigarette, there are lots of flavors, and then they'll say to themselves 'why would I turn to tobacco?' and they will get used to these flavors and will find tobacco cigarettes disgusting, which is good"* (Akre and Suris, 2017, p. 452). Although the results of the study provided unique contextual information, the results should be interpreted with caution, because the sample was small (n = 42) and non-representative.

Trends in E-Cigarette and Combustible Tobacco Cigarette Use in the Adolescent and Young Adult Population

Trends in the prevalence of e-cigarette use relative to combustible tobacco cigarette smoking over time may also shed light on whether and how e-cigarette use affects smoking. Holding all other factors constant, if e-cigarette use increased risk of smoking, then changes in the prevalence of e-cigarette use should parallel changes in the prevalence of smoking. If e-cigarette use prevented combustible tobacco cigarette smoking, changes in the prevalence of e-cigarette use and smoking over time should oppose each other. Evidence from the National Youth Tobacco Survey (NYTS) show that from 2011 to 2016, the past 30-day use of e-cigarettes increased (non-linearly) and combustible tobacco cigarette use decreased linearly in middle and high school students (Jamal et al., 2017) (see Figure 16-3).

The population-level ecological data are more consistent with the diversion hypothesis than the catalyst hypothesis and run counter to individual-level results, which predominately show that youth and young adults who use e-cigarettes are more likely to become ever smokers and past 30-day smokers. A more granular examination of the population-level data indicates that the pattern of trends in use for the two products are not unequivocally concordant. There is a non-linear trend for past 30-day e-cigarette use in NYTS high school students, which increased from 1.5 percent in 2011 to 16.0 percent in 2015 and then decreased to 11.3 percent in 2016. For past 30-day combustible tobacco cigarette use in the NYTS, use decreased from 15.8 percent in 2011 to 9.3 percent in 2015 and was 8.0 percent in 2016. Due to the methodological limitations of interpreting causality from this descriptive population-level trend analysis and the multitude of influences on population-level e-cigarette use (e.g., policy changes, cultural changes, historical cohort effects), the ecological analysis does not provide strong evidence to rule out a possible risk-enhancing effect of e-cigarette use on youth smoking. Some population-based ecological studies report that downward trends in smoking rates in youth

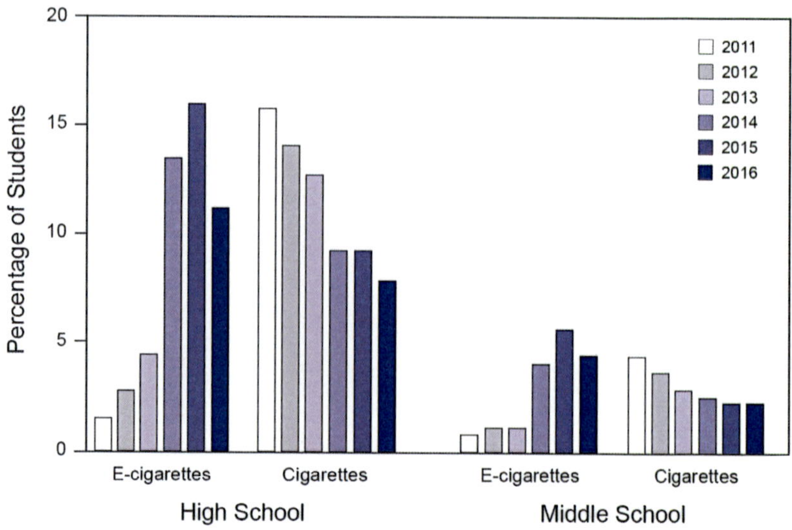

FIGURE 16-3 Past 30-day use of e-cigarettes and combustible tobacco cigarettes among high school and middle school students in the 2011–2016 National Youth Tobacco Survey.
SOURCE: Jamal et al., 2017.

across time stem back for decades. The rate of such reductions did not accelerate over the past several years after e-cigarette use was introduced into the U.S. market and became popular among youth (Barrington-Trimis et al., 2016a,b). In an analysis of NYTS data from 2004 to 2014, interrupted time series of ever (1 puff or more) and current (last 30 days) smoking comparing the rate of deceleration in combustible tobacco cigarette use before and after 2009 when e-cigarettes first became available showed no significant change in the overall linear trend in reduction in smoking by year before versus after 2009 (p = 0.57 and 0.23). Hence, the overall concordance in the ecological data is not clear. Overall, the population-based data broadly show opposing trends in e-cigarette and cigarette use prevalence across time among U.S. youth in recent years and thus do not provide confirmatory evidence of the epidemiological person-level positive associations of vaping and smoking.

Studies of the Association of E-Cigarette Use Policy Change and Youth Smoking

Three studies have examined whether changes in the prevalence of combustible tobacco cigarette use differ among youth who reside across different states as a function of when laws prohibiting sales of e-cigarettes to minors were enacted. The diversion model would hypothesize that magnitude of downward trends in smoking would be slowed before and after enactment of sales restrictions because youth would not have access to e-cigarettes as an alternative to satisfy exploratory drives and would be more likely to resort to smoking (Etter, 2017; Warner, 2016). The catalyst model would hypothesize that e-cigarette sales bans would accelerate downward trends in smoking by reducing the likelihood that one would be exposed to a product that increases risk of smoking (i.e., e-cigarettes). The findings differed across the three studies. The most recent article on the topic by Abouk and Adams (2017) concluded that e-cigarette sales restrictions were associated with reduced adolescent smoking through 2014, while two earlier articles by Friedman (2015) and Pesko and colleagues (2016) came to the opposite conclusion, that e-cigarette sales restrictions were associated with higher levels of adolescent smoking through 2013. Abouk and Adams (2017) noted that the analysis in their study was more "granular" because it took into account the exact month that e-cigarette bans went into place, while the other articles take into account year of the ban. Overall, the small and inconsistent evidence base on this topic fails to provide confirmatory evidence for or against individual-level associations found in the principal epidemiological data. Incidentally, a 2015 Institute of Medicine report addressing the effect of sales restrictions on youth tobacco use concluded that if bans effectively reduce availability of tobacco from commercial sources, the effect of this on use by youth is uncertain because of the continued availability of tobacco from non-commercial sources (IOM, 2015). Hence, these policy change studies provide minimal weight in interpreting the direction and causality of the association of e-cigarette use with youth smoking.

Analogous Studies Involving Other Tobacco Products and Studies of Associations of E-Cigarette Use with Other Risk Behaviors

Given that the catalyst model hypothesizes that e-cigarette use may increase smoking in youth by sensitizing youth to nicotine in a form that is more palatable and lacks aversive qualities of cigarettes (Schneider and Diehl, 2016), other products that share properties with e-cigarettes would also be expected to be associated with increased risk of smoking. Hookah waterpipe is one such product that mirrors e-cigarettes in that it also delivers nicotine, is available in sweet flavorings, and is less irritating to the airways due to water-based filtration and cooling of hookah smoke. Consistent with this notion, Soneji and colleagues (2017) found in a nationally representative sample of U.S. adolescents and young adult never smokers, hookah ever use at baseline was associated with cigarette smoking initiation (adjusted OR = 2.56; 95% CI = 1.46–4.47), past 30-day cigarette smoking (adjusted OR = 2.48; 95% CI = 1.01–6.06), and higher intensity of cigarette smoking (adjusted proportional OR = 2.55; 95% CI = 1.48–4.38) at a 1-year follow-up. In addition, e-cigarettes would be expected to increase risk of other combustible tobacco products per the catalyst hypothesis, which has been shown in several studies (Barrington-Trimis et al., 2016a; Leventhal et al., 2015). However, these studies can also be interpreted as providing evidence for the common liability model. Youth who have a liability to experiment with multiple tobacco products would show indiscriminate forms of poly-tobacco product use involving the use of multiple non-cigarette and cigarette products in various sequences. However, evidence showing that e-cigarette use is associated with later combustible tobacco cigarette use in samples excluding users of other tobacco products suggests that indiscriminate patterns of poly-tobacco product use are unlikely to explain the association (Leventhal et al., 2015; Loukas et al., 2018). Regardless, studies of associations involving analogous tobacco products can be interpreted as providing no evidence of *inverse* associations between use of analogous tobacco products with e-cigarettes and cigarettes, suggesting confirmatory evidence against the diversion hypothesis.

In addition to considering other tobacco products the committee considered associations of e-cigarette use with other risky behaviors. Some (but not all) of the putative mechanisms linking e-cigarette use with later smoking proposed by the catalyst hypothesis are expected to selectively increase risk of smoking and not impact likelihood of engaging in other risky behaviors (Schneider and Diehl, 2016). One longitudinal study of young adults in Los Angeles found that at 1-year follow-up, baseline past 30-day e-cigarette use was more strongly associated with past 30-day combustible tobacco cigarette (OR = 3.32; 95% CI = 1.55–7.10) than past 30-day cannabis use (OR = 1.97; 95% CI = 1.01–3.86) (Unger et al., 2016). The estimate appears larger for combustible tobacco cigarette than cannabis use; however, the confidence intervals for the estimates are overlapping with one another. Thus, this study provides suggestive evidence of specificity of the association from e-cigarette use to smoking aligned with the catalyst hypothesis and adds some further support to the conclusion from the primary review.

SYNTHESIS

Conclusion 16-1. There is ***substantial evidence*** *that e-cigarette use increases risk of ever using combustible tobacco cigarettes among youth and young adults.*

In the primary review of observational studies, there was consistent evidence from 10 of 10 studies[4] that the association between e-cigarette use and transition from never to ever combustible tobacco cigarette smoking was positive in direction. Results were consistent across a number of different methodologies, age ranges, research groups, and locations, and the associations were of considerable strength. While there were moderate to high attrition rates in most of these studies, analyses of attrition effects showed that the impact of attrition on the observed associations was modest. Across the studies, a wide range of covariates were adjusted for that spanned a number of sociodemographic, interpersonal, environmental, and intrapersonal factors, including use of other substances (see Table 16-1), which the committee considered a comprehensive selection of confounding factors. Use of tobacco products other than e-cigarettes and combustible tobacco cigarettes was adjusted for in several of the studies, and two studies reported positive associations of e-cigarette use and subsequent transition to ever smoking among baseline never users of any tobacco product. Covariate adjustment had non-uniform effects on the magnitude of associations, with some reports showing no effect of covariate adjustment and other studies showing a reduction in the estimate from unadjusted to adjusted models. However, the committee found no published reports of non-significant associations after adjusting for covariates. To the extent to which the adjusted covariates addressed the influence of confounders, it is unlikely that confounding entirely accounts for the association because reductions in estimates of association from unadjusted to adjusted models were not consistently observed in the literature. Only a small number of studies provide evidence to assess for the presence of a dose–response association between e-cigarette use and smoking initiation, but the results of these few studies suggested that higher levels of e-cigarette use were associated with increased odds of smoking in baseline non-smokers.

The primary evidence consisted of longitudinal cohort studies that assessed e-cigarette use at baseline and smoking at a future follow-up assessment among baseline never smokers. The committee deliberated at length regarding the strengths and weaknesses of this design and how it impacted interpretation of the evidence. Removal of baseline ever smokers from the analyses is critical for eliminating the possibility of reverse causation. However, this method also systematically alters the population under study in several ways, which could inflate the likelihood of finding

[4] As noted in the evidence review, one additional study published after the end of the committee's search dates for their systematic review that otherwise met the committee's inclusion criteria (Hammond et al., 2017) provides additional evidence of an association between e-cigarette use and subsequent ever smoking.

a positive association between e-cigarette use and ever smoking. Restriction to baseline never smokers removes youth and young adults who have highest liability for early-onset smoking. Because the diversion hypothesis would predict that protection against smoking initiation due to e-cigarette use would be most pronounced among those with highest liability for early-onset smoking, removing baseline smokers could restrict the capacity to detect diversion effects. The remaining sample of never smokers still likely retains some meaningful variation in liability for smoking onset that is not a consequence of e-cigarette use and due to other sources (e.g., social acceptance of smoking, residential proximity to tobacco product retailers). Such variance in smoking liability in the remaining sample of baseline never smokers could potentially influence e-cigarette use and thus confound associations between e-cigarette use and later transition to ever smoking. If, following the premises stated above, removal of baseline ever smokers were to significantly impact capacity to detect diversion effects, estimates of association between e-cigarette use and subsequent ever smoking would be expected to vacillate markedly across studies of populations that differ in liability for smoking. This was not the case. Robust positive associations between e-cigarette use in baseline never smokers and later ever smoking was observed in studies of young adolescents, older adolescents, and young adults, although these populations are known to differ in risk of smoking onset (Johnston et al., 2017). Different regions of the United States and other countries have unique tobacco product policies and sociocultural backdrops that may alter the availability and population-level risk of e-cigarette use or combustible tobacco cigarette use in each location. Associations between e-cigarette use and subsequent ever use of combustible tobacco products were observed in regional U.S. samples from California, Hawaii, Texas, and Virginia, and in nationally representative U.S. samples; and in Canadian, Scottish, and British samples. The overwhelming consistency of results across studies from different locations and across studies that differed in other ways (e.g., wording of survey questions; paper versus Internet survey; with versus without biochemical verification of self-reported smoking; length of follow-up) strengthened the committee's confidence in the robustness, validity, and causality of the association of e-cigarette use with transition from never to ever smoker status.

In the supplemental review, some results confirmed the primary evidence, whereas others did not. Studies of whether the association varied across moderator variables consistently supported the plausibility of the catalyst hypothesis. Eight longitudinal cohort studies found that e-cigarette use increases risk of ever smoking among youth with fewer traditional risk factors for smoking (e.g., fewer friends who smoke)—a subgroup of youth who would be expected to have low likelihood of becoming an ever smoker if e-cigarettes were not otherwise available. Other longitudinal evidence showed that e-cigarette use was associated with increased levels on mediator variables (e.g., more favorable perceptions of smoking) that are presumed by the catalyst hypothesis to channel the effect of e-cigarette use on to smoking. One study found that youth who vaped a higher concentration of nicotine were more likely to subsequently smoke at higher frequency and intensity levels, which further supports the catalyst hypothesis and suggests specificity of the association to nicotine and nicotine-containing products. Collectively, there was very strong evidence from longitudinal cohort studies of high plausibility that e-cigarette use may be a catalyst for smoking initiation, which strengthened the committee's confidence in a possible causal link from e-cigarette use to combustible tobacco cigarette ever use. By contrast, ecological trends in e-cigarette use and smoking prevalence in youth across time failed to provide confirmatory support that e-cigarette use causes smoking initiation, and, if anything, are more consistent with the notion that e-cigarette use is associated with reduced smoking. However, ecological studies of trends going back a decade found that the rate of reduction of smoking in U.S. youth has remained consistent and has not accelerated in recent years when e-cigarettes have become popular. In addition, the changes in the prevalence of tobacco product use by U.S. high school students from 2015 to 2016 declined substantially for e-cigarettes and marginally for combustible tobacco cigarettes, raising questions about whether there is a systematic concordance between e-cigarette and combustible tobacco cigarette use over time in the population. Results from studies of e-cigarette sales restrictions and analogous associations involving cigarette and non-cigarette tobacco products were found to provide negligible weight toward the overall conclusion. Suggestive evidence of specificity of the association of e-cigarette use with combustible tobacco cigarette use relative to cannabis use from one study added marginal weight to the conclusion that e-cigarette use increases risk of becoming an ever smoker. In sum, because the supplemental review provided strong evidence of plausibility and specificity of a possible causal effect of e-cigarette use on smoking, and did not find conclusive evidence to refute the catalyst explanation, the committee considered the overall body of evidence of a causal effect of e-cigarette use on risk of transition from never to ever smoking to be substantial.

> *Conclusion 16-2. Among youth and young adult e-cigarette users who ever use combustible tobacco cigarettes, there is* ***moderate evidence*** *that e-cigarette use increases the frequency and intensity of subsequent combustible tobacco cigarette smoking.*

Conclusion 16-3. Among youth and young adult e-cigarette users who ever use combustible tobacco cigarettes, there is ***limited evidence*** *that e-cigarette use increases, in the near term, the duration of subsequent combustible tobacco cigarette smoking.*

Primary review of the observational literature yielded several studies showing a positive association between e-cigarette–ever use and past 30-day smoking status, which is a weak proxy for patterns of smoking indicative of progression in frequency and intensity. Among studies better positioned to address progression in frequency and intensity, the evidence supported a positive association of more frequent e-cigarette use with progression in smoking frequency and intensity.[5] Dose–response associations were evident or suggestive across most analyses among those four studies. Two studies included multiple follow-up time points and addressed whether e-cigarette use is associated with longer duration of smoking. One study found that e-cigarette use was associated with an acceleration of smoking intensity over time. Another study showed that changes in smoking status across two follow-up times did not significantly differ between baseline e-cigarette–ever users compared with e-cigarette–never users. The supplemental review found that youth nonsmokers who vape higher concentrations of nicotine were more likely to subsequently smoke at higher frequency and intensity rates, which added weight to the plausibility that e-cigarette use affects progression of smoking in some manner. There were no reports across any of the studies reviewed by the committee showing that e-cigarette users were associated with lower likelihood or speed of progression of smoking frequency, intensity, or duration. Hence, it is highly unlikely that e-cigarette users who become ever smokers are overrepresented by youth who may just be temporarily experimenting at low levels of smoking.

REFERENCES

Abouk, R., and S. Adams. 2017. Bans on electronic cigarette sales to minors and smoking among high school students. *Journal of Health Economics* 54:17–24.

Akre, C., and J. C. Suris. 2017. Adolescents and young adults' perceptions of electronic cigarettes as a gateway to smoking: A qualitative study in Switzerland. *Health Education Research* 32(5):448–545.

Ambrose, B. K., H. R. Day, B. Rostron, K. P. Conway, N. Borek, A. Hyland, and A. C. Villanti. 2015. Flavored tobacco product use among U.S. youth aged 12–17 years, 2013–2014. *Journal of the American Medical Association* 314(17):1871–1873.

[5] As noted in the evidence review, one additional study published after the end of the committee's search dates for its systematic review that otherwise met the committee's inclusion criteria (Hammond et al., 2017) provides additional evidence of an association between e-cigarette use and progression to more frequent smoking.

Barrington-Trimis, J. L., R. Urman, K. Berhane, J. B. Unger, T. B. Cruz, M. A. Pentz, J. M. Samet, A. M. Leventhal, and R. McConnell. 2016a. E-cigarettes and future cigarette use. *Pediatrics* 138(1). doi.org/10.1542/peds.2016-0379 (accessed December 29, 2017).

Barrington-Trimis, J. L., R. Urman, A. M. Leventhal, W. J. Gauderman, T. B. Cruz, T. D. Gilreath, S. Howland, J. B. Unger, K. Berhane, J. M. Samet, and R. McConnell. 2016b. E-cigarettes, cigarettes, and the prevalence of adolescent tobacco use. *Pediatrics* 138(2). 10.1542/peds.2015-3983 (accessed December 29, 2017).

Best, C., F. Haseen, D. Currie, G. Ozakinci, A. M. MacKintosh, M. Stead, D. Eadie, A. MacGregor, J. Pearce, A. Amos, J. Frank, and S. Haw. 2017. Relationship between trying an electronic cigarette and subsequent cigarette experimentation in Scottish adolescents: A cohort study. *Tobacco Control* 20(1):140–144. doi: 10.1136/tobaccocontrol-2017-053691 (accessed February 2, 2018).

Bold, K. W., G. Kong, D. A. Cavallo, D. R. Camenga, and S. Krishnan-Sarin. 2016. E-cigarette susceptibility as a predictor of youth initiation of e-cigarettes. *Nicotine & Tobacco Research*. https://academic.oup.com/ntr/article-abstract/20/1/140/2754532 (accessed February 2, 2018).

Bold, K. W., G. Kong, D. R. Camenga, P. Simon, D. A. Cavallo, M. E. Morean, and S. Krishnan-Sarin. 2017. Trajectories of e-cigarette and conventional cigarette use among youth. *Pediatrics*. doi: 10.1542/peds.2017-1832 (accessed February 2, 2018).

CDC (Centers for Disease Control and Prevention). 2016. Quickstats: Cigarette smoking status among current adult e-cigarette users, age group—National Health Interview Survey, United States, 2015. *Morbidity and Mortality Weekly Report* 65(42):1177.

Chassin, L., P. J. Curran, C. C. Presson, S. J. Sherman, and R. J. Wirth. 2009. *Monograph 20: Phenotypes and endophenotypes: Foundations for genetic studies of nicotine use and dependence*. https://cancercontrol.cancer.gov/BRP/tcrb/monographs/20/m20_5.pdf (accessed December 20, 2017).

Conner, M., S. Grogan, R. Simms-Ellis, K. Flett, B. Sykes-Muskett, L. Cowap, R. I. Lawton, L. J. Armitage, D. Meads, C. Torgerson, R. West, and K. Siddiqi. 2017. Do electronic cigarettes increase cigarette smoking in U.K. adolescents? Evidence from a 12-month prospective study. *Tobacco Control*. http://tobaccocontrol.bmj.com/content/early/2017/07/28/tobaccocontrol-2016-053539 (accessed February 2, 2018).

Doran, N., K. Brikmanis, A. Petersen, K. Delucchi, W. K. Al-Delaimy, S. Luczak, M. Myers, and D. Strong. 2017. Does e-cigarette use predict cigarette escalation? A longitudinal study of young adult non-daily smokers. *Preventive Medicine* 100:279–284.

Dutra, L. M., S. A. Glantz, N. E. Lisha, and A. V. Song. 2017. Beyond experimentation: Five trajectories of cigarette smoking in a longitudinal sample of youth. *PLoS ONE* 12(2):e0171808. https://doi.org/10.1371/journal.pone.0171808 (accessed February 2, 2018).

Etter, J. F. 2017. Gateway effects and electronic cigarettes. *Addiction*. doi: 10.1111/add.13924 (accessed February 2, 2018).

Friedman, A. S. 2015. How does electronic cigarette access affect adolescent smoking? *Journal of Health Economics* 44:300–308.

Goldenson, N. I., A. M. Leventhal, M. D. Stone, R. S. McConnell, and J. L. Barrington-Trimis. 2017. Associations of e-cigarette nicotine concentration and subsequent cigarette smoking and vaping levels in adolescents. *JAMA Pediatrics* 171(12):1192–1199.

Hammond, D., J. L. Reid, A. G. Cole, and S. T. Leatherdale. 2017. Electronic cigarette use and smoking initiation among youth: A longitudinal cohort study. *Canadian Medical Association Journal* 189(43):E1328.

HHS (U.S. Department of Health and Human Services). 2012. *Preventing tobacco use among youth and young adults: A report of the Surgeon General.* Atlanta, GA: U.S. Department of Health and Human Services, Centers for Disease Control and Prevention, National Center for Chronic Disease Prevention and Health Promotion, Office on Smoking and Health.

HHS. 2014. *The health consequences of smoking—50 years of progress: A report of the Surgeon General.* Atlanta, GA: U.S. Department of Health and Human Services, Centers for Disease Control and Prevention, National Center for Disease Prevention and Health Promotion, Office on Smoking and Health.

HHS. 2016. *E-cigarette use among youth and young adults: A report of the Surgeon General.* Atlanta, GA: U.S. Department of Health and Human Services, Centers for Disease Control and Prevention, National Center for Chronic Disease Prevention and Health Promotion, Office on Smoking and Health.

Hornik, R. C., L. Gibson, and C. Lerman. 2016. *Pos5-30: Prediction of cigarette use from six-month prior electronic and combustible cigarette use for a U.S. national sample of 13-25 year olds* [abstract]. http://c.ymcdn.com/sites/www.srnt.org/resource/resmgr/Conferences/2016_Annual_Meeting/Program/SRNT_2016_Rapids_WEB2.pdf (accessed September 20, 2017).

IOM (Institute of Medicine). 2015. *Public health implications of raising the minimum age of legal access to tobacco products.* Washington, DC: The National Academies Press.

Jamal, A., B. A. King, L. J. Neff, J. Whitmill, S. D. Babb, and C. M. Graffunder. 2016. Current cigarette smoking among adults—United States, 2005–2015. *Morbidity and Mortality Weekly Report* 65(44):1205–1211.

Jamal, A., A. Gentzke, S. Hu, K. A. Cullen, B. J. Apelberg, D. M. Homa, and B. A. King. 2017. Tobacco use among middle and high school students—United States, 2011–2016. *Morbidity and Mortality Weekly Report* 66(23):597–603.

Johnston, L. D., P. M. O'Malley, R. Miech, J. G. Bachman, and J. E. Schulenberg. 2017. *Monitoring the Future national survey results on drug use, 1975–2016: Overview, key findings on adolescent drug use.* Ann Arbor: Institute for Social Research, University of Michigan. http://www.monitoringthefuture.org/pubs/monographs/mtf-overview2015.pdf (accessed February 2, 2018).

Kasza, K. A., B. K. Ambrose, K. P. Conway, N. Borek, K. Taylor, M. L. Goniewicz, K. M. Cummings, E. Sharma, J. L. Pearson, V. R. Green, A. R. Kaufman, M. Bansal-Travers, M. J. Travers, J. Kwan, C. Tworek, Y. C. Cheng, L. Yang, N. Pharris-Ciurej, D. M. van Bemmel, C. L. Backinger, W. M. Compton, and A. J. Hyland. 2017. Tobacco-product use by adults and youths in the United States in 2013 and 2014. *New England Journal of Medicine* 376(4):342–353.

Kong, G., M. E. Morean, D. A. Cavallo, D. R. Camenga, and S. Krishnan-Sarin. 2015. Reasons for electronic cigarette experimentation and discontinuation among adolescents and young adults. *Nicotine & Tobacco Research* 17(7):847–854.

Kozlowski, L. T., and K. E. Warner. 2017. Adolescents and e-cigarettes. Objects of concern may appear larger than they are. *Drug and Alcohol Dependence* 174:209–214.

Leventhal, A. M., D. R. Strong, M. G. Kirkpatrick, J. B. Unger, S. Sussman, N. R. Riggs, M. D. Stone, R. Khoddam, J. M. Samet, and J. Audrain-McGovern. 2015. Association of electronic cigarette use with initiation of combustible tobacco product smoking in early adolescence. *Journal of the American Medical Association* 314(7):700–707.

Leventhal, A. M., M. D. Stone, N. Andrabi, J. Barrington-Trimis, D. R. Strong, S. Sussman, and J. Audrain-McGovern. 2016. Association of e-cigarette vaping and progression to heavier patterns of cigarette smoking. *Journal of the American Medical Association* 316(18):1918–1920.

Loukas, A., C. N. Marti, M. Cooper, K. E. Pasch, and C. L. Perry. 2018. Exclusive e-cigarette use predicts cigarette initiation among college students. *Addictive Behaviors* 76(Supplement C):343–347.

Lydon, D. M., S. J. Wilson, A. Child, and C. F. Geier. 2014. Adolescent brain maturation and smoking: What we know and where we're headed. *Neuroscience & Biobehavioral Reviews* 45:323–342.

Miech, R., M. E. Patrick, P. M. O'Malley, and L. D. Johnston. 2016. What are kids vaping? Results from a national survey of U.S. adolescents. *Tobacco Control* 26(4):386–391.

Miech, R., M. E. Patrick, P. M. O'Malley, and L. D. Johnston. 2017. E-cigarette use as a predictor of cigarette smoking: Results from a 1-year follow-up of a national sample of 12th grade students. *Tobacco Control* 26:e106–e111. http://tobaccocontrol.bmj.com/content/26/e2/e106.info (accessed February 2, 2018).

Neff, L. J., R. A. Arrazola, R. S. Caraballo, C. G. Corey, S. Cox, B. A. King, C. J. Choiniere, and C. G. Husten. 2015. Frequency of tobacco use among middle and high school students—United States, 2014. *Morbidity and Mortality Weekly Report* 64(38):1061–1065.

Patel, D., K. C. Davis, S. Cox, B. Bradfield, B. A. King, P. Shafer, R. Caraballo, and R. Bunnell. 2016. Reasons for current e-cigarette use among U.S. adults. *Preventive Medicine* 93:14–20.

Pesko, M. F., J. M. Hughes, and F. S. Faisal. 2016. The influence of electronic cigarette age purchasing restrictions on adolescent tobacco and marijuana use. *Preventive Medicine* 87:207–212.

Phillips, C. V. 2015. Gateway effects: Why the cited evidence does not support their existence for low-risk tobacco products (and what evidence would). *International Journal of Environmental Research and Public Health* 12(5):5439–5464.

Primack, B. A., S. Soneji, M. Stoolmiller, M. J. Fine, and J. D. Sargent. 2015. Progression to traditional cigarette smoking after electronic cigarette use among U.S. adolescents and young adults. *JAMA Pediatrics* 169(11):1018–1023.

Primack, B. A., A. Shensa, J. E. Sidani, B. L. Hoffman, S. Soneji, M. J. Fine, J. Everette, and J. Sargent. 2016. *Initiation of cigarette smoking after e-cigarette use: A nationally representative study* [abstract]. http://www.sbm.org/UserFiles/file/2016AbstractSupplement.pdf (accessed September 20, 2017).

Sargent, J. D., J. Gabrielli, A. Budney, S. Soneji, and T. A. Wills. 2017. Adolescent smoking experimentation as a predictor of daily cigarette smoking. *Drug and Alcohol Dependence* 175:55–59.

Schneider, S., and K. Diehl. 2016. Vaping as a catalyst for smoking? An initial model on the initiation of electronic cigarette use and the transition to tobacco smoking among adolescents. *Nicotine & Tobacco Research* 18(5):647–653.

Selya, A. S., J. S. Rose, L. Dierker, D. Hedeker, and R. J. Mermelstein. 2017. Evaluating the mutual pathways among electronic cigarette use, conventional smoking and nicotine dependence. *Addiction* 113(2):325–333.

Soneji, S., J. L. Barrington-Trimis, T. A. Wills, A. M. Leventhal, J. B. Unger, L. A. Gibson, J. Yang, B. A. Primack, J. A. Andrews, R. A. Miech, T. R. Spindle, D. M. Dick, T. Eissenberg, R. C. Hornik, R. Dang, and J. D. Sargent. 2017. Association between initial use of e-cigarettes and subsequent cigarette smoking among adolescents and young adults: A systematic review and meta-analysis. *JAMA Pediatrics* 171(8):788–797.

Spindle, T. R., M. M. Hiler, M. E. Cooke, T. Eissenberg, K. S. Kendler, and D. M. Dick. 2017. Electronic cigarette use and uptake of cigarette smoking: A longitudinal examination of U.S. college students. *Addictive Behaviors* 67:66–72.

Unger, J. B., D. W. Soto, and A. Leventhal. 2016. E-cigarette use and subsequent cigarette and marijuana use among Hispanic young adults. *Drug and Alcohol Dependence* 163:261–264.

Warner, K. E. 2016. Frequency of e-cigarette use and cigarette smoking by American students in 2014. *American Journal of Preventive Medicine* 51(2):179–184.

Whiting, P., J. Savovic, J. P. Higgins, D. M. Caldwell, B. C. Reeves, B. Shea, P. Davies, J. Kleijnen, R. Churchill, and ROBIS group. 2016. ROBIS: A new tool to assess risk of bias in systematic reviews was developed. *Journal of Clinical Epidemiology* 69:225–234.

Wills, T. A., F. X. Gibbons, J. D. Sargent, and R. J. Schweitzer. 2016a. How is the effect of adolescent e-cigarette use on smoking onset mediated: A longitudinal analysis. *Psychology of Addictive Behaviors* 30(8):876–886.

Wills, T. A., R. Knight, J. D. Sargent, F. X. Gibbons, I. Pagano, and R. J. Williams. 2016b. Longitudinal study of e-cigarette use and onset of cigarette smoking among high school students in Hawaii. *Tobacco Control* 26(1):34–39.

Wills, T. A., J. D. Sargent, F. X. Gibbons, I. Pagano, and R. Schweitzer. 2016c. E-cigarette use is differentially related to smoking onset among lower risk adolescents. *Tobacco Control* 26(5):534–536.

Young, A. F., J. R. Powers, and S. L. Bell. 2006. Attrition in longitudinal studies: Who do you lose? *Australian and New Zealand Journal of Public Health* 30(4):353–361.

Zhuang, Y. L., S. E. Cummins, Y. S. J, and S. H. Zhu. 2016. Long-term e-cigarette use and smoking cessation: A longitudinal study with U.S. population. *Tobacco Control* 25(Supplement 1):i90–i95.

17

Smoking Cessation Among Adults

For both individuals and for public health, the central potential benefit of e-cigarettes is to promote smoking cessation among established cigarette smokers or at least to reduce smokers' exposure to combustible tobacco products. Although all tobacco use has health risks, the risk is highest when the user inhales the smoke produced by burning tobacco. Because e-cigarettes do not burn tobacco or generate smoke, the use of e-cigarettes likely confers a lower overall health risk than does smoking combustible tobacco products (see Chapter 18). Established combustible tobacco smokers who completely switch to using e-cigarettes therefore would be expected to reduce their tobacco-related health risks. Additional benefit would be expected if e-cigarette users subsequently stopped using both e-cigarettes and combustible tobacco products.

This section addresses the question: *Do e-cigarettes help smokers quit smoking combustible tobacco cigarettes?* In short, are e-cigarettes effective smoking cessation aids capable of increasing abstinence from combustible tobacco products compared with no treatment, a placebo treatment (usually a non-nicotine–containing e-cigarette), or a Food and Drug Administration (FDA)-approved smoking cessation aid such as a nicotine replacement product, varenicline, or bupropion?

A related but broader question is the following: *What is the impact of the availability of e-cigarettes on population smoking cessation rates?* The population impact of e-cigarettes will be a product not only of their effectiveness in an individual smoker but also of their reach, defined as the proportion of smokers who use them. E-cigarettes' current status as easily accessible consumer products may contribute to their appeal. If e-cigarettes have greater appeal to smokers than current FDA cessation aids, they could enhance population cessation rates simply by encouraging more current combustible tobacco cigarette smokers to make a quit attempt when they would not otherwise have attempted to quit tobacco.

CONCEPTUAL FRAMEWORK: PATTERNS OF E-CIGARETTE USE AMONG ESTABLISHED SMOKERS

Ultimately, the potential health benefit of e-cigarette use for cigarette smokers will depend on the characteristics of the smoker, the product (including both the e-cigarette device and e-liquid), and how the device is used. The pattern of e-cigarette use is likely to vary among individual smokers and over time as regular combustible tobacco cigarette smokers experiment with and perhaps transition to e-cigarettes. Figure 17-1 illustrates a conceptual model of these transitions.

The extent of risk reduction will depend on several factors that are defined by the answers to the following questions:

1. *Does the smoker switch completely to e-cigarettes (1a in Figure 17-1) or use both combustible tobacco cigarettes and e-cigarettes, a pattern referred to as dual use (1b in Figure 17-1)?* The extent of harm reduction should be much greater for a smoker who switches completely to e-cigarettes than for a smoker who uses e-cigarettes to replace

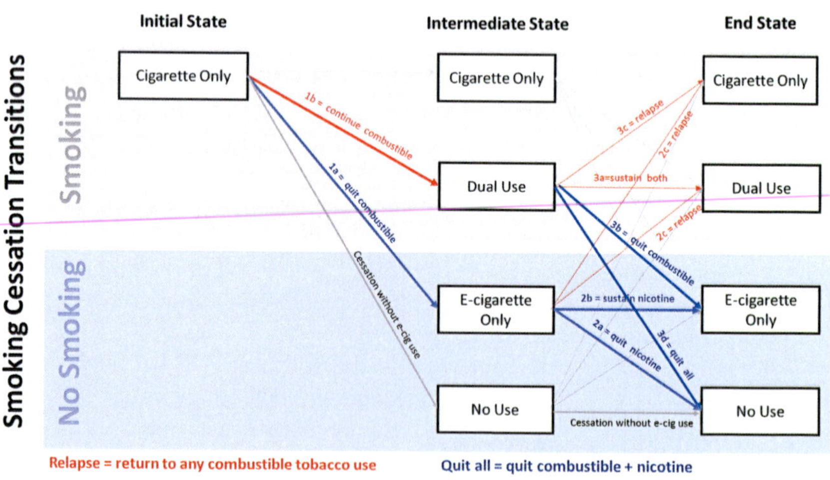

FIGURE 17-1 Conceptual framework of smoking cessation and e-cigarette use.

some, but not all, combustible tobacco cigarettes with e-cigarettes (dual use) because even small exposures to tobacco smoke increase health risks, especially the risk of cardiovascular disease (HHS, 2014). Because the risk of even small exposures to tobacco smoke may not be widely appreciated by the public, dual users may overestimate the degree to which they are reducing their tobacco-related risk and perhaps be less likely to continue efforts to stop combustible tobacco use altogether (Kasza et al., 2017).

2. *If the smoker switches completely to e-cigarettes, is the use of e-cigarettes:*
   a. *A temporary state leading to abstinence from both combustible tobacco cigarettes and e-cigarettes? (2a)*
   b. *A persistent state, in which exposure to e-cigarettes is sustained long-term? (2b)*
   c. *A temporary state followed by relapse to combustible tobacco products, with or without continued e-cigarette use? (2c)*

E-cigarettes should have the greatest benefit for the cigarette smoker who switches completely from combustible tobacco cigarettes to e-cigarettes or uses e-cigarettes for a limited time and then quits using both cigarettes and e-cigarettes (*2a* in Figure 17-1), producing abstinence from both tobacco smoke and nicotine, as well as any other potentially harmful constituents of e-cigarette aerosol. However, a complete switch from combustible tobacco cigarettes to e-cigarettes, with e-cigarette use persisting indefinitely, is still likely to reduce harm (*2b*). By contrast, a temporary switch to e-cigarettes followed by relapse to combustible tobacco use (*2c*) is unlikely to confer meaningful long-term reduction in health risk and could add whatever risk is conveyed by e-cigarette use.

3. *If the smoker becomes a dual user of cigarettes and e-cigarettes, is e-cigarette use:*
   a. *A persistent state of continued exposure to both tobacco smoke and to e-cigarette constituents? (3a)*
   b. *A temporary state en route to exclusive and persistent use of e-cigarettes? (3b)*
   c. *A temporary state followed by relapse to smoking combustible tobacco products? (3c)*
   d. *A temporary state on route to abstinence from all nicotine products? (3d)*

If dual use is a transitional state only, the extent of harm will depend on whether the individual returns to smoking only combustible tobacco cigarettes (relapse, *3c* in Figure 17-1); transitions completely to e-cigarettes, further reducing harm by reducing exposure to tobacco smoke (*3b*); continues dual use indefinitely (*3a*); or stops using both combustible tobacco cigarettes and e-cigarettes (*3d*). The last option, abstinence from tobacco smoke, nicotine, and other constituents of e-cigarette aerosol, is optimal. By contrast, a temporary switch to dual use followed by relapse to combustible tobacco use (*3c* in Figure 17-1) is likely to confer minimal long-term reduction in health risk.

Stopping smoking reduces the risk of tobacco-related diseases and extends life expectancy by up to a decade (Jha and Peto, 2014). The risks of cigarette smoking are well described, while the risks of e-cigarette use are just beginning to be assessed and much uncertainty remains. If e-cigarette use helps a smoker to completely quit combustible tobacco use (*2a* and *3d* in Figure 17-1), some degree of e-cigarette risk could still generate a net health benefit, as long as exposure to e-cigarettes is temporary and the benefit exceeds net short-term risk. However, if the final state is persistent e-cigarette use replacing combustible tobacco cigarette use (*2b* and *3b* in Figure 17-1), a lower level of e-cigarette risk would be required to generate an overall net benefit to the individual. Temporary e-cigarette use with return to combustible tobacco use (*2c* and *3c* in Figure 17-1) would likely have no net individual health benefit.

Currently, little information is available about the relative frequency at which smokers using e-cigarettes follow each path or about how the risks and benefits of each path compare. For the purposes of this chapter, the committee defines smoking cessation as stopping all combustible tobacco product use. It could be achieved following paths *2a*, *2b*, *3b*, or *3d* in Figure 17-1. This definition allows for sustained exposure to nicotine and other constituents in e-cigarettes. A more stringent criterion requiring nicotine abstinence from all sources is represented by paths *2a* and *3d* in Figure 17-1.

EVIDENCE REVIEW: LEVELS OF EVIDENCE AVAILABLE

The interpretation of epidemiological evidence must consider both its internal and external validity. Internal validity is a measure of how likely the finding of an association or causal relationship is accurate, which is determined by the degree to which a study minimizes systematic error (bias). Self-selection and confounding are important threats to internal validity. External validity addresses the extent to which a finding can be generalized to another context or to the general population.

To assess the efficacy of e-cigarettes for smoking cessation, the randomized controlled trial (RCT) provides the strongest study design to protect against threats to internal validity. Ideally, an RCT would enroll cigarette smokers seeking to quit and randomly assign them to switch from smoking combustible tobacco cigarettes to either using e-cigarettes or a comparison condition. The comparison condition could be no e-cigarettes (i.e., no treatment); a placebo (non-nicotine e-cigarette); an FDA-approved smoking-cessation pharmacotherapy, such as nicotine replacement, varenicline, or bupropion; or some other evidence-based cessation intervention, such as behavioral counseling. Each comparison condition would answer a slightly different variant of the question about e-cigarettes' effectiveness. Ideally, the RCT's primary outcome would be biochemically confirmed abstinence from combustible tobacco products 6 to 12 months later. Repeated assessments of adverse events occurring during the period of the study would allow for assessment of risks of e-cigarette use. As described below, the committee found that few RCTs have been conducted to address the question about effectiveness of e-cigarettes.

Prospective observational (cohort) studies offer less protection from threats to internal validity, but can provide valuable supporting evidence, especially when data from RCTs are limited (as in the current situation) or when randomization is unethical. A cohort study that could address the question could compare smokers who use e-cigarettes in a quit attempt with those who do not and assess the association between exposure to e-cigarettes and abstinence from tobacco products. An optimal prospective observational study design would identify and follow a large cohort of smokers who want to quit or are making a quit attempt, assess e-cigarette exposure in detail before the smoking cessation outcome is assessed, biochemically confirm self-reported tobacco abstinence, and adjust for multiple potential confounding factors associated with e-cigarette use and with smoking cessation. The limitation inherent in this study design is that smokers choose whether or not to use e-cigarettes. Those who do and do not choose to use e-cigarettes may differ in ways that independently influence a smoker's likelihood of success, confounding the observed association of e-cigarettes to quitting. Statistical methods can adjust for these factors, but unmeasured confounding remains a potential threat and makes it difficult to infer causality to an observed relationship between e-cigarette use and smoking cessation success.

Cross-sectional studies compare the prevalence of current or past e-cigarette use between current and former smokers. They provide a lower level of evidence and generally cannot be used to ascertain causality.

External validity depends on the representativeness of the study sample to the overall population to which a scientist or policy maker may wish to apply the study's findings. Studies that recruit or include nationally representative samples of smokers allow for broad generalizability of study findings and therefore maximize external validity. However, RCTs, which have the best internal validity, can rarely be conducted using large, nationally representative samples of individuals that maximize external validity. There is usually a trade-off of internal and external validity in any study. The committee considered both factors in its review of the evidence to address questions about the efficacy of e-cigarettes for smoking cessation.

The public health impact of an intervention is a broader question that is a function of both the intervention's efficacy and its reach (e.g., proportion of the at-risk population that uses it). As consumer products already easily accessible to smokers, e-cigarettes therefore have the potential to alter population cessation rates as a function of their efficacy as cessation aids and/or as a consequence of their appeal to smokers. RCTs measure the relative effectiveness of e-cigarettes in specific groups of smokers. However, the impact of e-cigarettes on population-level cessation rates will also depend on the proportion of smokers who use the products (i.e., reach) as well as characteristics of the products and how they are used (e.g., extent of nicotine delivery to the user). Population-level studies therefore provide an important additional type of evidence to evaluate in addressing the overall impact of e-cigarettes in a real-world setting. For studies of populations, prospective cohort and cross-sectional study designs are commonly used, with the former providing stronger internal validity to the latter.

EVIDENCE REVIEW: METHODS

The committee's initial scan of the evidence identified individual studies with varying designs and rigor and also identified multiple published reviews. Most of the latter were systematic reviews that summarized the evidence either qualitatively in a narrative format or quantitatively using meta-analysis. Many of them were very recent, having been published between 2016 and 2017. Given the availability of multiple recent systematic reviews, the committee chose as its principal strategy to conduct a review of the existing reviews.

Committee staff conducted a formal literature search to identify evidence reviews that were published through August 31, 2017, and that addressed the effectiveness of e-cigarettes for smoking cessation. The search strategy is described in Appendix B.

The search identified 21 review articles published between 2014 and 2017 (El Dib et al., 2017; Franck et al., 2014; Hajek et al., 2014; Harrell et al., 2014; Hartmann-Boyce et al., 2016; Heydari et al., 2014, 2017; Ioakeimidis et al., 2016; Kalkhoran and Glantz, 2016; Khoudigian et al., 2016; Knight-West and Bullen, 2016; Lam and West, 2015; MacDonald et al., 2016; Malas et al., 2016; McRobbie et al., 2014; Orr and Asal, 2014; Patnode et al., 2015; Rahman et al., 2014, 2015; Vanderkam et al., 2016; Waghel et al., 2015).

Table 17-1 summarizes characteristics of the studies that were identified by the literature search. One committee member reviewed the results and excluded four publications. One report (MacDonald et al., 2016) was a protocol for an ongoing review that was not yet completed. A second review was an earlier version of a review from the Cochrane Collaboration (McRobbie et al., 2014), whose update is included. Two reviews were excluded because they did not provide specific data on e-cigarettes and cessation; in both cases, the same lead author subsequently published a review of e-cigarettes and cessation that is included in this review (Heydari et al., 2017; Rahman et al., 2015).

One committee member reviewed each of the remaining 17 studies to determine whether they met criteria as systematic reviews, using criteria developed for a previous report (NASEM, 2017):

1. Does the article describe a search involving at least two databases?
2. Does the article describe a search involving appropriate search terms?
3. Does the article describe a search involving pre-specified eligibility criteria?
4. Does the article include a risk-of-bias discussion and/or quality assessment?
5. Does the article include a meta-analysis or qualitative synthesis of findings?

Of the remaining reviews, 17 met these criteria. Four were published in 2014, four in 2015, seven in 2016, and two in 2017. Six of the reviews conducted a formal meta-analysis, pooling data from at least some of the identified studies (El Dib et al., 2017; Hartmann-Boyce et al., 2016; Kalkhoran and Glantz, 2016; Khoudigian et al., 2016; Rahman et al., 2014; Vanderkam et al., 2016). Two other reviews cited the results of a meta-analysis that had previously been published elsewhere (Ioakeimidis et al., 2016; Knight-West and Bullen, 2016). All assessed a smoking cessation endpoint and some of them also assessed other endpoints such as smoking reduction (see Chapter 18 on Harm Reduction).

The scan of the studies that were not included in the systematic reviews and were published through August 31, 2017, identified several population studies, whose results are described below. No new RCTs were identified. Additional observational and cohort studies were identified, but their results were generally consistent with studies in the systematic reviews.

TABLE 17-1 Systematic Reviews of E-Cigarettes and Smoking Cessation Identified by Literature Search

Reference	Systematic Review	Meta-Analysis	Search Through	Studies Included
El Dib et al., 2017	Yes	Yes	12/29/2015 (updated until 5/2016)	12 (3 RCT, 9 cohort)
Franck et al., 2014	Yes	No	9/15/2013	7
Hajek et al., 2014	Yes	No	2/2014	Not specified
Harrell et al., 2014	Yes	No	11/2013	15
Hartmann-Boyce et al., 2016	Yes	Yes	1/2016	24 (3 RCT, 21 cohort)

Explicit Quality Assessment?	Conclusion Regarding E-Cigarettes and Cessation	Comments
Yes	"There is very limited evidence regarding the impact of e-cigarettes on tobacco smoking cessation, reduction or adverse effects: data from RCTs are of low certainty and observational studies of very low certainty.... This review underlines the need to conduct well-designed trials measuring biochemically validated outcomes and adverse effects" (El Dib et al., 2017, p. 1).	
Yes	"Given the limited available evidence on the risks and benefits of e-cigarette use, large, randomized, controlled trials are urgently needed to definitively establish their potential for smoking cessation" (Franck et al., 2014, p. 1945).	
No	None	Broad general review
No	"Data on the use of e-cigarettes for quitting smoking are suggestive but ultimately inconclusive" (Harrell et al., 2014, p. 381).	
Yes	"There is evidence from two trials that e-cigarettes help smokers to stop smoking in the long term compared with placebo e-cigarettes. However, the small number of trials, low event rates, and wide confidence intervals around the estimates mean that our confidence in the result is rated low" (Hartmann-Boyce et al., 2016, p. 2).	Update of 2014 Cochrane review (see McRobbie et al., 2014)

continued

TABLE 17-1 Continued

Reference	Systematic Review	Meta-Analysis	Search Through	Studies Included
Heydari et al., 2017	Yes	No	9/2014	69
Ioakeimidis et al., 2016	Yes	Yes (report result of other meta-analyses)	6/2015	2 RCT
Kalkhoran and Glantz, 2016	Yes	Yes	6/17/2015	20 (1 RCT, 1 NRCT, 15 cohort, 3 cross-sectional)
Khoudigian et al., 2016	Yes	Yes	5/2014	5

Explicit Quality Assessment?	Conclusion Regarding E-Cigarettes and Cessation	Comments
No	"Enough evidence to suggest that e-cigarettes are effective for quitting smoking is lacking, as is the evidence for the lack of their harm for respiratory system and thus being alternatives for smoking. However, further studies are needed" (Heydari et al., 2017, p. 27).	Non-standard methods to synthesize results
Yes	"Further research is needed to examine the longer term safety, potential for long-term use and efficacy as a cessation aid" (Ioakeimidis et al., 2016, p. 5).	
Yes	"As currently being used, e-cigarettes are associated with significantly less quitting among smokers" (Kalkhoran and Glantz, 2016, p. 2).	
Yes	"Limited low-quality evidence of a non-statistically significant trend toward smoking cessation in adults using nicotine e-cigarettes exists compared with other therapies or placebo. Larger, high-quality studies are needed to inform policy decisions" (Khoudigian et al., 2016, p. 257).	

continued

TABLE 17-1 Continued

Reference	Systematic Review	Meta-Analysis	Search Through	Studies Included
Knight-West and Bullen, 2016	Yes	Yes (report result of other meta-analyses)	9/2015	11 (3 RCT, 8 cohort)
Lam and West, 2015	Yes	No	2/2015	4
Malas et al., 2016	Yes	No	2/1/2016	62

Explicit Quality Assessment?	Conclusion Regarding E-Cigarettes and Cessation	Comments
No	"Collectively, these studies suggest modest cessation efficacy ... at least with the short-term use. More research, specifically well-conducted large efficacy trials comparing e-cigarettes with standard smoking cessation management (e.g., nicotine replacement therapy plus behavioral support) and long-term prospective studies for adverse events, is urgently needed to fill critical knowledge gaps on these products" (Knight-West and Bullen, 2016, p. 111).	
Yes	"Based on the current available literature, e-cigarettes may constitute an effective smoking cessation tool" (Lam and West, 2015, p. 98).	Limited to RCTs of e-cigarettes and cessation
Yes	"While inconclusive due to low quality, overall the existing literature suggests e-cigarettes may be helpful for some smokers for quitting or reducing smoking. However, more carefully designed and scientifically sound studies are urgently needed to establish unequivocally the long-term cessation effects of e-cigarettes" (Malas et al., 2016, p. 1926).	

continued

TABLE 17-1 Continued

Reference	Systematic Review	Meta-Analysis	Search Through	Studies Included
Orr and Asal, 2014	Yes	No	3/2014	6
Patnode et al., 2015	Yes (of reviews, not original studies)	No (for e-cigarettes)	3/1/2015	2
Rahman et al., 2015	Yes	Yes	5/2014	6 (2 RCT, 2 cohort, 2 cross-sectional)
Vanderkam et al., 2016	Yes	Yes	6/14/2015	13 (2 RCT, 2 NRCT, 9 cohort)

Explicit Quality Assessment?	Conclusion Regarding E-Cigarettes and Cessation	Comments
No	"There is limited evidence for the effectiveness of e-cigarettes in smoking cessation.... Additional well-designed, long-term cessation studies are warranted, especially in comparison to current FDA-approved products" (Orr and Asal, 2014, pp. 1502, 1505).	
Yes	"Only two trials addressed the efficacy and harms related to the use of electronic cigarettes and these trials suggested no benefit on smoking cessation among smokers intending to quit" (Patnode et al., 2015, p. v).	Review of reviews only. Done for the update of the U.S. Preventive Services Task Force review of smoking cessation therapies
Yes	"Use of e-cigarettes is associated with smoking cessation and reduction. More randomized controlled trials are needed to assess effectiveness against other cessation methods" (Rahman et al., 2015, p. 2).	Update of Rahman et al., 2014, a narrative review of multiple endpoints, not just tobacco cessation
Yes	"The use of electronic cigarettes with nicotine decreases tobacco consumption among regular smokers. Further studies are needed to specify electronic cigarettes' safety profile and its ability to cause a reduction in consumption and long-term cessation in smokers" (Vanderkam et al., 2016, p. 972).	Text in French. Primary outcome was smoking reduction, but cessation was a secondary outcome

continued

TABLE 17-1 Continued

Reference	Systematic Review	Meta-Analysis	Search Through	Studies Included
Waghel et al., 2015	Yes	No	5/2014	7
Excluded Reviews				
Heydari et al., 2014	Yes, but not specific to e-cigarettes	No	n/a	n/a
MacDonald et al., 2016	Yes	Not at present time	Ongoing	13 (in initial scoping of the literature in April 2014; ongoing at the time of publication)
McRobbie et al., 2014	Yes	Yes	7/2014	13 (2 RCT, 11 cohort)

Explicit Quality Assessment?	Conclusion Regarding E-Cigarettes and Cessation	Comments
No	"The limited evidence available supports that e-cigarettes may be effective as monotherapy for smoking cessation and reduction. However, superiority to nicotine replacement therapy was not proven" (Waghel et al., 2015, p. 8).	
n/a	n/a	Systematic review of all cessation methods, little focus on e-cigarettes
Yes	Ongoing project; no conclusions yet	Protocol paper for an ongoing meta-narrative review
yes	"There is evidence from two trials that e-cigarettes help smokers to stop smoking long-term compared with placebo e-cigarettes. However, the small number of trials, low event rates and wide confidence intervals around the estimates mean that our confidence in the result is rated 'low' by GRADE standards. The lack of difference between the effect of e-cigarettes compared with nicotine patches found in one trial is uncertain for similar reasons" (McRobbie et al., 2014, p. 2).	Updated as Hartmann-Boyce et al., 2016

continued

TABLE 17-1 Continued

Reference	Systematic Review	Meta-Analysis	Search Through	Studies Included
Rahman et al., 2014	Yes	No	1/2014	5 (for cessation endpoint)

NOTE: FDA = Food and Drug Administration; NRCT = non-randomized controlled trial; RCT = randomized controlled trial.

EVIDENCE REVIEW: RESULTS

Systematic Reviews

Overall, the reviews report on a small and overlapping evidence base. They consistently identified the same three RCTs whose characteristics and results are summarized in Table 17-2. The reviews also identified a few non-randomized interventional trials and a larger number of prospective observational trials and cross-sectional analyses. The reviews varied in the criteria used to include or exclude studies other than RCTs, with the result that the reviews summarized non-identical groups of observational cohort or cross-sectional studies. The committee reviewed in detail the most recent systematic reviews, defined as those published in 2016 or 2017, reasoning that these would be the most complete, and focused on those that conducted an independent formal meta-analysis. A total of five reviews met both criteria (El Dib et al., 2017; Hartmann-Boyce et al., 2016; Kalkhoran and Glantz, 2016; Khoudigian et al., 2016; Vanderkam et al., 2016). In addition, the committee examined in detail a 2016 systematic review that attempted a meta-analysis (Malas et al., 2016), but judged the studies to be too heterogeneous for this to be appropriate.

From this group, the committee identified two systematic reviews as those that provided the most comprehensive, most rigorous, and most recent summary of the available data (El Dib et al., 2017; Hartmann-Boyce et al., 2016). These two reviews were conducted independently by different groups of authors. Table 17-3 summarizes the two reviews' methods, results, and conclusions and illustrates that the two reviews shared many similarities. Both were systematic reviews with meta-analysis. The search strategy for each began with the results of the search done for the 2014 Cochrane Collaboration review (McRobbie et al., 2014) and updated it,

Explicit Quality Assessment?	Conclusion Regarding E-Cigarettes and Cessation	Comments
No	"E-cigarettes may have some potential as smoking cessation aids and, in the researchers' view, should therefore be subject to further research and regulation similar to other nicotine replacement therapies" (Rahman et al., 2014, p. 1).	Narrative review that aims to cover multiple topics, not just cessation. Excluded because authors published an updated review focused on cessation (Rahman et al., 2015)

adding studies that were published through December 2015 (El Dib et al., 2017) or January 2016 (Hartmann-Boyce et al., 2016). Both used comparable methods that are described in the *Cochrane Handbook* to screen studies, extract data, assess risk of bias, and assess the certainty of the overall body of evidence. Both included RCTs and prospective cohort studies that enrolled current combustible tobacco cigarette smokers regardless of intention to quit. They compared nicotine-containing e-cigarettes with non-nicotine e-cigarettes, other smoking cessation aids, or no aid. Both excluded cross-sectional studies. The primary measure of treatment effect was tobacco smoking cessation at the longest follow-up available (a minimum of 6 months) using biochemically validated cessation where available. There was general agreement about the results of the meta-analysis of RCTs and about the overall quality of the evidence. However, there were some differences between the methods used. The two reviews differed in their handling of missing outcome data in the statistical test used in the meta-analysis (fixed-effect or random-effect Mantel-Haenszel [MH] test), and the synthesis method used for non-randomized cohort studies (narrative review versus meta-analysis). They obtained similar results, but differed slightly in their interpretation of these results.

El Dib and colleagues (2017) conducted a systematic review and meta-analysis of the effect of e-cigarettes on tobacco use among cigarette smokers that was commissioned by the World Health Organization. The review compared nicotine-containing devices to non-nicotine e-cigarettes, no smoking cessation aid, or alternative smoking cessation aids. RCTs and prospective observational studies published up to December 2015 were screened independently by two independent reviewers who also extracted data and assessed studies' risk of bias. The review identified three eligible randomized trials with a total of 1,007 participants. Results

TABLE 17-2 Characteristics of Three Randomized Controlled Trials Testing the Efficacy of E-Cigarettes for Smoking Cessation

Reference	Country	No. of Subjects	Plan to Quit?	Study Arms	Duration of Treatment
Bullen et al., 2013 (ASCEND)	New Zealand	657	Yes	(1) INT:1st-generation e-cigarette (Elusion) (16 mg nicotine); (2) CTL: Placebo e-cigarette; (3) Active comparator: Nicotine patch (21 mg).	12 weeks
Caponnetto et al., 2013 (ECLAT)	Italy	300	No	(1) INT: 1st-generation e-cigarette (Categoria) (7.2 mg nicotine); (2) INT: Same e-cigarette (7.2 mg × 6 weeks, 5.2 mg × 6 weeks); (3) CTL: Placebo e-cigarette.	12 weeks
Adriaens et al., 2014	Belgium	50	No	(1) INT: 2nd generation (Joyetech, 18 mg/ml nicotine); (2) INT: 2nd generation (Kanger T2, 18 mg/ml nicotine); (3) CTL: Delayed e-cigarette (offered weeks 8–16).	8 weeks

[a] El Dib et al., 2017.
[b] Hartmann-Boyce et al., 2016.
NOTE: ASCEND = A Study of Cessation Using Electronic Nicotine Devices; CO = carbon monoxide; CTL = control; ECLAT = EffiCiency and Safety of an eLectronic CigAreTte; INT = intervention; RR = relative risk.

Behavioral Support	Outcome Assessment				Data Pooled for Meta-Analysis?[a,b]
	Follow-Up	Measure	Abstinence Rate	Difference	
Offered phone or text (few used). No training in use of e-cigarette.	6 months	CO-validated continuous abstinence	(1) INT = 7.3%; (2) CTL = 4.1%; (3) CTL = 5.8%.	1 versus 2: 7.3% versus 4.1%, RR = 1.77, 95% CI = 0.54–5.77 n = 362. 1 versus 3: 7.3% versus 5.8%, RR = 1.26, 95% CI = 0.68–2.34, n = 584.	Yes
No quit assistance or training in use of e-cigarette.	12 months	CO-validated continuous 6–12 months	(1) INT = 13%; (2) INT = 9%; (3) PCB = 4%.	Pooling INT 1 + 2, versus CTL: 11% versus 4%, RR = 2.75, 95% CI = 0.97–7.76, n = 300.	Yes
(1) and (2) Training in e-cigarette use; (3) No e-cigarette training.	2 months	CO-validated abstinence (no definition)	At 2 months: INT (1+2) = 34%; CTL = 0%.		No

TABLE 17-3 Selected Systematic Reviews: Part 1

Characteristic	Hartmann-Boyce et al., 2016 (Cochrane Collaboration)	El Dib et al., 2017 (WHO commissioned)
Study designs included	RCTs and prospective cohort studies	RCTs and prospective cohort studies
Participants	Current smokers Motivated or unmotivated to quit	Current cigarette smokers Motivated or unmotivated to quit
Interventions	E-cigarettes	E-cigarettes (with or without nicotine)
Comparison conditions	Placebo e-cigarettes, other smoking cessation aid, or no cessation aid	Placebo e-cigarettes, other smoking cessation aid, or no cessation aid
Search strategy: databases used	Updated results of 2014 Cochrane review using Cochrane Tobacco Addiction Group Specialized Register, Cochrane Central Register of Controlled Trials, MEDLINE, EMBASE, PsycINFO	Included results of 2014 Cochrane review, searched MEDLINE, CINHAL, EMBASE, CENTRAL, PsycINFO, Web of Science, ClinicalTrials.gov, PubMed
Search strategy: terms used	e-cig$ OR elect$ cigar$ OR electronic nicotine OR vape OR vaper OR vapers OR vaping	MeSH subject headings: electronic nicotine, smoking-cessation, tobacco-use-disorder, tobacco-smoking, quit
Literature search ended	January 2016	December 29, 2015 (updated until submission, May 2016)
Study selection and data extraction	Independently by two authors	Independently by three pairs of two authors
Risk of bias assessment	*Cochrane Handbook for Systematic Reviews of Interventions*[a]	Modified version of *Cochrane Handbook for Systematic Reviews of Interventions*[b] (RCTs); Ottawa-Newcastle instrument (cohort studies)[c]
Certainty of evidence assessment	GRADE methodology	GRADE methodology[d]
Outcome measures	Cessation at longest follow-up point (6-month minimum), prefer biochemically validated outcome measure	Tobacco smoking cessation at longest follow-up (6-month minimum), prefer biochemically validated measure; or 50 percent or more reduction in cigarette use

TABLE 17-3 Continued

Characteristic	Hartmann-Boyce et al., 2016 (Cochrane Collaboration)	El Dib et al., 2017 (WHO commissioned)
Measure of treatment effect	ITT analysis, calculate risk ratio at the longest follow-up	ITT analysis, calculate risk ratio at longest follow-up
Missing data	Missing outcome = smoker	Complete case analysis (excluded missing data); "worst case" sensitivity analysis done
RCTs		
Identified meeting criteria	3 (1,007 participants)	3 (1,007 participants)
Pooled for meta-analysis	2 (n = 662 subjects)	2 (n = 481 subjects)
Calculation of effect size	Fixed-effect Mantel-Haenszel model	Random-effect Mantel-Haenszel model
Result (smoking cessation): E-cigarette versus placebo e-cigarette E-cigarette versus nicotine patch	RR = 2.29, 95% CI = 1.05–4.96; RR = 1.26, 95% CI = 0.68–2.34; (1 study, no pooling)	RR = 2.03, 95% CI = 0.94–4.38; RR = 1.10, 95% CI = 0.60–2.03 (1 study, no pooling)
Result (50% reduction or more)	Not done	RR = 0.97, 95% CI = 0.57–1.66
Risk of bias in included studies	Low	Low
Overall quality of evidence (GRADE)	Low certainty (small number of studies)	Low certainty
Prospective Cohort Studies		
Identified meeting criteria	21	9 (13,115 participants)
Pooled for meta-analysis	0	8
Data synthesis method	Narrative review only	Random-effect Mantel-Haenszel model
Result (e-cigarette versus no e-cigarette)	Pooled analysis not done	OR = 0.74, 95% CI = 0.55–1.001, p = 0.051
Risk of bias in studies	High (selection bias)	High (missing data, imprecision in outcomes and prognostic factors)
Overall quality of evidence	Low certainty	Very low certainty

continued

TABLE 17-3 Continued

Characteristic	Hartmann-Boyce et al., 2016 (Cochrane Collaboration)	El Dib et al., 2017 (WHO commissioned)
Conclusions	"There is evidence from two trials that e-cigarettes help smokers to stop smoking in the long term compared with placebo e-cigarettes. However, the small number of trials, low event rates and wide confidence intervals around the estimates mean that our confidence in the result is rated low by GRADE standards. The lack of difference between the effect of e-cigarettes compared with nicotine patches found in one trial is uncertain for similar reasons."[e]	"Results from 2 RCTs suggest a possible increase in smoking cessation with ENDS in comparison with ENNDS...."[f] "There is very limited evidence regarding the impact of ENDS or ENNDS on tobacco smoking cessation, reduction or adverse effects: data from RCTs are of low certainty and observational studies of very low certainty ... from which no credible inferences can be drawn.... This review underlines the need to conduct well-designed trials measuring biochemically validated outcomes and adverse effects."[g]

[a] Higgins et al., 2011.

[b] El Dib et al., 2017. The authors (El Dib et al., 2017) cite the following reference, which has been modified: Guyatt, G. H., and J. W. Busse. n.d. *Modification of Cochrane tool to assess risk of bias in randomized controlled trials.* https://www.evidencepartners.com/resources/methodological-resources (accessed September 20, 2017).

[c] El Dib et al., 2017. The authors (El Dib et al., 2017) cite the following reference, which has been modified: Guyatt, G. H., and J. W. Busse. n.d. *Modification of Ottawa-Newcastle to assess risk of bias in nonrandomized trials.* https://www.evidencepartners.com/resources/methodological-resources (accessed September 20, 2017).

[d] Guyatt et al., 2011a–e.

[e] Hartmann-Boyce et al., 2016, p. 2.

[f] El Dib et al., 2017, p. 12.

[g] El Dib et al., 2017, p. 1.

NOTE: GRADE = Grading of Recommendations Assessment, Development, and Evaluation; ITT = intent-to-treat; OR = odds ratio; RCT = randomized controlled trial; RR = relative risk; WHO = World Health Organization.

from two of the three RCTs were appropriate for pooled analysis (Bullen et al., 2013; Caponnetto et al., 2013). The third was excluded because the effect of e-cigarettes versus no e-cigarettes could be compared for only 8 weeks (Adriaens et al., 2014). The treatment effect was calculated using the random-effect MH test and using complete case analysis (excluding cases with missing outcome data), producing a total sample of 481 participants. The result was a non-significant increase in smoking cessation with nicotine-containing e-cigarettes compared with non-nicotine e-cigarettes (RR = 2.03; 95% CI = 0.94–4.38; p = 0.07; quit rate = 11.7 percent nicotine, 6.3 percent non-nicotine; risk difference = 64/1,000 over 6 to 12 months). Combining the data on reduction in cigarettes per day, the two RCTs found no difference between the e-cigarette group and the non-nicotine e-cigarette group (RR = 0.97; 95% CI = 0.57–1.66; p = 0.92). The individual studies were judged to have low risk of bias, but the overall body of evidence was rated as low certainty due to the small number of trials and the extent of missing data.

The review also identified nine eligible cohort studies with a total of 13,115 participants. In contrast to the RCTs, combining the results from cohort studies produced a nearly significant reduction in quit rates with use of e-cigarettes compared with no use of e-cigarettes (OR = 0.74; 95% CI = 0.55–1.001; p = 0.051). Limitations of the cohort studies noted by the authors included the fact that not all participants were using e-cigarettes to quit. Additionally, missing outcome data and an imprecise assessment of prognostic factors and outcomes were judged to have produced a risk of bias. Consequently, the evidence provided by the cohort studies was judged to be very low certainty "from which no credible inferences can be drawn" (El Dib et al., 2017, p. 1). Because of the low-quality evidence, the review made no conclusion about the effectiveness of e-cigarettes as cessation aids. Instead, it identified the need for well-designed RCTs measuring biochemically validated outcomes to answer the question. In 2016, Hartmann-Boyce and colleagues updated the Cochrane Tobacco Addiction Group's 2014 systematic review and meta-analysis of the effectiveness of e-cigarettes for smoking cessation (Hartmann-Boyce et al., 2016; McRobbie et al., 2014). The authors identified RCTs in which current smokers (motivated or unmotivated to quit) were randomly assigned to e-cigarettes or to a control condition and followed for 6 months or longer. They also included prospective observational studies with at least 6-month follow-up. To assess treatment effect, authors used the most rigorous definition of tobacco abstinence available, ideally, biochemically validated abstinence. In contrast to the El Dib and colleagues (2017) review, the Hartmann-Boyce (2016) review included participants with missing outcome data as continued smokers for the pooled analysis. Standard Cochrane methods for screening studies and extracting data were used. Risk ratios and 95% CIs were calculated using a fixed-effect MH model for each study, and pooled where appropriate. The review identified 24 completed studies (3 RCTs and 21 cohort studies) and 27 ongoing studies. It specifically excluded cross-sectional studies that collected data at only one time point due to the potential for confounding and recall bias.

The same two RCTs that were judged appropriate for pooling by the El Dib and colleagues (2017) analysis were also pooled in the Hartmann-Boyce and colleagues (2016) analysis. Both studies compared nicotine-containing e-cigarettes with non-nicotine e-cigarettes. However, because Hartmann-Boyce included participants with missing data as smokers (rather than excluding them, as El Dib did), its pooled analysis had a larger combined sample size of 662 participants. In the meta-analysis of the two studies, e-cigarettes produced a higher smoking abstinence rate compared with non-nicotine–containing e-cigarettes and one that achieved statistical significance (RR = 2.29; 95% CI = 1.05–4.96; e-cigarette 9 percent versus placebo 4 percent). The one study that compared an e-cigarette to nicotine patch found no significant difference in 6-month abstinence rates (RR = 1.26; 95% CI = 0.68–2.34; 584 participants). Individual RCTs were assessed to be at low risk of bias but the overall quality of the evidence was rated as "low" or "very low" because of imprecision due to the small number of trials. The authors concluded that evidence from two trials indicated that "ECs help smokers to stop smoking in the long term compared with placebo ECs" (Hartmann-Boyce et al., 2016, p. 2), although they also acknowledged that their confidence in the result was low by GRADE standards. Only one trial compared e-cigarettes to a proven smoking cessation aid, nicotine patches. The authors interpreted the lack of difference between the effects of e-cigarettes and nicotine patches for cessation in that trial as inconclusive.

The Hartmann-Boyce review also described the non-randomized prospective observational studies it had identified, separating them into two categories, intervention versus non-intervention. Studies in which e-cigarettes were given to participant smokers as part of the study protocol were categorized as non-randomized intervention studies. Studies that simply recorded smokers' use of e-cigarettes at baseline and follow-up were termed "non-intervention studies." The review did not attempt to pool data from any of the non-randomized observational studies because, it stated, "these studies are heavily confounded due to the nature of their design" (Hartmann-Boyce et al., 2016, p. 8). Specifically, the authors noted that smokers who have already succeeded in quitting with e-cigarettes would not be eligible for non-randomized observational studies, which recruit only current smokers. They argued that enrolling only "e-cigarette treatment failures" into an e-cigarette intervention study would bias the result toward a null finding.

Summary of These Two Systematic Reviews

The two systematic reviews identified a similar group of studies and generally came to similar conclusions, specifically that the body of available evidence was small and that a critical need existed for additional evidence to provide definitive answers to the questions posed. However, the reviews differed slightly in their interpretation. The Cochrane review found a statistically significant effect of nicotine e-cigarettes compared with non-nicotine e-cigarettes and interpreted this as demonstrating a positive effect of e-cigarettes on quitting, albeit with low confidence that the estimate would not change when more evidence became available. It judged that the risk of confounding from observational data was so high that it did not pool those data. Using the same two RCTs, the El Dib review produced a similar but not quite significant effect of e-cigarettes versus non-nicotine e-cigarettes. El Dib and colleagues (2017) judged the low confidence in the evidence base and the opposite result of the cohort studies to be sufficient to preclude any conclusion about effectiveness of e-cigarettes at this time.

Other Systematic Reviews

Table 17-4 describes four of the five other systematic reviews that were published during 2016–2017 (Kalkhoran and Glantz, 2016; Khoudigian et al., 2016; Malas et al., 2016; Vanderkam et al., 2016). A fifth systematic review from this period is not discussed because it was of lower quality and used non-standard methods to summarize the search results (Heydari et al., 2017). In addition, Table 17-4 includes one earlier systematic review that included an independent meta-analysis (Rahman et al., 2015).

Khoudigian and colleagues (2016) conducted a systematic review and meta-analysis of RCTs and observational studies that were published through May 2014 and compared e-cigarettes with other non-randomized trials or placebo e-cigarettes. It included smokers regardless of their intention to quit smoking. The outcome of interest for this analysis was smoking abstinence for at least 6 months after the start of e-cigarette use. The literature search and data extraction were well conducted. The review identified five eligible studies, but only two of these had cessation outcomes. These were the same two RCTs that are included and pooled in the reviews described above (El Dib et al., 2017; Hartmann-Boyce et al., 2016). Pooling of these two studies produced a non-significant RR of 2.02 (95% CI = 0.97–4.21). Despite this, the authors observed that their results "suggest that the use of nicotine e-cigarettes increased the proportion of patients who stopped smoking, although this change was not statistically significant" (Khoudigian et al., 2016, p. 265). Overall, they concluded, "limited low-quality evidence of a non-statistically significant

TABLE 17-4 Selected Systematic Reviews: Part 2

Characteristic	Khoudigian et al., 2016	Malas et al., 2016
Study designs included	RCT and prospective cohort studies	RCTs, prospective cohort, experimental, and cross-sectional
Participants	Current smokers Motivated or unmotivated to quit	Current smokers Motivated or unmotivated to quit
Interventions	E-cigarettes (with nicotine)	E-cigarettes (with nicotine)
Comparison conditions	Placebo e-cigarettes or NRT	Not specified
Search strategy: databases used	MEDLINE, Embase, PsycINFO, Cochrane Central Registry of Controlled Trials; also found gray literature through searching websites of health technology assessment and related agencies, in addition to reports of major smoking cessation conference proceedings; also used Google for more Web-based materials	PubMed, MEDLINE, PsycINFO, CINAHL, ERIC, ROVER, Scopus, ISI Web of Science, Cochrane Library, Ontario Tobacco Research Unit library catalogue; gray literature identified using Grey Matters, OAIster, OpenGrey, NYAM website, Legacy Library, BIOSIS Previews, Conference Papers Index, ISI Proceedings, Dissertation Abstracts International, CIHI, GreyNet International
Search strategy: terms used	Searched controlled vocabularies (MeSH and EMTREE) and keywords on concept of "electronic cigarette" or "e-nicotine": 1. (electr*adj (cigar* or nicotine*)).mp 2. (e-cig* or ecig* or e-cigarette* or ecigarette*).mp 3. (e-nicotine* or enicotine*).mp 4. or/1-3	Electronic nicotine delivery system, ENDS, electronic cigarette, e-cigarette, e-cig, e-juice, e-liquid, e-hookah, cartomizer, alternative tobacco product, tobacco use cessation product, smoking cessation aid, vape, vaping, vaporizer, vape-pen
Literature search ended	May 2014	February 1, 2016

Kalkhoran et al., 2016	Vanderkam et al., 2016	Rahman et al., 2015
RCTs, prospective cohort, and cross-sectional studies	Interventional trials (RCTs and non-RCTs), prospective cohort	RCTs, prospective cohort, and cross-sectional studies
Current smokers Motivated or unmotivated to quit	Current smokers, 10 cigarettes per day or more, ages 18–60, no severe comorbidity or psychiatric illness	Current smokers Motivated or unmotivated to quit
E-cigarettes (with nicotine)	E-cigarettes (with nicotine)	E-cigarettes (with nicotine)
Not using e-cigarettes	Placebo e-cigarette	Placebo e-cigarette or other
PubMed, Web of Science Core Collection	MEDLINE, Cochrane	PubMed, Web of Knowledge, Scopus
Electronic cigarette, e-cigarette, electronic nicotine delivery, 1 or 2 or 3, stop, quit, cessation, abstain, abstinence, 5 or 6 or 7 or 8 or 9, 4 and 10	Electronic cigarette, electronic nicotine delivery device, electronic nicotine delivery system, vaping, e-cigarette	"electronic cigarettes OR e-cigarettes" AND "smoking cessation OR quit smoking"
June 17, 2015	June 14, 2015	May 2014

continued

TABLE 17-4 Continued

Characteristic	Khoudigian et al., 2016	Malas et al., 2016
Study selection and data extraction	2 authors	2 authors
Risk of bias assessment	Yes Cochrane Risk of Bias tool (RCTs); same criteria for controlled before–after studies, but "random sequence generation" and "allocation concealment" domains were reported as "high risk of bias"	Yes Modified version of QualSyst[a] tool by combining quantitative and qualitative checklists and revising criteria based on *Cochrane Handbook* guidelines
Outcome measures	Smoking abstinence for 6 months or more; also desire to smoke, number of cigarettes smoked, withdrawal symptoms	Smoking abstinence for 30 days; also reduction, withdrawal symptoms, craving
Studies identified	5 (4 RCTs [2 of which used in meta-analysis], 1 controlled before–after study)	62
Meta-analysis done	Yes (2 RCTs)	No (attempted, but data considered too heterogeneous)
Result (cessation): E-cigarette versus placebo e-cigarette	RR = 2.02; 95% CI = 0.97–4.21	n/a
E-cigarette versus no e-cigarette	n/a	n/a

Kalkhoran et al., 2016	Vanderkam et al., 2016	Rahman et al., 2015
1 author, with review by a second author	2 authors	2 authors
Yes ACROBAT-NRSI (observational) Cochrane Risk of Bias tool (clinical trials)	Yes Cochrane risk of bias tool	Yes Cochrane risk of bias tool (RCTs), Downs and Black instrument (observational studies)
Cigarette smoking abstinence of any duration. E-cigarette use explicitly allowed	Reduction of 50% in cigarettes/day for at least 3 months (primary outcome). Smoking abstinence for 3 months or more, validated biochemically (secondary outcome).	Smoking abstinence of any duration
38 (20 used in meta-analysis)	13 (2 RCTs used in meta-analysis)	6 (2 RCTs, 2 cohort, 2 cross-sectional)
Yes (20 studies: RCT, cohort, cross-sectional designs)	Yes (2 RCTs)	Yes (2 RCTs)
n/a	RR = 1.91; 95% CI = 0.93–3.89	RR = 2.29; 95% CI = 1.05–4.97
OR = 0.72; 95% CI = 0.57–0.91	n/a	n/a

continued

TABLE 17-4 Continued

Characteristic	Khoudigian et al., 2016	Malas et al., 2016
Conclusions	"Limited low-quality evidence of a non-statistically significant trend toward smoking cessation in adults using nicotine e-cigarettes exists compared with other therapies or placebo. Larger, high-quality studies are needed to inform policy decisions."[b]	"The results of this systematic review lead us to conclude that evidence for the effectiveness of e-cigarettes as a cessation aid is inconclusive. There is too much uncontrolled variation to allow for any general conclusion to be made."[c] "While inconclusive due to low quality, overall the existing literature suggests e-cigarettes may be helpful for some smokers for quitting or reducing smoking. However, more carefully designed and scientifically sound studies are urgently needed to establish unequivocally the long-term cessation effects of e-cigarettes"[d]

[a] Kmet et al., 2004.
[b] Khoudigian et al., 2016.
[c] Malas et al., 2016, p. 1931.
[d] Malas et al., 2016, p. 1926.
[e] Kalkhoran and Glantz, 2016, p. 2.
[f] Vanderkam et al., 2016, p. 972.

trend toward smoking cessation in adults using nicotine e-cigarettes exists compared with other therapies or placebo. Larger, high-quality studies are needed to inform policy decisions" (Khoudigian et al., 2016, p. 257). Overall, this review was carefully conducted, but did not identify studies published after May 2014.

Malas and colleagues (2016, p. 1927) conducted a systematic review of English-language studies containing "original data related to e-cigarettes and smoking cessation" that were identified from database searches through February 1, 2016, or a search of unpublished studies or abstracts (i.e., "gray literature"). Comparison conditions were not specified. Eligible study designs included RCTs, experimental studies, prospective observational studies, and cross-sectional studies. The primary outcome was cessation, defined as smoking abstinence or reduction with at least a

Kalkhoran et al., 2016	Vanderkam et al., 2016	Rahman et al., 2015
"As currently being used, e-cigarettes are associated with significantly less quitting among smokers."[e]	"The use of electronic cigarette with nicotine decreases tobacco consumption among regular smokers. Further studies are needed to specify an electronic cigarette's safety profile and its ability to cause a reduction in consumption and long-term cessation in smokers."[f]	"Use of e-cigarettes is associated with smoking cessation and reduction. More randomized controlled trials are needed to assess effectiveness against other cessation methods."[g] "Limitations: Included studies were heterogeneous, due to different study designs and gender variation."[h]

[g] Rahman et al., 2015, p. 2.
[h] Rahman et al., 2015, p. 2.
NOTE: NRT = nicotine replacement therapy; OR = odds ratio; RCT = randomized controlled trial; RR = relative risk.

30-day follow-up period. Identified studies underwent a systematic quality assessment and received a rating of weak, moderate, or strong. The review identified 11 relevant studies with moderate or strong results that enrolled smokers from the general population. The authors summarized the studies qualitatively and attempted to do a quantitative synthesis, combining all study designs, but they concluded it could not be done due to heterogeneity of outcome measures and study designs. They stated, "The results of this systematic review lead us to conclude that evidence for the effectiveness of e-cigarettes as a cessation aid is inconclusive. There is too much uncontrolled variation to allow for any general conclusion to be made" (Malas et al., 2016, p. 1931). The authors identified an urgent need for "more carefully designed and scientifically sound studies ... to establish unequivocally the long-term cessation effects of e-cigarettes and to better understand how and when e-cigarettes may be helpful" (Malas et al., 2016, p. 1926).

Kalkhoran and Glantz (2016) conducted a systematic review and meta-analysis of English-language studies that assessed the relationship between e-cigarette use and cigarette smoking cessation among adult smokers, regardless of their interest in quitting smoking. They included RCTs and non-RCTs, cohort studies, and cross-sectional studies that were identified by a search ending June 17, 2015. The authors also monitored the literature for studies published before publication of their paper in January 2016 and added two studies. Outcomes were either self-reported or biochemically confirmed combustible tobacco cigarette smoking abstinence, with no required minimum duration of abstinence required. E-cigarette use was permitted under the definition of smoking abstinence. A total of 38 eligible studies were identified. They were heterogeneous in study design, duration, and definition of the e-cigarette exposure measure and the smoking cessation outcome. Twenty studies with control groups were included in a random-effects meta-analysis that found a negative effect of e-cigarette use on cessation (OR = 0.72; 95% CI = 0.57–0.91). Unlike other meta-analyses that separated RCTs and observational studies, this meta-analysis combined all study designs (15 cohort studies, 3 cross-sectional studies, and 2 clinical trials [only 1 randomized]). Sensitivity analyses compared the results of meta-analyses stratified by several factors, including interest in quitting, study design (clinical trial versus observational, longitudinal versus cross-sectional), biochemical verification, and recent e-cigarette use. The ORs generated in the sensitivity analysis for each of the different factors were not statistically significantly different from one another. The authors concluded, "As currently being used, e-cigarettes are associated with significantly less quitting among smokers" (Kalkhoran and Glantz, 2016, p. 2). They suggest that one explanation may be that e-cigarettes are used differently in a controlled clinical trial than in the real world, where e-cigarettes are readily available consumer products without clear instructions for use. They suggest that the results of observational trials provide insight into the effect of real-world e-cigarette use on cessation.

Vanderkam and colleagues (2016) conducted a systematic review and meta-analysis of randomized and non-randomized intervention trials and prospective cohort studies that were published up to June 14, 2015. They compared nicotine-containing e-cigarettes to non-nicotine–containing e-cigarettes. The primary endpoint was 50 percent reduction of combustible tobacco cigarettes or more for at least 3 months, confirmed by a biochemical measure. However, they also included as a secondary measure of smoking cessation for at least 3 months, confirmed by biomarker. Their search identified 13 papers, of which 2 were the same 2 RCTs identified by other reviews (El Dib et al., 2017; Hartmann-Boyce et al., 2016; Khoudigian et al., 2016). In these authors' hands, pooling the cessation data produced a non-significant effect of e-cigarettes over placebo e-cigarettes (RR = 1.91; 95% CI = 0.93–3.89). They did find a significant increase in the proportion of smokers with a validated self-report of 50 percent or greater reduction in daily cigarette consumption (RR = 1.30; 95% CI = 1.02–1.66). The authors concluded that evidence was insufficient to determine effectiveness of e-cigarettes for quitting smoking.

The committee identified only one earlier systematic review that included a meta-analysis. Rahman and colleagues (2015) reviewed controlled trials, prospective cohort studies, and cross-sectional studies of e-cigarette use that were published up to May 2014. The review included studies that compared current smokers (variously defined and irrespective of interest in quitting) who used e-cigarettes for at least 3 months with those who used any other method. The outcome measure was smoking cessation, not necessarily biochemically validated. The search and data extraction were carefully done and risk of bias was assessed. The search identified six studies, including the same two RCTs (Bullen et al., 2013; Caponnetto et al., 2013) that were identified in other reviews. A meta-analysis of these two studies, including missing data on smokers and using a random-effects MH test, produced an identical relative risk of quitting as that reported in the Hartmann-Boyce and colleagues (2016) review (RR = 2.29; 95% CI = 1.05–4.96). However, Rahman and colleagues' interpretation of this finding was stated more positively than that of the Hartmann-Boyce and colleagues (2016) review; they concluded that the "use of e-cigarettes is associated with smoking cessation and reduction" (Rahman et al., 2015, p. 2). However, the review did acknowledge the small size and heterogeneity of the evidence base and called for more RCTs to be done to answer the question. Additionally, reduction in rate of smoking does not ensure reduction in tobacco-related harm.

Evaluation of the Evidence from Systematic Reviews

Overall, the systematic reviews identified by the committee generally came to similar conclusions, despite some methodological differences in the conduct of the meta-analyses. Table 17-1 includes the verbatim conclusions of all the systematic reviews to illustrate this similarity. Furthermore, the same two RCTs were consistently identified by most authors and were included in a formal meta-analysis by five of the systematic reviews. Both RCTs compared nicotine-containing e-cigarettes to non-nicotine placebo e-cigarettes. The relative risks generated in the meta-analyses ranged from 1.91 to 2.29, with 95% confidence limits falling near a relative risk of 1.0 in all cases. In two reviews (Hartmann-Boyce et al., 2016; Rahman et al., 2015), the 95% CI around the estimate excluded 1.0, indicating that the superiority of e-cigarettes over placebo e-cigarettes was statistically significant, but in three other reviews, the 95% CI included 1.0, ranging from 0.93 to 0.97, thereby missing statistical significance. Although this difference led to slightly different interpretations, all reviews agreed that their confidence in their conclusion was low and that additional evidence might shift their conclusions.

In contrast to RCTs, different groups of observational studies, primarily longitudinal cohort studies, were included in the systematic reviews. Only two systematic reviews conducted a meta-analysis of the cohort studies that they had identified (El Dib et al., 2017; Kalkhoran and Glantz, 2016). In contrast to the results of meta-analyses of RCTs, both meta-analyses of cohort studies found a negative association between e-cigarette use and cessation. Most other systematic reviews provided only a narrative summary of their observational studies. This summary identified limitations that may account for some of the discrepancy. These limitations include imprecision in measurement of e-cigarette exposure, inclusion of smokers not using e-cigarettes to quit, limited adjustment for confounding factors, and variable outcome measures of cessation (Levy et al., 2017).

In particular, observational studies included in systematic reviews consistently noted an apparent association between the measure of exposure to e-cigarettes and likelihood of smoking cessation. Several observational studies found an association between frequent (i.e., daily or at least 20 of the past 30 days) e-cigarette use and smoking cessation success (Beard et al., 2015; Biener and Hargraves, 2015; Brose et al., 2015; Hitchman et al., 2015) or quit attempts made (Brose et al., 2015), while measures of less frequent e-cigarette use were associated with less smoking cessation than non-use of e-cigarettes (Beard et al., 2016; Biener and Hargraves, 2015; Brose et al., 2015; Hitchman et al., 2015).

In summary, the existing systematic reviews consistently agreed that the available evidence base was insufficient to definitively answer the question of whether e-cigarettes helped smokers to quit. They uniformly identified the urgent need for additional studies of high scientific quality, especially RCTs.

Effect of E-Cigarettes on Population-Level Cessation Rates

The committee identified only a small number of studies that enrolled nationally representative samples of individuals to assess the effect of e-cigarette availability on population cessation rates. Available studies used prospective cohort or repeat cross-sectional study designs. No RCTs are available. Few studies are available because e-cigarettes have been broadly available consumer products for only a few years and national surveys, from which study data were drawn, started to collect data on e-cigarette use only recently.

The most recent and largest study in the United States provides evidence of an association between e-cigarette use and smoking cessation rates at the population level. Zhu and colleagues (2017) analyzed data from five waves (i.e., repeated cross-sections) of the large, nationally representative U.S. Current Population Survey–Tobacco Use Supplement (CPS-TUS). The authors used these cross-sectional data to create a retrospective cohort of individuals who reported having been smokers one year prior to the survey. The analysis compared the quit rate (defined as the proportion who reported having been abstinent for at least 3 months at the time of the survey among those who were smoking 1 year earlier) between those who had ever used or currently used (defined as now used every day or some days) an e-cigarette. In the most recent survey of more than 160,000 respondents conducted in 2014–2015, smokers who used e-cigarettes in the previous 12 months were more likely to have made a quit attempt during that period and to have achieved at least 3 months of tobacco cessation than smokers who were not e-cigarette users.

In the same publication, Zhu and colleagues (2017) also used repeated cross-sectional CPS-TUS surveys to examine the population-level rates of making a quit attempt in the past year and of quitting smoking. Both measures increased significantly in 2014–2015 after remaining stable in four previous surveys beginning in 2001–2002. The population-level smoking cessation rate increased by 1.1 percentage points (4.5 percent to 5.6 percent) between 2010–2011 and 2014–2015. This coincided with the increase in e-cigarette use in the population, but it could also have been the result of other broad population-level influences on smoking cessation rates. The authors carefully considered concurrent factors, including an increase in federal tobacco excise tax in 2009 and annual national media campaigns beginning in 2012. They argue that these are not likely to have caused the change in quit rates. The study findings are consistent with findings of a study from England that also analyzed repeated cross-sections of nationally representative population samples (Beard et al., 2016). That study found a higher success rate of quit attempts among smokers who used e-cigarettes during a quit attempt, compared with those who did not use e-cigarettes during a quit attempt. It did not, however, find an association between e-cigarette use and the likelihood of a smoker making a quit attempt, as the Zhu and colleagues (2017) study did. It may also have been confounded by secular changes in the availability of treatment in the National Health Service (Britton, 2016).

Like Zhu and colleagues (2017), Levy and colleagues (2017) also analyzed data from the cross-sectional 2014–2015 CPS-TUS. They retrospectively created a cohort of individuals who were smoking 1 year prior to the survey. Their analysis focused on the relationship between the frequency of e-cigarette use at the time of the survey and two outcomes: (1) having made a quit attempt in the past year, and (2) having been abstinent from cigarettes for at least 3 months at the time of the survey if a quit attempt was made. Using multiple logistic regression analysis, the authors found consistent evidence between the frequency of e-cigarette use and both outcomes. Having made a quit attempt in the past year was associated with having ever used or currently using e-cigarettes, and the strength of this association increased with increasing number of days of e-cigarette use in the 30 days before the survey was conducted. Furthermore, among smokers who had made a quit attempt in the past year, the likelihood of having quit for 3 months or more at the time of the survey was significantly associated with current e-cigarette use. The strength of the relationship increased in a dose–response relationship with the number of days of e-cigarette use in the past 30 days. The adjusted odds ratio (AOR) for smokers who had used e-cigarettes on 20 or more days in the past 30 days (versus no use) was 2.81 (95% CI = 2.26–3.49), compared with 1.59 (95% CI = 1.31–1.92) for 5 or more days of use and 1.22 (95% CI = 1.02–1.46) for any number of days of current use. By contrast, there was an inverse relationship between being abstinent and ever use of an e-cigarette (AOR = 0.80; 95% CI = 0.69–0.92).

Giovenco and Delnevo (2018) used a similar approach to analyze a different large nationally representative annual cross-sectional survey, the National Health Interview Survey. They pooled data from the 2014 and 2015 surveys, which were the first to collect data on e-cigarette use. They constructed a retrospective cohort by including current smokers and any former smoker who quit in 2010 or later. They chose this date because e-cigarettes were rarely used in the United States prior to that date. Among this group of current and former smokers, daily e-cigarette users at the time of the survey (2014–2015) were more likely to be former smokers than e-cigarette–never users (52 percent versus 28 percent, adjusted prevalence ratio [aPR] = 3.15; 95% CI = 2.66–3.73). By contrast, those who previously tried e-cigarettes but did not use them currently and those who used them on only some days were less likely to be former smokers at the time of the survey than those who never used e-cigarettes (aPR = 0.67 [95% CI = 0.61–0.75] and 0.38 [95% CI = 0.32–0.47], respectively).

Recall bias of e-cigarette use and quit attempts is a limitation of the Giovenco and Delnevo (2018), Levy and colleagues (2017), and Zhu and colleagues (2017) studies' retrospective cohort design, as the authors acknowledge. They also recognize that reverse causation (i.e., quitting led to e-cigarette use to prevent relapse) also cannot be excluded. Other limitations include lack of information on potential confounders such as the type of e-cigarette used, the reason for e-cigarette use, or factors reflecting motivation or confidence in the ability to quit or past quit attempts. For example, smokers who use e-cigarettes daily could also be the ones most motivated to quit and therefore most likely to succeed. A strength of the Giovenco and Delnevo (2018) study was its unique ability to adjust for one potential confounder, serious psychological distress, which is associated with a lower success in quit attempts. This information is rarely available from population-based surveys. Using the stronger prospective longitudinal cohort design that avoids recall bias and reverse causation, Zhuang and colleagues (2016) conducted a U.S. population-based study of 2,028 smokers who were interviewed in 2012 and followed for 2 years. Smokers who reported using e-cigarettes at both points were defined as long-term users, while smokers reporting use at only one time were defined as short-term users. Long-term e-cigarette users had a higher cessation rate at 2 years compared with short-term e-cigarette users or non-users (42.4 percent versus 14.2 percent versus 15.6 percent). The difference in cessation rates between long-term users and either short-term or non-users was statistically significant after multivariable adjustment, suggesting that long-term but not short-term e-cigarette use promotes smoking cessation.

Shi and colleagues (2016) also conducted a prospective longitudinal population-based study to examine the relationship between e-cigarette use and smoking cessation, but found a different result. A nationally representative cohort of 2,454 smokers responding to the 2010 CPS-TUS was contacted 1 year later. The analysis found a negative association between ever use of e-cigarettes and quitting smoking for at least 1 month at follow-up. However, the measure of e-cigarette use was limited to ever use. No more detail about the intensity or duration of use, which the Zhuang and colleagues (2016) study suggests may be important factors, was available. Furthermore, the authors point out that only first-generation e-cigarettes were available to U.S. smokers at the time of the study. These may have been less effective for cessation because they delivered less nicotine to the user than do later-generation devices.

SYNTHESIS

There is general agreement that the number, size, and quality of studies for judging the effectiveness of e-cigarettes as cessation aids in comparison with cessation aids of proven efficacy are limited, and therefore there is insufficient evidence to permit a definitive conclusion at this time. Not only are existing studies limited in number, but the randomized trials provide a limited range of treatment comparisons. Interpretation of relevant observational studies on the topic of the effectiveness of e-cigarettes as cessation aids is complicated by the fact that they generally do not account for important covariates that may affect the success of e-cigarettes as cessation aids. These covariates include (1) the e-cigarette product (e.g., type of device, nicotine content and delivery, flavorings or other contents of the e-liquid), (2) pattern of current use (e.g., frequency of use, duration of use), and (3) user characteristics (particularly interest in quitting and prior history of e-cigarette use, but also demographics and smoking history) (Malas et al., 2016). By contrast, some of the more recently published (e.g., since 2016) cohort studies and nationally representative cross-sectional studies have included one key variable, the frequency of e-cigarette use. Based on this rationale, as described below, the evidence from more recent cohort studies and cross-sectional studies provides the foundation for the committee's conclusion about the frequency of e-cigarette use in relation to likelihood of smoking cessation. Future studies, both observational and experimental, will be strengthened by carefully measuring characteristics of the e-cigarette product, the pattern of use, and characteristics of the users.

Within the current body of evidence, different study designs have produced conflicting findings. The results of the few RCTs, the study design with the least risk of bias and greatest internal validity, suggest a possible though not definitively positive association with quitting smoking (Adriaens et al., 2014; Bullen et al., 2013; Caponnetto et al., 2013) (see Table 17-2). In these trials, the strongest results were observed in the trials that compared the efficacy of a nicotine-containing e-cigarette with a non-nicotine placebo e-cigarette. Two RCTs addressed this narrow question about the marginal benefit of having nicotine in a vaping device. Both trials compared a nicotine-containing e-cigarette with an e-cigarette without nicotine (Bullen et al., 2013; Caponnetto et al., 2013). They found consistent results that were statistically significant in one of two meta-analyses that pooled data from the two trials (El Dib et al., 2017; Hartmann-Boyce et al., 2016). There are no opposing findings from RCTs. The committee also considered the substantial body of RCT evidence demonstrating the efficacy of nicotine replacement products compared with placebo products as smoking cessation aids as evidence that provided plausibility for the role of nicotine in enhancing the likelihood of smoking cessation. The combination of RCT evidence and indirect supportive evidence was judged by the committee to provide moderate evidence that e-cigarettes with nicotine are more effective than e-cigarettes without nicotine for smoking cessation.

While scientifically valuable, this evidence does not address a question that is more relevant to public health: how do e-cigarettes with or without nicotine compare to proven FDA-approved cessation aids or to no specific treatment among smokers who are trying to quit? Only one trial has compared an e-cigarette to a nicotine patch (Bullen et al., 2013). No statistically significant difference in quit rates was observed in that trial, and the absolute quit rates were low in all groups. Without replication, this trial by itself provides insufficient evidence at present to support a conclusion of the relative effectiveness of e-cigarettes versus other cessation aids among smokers who are motivated to quit. This is a question of critical public health importance that deserves priority for federal funding agencies. A separate key question for public health impact is whether the availability of e-cigarettes induces more smokers to try to quit, because smokers perceive e-cigarettes to be a more appealing option than FDA-approved cessation aids.

An important note is that characteristics of the study design of the few published RCTs may have minimized the potential effectiveness of e-cigarettes as cessation aids. First, participants in two of three trials were not limited to smokers who wanted to quit smoking. One trial specifically recruited smokers not intending to quit (Caponnetto et al., 2013). An e-cigarette may be more effective in helping smokers who are motivated to quit, although this is a hypothesis that requires testing. Second, the existing RCTs used early e-cigarette models with low nicotine content and poor battery life that likely produced insufficient nicotine delivery. Newer-generation e-cigarettes, which deliver higher doses of nicotine to the user, may be more effective than first-generation devices, which are the ones that have largely been studied in clinical trials. Studies with newer e-cigarettes might produce larger effects, although this remains to be demonstrated. Third, the amount of behavioral support (including instruction in proper use of the product) may affect the effectiveness of e-cigarettes, but existing trials have offered low levels of behavioral support, which might have increased cessation rates of both e-cigarettes and other methods tested (Malas et al., 2016).

RCTs are superior to observational studies with respect to internal validity, but a strength of observational studies is that they reflect the effectiveness of e-cigarettes as they are being used in real-world settings, rather than how a specific device would perform under controlled or optimal conditions. Observational studies reflect how e-cigarettes are actually being used in the population, where they are consumer products sold without specific instructions to aid cessation. The evidence from observational studies is discrepant between studies published through 2015 and those published subsequently. The results of cohort studies have produced mixed results, but the associations in cohort studies published prior to 2016 generally indicate that e-cigarette users are less likely than non-users of combustible tobacco cigarettes to quit smoking. The two systematic reviews that included cohort studies published between 2013 and 2015 in meta-analyses each found a negative association between e-cigarette use and cessation, with ORs of 0.74 and 0.72, respectively (El Dib et al., 2017; Kalkhoran and Glantz, 2016). In one case (El Dib et al., 2017), the result was not statistically significant. The disparate results of data from RCTs and cohort studies published prior to 2016 are striking and contribute to the uncertainty about the overall effect of e-cigarettes on cessation.

One potential explanation for the discrepancy is a difference between observational studies and RCTs in the measurement of e-cigarette use. As described above, the measurement of e-cigarette exposure in most of the cohort studies is relatively blunt. It is often a dichotomous measure such as "ever use" versus "never use" that cannot account for individual differences in the intensity or frequency of use or in the type of device used. The exposure measured in these earlier cohort studies is likely to have been less frequent or intensive that those in the RCTs. Another important reason for the discrepancy is bias in cohort studies due to self-selection. This would occur if the smokers who choose to use e-cigarettes are less likely to succeed because of stronger nicotine dependence, less access to or interest in using effective smoking cessation medications, having failed to quit after having exhausted all other smoking cessation aids, or other factors that could bias relative risk estimates of associations with e-cigarette use toward less favorable cessation outcomes. Furthermore, the motivation for e-cigarette use (e.g., to quit smoking or to be a dual user) was usually not measured in the older cohort studies. While a number of cohort studies used multivariable analysis to attempt to adjust for these factors, unmeasured confounding is always a threat to internal validity in observational studies. Notably, an analogous discrepancy exists between the results of RCTs and cohort studies regarding the effectiveness of nicotine replacement products, but because these products were consistently shown to be efficacious in numerous RCTs the efficacy of these products is well established (Fiore et al., 2008; Stead et al., 2012; USPSTF, 2015).

Observational data may largely reflect dual or intermittent use of e-cigarettes. This pattern may not contribute to cessation success any more than does poor adherence to FDA-approved cessation medications. Most cohort and cross-sectional studies published through 2015 have not characterized patterns of use sufficiently to allow stratified analysis by this or similar factors. Further complicating the interpretation of observational studies is the fact that real-world use of e-cigarettes changed during the period of time when the studies were conducted because e-cigarette have been evolving as consumer products. The committee thus gave greater weight to more recently published data from both prospective cohort and cross-sectional studies that measured frequency of e-cigarette use. With respect to prospective cohort studies, a population-based prospective longitudinal study found persistent e-cigarette use to be associated with cessation while short-term use was not (Zhuang et al., 2016). Other prospective longitudinal studies report that daily or very frequent e-cigarette use may be associated with cessation while intermittent use may not (Biener and Hargraves, 2015; Brose et al., 2015; Delnevo et al., 2016; Hitchman et al., 2015; Levy et al., 2017; Malas et al., 2016). Furthermore, several recent cross-sectional studies using nationally representative population-based samples of adults measured exposure frequency in even finer detail (e.g., number of days of use in a defined time period). Four of five studies analyzing U.S. population samples found an association between more frequent e-cigarette use and smoking cessation. The importance of the measurement limitations in the older studies is highlighted by the fact that even within these U.S. cross-sectional studies, when the measures of "ever use" or "intermittent use" of e-cigarettes were considered, several of the studies showed an inverse relationship between these measures of e-cigarette use and cessation.

The committee judged the results from more recent observational studies to be biologically plausible, as these findings are conceptually consistent with the large body of evidence that smokers trying to quit benefit from adequate nicotine replacement to reduce nicotine withdrawal symptoms. More frequent use of an e-cigarette (or a licensed short-acting nicotine replacement product) should deliver more nicotine. Furthermore, substantial evidence exists to associate higher cessation rates with better adherence to FDA-approved cessation aids among smokers who are attempting to quit.

Based on this biological plausibility and the strong, consistent body of evidence from higher-quality studies published more recently that overcome measurement limitations of studies published in the past, the committee concluded that there was moderate evidence that more frequent use of e-cigarettes is associated with quitting smoking. Observational studies are inherently limited for causal inferences due to the potential for selection bias and unmeasured confounding. The committee gave greater weight to the evidence from RCTs but acknowledged the overall evidence from observational studies in describing the strength of its overall conclusion on the effectiveness of e-cigarettes as a cessation aid. In combination with the limited evidence from RCTs, this body of observational evidence also contributed to the committee's judgment that the total body of evidence that e-cigarettes may be an effective smoking cessation aid was limited.

Future cohort studies will be most useful if they measure more detailed information about e-cigarette use. Factors likely to be important include the type of e-cigarette product (first-generation versus second- and later-generation devices), the frequency of use (daily/regularly or not), the method of use (complete switch to e-cigarettes versus dual use), and the goal of use (to quit smoking versus primarily to reduce number of combustible tobacco cigarettes smoked or otherwise reduce harm without quitting). For both randomized trials and observational studies, critical modifiers of the association of e-cigarette use and smoking cessation may exist, such that certain patterns of use or types of e-cigarettes may be more effective as cessation aids than others.

CONCLUSIONS

Conclusion 17-1. Overall, there is ***limited evidence*** *that e-cigarettes may be effective aids to promote smoking cessation.*

Conclusion 17-2. There is ***moderate evidence*** *from randomized controlled trials that e-cigarettes with nicotine are more effective than e-cigarettes without nicotine for smoking cessation.*

Conclusion 17-3. There is ***insufficient evidence*** *from randomized controlled trials about the effectiveness of e-cigarettes as cessation aids compared with no treatment or to Food and Drug Administration–approved smoking cessation treatments.*

Conclusion 17-4. While the overall evidence from observational trials is mixed, there is ***moderate evidence*** *from observational studies that more frequent use of e-cigarettes is associated with an increased likelihood of cessation.*

REFERENCES

Adriaens, K., D. Van Gucht, P. Declerck, and F. Baeyens. 2014. Effectiveness of the electronic cigarette: An eight-week Flemish study with six-month follow-up on smoking reduction, craving and experienced benefits and complaints. *International Journal of Environmental Research & Public Health* 11(11):11220–11248.

Beard, E., J. Brown, A. McNeill, S. Michie, and R. West. 2015. Has growth in electronic cigarette use by smokers been responsible for the decline in use of licensed nicotine products? Findings from repeated cross-sectional surveys. *Thorax* 70(10):974–978.

Beard, E., R. West, S. Michie, and J. Brown. 2016. Association between electronic cigarette use and changes in quit attempts, success of quit attempts, use of smoking cessation pharmacotherapy, and use of stop smoking services in England: Time series analysis of population trends. *BMJ* 354:i4645. https://doi.org/10.1136/bmj.i4645 (accessed February 9, 2018.

Biener, L., and J. L. Hargraves. 2015. A longitudinal study of electronic cigarette use among a population-based sample of adult smokers: Association with smoking cessation and motivation to quit. *Nicotine & Tobacco Research* 17(2):127–133.

Britton, J. 2016. Electronic cigarettes and smoking cessation in England. *BMJ* 354:i4819. https://doi.org/10.1136/bmj.i4819 (accessed February 9, 2018).

Brose, L. S., S. C. Hitchman, J. Brown, R. West, and A. McNeill. 2015. Is the use of electronic cigarettes while smoking associated with smoking cessation attempts, cessation and reduced cigarette consumption? A survey with a 1-year follow-up. *Addiction* 110(7):1160–1168.

Bullen, C., C. Howe, M. Laugesen, H. McRobbie, V. Parag, J. Williman, and N. Walker. 2013. Electronic cigarettes for smoking cessation: A randomised controlled trial. *Lancet* 382(9905):1629–1637.

Caponnetto, P., D. Campagna, F. Cibella, J. B. Morjaria, M. Caruso, C. Russo, and R. Polosa. 2013. Efficiency and safety of an electronic cigarette (ECLAT) as tobacco cigarettes substitute: A prospective 12-month randomized control design study. *PLoS ONE* 8(6):e66317. https://doi.org/10.1371/journal.pone.0066317 (accessed February 9, 2018).

Delnevo, C. D., D. P. Giovenco, M. B. Steinberg, A. C. Villanti, J. L. Pearson, R. S. Niaura, and D. B. Abrams. 2016. Patterns of electronic cigarette use among adults in the United States. *Nicotine & Tobacco Research* 18(5):715–719.

El Dib, R., E. A. Suzumura, E. A. Akl, H. Gomaa, A. Agarwal, Y. Chang, M. Prasad, V. Ashoorion, D. Heels-Ansdell, W. Maziak, and G. Guyatt. 2017. Electronic nicotine delivery systems and/or electronic non-nicotine delivery systems for tobacco smoking cessation or reduction: A systematic review and meta-analysis. *BMJ Open* 7(2):e012680. https://doi.org/10.1136/bmjopen-2016-012680 (accessed February 9, 2018).

Fiore, M. C., C. R. Jaen, and T. B. Baker. 2008. *Clinical practice guideline: Treating tobacco use and dependence: 2008 update*. Rockville, MD: U.S. Department of Health and Human Services, Public Health Service.

Franck, C., T. Budlovsky, S. B. Windle, K. B. Filion, and M. J. Eisenberg. 2014. Electronic cigarettes in North America: History, use, and implications for smoking cessation. *Circulation* 129(19):1945–1952.

Giovenco, D. P., and C. D. Delnevo. 2018. Prevalence of population smoking cessation by electronic cigarette use status in a national sample of recent smokers. *Addictive Behaviors* 76:129–134.

Guyatt, G. H., A. D. Oxman, R. Kunz, J. Brozek, P. Alonso-Coello, D. Rind, P. J. Devereaux, V. M. Montori, B. Freyschuss, G. Vist, R. Jaeschke, J. W. Williams, Jr., M. H. Murad, D. Sinclair, Y. Falck-Ytter, J. Meerpohl, C. Whittington, K. Thorlund, J. Andrews, and H. J. Schunemann. 2011a. GRADE guidelines 6. Rating the quality of evidence—Imprecision. *Journal of Clinical Epidemiology* 64(12):1283–1293.

Guyatt, G. H., A. D. Oxman, R. Kunz, J. Woodcock, J. Brozek, M. Helfand, P. Alonso-Coello, Y. Falck-Ytter, R. Jaeschke, G. Vist, E. A. Akl, P. N. Post, S. Norris, J. Meerpohl, V. K. Shukla, M. Nasser, H. J. Schunemann, and GRADE Working Group. 2011b. GRADE guidelines: 8. Rating the quality of evidence—Indirectness. *Journal of Clinical Epidemiology* 64(12):1303–1310.

Guyatt, G. H., A. D. Oxman, R. Kunz, J. Woodcock, J. Brozek, M. Helfand, P. Alonso-Coello, P. Glasziou, R. Jaeschke, E. A. Akl, S. Norris, G. Vist, P. Dahm, V. K. Shukla, J. Higgins, Y. Falck-Ytter, H. J. Schunemann, and GRADE Working Group. 2011c. GRADE guidelines: 7. Rating the quality of evidence—Inconsistency. *Journal of Clinical Epidemiology* 64(12):1294–1302.

Guyatt, G. H., A. D. Oxman, V. Montori, G. Vist, R. Kunz, J. Brozek, P. Alonso-Coello, B. Djulbegovic, D. Atkins, Y. Falck-Ytter, J. W. Williams, Jr., J. Meerpohl, S. L. Norris, E. A. Akl, and H. J. Schunemann. 2011d. GRADE guidelines: 5. Rating the quality of evidence—Publication bias. *Journal of Clinical Epidemiology* 64(12):1277–1282.

Guyatt, G. H., A. D. Oxman, G. Vist, R. Kunz, J. Brozek, P. Alonso-Coello, V. Montori, E. A. Akl, B. Djulbegovic, Y. Falck-Ytter, S. L. Norris, J. W. Williams, Jr., D. Atkins, J. Meerpohl, and H. J. Schunemann. 2011e. GRADE guidelines: 4. Rating the quality of evidence—Study limitations (risk of bias). *Journal of Clinical Epidemiology* 64(4):407–415.

Hajek, P., J. F. Etter, N. Benowitz, T. Eissenberg, and H. McRobbie. 2014. Electronic cigarettes: Review of use, content, safety, effects on smokers and potential for harm and benefit. *Addiction* 109(11):1801–1810.

Harrell, P. T., V. N. Simmons, J. B. Correa, T. A. Padhya, and T. H. Brandon. 2014. Electronic nicotine delivery systems ("e-cigarettes"): Review of safety and smoking cessation efficacy. *Otolaryngology—Head and Neck Surgery (United States)* 151(3):381–393.

Hartmann-Boyce, J., H. McRobbie, C. Bullen, R. Begh, L. F. Stead, and P. Hajek. 2016. Electronic cigarettes for smoking cessation. *Cochrane Database of Systematic Reviews* 9:CD010216.

Heydari, G., M. Masjedi, A. E. Ahmady, S. J. Leischow, H. A. Lando, M. B. Shadmehr, and L. Fadaizadeh. 2014. A comparative study on tobacco cessation methods: A quantitative systematic review. *International Journal of Preventive Medicine* 5(6):673–678.

Heydari, G., A. E. Ahmady, F. Chamyani, M. Masjedi, and L. Fadaizadeh. 2017. Electronic cigarette, effective or harmful for quitting smoking and respiratory health: A quantitative review papers. *Lung India* 34(1):25–28.

HHS (U.S. Department of Health and Human Services). 2014. *The health consequences of smoking—50 years of progress: A report of the Surgeon General.* Atlanta, GA: U.S. Department of Health and Human Services, Centers for Disease Control and Prevention, National Center for Disease Prevention and Health Promotion, Office on Smoking and Health.

Higgins, J. P., D. G. Altman, P. C. Gotzsche, P. Juni, D. Moher, A. D. Oxman, J. Savovic, K. F. Schulz, L. Weeks, J. A. Sterne, Cochrane Bias Methods Group, and Cochrane Statistical Methods Group. 2011. The Cochrane Collaboration's tool for assessing risk of bias in randomised trials. *BMJ* 343:d5928. https://doi.org/10.1136/bmj.d5928 (accessed February 9, 2018).

Hitchman, S. C., L. S. Brose, J. Brown, D. Robson, and A. McNeill. 2015. Associations between e-cigarette type, frequency of use, and quitting smoking: Findings from a longitudinal online panel survey in Great Britain. *Nicotine & Tobacco Research* 17(10):1187–1194.

Ioakeimidis, N., C. Vlachopoulos, and D. Tousoulis. 2016. Efficacy and safety of electronic cigarettes for smoking cessation: A critical approach. *Hellenic Journal of Cardiology* 57(January–February):1–6.

Jha, P., and R. Peto. 2014. Global effects of smoking, of quitting, and of taxing tobacco. *New England Journal of Medicine* 370(1):60–68.

Kalkhoran, S., and S. A. Glantz. 2016. E-cigarettes and smoking cessation in real-world and clinical settings: A systematic review and meta-analysis. *The Lancet Respiratory Medicine* 4(2):116–128.

Kasza, K. A., B. K. Ambrose, K. P. Conway, N. Borek, K. Taylor, M. L. Goniewicz, K. M. Cummings, E. Sharma, J. L. Pearson, V. R. Green, A. R. Kaufman, M. Bansal-Travers, M. J. Travers, J. Kwan, C. Tworek, Y. C. Cheng, L. Yang, N. Pharris-Ciurej, D. M. van Bemmel, C. L. Backinger, W. M. Compton, and A. J. Hyland. 2017. Tobacco-product use by adults and youths in the United States in 2013 and 2014. *New England Journal of Medicine* 376(4):342–353.

Khoudigian, S., T. Devji, L. Lytvyn, K. Campbell, R. Hopkins, and D. O'Reilly. 2016. The efficacy and short-term effects of electronic cigarettes as a method for smoking cessation: A systematic review and a meta-analysis. *International Journal of Public Health* 61(2):257–267.

Kmet, L. M., R. C. Lee, and L. S. Cook. 2004. *HTA Initiative #13: Standard quality assessment criteria for evaluating primary research papers from a variety of fields.* Edmonton, Alberta: Alberta Heritage Foundation for Medical Research.

Knight-West, O., and C. Bullen. 2016. E-cigarettes for the management of nicotine addiction. *Substance Abuse and Rehabilitation* 7:111–118.

Lam, C., and A. West. 2015. Are electronic nicotine delivery systems an effective smoking cessation tool? *Canadian Journal of Respiratory Therapy* 51(4):93–98.

Levy, D. T., Z. Yuan, Y. Luo, and D. B. Abrams. 2017. The relationship of e-cigarette use to cigarette quit attempts and cessation: Insights from a large, nationally representative U.S. survey. *Nicotine & Tobacco Research*. https://doi.org/10.1093/ntr/ntx166 (accessed February 9, 2018).

MacDonald, M., R. O'Leary, T. Stockwell, and D. Reist. 2016. Clearing the air: Protocol for a systematic meta-narrative review on the harms and benefits of e-cigarettes and vapour devices. *Systematic Reviews* 5(1):85. https://doi.org/10.1186/s13643-016-0264-y (accessed February 9, 2018).

Malas, M., J. van der Tempel, R. Schwartz, A. Minichiello, C. Lightfoot, A. Noormohamed, J. Andrews, L. Zawertailo, and R. Ferrence. 2016. Electronic cigarettes for smoking cessation: A systematic review. *Nicotine & Tobacco Research* 18(10):1926–1936.

McRobbie, H., C. Bullen, J. Hartmann-Boyce, and P. Hajek. 2014. Electronic cigarettes for smoking cessation and reduction. *Cochrane Database of Systematic Reviews* 12:CD010216.

NASEM (National Academies of Sciences, Engineering, and Medicine). 2017. *The health effects of cannabis and cannabinoids: The current state of evidence and recommendations for research.* Washington, DC: The National Academies Press.

Orr, K. K., and N. J. Asal. 2014. Efficacy of electronic cigarettes for smoking cessation. *Annals of Pharmacotherapy* 48(11):1502–1506.

Patnode, C. D., J. T. Henderson, J. H. Thompson, C. A. Senger, S. P. Fortmann, and E. P. Whitlock. 2015. Behavioral counseling and pharmacotherapy interventions for tobacco cessation in adults, including pregnant women: A review of reviews for the U.S. Preventive Services Task Force. *Annals of Internal Medicine* 163(8):608–621.

Rahman, M. A., N. Hann, A. Wilson, and L. Worrall-Carter. 2014. Electronic cigarettes: Patterns of use, health effects, use in smoking cessation and regulatory issues. *Tobacco Induced Diseases* 12(1):21. https://doi.org/10.1186/1617-9625-12-21 (accessed February 9, 2018).

Rahman, M. A., N. Hann, A. Wilson, G. Mnatzaganian, and L. Worrall-Carter. 2015. E-cigarettes and smoking cessation: Evidence from a systematic review and meta-analysis. *PLoS ONE* 10(3):e0122544. https://doi.org/10.1371/journal.pone.0122544 (accessed February 7, 2018).

Shi, Y. Y., J. P. Pierce, M. White, M. Vijayaraghavan, W. Compton, K. Conway, A. M. Hartman, and K. Messer. 2016. E-cigarette use and smoking reduction or cessation in the 2010/2011 TUS-CPS longitudinal cohort. *BMC Public Health* 16:1105. https://doi.org/10.1186/s12889-016-3770-x (accessed February 9, 2018).

Stead, L. F., R. Perera, C. Bullen, D. Mant, J. Hartmann-Boyce, K. Cahill, and T. Lancaster. 2012. Nicotine replacement therapy for smoking cessation. *Cochrane Database Systematic Reviews* 11:CD000146.

USPSTF (U.S. Preventive Services Task Force). 2015. Behavioral and pharmacotherapy interventions for tobacco smoking cessation in adults, including pregnant women: U.S. Preventive Services Task Force recommendation statement. *Annals of Internal Medicine* 163(8):622–634.

Vanderkam, P., R. Boussageon, M. Underner, N. Langbourg, Y. Brabant, P. Binder, B. Freche, and N. Jaafari. 2016. Efficacy and security of electronic cigarette for tobacco harm reduction: Systematic review and meta-analysis. *Presse Medicale* 45(11):971–985.

Waghel, R. C., D. M. Battise, and M. L. Ducker. 2015. Effectiveness of electronic cigarettes as a tool for smoking cessation or reduction. *Journal of Pharmacy Technology* 31(1):8–12.

Zhu, S. H., Y. L. Zhuang, S. Wong, S. E. Cummins, and G. J. Tedeschi. 2017. E-cigarette use and associated changes in population smoking cessation: Evidence from U.S. current population surveys. *BMJ* 358:j3262. https://doi.org/10.1136/bmj.j3262 (accessed February 7, 2018).

Zhuang, Y. L., S. E. Cummins, J. Y. Sun, and S. H. Zhu. 2016. Long-term e-cigarette use and smoking cessation: A longitudinal study with U.S. population. *Tobacco Control* 25:i90–i95. http://dx.doi.org/10.1136/tobaccocontrol-2016-053096 (accessed February 7, 2018).

18

Harm Reduction

The adverse health consequences of combustible tobacco use have been documented extensively (HHS, 2014), and a major goal of tobacco control efforts is to reduce their health burden (Healthy People 2020, 2017). As described in the previous two chapters, primary strategies to achieve this goal are to prevent youth and young adults from starting smoking and to help current smokers quit expeditiously. Despite these efforts and in spite of successes to reduce initiation and increase cessation, a substantial portion of Americans still become regular smokers. Some of these regular smokers are unwilling to quit and, even among those who want to quit, some have serious difficulty quitting. For these populations who continue to expose themselves and others to harm from combustible tobacco use, it is appropriate to consider strategies that minimize or reduce but not eliminate harm from smoking.

The preceding chapters of this report describe the potential harms of e-cigarette use. Section I presents the evidence on known health effects of individual constituents present in e-cigarette liquids and aerosols. Section II presents the evidence on the health consequences of e-cigarettes on mental and physical health outcomes. By contrast to these earlier chapters, this chapter examines the potential harms of e-cigarettes relative to those of combustible tobacco cigarettes. In so doing, the committee applies a harm reduction approach. Broadly, harm reduction policies attempt to diminish the damaging effects of a particular behavior without aiming to eliminate the behavior itself. Thus, harm reduction policies and interventions consider a broader set of outcomes than would be considered in an approach that aims solely to reduce prevalence.

Applied to tobacco, a harm reduction approach would aim to reduce but not eliminate tobacco-related health risks at the individual and population levels (IOM, 2001; Zeller et al., 2009). The most effective strategies are those that prevent initiation among non-users, promote cessation among current users, and prevent secondhand and thirdhand exposure among non-smokers. Indeed, cessation of any form of tobacco or nicotine-containing product use is currently considered the only guaranteed way to reduce tobacco-related health risks (IOM, 2001). A tobacco harm reduction approach also considers strategies that would reduce tobacco-related health risks while assuming continued use of tobacco or nicotine-containing products (i.e., those that reduce risks without reducing prevalence of tobacco use or exposure to nicotine). Because tobacco control efforts have focused on promoting abstinence from tobacco products, there is currently little evidence on the effectiveness of interventions to reduce harm from continued tobacco use (IOM, 2001). To date, most tobacco control interventions such as nicotine replacement therapy (NRT) are intended for short-term use and not considered long-term substitutes for smoking. A Cochrane review assessing such interventions concluded that using NRT could help smokers unwilling to quit to reduce their cigarette smoking in the short term and to quit in the longer term (Lindson-Hawley et al., 2016). Although tobacco harm reduction strategies could support smoking reduction, the health benefits of doing so remain unclear. Nevertheless, if e-cigarettes confer lower health risks compared with combustible tobacco cigarettes, encouraging use of this reduced-risk product rather than encouraging complete abstinence only could have public health benefits. As suggested by the Cochrane review's conclusions, this approach might be especially salient for combustible tobacco cigarette smokers who are unable or unwilling to quit.

Although e-cigarettes have not been theoretically or experimentally proven to be safe, evidence reviewed in the previous chapters of this report suggest that they may be less harmful alternatives to combustible tobacco cigarettes in at least some scenarios. Some users perceive e-cigarettes to be less harmful than combustible tobacco cigarettes, although the proportion of U.S. adults who consider them to be as harmful as combustible tobacco cigarettes has increased over time (Majeed et al., 2016). These devices are also often advertised as less harmful products because they are believed to contain fewer and less toxic inhaled compounds than combustible tobacco cigarettes. If less harmful, their effectiveness at reducing tobacco-related harms will also depend on their reach. Because of their sensory and behavioral similarities to combustible tobacco cigarettes, e-cigarettes may be more appealing than NRT for both smoking cessation and tobacco harm reduction, and therefore could have greater reach by attracting smokers who are unwilling or unsuccessful at using other approaches. Consequently, e-cigarettes could be an appropriate tool for tobacco harm reduction. Because the efficacy of e-cigarettes to actually reduce harm remains unclear, some researchers have raised concerns about using e-cigarettes for tobacco harm reduction. These concerns include the promotion of continued use of a substance with its own potential health risks (including uncertainty about long-term health risks), the possibility of increasing use of conventional tobacco products through both initiation and relapse, and concerns about questionable terms of engagement with the tobacco industry (McKee and Capewell, 2015).

The extent of risk reduction when transitioning from combustible tobacco cigarette smoking to e-cigarette use will depend on whether an individual switches completely or in part. Those who switch completely would be expected to accrue greater reductions compared with those who continue any smoking. Furthermore, due to the health risks of combustible tobacco smoke from even low levels of use, e-cigarette use among those who continue to smoke (concurrent e-cigarette and combustible tobacco cigarette use, i.e., dual use) may only confer benefits if dual use is merely a transitional state, after which a user transitions completely to e-cigarettes (i.e., quits combustible tobacco cigarettes). E-cigarette use would likely confer little long-term reduction in tobacco-related harm if an individual returns (relapses) to smoking only combustible tobacco cigarettes; it would be more worrisome if e-cigarettes increased likelihood of relapse.

In assessing the harm reduction potential of e-cigarettes among users, the committee therefore considered effects in two populations: smokers who switched to e-cigarette use alone and smokers who use e-cigarettes concurrently with combustible tobacco cigarettes. For smokers who transition completely to e-cigarette use, the committee sought to determine the effects on their health risk profile. The committee uses the term "health risk profile" to capture the various individual health effects and outcomes (e.g., cardiovascular, respiratory, oral) taken together. Overall risk profile is a cumulative product of various individual health risks. In other words, whereas the chapters in Section II examine effects on individual health outcomes from e-cigarette use among naïve users as well as current and former smokers, this chapter focuses on aggregate health effects. For dual users, the committee also sought to determine the reduction in the health risk profile. However, because the greatest reductions in health risk are expected to occur if they eventually quit combustible tobacco cigarette smoking, the committee sought to determine the influence of dual use on subsequent smoking cessation.

The committee also considered effects on non-smokers passively exposed to e-cigarette aerosols compared with combustible tobacco smoke. Exposure of bystanders to environmental combustible tobacco smoke is associated with an increased risk of respiratory and cardiovascular conditions. Smoking cessation among household members is the only effective way of reducing risks from secondhand and thirdhand exposure to potentially toxic chemicals among passive smokers. Similar to the harm reduction strategy among active smokers, changing smoking practices by switching to e-cigarettes in indoor environments may reduce but not eliminate passive exposure to combustible tobacco smoke constituents, especially when smoking cessation is not possible. The committee therefore sought to determine the effectiveness of substituting combustible tobacco cigarettes with e-cigarettes on changes in health effects and exposure to toxicants among non-smokers passively exposed to e-cigarette aerosols compared with tobacco smoke.

EVIDENCE REVIEW: LEVELS OF EVIDENCE AVAILABLE

The committee drew upon comparisons of evidence from several points along the causal pathway between e-cigarettes or combustible tobacco cigarettes and health outcomes. These include evidence on the exposure to toxicants present in e-cigarette aerosols compared with those in cigarette smoke; nicotine and toxicant exposures in e-cigarette users as an intermediate outcome; and comparisons of effects on any health outcome from e-cigarette use compared with combustible tobacco cigarette smoking. Because multiple studies were available comparing e-cigarettes with combustible tobacco cigarettes for each step in the causal pathway, in this section, the committee discusses evidence by establishing likely exposures from the two products and moves down the causal chain to show how these exposures might shape health effects differently. The committee begins by drawing upon studies examining individual constituents discussed in Chapter 5 and highlights studies that directly compared emissions from e-cigarette devices and combustible tobacco cigarettes. The committee then reviews evidence on nicotine and other toxicant exposures among combustible tobacco cigarette smokers who completely switched to e-cigarettes. The optimal study design would include baseline data collection from subjects at the time of combustible tobacco cigarette use and follow-up evaluation after complete and partial substitution of combustible tobacco cigarettes with e-cigarettes. The committee also reviewed studies with cross-sectional designs, when exposure to nicotine and toxicants was compared among e-cigarette users, combustible tobacco cigarette smokers, and dual users of both products. The committee proceeds by discussing evidence comparing e-cigarette and combustible tobacco cigarette use on health outcomes. The optimal study design should include baseline collection of clinically relevant health outcomes from subjects at the time of combustible tobacco cigarette use and follow-up evaluation after sufficient time of complete and partial substitution of combustible cigarettes with e-cigarettes. The committee also reviewed cross-sectional studies, when clinically relevant health outcomes were compared among e-cigarette users, combustible tobacco cigarette smokers, and dual users of both products. The committee then turns to supporting evidence on toxicity from animal and in vitro studies.

Epidemiological studies and randomized controlled trials (RCTs) evaluating the long-term health effects of exclusive e-cigarette use as well as reducing the frequency and number of combustible tobacco cigarettes smoked with concurrent combustible tobacco cigarette smoking and e-cigarette use (dual use) would provide the strongest evidence of harm reduction in these populations of users. As in the section on health effects (Section II), in their absence, the committee looks further up the causal pathway to epidemiological evidence on intermediate outcomes, including biomarkers of disease as well as evidence on exposure levels (i.e., studies that look at changes and differences in biomarkers levels). Furthermore, given that the greatest health benefits are likely to occur if dual use represents a temporary transitional stage before combustible tobacco cigarette users transition to e-cigarette use alone, the committee draws upon evidence of e-cigarette studies examining whether dual use increases likelihood of smoking cessation.

For studies on the effects of switching from combustible tobacco cigarettes to e-cigarettes to reduce harm from passive exposures, RCTs, and longitudinal observational studies that follow household members of combustible tobacco cigarette smokers who switch to e-cigarettes completely would provide the strongest evidence. In their absence, the committee draws inferences from studies that examine exposure to toxicants from passive exposure to e-cigarette aerosols compared with combustible tobacco smoke.

EVIDENCE REVIEW: METHODS

The committee identified four studies comparing toxicant levels in e-cigarette aerosols and combustible tobacco cigarette smoke (Goniewicz et al., 2014; Margham et al., 2016; Tayyarah and Long, 2014; Williams et al., 2013). One study compared potentially toxic substances from different e-cigarette models and combustible tobacco cigarettes based on published literature (Goniewicz et al., 2014). Three laboratory studies compared e-cigarette aerosols to combustible tobacco cigarette smoke (Margham et al., 2016; Tayyarah and Long, 2014; Williams et al., 2013).

To assess effects in smokers who transition completely from combustible tobacco cigarettes to e-cigarettes, the committee identified studies that prospectively evaluated changes in health outcomes. Because the committee was interested in the overall health risk from e-cigarette use, the committee included literature on all health outcomes among former smokers who use e-cigarettes. Only studies that included e-cigarette exposure as the treatment condition and combustible tobacco cigarette exposure as a positive control were included. Studies that calculated potential risk levels from known risks of toxicants in e-cigarettes and combustible tobacco cigarettes from other settings (e.g., environmental or occupational exposures) were excluded. The committee identified both longitudinal observational studies and crossover experimental studies (n = 15 total). Because a fair number of studies met these criteria, the committee excluded cross-sectional studies and case reports, which are weaker study designs, from this analysis. The committee also drew on analogous data from in vivo animal and in vitro studies comparing the toxicity of e-cigarettes and combustible tobacco cigarettes. The committee limited studies to those that used the same models and experiment settings to expose cells or animals to both e-cigarette aerosols and combustible tobacco cigarette smoke. As with human studies, each study included in this review assessed harmful effects of e-cigarette aerosols with combustible tobacco smoke as a positive control. The committee identified 27 in vitro studies (Anderson et al., 2016; Anthérieu et al., 2017; Aufderheide and Emura, 2017; Aug et al., 2015; Azzopardi et al., 2016; Banerjee et al., 2017; Barber et al., 2016; Breheny et al., 2017; Carson et al., 2017; Cervellati et al., 2014; Farsalinos et al., 2013; Fields et al., 2017; Haswell et al., 2017; Hom et al., 2016; Leigh et al., 2016; Misra et al., 2014; Moses et al., 2017; Neilson et al., 2015; Putzhammer et al., 2016; Romagna et al., 2013; Rubenstein et al., 2015; Scheffler et al., 2015; Shen et al., 2016; Taylor et al., 2016; Teasdale et al., 2016; Thorne et al., 2016, 2017) and 5 in vivo animal studies (Larcombe et al., 2017; Palpant et al., 2015; Parker and Rayburn, 2017; Ponzoni et al., 2015; Rau et al., 2017).

To assess whether e-cigarettes may reduce harm among dual users, the committee sought to identify studies on the health risk profile in dual users, including exposure to nicotine and toxicants, intermediate outcomes, and distal health outcomes. Only studies that aimed for direct comparison of the outcomes between groups of smokers and e-cigarette users were included in the review. The studies included in the review should have recruited and measured outcomes at the same time, using the same analytical methods and clinical tools. Studies that measured outcomes only in e-cigarette users and compared results with historical data collected in different studies were excluded. The committee identified one study reporting nicotine exposure (Jorenby et al., 2017) and two studies reporting dependence symptoms (Jorenby et al., 2017; Loukas et al., 2016).

The committee identified no studies on the long-term health effects of using e-cigarettes concurrently with combustible tobacco cigarettes. However, because the greatest health benefits are likely to occur if smokers transition to e-cigarette use alone, the committee also identified studies on whether using e-cigarettes while also smoking combustible tobacco cigarettes is associated with greater likelihood of combustible tobacco cigarette smoking cessation. The committee identified two longitudinal observational studies (Etter and Bullen, 2014; Manzoli et al., 2015, 2017), one 26-day laboratory study (Jorenby et al., 2017), and one cross-sectional study (Loukas et al., 2016).

Finally, to assess whether changing smoking practices by switching to e-cigarettes in indoor environments may reduce passive exposure to combustible tobacco smoke constituents among non-smokers, the committee sought to identify studies examining changes in health effects and exposure to toxicants from passive exposure to e-cigarette aerosols compared with combustible tobacco smoke. Only studies that aimed for direct comparison of the environmental exposure levels between secondhand (and thirdhand) emissions from e-cigarettes and combustible tobacco cigarettes were included in the review. The same inclusion criteria applied to studies that evaluated biomarkers of exposure in persons passively exposed to aerosols emitted from e-cigarettes or environmental tobacco smoke. The studies included in the review should have used the same analytical methods to assess secondhand exposure from the two products. Studies that assessed secondhand exposure only in e-cigarette exposure conditions and compared results with historical data collected in different studies or with different methods were excluded from review. The committee identified no studies on intermediate or distal health outcomes related to passive exposures to e-cigarette aerosols compared with combustible tobacco smoke. In their absence, the committee identified four studies comparing passive exposures (Ballbè et al., 2014; Bush and Goniewicz, 2015; Czogała et al., 2014; Flouris et al., 2012).

EVIDENCE REVIEW: RESULTS

Comparison of Toxic Levels in E-Cigarettes and Combustible Tobacco Cigarettes

E-cigarette liquids can expose users to toxicants through solvents (propylene glycol [PG] and glycerol), flavorings, and other additives; heating and aerosolizing e-liquids can generate additional toxicants. Although some of these toxicants are also found in combustible tobacco cigarettes, they are generally at much lower levels in e-cigarettes. Carbon monoxide (CO), for example, is present in combustible tobacco smoke and delivered to smokers, but is absent from e-cigarette aerosol (Vansickel et al., 2010). The physicochemical composition of an e-cigarette aerosol may be a key driver behind functional impairments. While e-cigarettes seem to be a promising harm reduction tool for smokers of combustible tobacco, evidence suggests that using these products could result in repeated inhalation of respiratory toxicants, irritants, and sensitizers. In other words, whereas evidence reviewed in Chapter 4 on nicotine and Chapter 5 on other constituents and metals in e-cigarettes examined effects of acute exposures from individual constituents, this chapter examines effects of periodic exposures over time to e-cigarette aerosols as a whole. To that end, this section reviews studies that directly compared emissions of harmful and potentially harmful chemicals from e-cigarette devices and from combustible tobacco cigarettes.

Reducing the quantity of tobacco a person uses and reducing the potentially toxic substances in tobacco products (such as in pharmaceutical nicotine and in potential reduced-exposure tobacco products) are strategies for reducing exposure to toxicants from smoking. Most studies evaluating toxicant levels in e-cigarettes have focused on liquid composition, showing that the levels of toxic chemicals present in liquids are far lower than in combustible tobacco cigarettes. Compared with combustible tobacco smoke, e-cigarette aerosol is simpler in composition and primarily composed of homogeneous particles with very low levels of volatile species suspended in air. Additionally, e-cigarette aerosol contains substantially lower levels of toxicants than combustible tobacco cigarette smoke.

Using data available in the literature, Goniewicz and colleagues (2014) compared the content of harmful substances among several models of e-cigarettes and combustible tobacco cigarettes. To compare levels of selected toxicants in e-cigarette aerosol and combustible tobacco cigarette mainstream smoke, the authors assumed that e-cigarette users take an average of 15 puffs during one session of product use, which would correspond to smoking one combustible tobacco cigarette. As shown in Table 18-1, levels of selected toxic compounds found in combustible tobacco cigarette smoke were from 9- to 450-fold higher than levels in e-cigarette aerosol. The results of the study support the proposition that the aerosol emitted from an e-cigarette is less injurious than the smoke from combustible tobacco cigarettes. Thus, one would expect that if a person switched from combustible tobacco cigarettes to e-cigarettes, exposure to toxic chemicals and related adverse health effects would be reduced. This hypothesis has been confirmed in several studies involving people using e-cigarette devices.

Margham and colleagues (2016) examined 150 chemicals emitted from an e-cigarette (Vype ePen), a reference combustible tobacco cigarette (Ky3R4F), and laboratory air (method blanks). Of the chemicals

TABLE 18-1 Comparison of Toxicant Levels Among Combustible Tobacco Cigarette Smoke and E-Cigarette Aerosol

Toxic Compound	Combustible Tobacco Cigarette (μg in mainstream smoke)	E-Cigarette (μg per 15 puffs)	Average Ratio (combustible tobacco cigarette versus e-cigarette)
Formaldehyde	1.6–52	0.20–5.61	9
Acetaldehyde	52–140	0.11–1.36	450
Acrolein	2.4–62	0.07–4.19	15
Toluene	8.3–70	0.02–0.63	120
NNN	0.0005–0.19	0.00008–0.00043	380
NNK	0.012–0.11	0.00011–0.00283	40

NOTE: NNK = 4-(methylnitrosamino)-1-(3-pyridyl)-1-butanone; NNN = *N*′-nitrosonornicotine.
SOURCE: Goniewicz et al., 2014.

examined, only 25 were detected; 104 chemicals were not detected and 21 were present due to laboratory background. Of those detected in the aerosol, the e-cigarette generated 16 (either in whole or in part), and 9 were present at levels too low to be quantified. The chemicals detected included e-liquid constituents (nicotine, PG, and glycerol), and eight thermal decomposition products of PG or glycerol. By contrast, approximately 100 chemicals were detected in mainstream combustible tobacco cigarette smoke. The authors concluded that, on a per-puff basis and depending on the regulatory list considered and the puffing method used, the toxicants emitted were from 82 to more than 99 percent lower in the e-cigarette aerosol than from the combustible tobacco cigarette smoke.

A study by Tayyarah and Long (2014) found that aerosol nicotine for the e-cigarette samples (blu and SKYCIG brands) was 85 percent lower than the nicotine yield for the combustible tobacco cigarettes. The authors also found that the mainstream combustible tobacco cigarette smoke contained approximately 1,500 times more harmful and potentially harmful constituents (HPHCs) compared with e-cigarette aerosol or room air. The deliveries of HPHCs tested for these e-cigarette products were more similar to the air blanks rather than to deliveries from combustible tobacco cigarettes; the HPHCs detected in combustible tobacco cigarette smoke were either not detected or detected at trace levels in the e-cigarette aerosols.

Williams and colleagues (2013) compared the concentrations of various metals in the aerosol generated from an e-cigarette cartomizer from a leading manufacturer (10 puffs) with the concentrations in the mainstream smoke from one combustible tobacco cigarette. For 11 metals for which data were available for combustible tobacco cigarette smoke, the concentration of elements in the e-cigarette aerosol was higher for four elements (aluminum, iron, nickel, and sodium), within the combustible tobacco smoke range for five elements (chromium, copper, lead, magnesium, and manganese), and lower for two elements (potassium and zinc).

Synthesis

Although a limited number of laboratory studies compared emissions of harmful and potentially harmful chemicals from e-cigarette devices and from combustible tobacco cigarettes, laboratory studies reviewed above and in Chapter 5 overall found that an aerosol emitted from e-cigarettes is substantially less complex than tobacco smoke. Although several potentially toxic substances have been identified in e-cigarette aerosol, the amounts emitted from e-cigarettes under typical conditions of use are significantly lower compared with levels measured in combustible tobacco smoke. Thus, as the committee concluded in Chapter 5, *there is **substantial evidence** that except for nicotine, under typical conditions of use, exposure to potentially toxic substances from e-cigarettes is significantly lower compared with combustible tobacco cigarettes* (see Conclusion 5-3).

Harm Reduction in Smokers Who Switched from Combustible Tobacco Cigarettes to E-Cigarettes

Comparison of Nicotine and Toxicant Exposure

Whether e-cigarettes will substitute for combustible tobacco cigarettes depends, in part, on if they yield effects approximating the combustible tobacco cigarette effects thought to cause dependent cigarette use, including delivery of similar levels of nicotine. Potential harm reduction will be at least partially determined by the magnitude of reduction in exposure to harmful and potentially harmful toxicants as compared with exposure from tobacco smoking. Below, the committee reviews cross-sectional and longitudinal studies that compared exposure to nicotine and toxicants in tobacco smokers who substituted e-cigarettes for their combustible tobacco cigarettes.

Adriaens and colleagues (2014) conducted an RCT with 8 months follow-up on the effects on smoking behavior of providing e-cigarettes (Joyetech eGo-C and Kanger T2-CC brands) to combustible tobacco cigarette smokers. The researchers recruited participants who were willing to try a less harmful alternative, but did not intend to quit. Participants (n = 48) were randomized into two e-cigarette groups and one control group. Over the first 2 months of the study during which laboratory studies were conducted, participants in the e-cigarette groups were provided with e-cigarettes to use, while participants in the control group continued smoking combustible tobacco cigarettes. After 8 weeks, the investigators also gave the control group e-cigarettes (same brands and types as those in the two e-cigarette groups). During the laboratory studies in the first 2-month period of the study, investigators examined craving and withdrawal symptoms in the lab. For 8 months after providing participants with e-cigarettes, the investigators assessed effects on smoking behavior, as well as benefits of and complaints about using an e-cigarette. At 3 months after the last lab session (5 months from the start of the study when the e-cigarette groups were given e-cigarettes; 3 months from when the control group was given e-cigarettes), 38 percent of participants across all groups (37 percent in the e-cigarette groups combined and 39 percent in the control group) reported complete abstinence from smoking, 6 percent showed a reduction in smoking of more than 80 percent, and another 10 percent showed a reduction of more than 50 percent. At the same time, 46 percent of participants were smoking 50 percent or more of their number of combustible tobacco cigarettes at baseline (including participants with missing data). Of note, in the control group, there were no significant changes in smoking behavior over the first 2 months of the study (during which they monitored behavior but were not provided e-cigarettes). At follow-up 6 months after the last laboratory session (8 months after the start of the study), 21 percent of participants across all groups (19 percent of the e-cigarette groups combined and 25 percent of the control group) reported complete abstinence from smoking, 15 percent showed a reduction in combustible tobacco cigarette use of more than 80 percent, and another 8 percent showed a reduction of more than 50 percent; 56 percent reported smoking 50 percent or more of their number of combustible tobacco cigarettes at baseline (including missing data). Reduction in smoking was consistent with decreased levels of expired CO. There were no significant differences in saliva cotinine levels among groups either during the laboratory sessions (during which the control group was smoking combustible tobacco cigarettes exclusively) or at follow-up. Together, these results suggest that e-cigarettes may help promote smoking reduction or cessation even among smokers who do not intend to quit, and also that e-cigarette users (both exclusive and dual) can self-titrate nicotine intake from e-cigarettes with some practice.

Cravo and colleagues (2016) conducted a randomized, parallel group clinical study to evaluate the safety profile of an e-cigarette product (2.0 percent nicotine, developed by Fontem Ventures B.V., Amsterdam, the Netherlands) in 420 smokers of combustible tobacco cigarettes switching to use the e-cigarette product for 12 weeks. Urine nicotine equivalents decreased by up to 33.8 percent in e-cigarette product subjects and three biomarkers of exposure to toxicants known to be present in combustible tobacco cigarette smoke (benzene, acrolein, and 4-[methylnitrosamino]-1-[3-pyridyl]-1-butanone [NNK]) also decreased. The decrease in nicotine equivalents coincided with an increase in nicotine withdrawal symptoms, measured by a questionnaire, which subsided after 2 weeks.

A 5-day study randomized 105 clinically confirmed smokers into one of seven groups: three exclusive e-cigarette use groups (blu e-cigarettes in rechargeable tobacco, rechargeable cherry, and disposable cherry), three dual-use groups (one of the three blu e-cigarettes and continued combustible tobacco cigarette smoking), and one group that abstained from all nicotine and tobacco products (cessation) (D'Ruiz et al., 2016; O'Connell et al., 2016). The investigators assessed blood, urine, and exhaled breath biomarkers of exposure of toxicants believed to contribute to smoking-related disease at baseline and 5-day follow-up. They found that subjects switching to e-cigarettes (either partially or completely) had significantly lower levels (29–95 percent) of urinary biomarkers of exposure. All groups experienced significant decreases in exhaled CO (27–89 percent), and nicotine equivalents decreased by 25–40 percent. Dual users who reported that they substituted half of their daily combustible tobacco cigarette consumption with e-cigarettes experienced 7–38 percent reductions, but had increases (1–20 percent) in nicotine equivalents. Reductions were broadly proportional to the reduced numbers of combustible tobacco cigarettes smoked. At follow-up, blood nicotine biomarker levels were lower in the cessation (75–96 percent) and e-cigarette use groups (11–83 percent), but there were no significant reductions among dual users. All subjects experienced significant decreases in exhaled CO; reductions of 88–89 percent were observed among the cessation and exclusive e-cigarette use groups and from 27 percent to 32 percent among dual users. Exhaled nitric oxide (NO) increased (46–63 percent) in the cessation and e-cigarette groups, but there were only minimal changes among dual users (O'Connell et al., 2016).

Using a longitudinal within-subjects observational design, Goniewicz and colleagues (2017), evaluated the effects of switching from combustible tobacco cigarettes to e-cigarettes on nicotine delivery and exposure to selected carcinogens and toxicants. The authors measured metabolites of nicotine and major carcinogens and toxicants present in combustible tobacco smoke and combustible tobacco smoke exposure biomarkers (including NNK, 1,3-butadiene, crotonaldehyde, acrolein, benzene, acrylamide, acrylonitrile, ethylene oxide, propylene oxide, naphthalene, fluorene, phenanthrene, and pyrene) in the urine samples of 20 smokers collected before and after switching to pen-style M201 e-cigarettes for 2 weeks. One week after participants switched from combustible tobacco cigarettes to e-cigarettes, levels of total nicotine and some polycyclic aromatic hydrocarbon metabolites did not change, but all other biomarkers significantly decreased ($p < 0.05$). The greatest reductions were seen in metabolites of 1,3-butadiene, benzene, and acrylonitrile. Total 4-(methylnitrosamino)-1-(3-pyridyl)-1-butanol, known as NNAL (a metabolite of a tobacco-specific nitrosamine [TSNA], NNK), declined by 57 percent after 1 week and 64 percent after 2 weeks. Levels of 3-hydroxyfluorene declined by 46 percent after 1 week and 34 percent after 2 weeks. Results from this study are shown in Figure 18-1.

Hecht and colleagues (2015) analyzed urine samples from 28 e-cigarette users who had not smoked combustible tobacco cigarettes for at least 2 months for toxicant and carcinogen metabolites, including 1-hydroxypyrene (1-HOP), NNAL and its glucuronides (total NNAL), 3-hydroxypropylmercapturic acid (3-HPMA, the primary metabolite of acrolein), 2-hydroxypropylmercapturic acid (2-HPMA), 3-hydroxy-1-methylpropylmercapturic acid (HMPMA), *S*-phenylmercapturic acid (SPMA), nicotine,

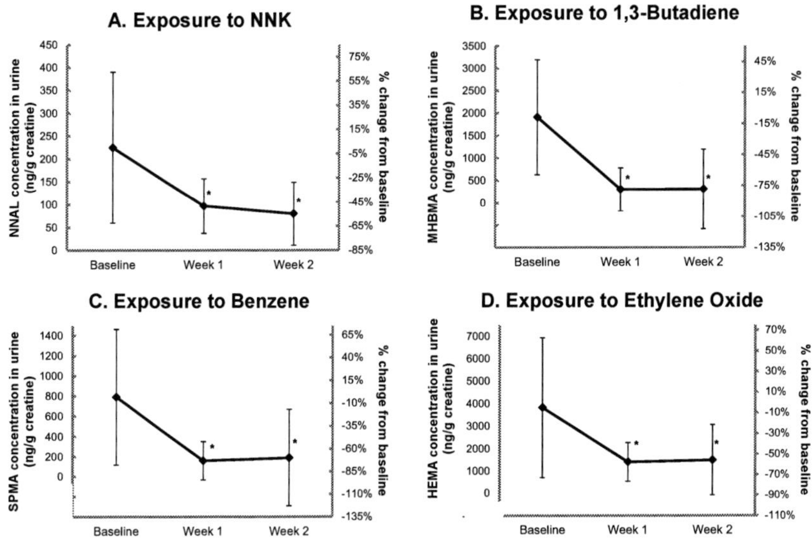

FIGURE 18-1 Changes in select carcinogen levels over 2 weeks of electronic cigarette use among 20 smokers (mean ± SD).
NOTES: *Denotes statistically significant differences from baseline according to repeated-measure analysis of variance ($p < 0.05$). HEMA = 2-hydroxyethylmercapturic acid; MHBMA = 2-hydroxy-3-buten-1-yl-mercapturic acid; NNAL = 4-(methylnitrosamino)-1-(3-pyridyl)-1-butanol; NNK = 4-(methylnitrosamino)-1-(3-pyridyl)-1-butanone; SPMA = *S*-phenylmercapturic acid.
SOURCE: Goniewicz et al., 2017.

and cotinine. The authors compared these samples to previous analyses of combustible tobacco cigarette smokers' urine using similar, validated methods. These comparisons showed that samples from e-cigarette users had significantly lower levels of 1-HOP, total NNAL, 3-HPMA, 2-HPMA, HMPMA, and SPMA. However, levels of nicotine and cotinine in e-cigarette users were significantly lower compared with combustible tobacco cigarette smokers in one study but not another.

McRobbie and colleagues (2015) measured exposure to CO, urinary cotinine (as a nicotine metabolite), and urinary 3-HPMA before and after 4 weeks of e-cigarette use (Green Smoke cigalike device, labeled 2.4 percent nicotine) in 40 smokers. Four weeks after quitting, 33 participants reported using e-cigarettes, 48 percent reported abstaining from combustible tobacco cigarettes and exclusively using e-cigarettes in the week prior, and 52 percent reported using both e-cigarettes and combustible tobacco cigarettes (dual use). CO levels were significantly reduced among e-cigarette–only users (80 percent decrease) and dual users (52 percent decrease). Cotinine levels also declined, but to a lesser extent (17 percent decrease among exclusive e-cigarette users and 44 percent decrease among dual users). Mean 3-HPMA levels decreased 79 percent among exclusive e-cigarette users and by 60 percent in dual users.

Pulvers and colleagues (2016) enrolled 40 combustible tobacco cigarette smokers (with 1 year or more of smoking) interested in switching to e-cigarettes in a 4-week observational study. The researchers provided participants with an e-Go C non-variable battery e-cigarette and refillable atomizers in a choice of eight flavors with 12 mg or 24 mg nicotine and measured urinary cotinine, NNAL, and eight volatile organic compounds (VOCs) that are known toxic constituents of combustible tobacco cigarettes at baseline and week 4. All participants with follow-up data (92.5 percent) reported using the study e-cigarette. At week 2, 40 percent reported abstaining from combustible tobacco cigarettes. At week 4, 15 percent had remained abstinent. At 4 weeks, there were no significant changes in nicotine intake ($p = 0.90$), but CO ($p < 0.001$), NNAL ($p < 0.01$), and metabolites of benzene ($p < 0.01$) and acrylonitrile ($p = 0.001$) decreased significantly. Smokers switching exclusively to e-cigarettes for at least half of the study period demonstrated significant reductions in metabolites of ethylene oxide ($p = 0.03$) and acrylamide ($p < 0.01$).

Shahab and colleagues (2017) compared biomarkers of exposure to nicotine and potentially toxic and carcinogenic chemicals among exclusive combustible tobacco cigarette smokers, former smokers with long-term exclusive e-cigarette use, former smokers with long-term exclusive NRT use, long-term dual users of both combustible tobacco cigarettes and e-cigarettes, and long-term users of both combustible tobacco cigarettes and NRT ($n = 36$ or 37 per group; total $n = 181$). Participants provided urine and saliva samples, which were analyzed for biomarkers of nicotine, TSNAs, and VOCs. There were no differences in salivary or urinary biomarkers of nicotine intake after controlling for confounders. Levels of metabolites of TSNAs (including NNAL) and VOCs (including metabolites of the toxicants acrolein, acrylamide, acrylonitrile, 1,3-butadiene, and ethylene oxide) were significantly lower among exclusive e-cigarette and exclusive NRT users than for exclusive combustible tobacco cigarette smokers, dual combustible tobacco cigarette–e-cigarette users, and dual combustible tobacco cigarette–NRT users. The e-cigarette–only users had significantly lower NNAL levels than all other groups. Levels of TSNA and VOC metabolites were similar among combustible tobacco cigarette–only, dual combustible tobacco cigarette–NRT users, and dual combustible tobacco cigarette–e-cigarette users. Results from this study are shown in Figure 18-2.

van Staden and colleagues (2013) used a single group within-subject design to examine effects of switching from combustible tobacco cigarettes to e-cigarettes (Twisp brand) for 2 weeks among 13 participants (median age = 38 years, range = 23–46, median cigarettes per day = 20, range = 12–30). At baseline (before using e-cigarettes) and 2-week follow-up, the researchers measured arterial carboxyhaemoglobin (COHb), venous COHb, and venous cotinine levels and asked the participants to complete a questionnaire reporting perceptions of their health and

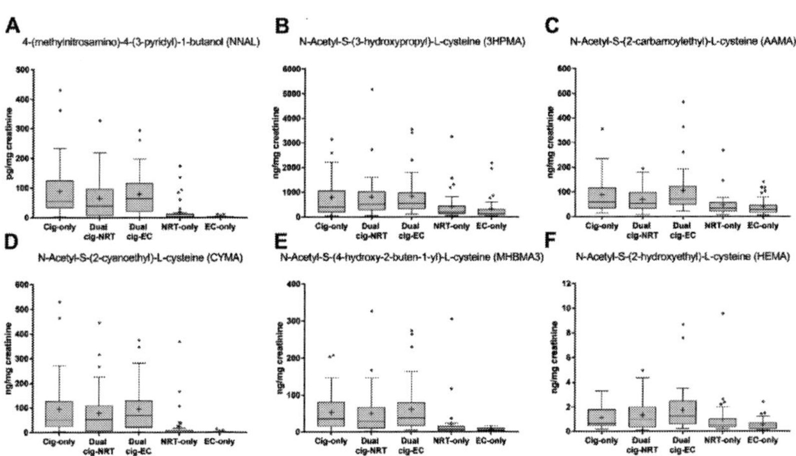

FIGURE 18-2 Urinary metabolite levels for selected toxins and carcinogens, by group.
NOTE: EC = e-cigarette; NRT = nicotine replacement therapy.
SOURCE: Shahab et al., 2017.

lifestyle. After 2 weeks of e-cigarette use, COHb levels were significantly lower (percent mean ± SD for both arterial COHb and venous COHb after 2 weeks of e-cigarette use compared with baseline [arterial: 4.66 ± 1.99 at baseline versus 2.46 ± 1.35 at 2-week follow-up, p = 0.014; venous: 4.37 ± 2.1 at baseline versus 2.50 ± 1.23 at follow-up, p = 0.018]). The authors also found a significant decrease in cotinine levels (p = 0.001) and a significant increase in oxygen saturation (p = 0.002). Most participants reported perceiving improvements in their health and lifestyle measures.

A cross-sectional study by Martin and colleagues (2016) compared immune gene expression profiles in superficial nasal scrape biopsies collected from non-smokers (n = 13), combustible tobacco cigarette smokers (n = 14), and e-cigarette users (n = 12), and analyzed them using the nCounter human immunology V2 expression panel. The researchers determined smoking status by taking smoking histories and from a 3- to 4-week smoking diary, which was biochemically confirmed with serum cotinine and urinary NNAL. Results showed that all genes with decreased expression in combustible tobacco cigarette smokers (n = 53) were also decreased in e-cigarette smokers. Moreover, compared with combustible tobacco cigarette smokers, e-cigarette users showed more gene expression changes and stronger levels of suppression in a gene-by-gene comparison. In genes common with those changed in smokers, e-cigarette users showed greater suppression, especially for expression of transcription factors. For example, *EGR1* was functionally associated with decreased expression of 18 target genes in e-cigarette users compared with only 5 target genes in combustible tobacco cigarette smokers.

Synthesis Several cross-sectional and longitudinal studies compared exposure to nicotine and toxicants in smokers who substituted e-cigarettes for their combustible tobacco cigarettes. All studies showed that smokers who substituted their tobacco cigarettes with e-cigarettes had significantly reduced levels of biomarkers of exposure to potentially toxic chemicals. Nicotine intake from e-cigarette devices among ex-smokers who were experienced e-cigarette users was comparable to that from tobacco cigarettes. Except for nicotine, exposure to potentially toxic substances from using e-cigarettes was significantly lower compared with smoking combustible tobacco cigarettes.

Conclusion 18-1. There is ***conclusive evidence*** *that completely substituting e-cigarettes for combustible tobacco cigarettes reduces users' exposure to numerous toxicants and carcinogens present in combustible tobacco cigarettes.*

Health Risk Profile

In the same 8-month follow-up study by Adriaens and colleagues (2014) described in the harm reduction section above of smokers not intending to quit (n = 48), who were randomized to three e-cigarette–only groups, three dual-use groups, and a control group (cessation from nicotine and tobacco for 8 weeks, followed by switching to the same type of e-cigarettes as the e-cigarette groups), the authors also assessed benefits of and complaints about using e-cigarettes and smoking combustible tobacco cigarettes. Participants reported these benefits and complaints in online diaries. Adverse events included in the reported complaints included dry mouth/throat, mouth/throat irritation, dizziness, headache, nausea, increased heart rate/palpitations, and increased weight. Participants also reported concerns about health risks. Benefits included pleasant sensation when inhaling, improved breathing, pleasant taste when inhaling, less coughing or sore throat, improved health and fitness, improved taste and smell, less unpleasant smells, and improved sleep. E-cigarette users were also asked about the pleasure of e-cigarette use, decreased desire for combustible tobacco cigarettes, fresher breath, and a device that can be used in more places. At the beginning of the study, the control group reported more complaints about their combustible tobacco cigarettes than the e-cigarette groups did about their e-cigarettes, but this difference disappeared at follow-up. This change may be attributable to the fact that the control group switched to the e-cigarettes after 8 weeks. Participants in the e-cigarette groups also reported more benefits experienced from the e-cigarette than the control group experienced from combustible tobacco cigarettes. Results also showed an increase in experienced benefits among e-cigarette users over the course of the study, which may reflect a learning effect.

In a single-blind, crossover study, Carnevale and colleagues (2016) compared the effects of e-cigarettes and combustible tobacco cigarettes on oxidative stress and endothelial cell function in healthy adult smokers (n = 20) and non-smokers (n = 20). Participants were matched for age and sex. First, all subjects smoked combustible tobacco cigarettes. After 1 week, the subjects switched to smoking an e-cigarette with the same labeled nicotine content as contained in the combustible tobacco cigarettes. Immediately before and after smoking, blood samples were drawn and markers of oxidative stress, nitric oxide bioavailability, and vitamin E levels were measured. Flow-mediated dilation (FMD), a marker of endothelial function in humans, was also measured. Levels of soluble NOX2-derived peptide and 8-*iso*-prostaglandin F2α and a significant decrease in nitric oxide bioavailability, vitamin E levels, and FMD increased significantly after both e-cigarette use and combustible tobacco smoking. Generalized estimating equation analysis confirmed that smoking affected all markers of oxidative stress and FMD and showed that the biological effects of e-cigarettes compared with combustible tobacco cigarettes on vitamin E levels and FMD were not statistically different. However, e-cigarettes showed a lesser impact than combustible tobacco cigarettes on levels of soluble NOX2-derived peptide, 8-*iso*-prostaglandin F2α, and nitric oxide bioavailability.

Cibella and colleagues (2016) conducted a 1-year randomized controlled trial to evaluate changes in spirometric indexes and respiratory symptoms. Participants (n = 300) were smokers invited to substitute their combustible tobacco cigarettes with e-cigarettes wholly (to quit) or in part (to reduce their smoking), and were given e-cigarettes with 2.4 percent, 1.8 percent, or 0 percent nicotine. Participants were classified as quitters (those who completely switched from combustible tobacco cigarettes to e-cigarettes), reducers (those who substituted some of their smoking with e-cigarettes and reduced their combustible tobacco cigarette consumption), and failures (those with no changes in smoking). The authors found no significant differences in spirometric indexes (forced expiratory volume [FEV1], forced vital capacity [FVC], and FEV1/FVC ratio) among the groups, except for forced expiratory flow 25–75 percent, which significantly increased over the time among those who quit smoking (85.7 ± 15.6 percent at baseline to 100.8 ± 14.6 percent at follow-up, p = 0.034). Among all participants, 43.1 percent reported having cough or phlegm and 34.8 percent reported shortness of breath at baseline. The prevalence of these symptoms decreased substantially over follow-up visits. No participants who reduced their smoking by substituting some of their smoking with e-cigarette use reported shortness of breath at any follow-up visit (week 12, 24, and 52), and participants who switched completely reported neither symptom at any follow-up.

Cravo and colleagues (2016) conducted a randomized, parallel group clinical study to evaluate the safety profile of an e-cigarette product (2.0 percent nicotine, developed by Fontem Ventures B.V., Amsterdam, the Netherlands) in 420 smokers of combustible tobacco cigarettes switching to use the e-cigarette product for 12 weeks. During the study, no clinically significant product-related findings were observed in terms of vital signs, electrocardiogram, lung function tests, and standard clinical laboratory parameters. Adverse events (AEs) reported by e-cigarette product subjects were more frequent during the first week after switching to the e-cigarette product. The frequency of AEs decreased thereafter, and out of a total of 1,515 reported AEs, 495 were judged as being related to nicotine withdrawal symptoms. The most frequently stated AEs were headache, sore throat, desire to smoke, and cough reported by 47.4 percent, 27.8 percent, 27.5 percent, and 17.0 percent of subjects, respectively.

D'Ruiz and colleagues (2015) conducted a randomized, partially single-blinded, crossover study on the nicotine pharmacokinetics, effects on smoking urge, tolerability of, and AEs from using e-cigarettes compared with combustible tobacco cigarettes. Thirty-eight adult smokers (averaging 10 or more cigarettes per day, biochemically confirmed with urine cotinine and CO) were given two of the study e-cigarette products (non-menthol and menthol flavors with 2.4 percent nicotine, glycerol-based e-liquid) to practice using the devices for a 7-day at-home period. Of these 38 participants, 24 were randomly selected for enrollment in the 11-day trial, during which they were randomized to one of six product usage sequences. Products used were a combustible tobacco cigarette or a commercially available, rechargeable e-cigarette (3.7 nominal volts, 3-Ω resistance) containing one of five e-liquids:

1. Commercial product in classic tobacco flavor with 1.6 percent nicotine in a 50 percent glycerol/20 percent PG base;
2. Commercial product in classic tobacco flavor with 1.6 percent nicotine in a 75 percent glycerol base;
3. Non-commercial product in classic tobacco flavor with 2.4 percent nicotine in a 75 percent glycerol base;
4. Non-commercial product in classic tobacco flavor with 2.4 percent nicotine in a 50 percent glycerol/20 percent PG base; and
5. Non-commercial product in menthol flavor with 75 percent glycerol base.

On product use days, subjects participated in 90-minute exposure sessions (30 minutes controlled followed by 1 hour ad lib use). None of the participants reported serious AEs or discontinued the study owing to AEs. Eighteen of the 38 total subjects provided with a study product reported minor AEs such as cough (20 reports by 11 subjects, more commonly among e-cigarette users than smokers), throat irritation (8 reports by 5 subjects), headache (6 reports by 5 subjects), and dizziness (5 reports by 4 subjects). All of the AEs resolved without sequelae.

The authors also investigated the acute effects of e-cigarettes on blood pressure and heart rate compared with the effects of combustible tobacco cigarette smoking (Yan and D'Ruiz, 2015). On product use days, they measured participants' (n = 23) systolic and diastolic blood pressure approximately 30 minutes before the controlled session and approximately 20 minutes after the end of the ad lib session. The heart rate and systolic and diastolic blood pressure were significantly elevated after use of Marlboro cigarettes, but the elevation was less after use of most of the e-cigarettes.

In another study, D'Ruiz and colleagues (2017) measured cardiovascular physiology (systolic and diastolic blood pressure and heart rate), pulmonary function (FVC, FEV1, and exhaled CO and NO), and AEs in 105 clinically confined subjects who were randomized into groups that either completely or partially switched from combustible tobacco cigarettes to e-cigarettes (blu) or completely discontinued using tobacco and nicotine products altogether. Use of the e-cigarettes for 5 days under the various study conditions did not lead to higher blood pressure or heart rate values, negative respiratory health outcomes, or serious adverse health events. Reductions in blood pressure and heart rate vital signs were observed in most of the participants who either ceased tobacco and nicotine product use altogether or switched completely to using e-cigarettes. Pulmonary function tests showed small but non-statistically significant improvements in FVC and FEV1 measurements in most use groups. Statistically significant ($p < 0.05$) benefits associated with smoking reduction were also noted in exhaled CO and NO levels. All study products were well tolerated.

Flouris and colleagues (2012) evaluated the acute effect of e-cigarette use and combustible tobacco cigarette smoking on complete blood count (CBC) markers in smokers ($n = 15$, eight men, averaging 15 or more cigarettes per day). Subjects participated in three 30-minute experimental sessions (e-cigarette use, combustible tobacco cigarette smoking, and control) in random order, with a minimum wash-out period of 7 days. For the e-cigarette session, the authors provided an e-cigarette device (Giant, Nobacco, G.P., Greece) containing tobacco-flavored e-liquid with 11 mg/ml nominal nicotine concentration in a base of greater than 60 percent PG and instructed participants to take a number of puffs (calculated for each participant based on his or her combustible tobacco cigarette consumption). Participants smoked two cigarettes of their own brand for the smoking session and smoked a sham (unlit) cigarette of their own brand for the control session. Blood samples were collected before, immediately after, and 1 hour after each experimental session. The authors found that CBC indexes remained unchanged during the control session and the e-cigarette exposure sessions ($p > 0.05$), whereas combustible tobacco cigarette smoke exposure increased white blood cell, lymphocyte, and granulocyte counts for at least 1 hour ($p < 0.05$).

From the same experimental setup, the researchers (Poulianiti et al., 2016) also examined the acute effects of e-cigarette use and combustible tobacco cigarette smoking on selected redox status markers. The researchers assessed total antioxidant capacity (TAC), catalase activity (CAT), and reduced glutathione (GSH) in the blood samples collected prior to, immediately after, and 1 hour after exposure. Results showed that TAC, CAT, and GSH remained similar to baseline levels immediately after and 1 hour after exposure ($p > 0.05$) to e-cigarette, combustible tobacco cigarette, and control conditions.

In a number of studies, Polosa and colleagues (2014a,b, 2016b,c) retrospectively assessed changes in respiratory and asthma symptoms (changes in spirometry data, airway hyperresponsiveness [AHR], asthma exacerbations, and subjective asthma control) from baseline (prior to switching) over 1-year follow-up (with visits at 6 and 12 months). Participants were 18 asthmatic smokers (10 single users, 8 dual users) who switched to e-cigarettes (Polosa et al., 2014a). Overall spirometry data, asthma control, and AHR improved significantly among both exclusive combustible tobacco cigarette smokers and dual users at baseline (Polosa et al., 2014a). Figure 18-3 shows the results for FEV1 at the four assessment points. Participants reported fewer asthma exacerbations, but the reduction did not reach statistical significance. They also reported no severe AEs.

Polosa and colleagues (2016a) reviewed medical records to evaluate changes in resting blood pressure and blood pressure control among hypertensive current and former smokers who reported using e-cigarettes daily at two consecutive visits (n = 43) compared with a control group of combustible tobacco cigarette smokers (n = 46). The authors observed a marked reduction in combustible tobacco cigarette smoking in those who had switched to e-cigarettes (both completely and partly), whereas no such change was observed in the control group. Among e-cigarette users, smoking reduction was associated with significant reductions in median

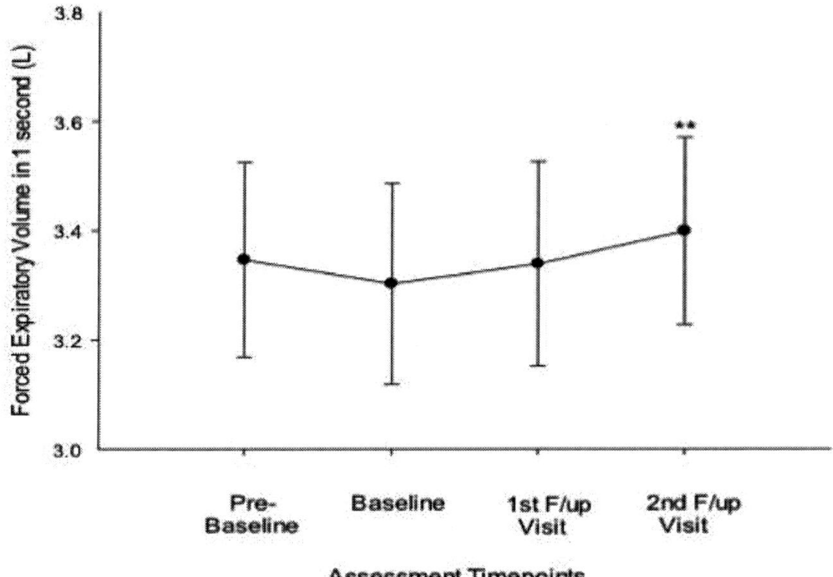

FIGURE 18-3 Forced expiratory volume (FEV1) at the four time points of assessment for all 18 patients.
NOTES: All data expressed as mean, and error bars are standard error of the mean. ** = $p \leq 0.01$.
SOURCE: Polosa et al., 2014a.

(25th, 75th centile) systolic blood pressure (140 [134.5, 144] to 130 [123.5, 138.5] mmHg; $p < 0.001$) and diastolic blood pressure (86 [78, 90] to 80 [74.5, 90] mmHg; $p = 0.006$) at 12-month follow-up compared with baseline. No significant changes were observed in the control group. Figure 18-4 illustrates the changes in diastolic blood pressure among e-cigarette users and controls (combustible tobacco cigarette smokers).

In another study, Polosa and colleagues (2016c) retrospectively reviewed medical records of current and former smokers with chronic obstructive pulmonary disease (COPD) who reported using e-cigarettes daily on three visits (baseline, 12-month follow-up, and 24-month follow-up) to examine changes in respiratory outcomes. Regularly smoking COPD patients (n = 24) were included as a reference group. Among exclusive e-cigarette users, the authors observed a significant reduction in COPD exacerbations, with their mean (± SD) severity score decreasing from 2.3 (±1) at baseline to 1.8 (±1; $p = 0.002$) at 12-month follow-up and 1.4 (± 0.9; $p < 0.001$) at 24-month follow-up (see Figure 18-5). The authors

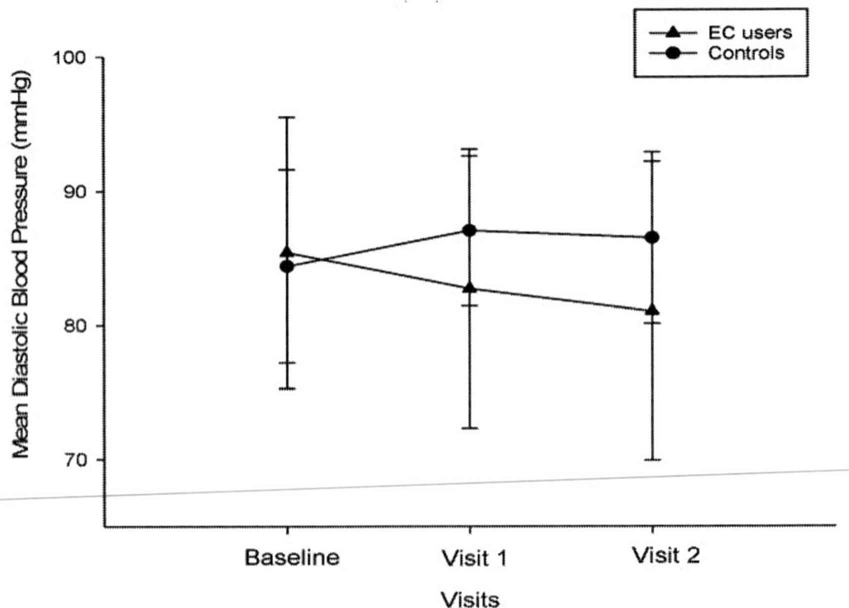

FIGURE 18-4 Changes in diastolic blood pressure from baseline, follow-up 1 (6 ± 1 month) and follow-up 2 (12 ± 2 months) separately for e-cigarette users (exclusive and dual) and exclusive combustible tobacco cigarette smokers (control group).
NOTES: All data expressed as mean, and error bars are standard error of the mean. EC = e-cigarette; mmHg = millimeters of mercury.
SOURCE: Polosa et al., 2016a.

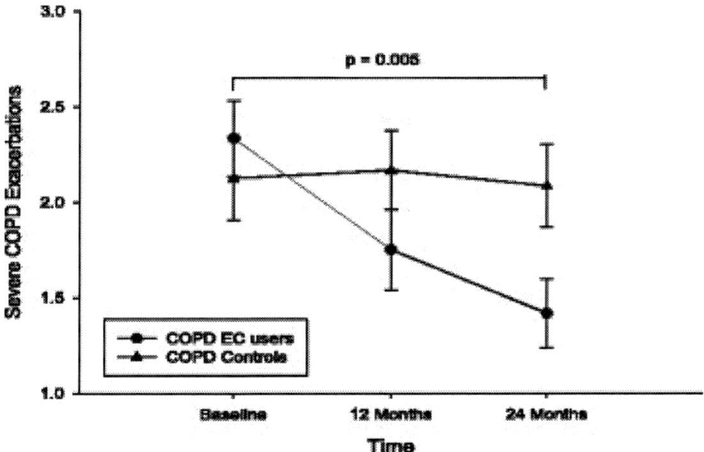

FIGURE 18-5 Changes in the number of chronic obstructive pulmonary disease exacerbations from baseline, at follow-up visit 1 (12 ± 1.5 months) and visit 2 (24 ± 2.5 months) separately for e-cigarette users and controls.
NOTES: All data expressed as mean, and error bars are standard deviation of the mean. The p-value is an overall comparison of both groups over the 24-month period. COPD = chronic obstructive pulmonary disease; EC = e-cigarette.
SOURCE: Polosa et al., 2016c.

also observed a significant reduction in COPD exacerbations among dual users. In addition, COPD symptoms and ability to perform physical activities improved at both follow-ups among e-cigarette users, whereas no changes were observed among the control group (exclusive smokers).

Szołtysek-Bołdys and colleagues (2014) examined the effects of e-cigarettes on acute cardiovascular outcomes compared with combustible tobacco smoking. Participants were smokers (n = 15 women) who smoked five or more combustible tobacco cigarettes per day for at least 2 years. The authors measured arterial stiffness (stiffness index and reflection index), systolic and diastolic blood pressure, and heart rate before and after smoking a combustible tobacco cigarette (filtered, "slim" cigarette with manufacturer-defined 0.7 mg nicotine) and using an e-cigarette (Ego-3, Volish Ltd., Poland with Crystal 2 clearomizer, 2.4-Ω heating coil, 3.4-V battery and e-liquid with 24 mg/ml nicotine). The authors observed no significant changes in arterial stiffness before and after smoking a combustible tobacco cigarette (stiffness index: 6.75 m/s [95% CI = 6.66–6.85] after versus 6.56 m/s [95% CI = 6.46–6.65] before, p = 0.0056; reflection index: 54.0 percent [95% CI = 51.5–56.7] after versus 49.6 percent [95% CI = 47.5–51.8] after, p = 0.010). They observed no significant changes in arterial stiffness after e-cigarette use, compared with before use. Systolic and diastolic blood pressure and heart rate increased after use of both products, but the changes did not meet statistical significance.

Tatullo and colleagues (2016) conducted a clinical observational pilot study involving 110 smokers who switched to e-cigarettes. Smokers were divided into two groups, according to the number of years of combustible tobacco cigarette smoking: group 1 (less than 10 years of combustible tobacco cigarette smoking) and group 2 (more than 10 years). Patients were subjected to oral examinations to investigate plaque index, bleeding index, and papillary bleeding index. A questionnaire was distributed to self-assess the variations of some parameters of general health and to self-assess the need to smoke combustible tobacco cigarettes. At the end of the study, authors registered a progressive improvement in the periodontal indexes, as well as in the general health perception.

In a pilot study, Wadia and colleagues (2016) compared the gingival health (bleeding on probing to assess gingival inflammation) among 20 established smokers who substituted e-cigarettes for smoking combustible tobacco cigarettes for 2 weeks. The authors found a statistically significant increase in gingival inflammation after 2 weeks of using e-cigarettes instead of their usual combustible tobacco cigarettes.

Toxicity in In Vitro and Animal Studies

The committee reviewed in vitro and animal studies that directly compared effects of exposure to aerosols from e-cigarettes to effects of combustible tobacco cigarette smoke exposure. Table 18-2 compares characteristics of in vitro studies on the toxic effect of e-cigarettes compared with combustible tobacco cigarette studies. Table 18-3 compares characteristics of in vivo animal studies on the toxic effect of e-cigarettes compared with combustible tobacco cigarette studies. As the tables illustrate, the majority of studies (21 of 27 in vitro studies and 3 of 5 in vivo animal studies) favored e-cigarettes as products less harmful than combustible tobacco cigarettes. No studies found e-cigarettes to be more harmful than combustible tobacco cigarettes.

Synthesis

The health effects of using e-cigarettes are still not well understood, but current evidence points to e-cigarettes being less harmful than combustible tobacco cigarettes. All but one of the human studies reviewed showed significant short-term improvements in health outcomes in smokers who switched from combustible tobacco cigarettes to e-cigarettes. Although most of the reviewed studies included relatively small numbers of subjects, the health improvement after this transition

TABLE 18-2 Comparison of In Vitro Studies That Compared Toxicity of E-Cigarettes and Combustible Tobacco Cigarettes

		Harmful Effects of E-Cigarettes Versus Combustible Tobacco Cigarettes		
Reference	Study Measures and Outcomes	Favors E-Cigarettes as Less Harmful	Similar Harm	Favors Combustible Tobacco Cigarettes as Less Harmful
Anderson et al., 2016	Reactive oxygen species, DNA damage, cell viability, and markers of programmed cell death pathways in HUVECs	✓		
Anthérieu et al., 2017	Viability, oxidative stress, and secretion of inflammatory mediators by human bronchial epithelial BEAS-2B cells	✓		
Aufderheide and Emura, 2017	Morphological alterations (histopathology) of differentiated immortalized primary NHBE cells (CL-1548)		✓	
Aug et al., 2015	Metabolome of HBECs		✓	
Azzopardi et al., 2016	Cytotoxicity test with H292 human bronchial epithelial cells	✓		
Banerjee et al., 2017	Transcriptomic perturbations in lung epithelial tissue (MucilAir)	✓		
Barber et al., 2016	Inflammatory processes, viability, density, and metabolic activity of HUVECs		✓	
Breheny et al., 2017	Carcinogenic potential with cell transformation assays in mouse fibroblast cells (Bhas 42)	✓		

continued

TABLE 18-2 Continued

		Harmful Effects of E-Cigarettes Versus Combustible Tobacco Cigarettes		
Reference	Study Measures and Outcomes	Favors E-Cigarettes as Less Harmful	Similar Harm	Favors Combustible Tobacco Cigarettes as Less Harmful
Carson et al., 2017	Ciliary function and secretion, cellular and exogenous NO concentrations in airway epithelial cultures from non-smoking human subjects		✓	
Cervellati et al., 2014	Cytotoxicity, ultrastructural morphology, and pro-inflammatory cytokines in skin (HaCaT) and lung (A549) cells	✓		
Farsalinos et al., 2013	Cytotoxicity in myocardial cells (H9c2)	✓		
Fields et al., 2017	Viability, barrier integrity, and gene promoter/expression regulation in human airway culture (EpiAirway)	✓		
Haswell et al., 2017	Transcriptional response in differentiated reconstituted human airway epithelia (MucilAir)	✓		
Hom et al., 2016	Platelets from healthy volunteers (n = 50) were exposed to combustible tobacco smoke extracts and e-cigarette aerosol extracts, and changes in platelet activation, adhesion, aggregation, and inflammation were evaluated		✓	
Leigh et al., 2016	Cell viability, metabolic activity, and release of inflammatory mediators (cytokines) in H292 human bronchial epithelial cells	✓		

Misra et al., 2014	Cytotoxicity, mutagenicity, genotoxicity, and inflammatory responses in human lung epithelial carcinoma cells (A549)	✓	
Moses et al., 2017	Gene expression profiling in primary HBEC cells	✓	
Neilson et al., 2015	Cytotoxicity in human 3D reconstructed airway tissues	✓	
Putzhammer et al., 2016	Cell death induction, proliferation rates, occurrence of intracellular reactive oxygen species, cell morphology in HUVECs	✓	
Romagna et al., 2013	Cell viability in murine fibroblasts (3T3)	✓	
Rubenstein et al., 2015	Kupffer cell complement receptor expression, oxidative stress production, cytokine release and viability, and density		✓
Scheffler et al., 2015	Cell viability and histology of immortalized normal human bronchial epithelial cell (NHBE48)	✓	
Shen et al., 2016	Transcriptomes of differentiated human bronchial epithelial cells	✓	
Taylor et al., 2016	Oxidative stress, apoptotic and necrotic responses in human bronchial epithelial cells	✓	
Teasdale et al., 2016	Stress response in human coronary artery endothelial cells	✓	
Thorne et al., 2016	Mutagenicity test with *Salmonella typhimurium* strains TA98 and TA100	✓	
Thorne et al., 2017	Induction of double-strand DNA damage in vitro using human lung epithelial cells (BEAS-2Bs)	✓	

NOTE: HBEC = human bronchial epithelial cell; HUVEC = human umbilical vein endothelial cell; NHBE = normal human bronchial epithelial.

TABLE 18-3 Comparison of Animal Studies That Compared Toxicity of E-Cigarettes and Combustible Tobacco Cigarettes

		Harmful Effects of E-Cigarettes Versus Combustible Tobacco Cigarettes		
Reference	Study Measures and Outcomes	Favors E-Cigarettes as Less Harmful	Similar Harm	Favors Combustible Tobacco Cigarettes as Less Harmful
Larcombe et al., 2017	Pulmonary inflammation, lung volume, lung mechanics, and responsiveness to methacholine were measured in female BALB/c mice exposed for 8 weeks to tobacco smoke or one of four types of e-cigarette aerosol		✓	
Palpant et al., 2015	Developmental effects in vivo with zebrafish (*Danio rerio*) and cardiac differentiation of human embryonic stem cells	✓		
Parker et al., 2017	Developmental toxicities using the FETAX	✓		
Ponzoni et al., 2015	Body weight, food intake, and the signs of mecamylamine-precipitated and spontaneous withdrawal episodic memory and emotional responses in male BALB/c mice	✓		
Rau et al., 2017	Skin flap survival (microcirculation and perfusion) in rats		✓	

NOTE: FETAX = frog embryo teratogenesis assay–*Xenopus*.

from smoking combustible tobacco cigarettes to using e-cigarettes was consistent across all studies and was observed for respiratory, cardiovascular, and oral health outcomes. In several studies, smokers also self-reported improvement in health after switching to e-cigarettes. Although in vitro and animal studies that compared acute effects of exposure to e-cigarette aerosols with effects caused by combustible tobacco smoke provided mixed results, the majority of studies favored e-cigarettes as less harmful products than combustible tobacco cigarettes. Moreover, although some studies found similar harm from e-cigarettes, no studies found that e-cigarettes were *more* harmful than combustible tobacco cigarettes among combustible tobacco cigarette smokers who switched to exclusive e-cigarette use. E-cigarettes might be considered as a harm reduction tool for tobacco smokers if their efficacy in reducing health risk is supported by epidemiological studies and proven in well-performed epidemiological studies and RCTs.

Conclusion 18-2. There is ***substantial evidence*** *that completely switching from regular use of combustible tobacco cigarettes to e-cigarettes results in reduced short-term adverse health outcomes in several organ systems.*

Harm Reduction in Smokers Who Use E-Cigarettes Concurrently with Combustible Tobacco Cigarettes (Dual Users)

Health Risk Profile and Smoking Cessation

People who smoke combustible tobacco cigarettes may switch to other tobacco products (e.g., chewing tobacco) or use products concurrently (dual users) when attempting to quit smoking (Messer et al., 2015; Popova and Ling, 2013). This, however, is not a proven method for combustible tobacco cigarette cessation, conceivably because nicotine dependence persists while using these other products (Dunbar et al., 2016; Popova and Ling, 2013). For example, a recent study using data from the 2010–2011 Tobacco Use Supplement to the Current Population Survey found that although dual users were more likely to attempt to quit than those who smoked only combustible tobacco cigarettes, they reverted back to smoking more quickly (Messer et al., 2015). The study found no significant difference in the proportion of dual users and exclusive combustible tobacco cigarette smokers who abstained from combustible tobacco cigarettes in the last 30 days (Messer et al., 2015). In this sample, lower combustible tobacco cigarette consumption was the best predictor of abstinence from combustible tobacco cigarette smoking (Messer et al., 2015). These results have implications for clinicians advising patients attempting to quit smoking combustible tobacco cigarettes (Dunbar et al., 2016).

Etter and Bullen (2014) used longitudinal Internet surveys to assess changes in tobacco use among e-cigarette users (including those using other tobacco products concurrently) over 12 months between 2011 and 2013. The authors recruited participants through e-cigarette and smoking cessation websites. In the recruited cohort, e-cigarette and tobacco use was assessed at baseline (n = 733), after 1 month (n = 477), and after 1 year (n = 367). Among dual users of e-cigarettes and combustible tobacco cigarettes at baseline, 22 percent reported abstaining from smoking in the previous 7 days after 1 month and 46 percent after 1 year. Dual users who were still smoking at follow-up reported a temporary reduction in combustible tobacco cigarette smoking at 1 month (average cigarettes per day declined from 11.3 to 6.0, p = 0.006). However, results showed no changes in smoking between baseline and 1-year follow-up.

Jorenby and colleagues (2017) conducted a 26-day study examining tobacco use behaviors among dual users (n = 74) compared with exclusive combustible tobacco cigarette smokers (n = 74). Subjects participated in 1 week of ad lib use, 1 week of 75 percent combustible tobacco smoking reduction (dual users were free to use their e-cigarettes as they wished), followed by another week of ad lib use, and finally 3 days of abstinence. The authors also measured CO and urinary nicotine and cotinine. Results showed that combustible tobacco cigarette consumption did not differ between dual users and exclusive smokers during ad lib periods. However, dual users quadrupled their e-cigarette use during smoking reduction periods. Dual users were significantly more likely to maintain 100 percent reduction (97.1 percent versus 81.2 percent). Nicotine levels were higher among women dual users.

Loukas and colleagues (2016) examined patterns of tobacco and e-cigarette use, quit attempts, and dependence symptoms among college students (n = 5,468, age 18–29). The study found that poly-tobacco product use is associated with some indicators of dependence, but not with smoking cessation attempts.

Manzoli and colleagues (2015, 2017) evaluated e-cigarette efficacy and safety at 12 and 24 months using data from a prospective cohort study of 1,355 subjects, including 343 users of e-cigarettes only and 319 dual users of tobacco and e-cigarettes. Most dual users at baseline abandoned e-cigarettes and continued to smoke tobacco. At 12 months, 21.9 percent of dual users quit combustible tobacco smoking while 20.5 percent of those who only smoked combustible tobacco cigarettes quit smoking. After 24 months, 26.0 percent of dual users quit smoking while 23.1 percent of those who only smoke combustible tobacco cigarettes quit smoking.

Synthesis

Dual use of combustible tobacco cigarettes and e-cigarettes is highly prevalent among adults and youth; however, there is limited evidence about dual users' patterns of use and smoking cessation attempts. The studies reviewed show that, on average, dual users do not smoke fewer combustible tobacco cigarettes than those who smoke only combustible tobacco cigarettes; however, among dual users, e-cigarettes may help maintain smoking reduction. There is a lack of evidence on exposure levels to nicotine and toxicants and health outcomes among dual users who do not reduce combustible tobacco cigarette use. It is very unlikely that those smokers who do not reduce smoking after initiating e-cigarette use will reduce health risks of smoking and they may also be exposed to additional adverse health effects of e-cigarettes. A better understanding of the patterns and differing contexts of dual use of e-cigarettes and combustible tobacco cigarettes is needed to inform public policy on adult and youth e-cigarette use and combustible tobacco cigarette smoking.

Conclusion 18-3. There is ***no available evidence*** *whether or not long-term e-cigarette use among smokers (dual use) changes morbidity or mortality compared with those who only smoke combustible tobacco cigarettes.*

Conclusion 18-4. There is ***insufficient evidence*** *that e-cigarette use changes short-term adverse health outcomes in several organ systems in smokers who continue to smoke combustible tobacco cigarettes (dual users).*

Harm Reduction from Passive Exposure to E-Cigarette Aerosol Compared with Combustible Tobacco Cigarette Smoke Among Non-Users

As described in the committee's discussion of secondhand exposures to e-cigarette aerosol compared with ambient air (see Chapter 3), the Surgeon General and the World Health Organization Framework Convention on Tobacco Control have indicated that there is no risk-free level of exposure to secondhand tobacco smoke (HHS, 2006; WHO, 2003). Additionally, just as quitting smoking is the only guaranteed way to reduce tobacco-related harms, eliminating exposure from indoor spaces is the most effective intervention to prevent secondhand tobacco smoke exposure. Due to the involuntary nature of secondhand exposure, such strategies are particularly important to reduce exposures to vulnerable populations, such as children, pregnant women, the elderly, and individuals with cardiorespiratory disease. Because eliminating exposure to passive combustible tobacco cigarette smoke in the indoor environment has been the traditional focus of tobacco control, whether replacing smoking by e-cigarette use in indoor environments is a possible strategy to reduce risk of health effects among those involuntarily exposed to secondhand smoke is an effective harm reduction strategy is unknown. This may be especially important to reduce harm for non-smoking household members of smokers who are unable or unwilling to quit using other evidence-based smoking cessation methods. In this section, the committee reviews evidence on whether changing smoking practices by switching to e-cigarettes in indoor environments may reduce passive exposure to combustible tobacco smoke constituents. The committee did not identify evidence on clinically relevant health outcomes of passive exposure to e-cigarettes. In the absence of such direct literature, the committee draws upon four studies assessing exposure among non-smokers to emissions from e-cigarettes compared with combustible tobacco cigarettes.

In the same study described earlier in the chapter regarding effects of active e-cigarette use on CBC markers compared with effects of active smoking, Flouris and colleagues (2012) also evaluated the effect of passive exposure on CBC markers in 15 never smokers. Never smokers underwent three 30-minute experimental exposure sessions: a control session, a passive combustible tobacco cigarette exposure session, and a passive e-cigarette exposure session (Giant brand, Nobacco G.P., Greece filled with tobacco-flavored nicotine-containing 11-mg/ml solution). CBC indexes remained unchanged during the control session and the passive e-cigarette exposure sessions ($p > 0.05$). By contrast, passive combustible tobacco smoke exposure increased white blood cell, lymphocyte, and granulocyte counts for at least 1 hour in never smokers ($p < 0.05$). The authors also examined effects on antioxidant response, and found no changes in TAC, CAT, and GSH before, immediately after, and 1 hour after exposure to any condition (e-cigarette aerosol, combustible tobacco smoke, and control) (Poulianiti et al., 2016).

Ballbè and colleagues (2014) conducted an observational study to characterize passive exposure to nicotine from e-cigarettes and combustible tobacco cigarettes among non-smokers ($n = 54$) from home settings with different tobacco use conditions. Twenty-five participants lived in homes with smokers, 5 lived with nicotine-containing e-cigarette users, and 24 lived in homes with no combustible tobacco cigarette smokers or e-cigarette users (control homes). All participants passively exposed to e-cigarettes reported more than 2 hours of exposure per day, while 17 of the 25 participants passively exposed to tobacco smoke reported less than 2 hours of exposure per day. Airborne nicotine at home and biomarkers of nicotine exposure (salivary and urinary cotinine) were measured. Airborne nicotine was significantly higher (5.7 times) in homes with smokers than in homes with e-cigarette users. Airborne nicotine (geometric means [geometric standard deviation, GSD]) was 0.74 $\mu g/m^3$ (GSD = 4.05) in homes with smokers and 0.13 $\mu g/m^3$ (GSD = 2.4) in homes with e-cigarette users. Salivary cotinine concentrations were also significantly higher among non-smokers passively exposed to tobacco smoke compared with those passively exposed to e-cigarettes. Salivary cotinine was 0.38 ng/ml (GSD = 2.34) in the smokers' homes compared with 0.19 ng/ml (GSD = 2.17) in the e-cigarettes users' homes.

Czogała and colleagues (2014) compared secondhand exposure among aerosols from three e-cigarette models (Colins Age with Camel High cartomizer with 11 mg nicotine [Colins Poland], Dekang 510 Pen with SGC Regular cartridge with 18 mg nicotine [Ecigars Polska], and Mild M201 Pen with Marlboro cartridge with 19 mg nicotine [Mild Poland]) and combustible tobacco smoke generated by a smoking machine and by five dual users. Nicotine was measured over 1-hour exposure using gas chromatography with nitrogen–phosphorus detector following active sampling on XAD-4 sorption tubes (SKC Inc.) according to the National Institute of Occupational Safety and Health reference method 2551. Results showed that e-cigarettes are a source of secondhand exposure to nicotine, but not CO, and VOCs. The average concentration of airborne nicotine over 1 hour from smoking combustible tobacco cigarettes was 10 times higher than from e-cigarettes (31.60 ± 6.91 versus 3.32 ± 2.49 $\mu g/m^3$, respectively; $p = 0.0081$; see Figure 18-6). Similarly, the mean $PM_{2.5}$ concentration from tobacco smoke was seven times higher compared with that from e-cigarettes (819.3 ± 228.6 versus 151.7 ± 86.8 $\mu g/m^3$, respectively; $p = 0.0081$). The number of aerosol particles ($PM_{2.5}$) generated directly by the e-cigarette user was higher than generated by a smoking machine, suggesting that examining aerosols exhaled by users may be more appropriate than those produced by smoking machines.

In a pilot study, Bush and Goniewicz (2015) measured nicotine on the household surfaces in homes of e-cigarette users (n = 8), combustible tobacco cigarette smokers (n = 6), and non-users of either product (n = 8) in western New York. The e-cigarette users estimated that they puffed on their own devices from 50 to 500 times per day in their home and reported that the nicotine concentration in their e-liquids ranged from 10 to 15 mg/ml. Investigators took surface wipe samples from the floor, wall, and window. They then extracted nicotine from the wipes and analyzed the extract using gas chromatography. Results showed that detectable levels of nicotine were found on surfaces of half of the e-cigarette users' homes, whereas it was found on surfaces in all of the smokers' homes. Additionally, in homes of e-cigarette users where nicotine was found on surfaces, the nicotine levels were significantly lower than in combustible tobacco

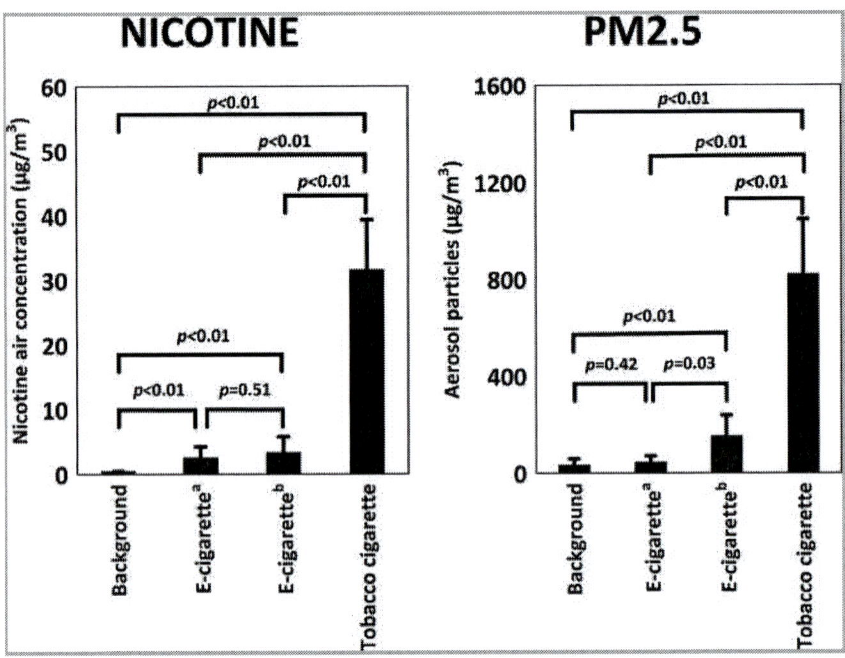

FIGURE 18-6 Comparison of indoor air nicotine (left) and aerosol particle (right) concentrations released from e-cigarette with background values and combustible tobacco cigarette smoking.

[a] Aerosol generated with smoking machine (Study 1).

[b] Aerosol exhaled by users (Study 2).

NOTE: $PM_{2.5}$ = particulate matter 2.5 micrometers or less in diameter.

SOURCE: Czogała et al., 2014.

cigarette smokers' homes (average concentration 7.7 ± 17.2 versus 1,303 ± 2,676 μg/m^2; $p < 0.05$).

Synthesis

The committee identified a limited number of studies that compared secondhand exposure to e-cigarette emissions to combustible tobacco cigarette smoke. The committee did not identify any long-term studies comparing health effects resulting from passive exposure to secondhand aerosol from e-cigarettes with effects in non-smokers passively exposed to tobacco smoke. In general, the studies reviewed show that using an e-cigarette in indoor environments may involuntarily expose non-users to nicotine and particulates, but at lower levels compared with exposure to secondhand tobacco smoke from combustible tobacco cigarettes. Secondhand exposure to toxic tobacco-specific combustion products is substantially reduced from e-cigarettes compared with combustible tobacco cigarettes. Of note, the effects of these reduced exposures on health remain unknown. Due to the involuntary nature of secondhand exposure and because even low levels of particulate matter may confer health risks, vulnerable populations such as children, pregnant women, the elderly, and individuals with cardiorespiratory diseases may still be at special risk.

*Conclusion 18-5. There is **moderate evidence** that secondhand exposure to nicotine and particulates is lower from e-cigarettes compared with combustible tobacco cigarettes.*

REFERENCES

Adriaens, K., D. Van Gucht, P. Declerck, and F. Baeyens. 2014. Effectiveness of the electronic cigarette: An eight-week Flemish study with six-month follow-up on smoking reduction, craving and experienced benefits and complaints. *International Journal of Environmental Research & Public Health* 11(11):11220–11248.

Anderson, C., A. Majeste, J. Hanus, and S. Wang. 2016. E-cigarette aerosol exposure induces reactive oxygen species, DNA damage, and cell death in vascular endothelial cells. *Toxicological Sciences* 154(2):332–340.

Anthérieu, S., A. Garat, N. Beauval, M. Soyez, D. Allorge, G. Garçon, and J. M. Lo-Guidice. 2017. Comparison of cellular and transcriptomic effects between electronic cigarette vapor and cigarette smoke in human bronchial epithelial cells. *Toxicology in Vitro* 45(Part 3):417–425.

Aufderheide, M., and M. Emura. 2017. Phenotypical changes in a differentiating immortalized bronchial epithelial cell line after exposure to mainstream cigarette smoke and e-cigarette vapor. *Experimental and Toxicologic Pathology* 69(6):393–401.

Aug, A., S. Altraja, K. Kilk, R. Porosk, U. Soomets, and A. Altraja. 2015. E-cigarette affects the metabolome of primary normal human bronchial epithelial cells. *PLoS ONE* 10(11):e0142053. https://doi.org/10.1371/journal.pone.0142053 (accessed February 7, 2018).

Azzopardi, D., K. Patel, T. Jaunky, S. Santopietro, O. M. Camacho, J. McAughey, and M. Gaça. 2016. Electronic cigarette aerosol induces significantly less cytotoxicity than tobacco smoke. *Toxicology Mechanisms and Methods* 26(6):477–491.

Ballbè, M., J. M. Martínez-Sánchez, X. Sureda, M. Fu, R. Pérez-Ortuño, J. A. Pascual, E. Saltó, and E. Fernández. 2014. Cigarettes vs. e-cigarettes: Passive exposure at home measured by means of airborne marker and biomarkers. *Environmental Research* 135:76–80.

Banerjee, A., L. E. Haswell, A. Baxter, A. Parmar, D. Azzopardi, S. Corke, D. Thorne, J. Adamson, J. Mushonganono, M. Gaça, and E. Minet. 2017. Differential gene expression using RNA sequencing profiling in a reconstituted airway epithelium exposed to conventional cigarette smoke or electronic cigarette aerosols. *Applied In Vitro Toxicology* 3(1):84–98.

Barber, K. E., B. Ghebrehiwet, W. Yin, and D. A. Rubenstein. 2016. Endothelial cell inflammatory reactions are altered in the presence of e-cigarette extracts of variable nicotine. *Cellular and Molecular Bioengineering* 10(1):124–133.

Breheny, D., O. Oke, K. Pant, and M. Gaça. 2017. Comparative tumor promotion assessment of e-cigarette and cigarettes using the in vitro Bhas 42 cell transformation assay. *Environmental and Molecular Mutagenesis* 58(4):190–198.

Bush, D., and M. L. Goniewicz. 2015. A pilot study on nicotine residues in houses of electronic cigarette users, tobacco smokers, and non-users of nicotine-containing products. *International Journal of Drug Policy* 26(6):609–611.

Carnevale, R., S. Sciarretta, F. Violi, C. Nocella, L. Loffredo, L. Perri, M. Peruzzi, A. G. M. Marullo, E. De Falco, I. Chimenti, V. Valenti, G. Biondi-Zoccai, and G. Frati. 2016. Acute impact of tobacco vs. electronic cigarette smoking on oxidative stress and vascular function. *Chest* 150(3):606–612.

Carson, J. L., L. Zhou, L. Brighton, K. H. Mills, H. Zhou, I. Jaspers, and M. Hazucha. 2017. Temporal structure/function variation in cultured differentiated human nasal epithelium associated with acute single exposure to tobacco smoke or e-cigarette vapor. *Inhalation Toxicology* 29(3):137–144.

Cervellati, F., X. M. Muresan, C. Sticozzi, R. Gambari, G. Montagner, H. J. Forman, C. Torricelli, E. Maioli, and G. Valacchi. 2014. Comparative effects between electronic and cigarette smoke in human keratinocytes and epithelial lung cells. *Toxicology in Vitro* 28(5):999–1005.

Cibella, F., D. Campagna, P. Caponnetto, M. D. Amaradio, M. Caruso, C. Russo, D. W. Cockcroft, and R. Polosa. 2016. Lung function and respiratory symptoms in a randomized smoking cessation trial of electronic cigarettes. *Clinical Science* 130(21):1929–1937.

Cravo, A. S., J. Bush, G. Sharma, R. Savioz, C. Martin, S. Craige, and T. Walele. 2016. A randomised, parallel group study to evaluate the safety profile of an electronic vapour product over 12 weeks. *Regulatory Toxicology and Pharmacology* 81 (Supplement 1):S1–S14. https://doi.org/10.1016/j.yrtph.2016.10.003 (accessed February 7, 2018).

Czogała, J., M. L. Goniewicz, B. Fidelus, W. Zielinska-Danch, M. J. Travers, and A. Sobczak. 2014. Secondhand exposure to vapors from electronic cigarettes. *Nicotine & Tobacco Research* 16(6):655–662.

D'Ruiz, C. D., D. W. Graff, and X. S. Yan. 2015. Nicotine delivery, tolerability and reduction of smoking urge in smokers following short-term use of one brand of electronic cigarettes. *BMC Public Health* 15:991. https://doi.org/10.1186/s12889-015-2349-2 (accessed February 7, 2018).

D'Ruiz, C. D., D. W. Graff, and E. Robinson. 2016. Reductions in biomarkers of exposure, impacts on smoking urge and assessment of product use and tolerability in adult smokers following partial or complete substitution of cigarettes with electronic cigarettes. *BMC Public Health* 16(1):543.

D'Ruiz, C. D., G. O'Connell, D. W. Graff, and X. S. Yan. 2017. Measurement of cardiovascular and pulmonary function endpoints and other physiological effects following partial or complete substitution of cigarettes with electronic cigarettes in adult smokers. *Regulatory Toxicology and Pharmacology* 87:36–53.

Dunbar, M. S., W. G. Shadel, J. S. Tucker, and M. O. Edelen. 2016. Use of and reasons for using multiple other tobacco products in daily and nondaily smokers: Associations with cigarette consumption and nicotine dependence. *Drug and Alcohol Dependence* 168:156–163.

Etter, J. F., and C. Bullen. 2014. A longitudinal study of electronic cigarette users. *Addictive Behaviors* 39(2):491–494.

Farsalinos, K. E., G. Romagna, E. Allifranchini, E. Ripamonti, E. Bocchietto, S. Todeschi, D. Tsiapras, S. Kyrzopoulos, and V. Voudris. 2013. Comparison of the cytotoxic potential of cigarette smoke and electronic cigarette vapour extract on cultured myocardial cells. *International Journal of Environmental Research and Public Health* 10(10):5146–5162.

Fields, W., A. Maione, B. Keyser, and B. Bombick. 2017. Characterization and application of the Vitrocell VC1 smoke exposure system and 3D EpiAirway models for toxicological and e-cigarette evaluations. *Applied In Vitro Toxicology* 3(1):68–83.

Flouris, A. D., K. P. Poulianiti, M. S. Chorti, A. Z. Jamurtas, D. Kouretas, E. O. Owolabi, M. N. Tzatzarakis, A. M. Tsatsakis, and Y. Koutedakis. 2012. Acute effects of electronic and tobacco cigarette smoking on complete blood count. *Food and Chemical Toxicology* 50(10):3600–3603.

Goniewicz, M. L., J. Knysak, M. Gawron, L. Kosmider, A. Sobczak, J. Kurek, A. Prokopowicz, M. Jablonska-Czapla, C. Rosik-Dulewska, C. Havel, P. Jacob, and N. Benowitz. 2014. Levels of selected carcinogens and toxicants in vapour from electronic cigarettes. *Tobacco Control* 23(2):133–139.

Goniewicz, M. L., M. Gawron, D. M. Smith, M. Peng, P. Jacob, 3rd, and N. L. Benowitz. 2017. Exposure to nicotine and selected toxicants in cigarette smokers who switched to electronic cigarettes: A longitudinal within-subjects observational study. *Nicotine & Tobacco Research* 19(2):160–167.

Haswell, L. E., A. Baxter, A. Banerjee, I. Verrastro, J. Mushonganono, J. Adamson, D. Thorne, M. Gaça, and E. Minet. 2017. Reduced biological effect of e-cigarette aerosol compared to cigarette smoke evaluated in vitro using normalized nicotine dose and RNA-seq-based toxicogenomics. *Scientific Reports* 7(1):888. https://doi.org/10.1038/s41598-017-00852-y (accessed February 7, 2018).

Healthy People 2020. 2017. *Tobacco: Overview and impact*. https://www.healthypeople.gov/2020/leading-health-indicators/2020-lhi-topics/Tobacco (accessed November 29, 2017).

Hecht, S. S., S. G. Carmella, D. Kotandeniya, M. E. Pillsbury, M. Chen, B. W. Ransom, R. I. Vogel, E. Thompson, S. E. Murphy, and D. K. Hatsukami. 2015. Evaluation of toxicant and carcinogen metabolites in the urine of e-cigarette users versus cigarette smokers. *Nicotine & Tobacco Research* 17(6):704–709.

HHS (U.S. Department of Health and Human Services). 2006. *The health consequences of involuntary exposure to tobacco smoke: A report of the Surgeon General*. Atlanta, GA: U.S. Department of Health and Human Services, Centers for Disease Control and Prevention, National Center for Disease Prevention and Health Promotion, Office on Smoking and Health.

HHS. 2014. *The health consequences of smoking—50 years of progress: A report of the Surgeon General*. Atlanta, GA: U.S. Department of Health and Human Services, Centers for Disease Control and Prevention, National Center for Disease Prevention and Health Promotion, Office on Smoking and Health.

Hom, S., L. Chen, T. Wang, B. Ghebrehiwet, W. Yin, and D. A. Rubenstein. 2016. Platelet activation, adhesion, inflammation, and aggregation potential are altered in the presence of electronic cigarette extracts of variable nicotine concentrations. *Platelets* 27(7):694–702.

IOM (Institute of Medicine). 2001. *Clearing the smoke: Assessing the science base for tobacco harm reduction*. Washington, DC: National Academy Press.

Jorenby, D. E., S. S. Smith, M. C. Fiore, and T. B. Baker. 2017. Nicotine levels, withdrawal symptoms, and smoking reduction success in real world use: A comparison of cigarette smokers and dual users of both cigarettes and e-cigarettes. *Drug and Alcohol Dependence* 170:93–101.

Larcombe, A. N., M. A. Janka, B. J. Mullins, L. J. Berry, A. Bredin, and P. J. Franklin. 2017. The effects of electronic cigarette aerosol exposure on inflammation and lung function in mice. *American Journal of Physiology: Lung Cellular and Molecular Physiology* 313(1):L67–L79.

Leigh, N. J., R. I. Lawton, P. A. Hershberger, and M. L. Goniewicz. 2016. Flavourings significantly affect inhalation toxicity of aerosol generated from electronic nicotine delivery systems (ENDS). *Tobacco Control* 25:ii81–ii87. https://doi.org/10.1136/tobaccocontrol-2016-053205 (accessed February 7, 2018).

Lindson-Hawley, N., J. Hartmann-Boyce, T. R. Fanshawe, R. Begh, A. Farley, and T. Lancaster. 2016. Interventions to reduce harm from continued tobacco use. *Cochrane Database of Systematic Reviews* 10:CD005231.

Loukas, A., S. Chow, K. E. Pasch, X. Li, J. T. Hinds, III, C. N. Marti, M. B. Harrell, M. R. Creamer, and C. L. Perry. 2016. College students' polytobacco use, cigarette cessation, and dependence. *American Journal of Health Behavior* 40(4):514–522.

Majeed, B. A., S. R. Weaver, K. R. Gregory, C. F. Whitney, P. Slovic, T. F. Pechacek, and M. P. Eriksen. 2016. Changing perceptions of harm of e-cigarettes among U.S. adults, 2012–2015. *American Journal of Preventive Medicine* 52(3):331–338.

Manzoli, L., M. E. Flacco, M. Fiore, C. La Vecchia, C. Marzuillo, M. R. Gualano, G. Liguori, G. Cicolini, L. Capasso, C. D'Amario, S. Boccia, R. Siliquini, W. Ricciardi, and P. Villari. 2015. Electronic cigarettes efficacy and safety at 12 months: Cohort study. *PLoS ONE* 10(6):e0129443. https://doi.org/10.1371/journal.pone.0129443 (accessed February 7, 2018).

Manzoli, L., M. E. Flacco, M. Ferrante, C. La Vecchia, R. Siliquini, W. Ricciardi, C. Marzuillo, P. Villari, and M. Fiore. 2017. Cohort study of electronic cigarette use: Effectiveness and safety at 24 months. *Tobacco Control* 26(3):284–292.

Margham, J., K. McAdam, M. Forster, C. Liu, C. Wright, D. Mariner, and C. Proctor. 2016. Chemical composition of aerosol from an e-cigarette: A quantitative comparison with cigarette smoke. *Chemical Research in Toxicology* 29(10):1662–1678.

Martin, E. M., P. W. Clapp, M. E. Rebuli, E. A. Pawlak, E. Glista-Baker, N. L. Benowitz, R. C. Fry, and I. Jaspers. 2016. E-cigarette use results in suppression of immune and inflammatory-response genes in nasal epithelial cells similar to cigarette smoke. *American Journal of Physiology: Lung Cellular and Molecular Physiology* 311(1):L135–L144.

McKee, M., and S. Capewell. 2015. Evidence about electronic cigarettes: A foundation built on rock or sand? *BMJ* 351:h4863. https://doi.org/10.1136/bmj.h4863 (accessed February 7, 2018).

McRobbie, H., A. Phillips, M. L. Goniewicz, K. M. Smith, O. Knight-West, D. Przulj, and P. Hajek. 2015. Effects of switching to electronic cigarettes with and without concurrent smoking on exposure to nicotine, carbon monoxide, and acrolein. *Cancer Prevention Research* 8(9):873–878.

Messer, K., M. Vijayaraghavan, M. M. White, Y. Shi, C. Chang, K. P. Conway, A. Hartman, M. J. Schroeder, W. M. Compton, and J. P. Pierce. 2015. Cigarette smoking cessation attempts among current U.S. smokers who also use smokeless tobacco. *Addictive Behaviors* 51:113–119.

Misra, M., R. D. Leverette, B. T. Cooper, M. B. Bennett, and S. E. Brown. 2014. Comparative in vitro toxicity profile of electronic and tobacco cigarettes, smokeless tobacco and nicotine replacement therapy products: E-liquids, extracts and collected aerosols. *International Journal of Environmental Research & Public Health* 11(11):11325–11347.

Moses, E., T. Wang, S. Corbett, G. R. Jackson, E. Drizik, C. Perdomo, C. Perdomo, E. Kleerup, D. Brooks, G. O'Connor, S. Dubinett, P. Hayden, M. E. Lenburg, and A. Spira. 2017. Molecular impact of electronic cigarette aerosol exposure in human bronchial epithelium. *Toxicological Sciences* 155(1):248–257.

Neilson, L., C. Mankus, D. Thorne, G. Jackson, J. DeBay, and C. Meredith. 2015. Development of an in vitro cytotoxicity model for aerosol exposure using 3D reconstructed human airway tissue; application for assessment of e-cigarette aerosol. *Toxicology in Vitro* 29(7):1952–1962.

O'Connell, G., D. W. Graff, and C. D. D'Ruiz. 2016. Reductions in biomarkers of exposure (BOE) to harmful or potentially harmful constituents (HPHCs) following partial or complete substitution of cigarettes with electronic cigarettes in adult smokers. *Toxicology Mechanisms and Methods* 26(6):443–454.

Palpant, N. J., P. Hofsteen, L. Pabon, H. Reinecke, and C. E. Murry. 2015. Cardiac development in zebrafish and human embryonic stem cells is inhibited by exposure to tobacco cigarettes and e-cigarettes. *PLoS ONE* 10(5):e0126259. https://doi.org/10.1371/journal.pone.0126259 (accessed February 7, 2018).

Parker, T. T., and J. Rayburn. 2017. A comparison of electronic and traditional cigarette butt leachate on the development of *Xenopus laevis* embryos. *Toxicology Reports* 4:77–82.

Polosa, R., J. Morjaria, P. Caponnetto, M. Caruso, S. Strano, E. Battaglia, and C. Russo. 2014a. Effect of smoking abstinence and reduction in asthmatic smokers switching to electronic cigarettes: Evidence for harm reversal. *International Journal of Environmental Research and Public Health* 11(5):4965–4977.

Polosa, R., J. B. Morjaria, P. Caponnetto, D. Campagna, C. Russo, A. Alamo, M. D. Amaradio, and A. Fisichella. 2014b. Effectiveness and tolerability of electronic cigarette in real-life: A 24-month prospective observational study. *Internal and Emergency Medicine* 9(5):537–546.

Polosa, R., J. B. Morjaria, P. Caponnetto, E. Battaglia, C. Russo, C. Ciampi, G. Adams, and C. M. Bruno. 2016a. Blood pressure control in smokers with arterial hypertension who switched to electronic cigarettes. *International Journal of Environmental Research and Public Health* 13(11):E1123. https://doi.org/10.3390/ijerph13111123 (accessed February 7, 2018).

Polosa, R., J. B. Morjaria, P. Caponnetto, M. Caruso, D. Campagna, M. D. Amaradio, G. Ciampi, C. Russo, and A. Fisichella. 2016b. Persisting long term benefits of smoking abstinence and reduction in asthmatic smokers who have switched to electronic cigarettes. *Discovery Medicine* 21(114):99–108.

Polosa, R., J. B. Morjaria, P. Caponnetto, U. Prosperini, C. Russo, A. Pennisi, and C. M. Bruno. 2016c. Evidence for harm reduction in COPD smokers who switch to electronic cigarettes. *Respiratory Research* 17(1):166. https://doi.org/10.1186/s12931-016-0481-x (accessed February 7, 2018).

Ponzoni, L., M. Moretti, M. Sala, F. Fasoli, V. Mucchietto, V. Lucini, G. Cannazza, G. Gallesi, C. N. Castellana, F. Clementi, M. Zoli, C. Gotti, and D. Braida. 2015. Different physiological and behavioural effects of e-cigarette vapour and cigarette smoke in mice. *European Neuropsychopharmacology* 25(10):1775–1786.

Popova, L., and P. M. Ling. 2013. Alternative tobacco product use and smoking cessation: A national study. *American Journal of Public Health* 103(5):923–930.

Poulianiti, K., C. Karatzaferi, A. D. Flouris, I. G. Fatouros, Y. Koutedakis, and A. Z. Jamurtas. 2016. Antioxidant responses following active and passive smoking of tobacco and electronic cigarettes. *Toxicology Mechanisms and Methods* 26(6):455–461.

Pulvers, K., A. S. Emami, N. L. Nollen, D. R. Romero, D. R. Strong, N. L. Benowitz, and J. S. Ahluwalia. 2016. Tobacco consumption and toxicant exposure of cigarette smokers using electronic cigarettes. *Nicotine & Tobacco Research* 20(2):206–214.

Putzhammer, R., C. Doppler, T. Jakschitz, K. Heinz, J. Forste, K. Danzl, B. Messner, and D. Bernhard. 2016. Vapours of U.S. and E.U. market leader electronic cigarette brands and liquids are cytotoxic for human vascular endothelial cells. *PLoS ONE* 11(6):e0157337. https://doi.org/10.1371/journal.pone.0157337 (accessed February 7, 2018).

Rau, A. S., V. Reinikovaite, E. P. Schmidt, L. Taraseviciene-Stewart, and F. W. Deleyiannis. 2017. Electronic cigarettes are as toxic to skin flap survival as tobacco cigarettes. *Annals of Plastic Surgery* 79(1):86–91.

Romagna, G., E. Allifranchini, E. Bocchietto, S. Todeschi, M. Esposito, and K. E. Farsalinos. 2013. Cytotoxicity evaluation of electronic cigarette vapor extract on cultured mammalian fibroblasts (ClearStream-LIFE): Comparison with tobacco cigarette smoke extract. *Inhalation Toxicology* 25(6):354–361.

Rubenstein, D. A., S. Hom, B. Ghebrehiwet, and W. Yin. 2015. Tobacco and e-cigarette products initiate Kupffer cell inflammatory responses. *Molecular Immunology* 67(2):652–660.

Scheffler, S., H. Dieken, O. Krischenowski, and M. Aufderheide. 2015. Cytotoxic evaluation of e-liquid aerosol using different lung-derived cell models. *International Journal of Environmental Research and Public Health* 12(10):12466–12474.

Shahab, L., M. L. Goniewicz, B. C. Blount, J. Brown, A. McNeill, K. U. Alwis, J. Feng, L. Wang, and R. West. 2017. Nicotine, carcinogen, and toxin exposure in long-term e-cigarette and nicotine replacement therapy users: A cross-sectional study. *Annals of Internal Medicine* 166(6):390–400.

Shen, Y., M. J. Wolkowicz, T. Kotova, L. Fan, and M. P. Timko. 2016. Transcriptome sequencing reveals e-cigarette vapor and mainstream-smoke from tobacco cigarettes activate different gene expression profiles in human bronchial epithelial cells. *Scientific Reports* 6:23984. https://doi.org/10.1038/srep23984 (accessed February 7, 2018).

Szołtysek-Bołdys, I., A. Sobczak, W. Zieli ska-Danch, A. Bartoń, B. Koszowski, and L. Kośmider. 2014. Influence of inhaled nicotine source on arterial stiffness. *Przegląd lekarski* 71(11):572–575.

Tatullo, M., S. Gentile, F. Paduano, L. Santacroce, and M. Marrelli. 2016. Crosstalk between oral and general health status in e-smokers. *Medicine (United States)* 95(49):e5589. https://doi.org/10.1097/MD.0000000000005589 (accessed February 7, 2018).

Taylor, M., T. Carr, O. Oke, T. Jaunky, D. Breheny, F. Lowe, and M. Gaça. 2016. E-cigarette aerosols induce lower oxidative stress in vitro when compared to tobacco smoke. *Toxicology Mechanisms and Methods* 26(6):465–476.

Tayyarah, R., and G. A. Long. 2014. Comparison of select analytes in aerosol from e-cigarettes with smoke from conventional cigarettes and with ambient air. *Regulatory Toxicology and Pharmacology* 70(3):704–710.

Teasdale, J. E., A. C. Newby, N. J. Timpson, M. R. Munafo, and S. J. White. 2016. Cigarette smoke but not electronic cigarette aerosol activates a stress response in human coronary artery endothelial cells in culture. *Drug and Alcohol Dependence* 163:256–260.

Thorne, D., I. Crooks, M. Hollings, A. Seymour, C. Meredith, and M. Gaça. 2016. The mutagenic assessment of an electronic-cigarette and reference cigarette smoke using the Ames assay in strains TA98 and TA100. *Mutation Research—Genetic Toxicology and Environmental Mutagenesis* 812:29–38.

Thorne, D., S. Larard, A. Baxter, C. Meredith, and M. Gaça. 2017. The comparative in vitro assessment of e-cigarette and cigarette smoke aerosols using the γ-H2AX assay and applied dose measurements. *Toxicology Letters* 265:170–178.

van Staden, S. R., M. Groenewald, R. Engelbrecht, P. J. Becker, and L. T. Hazelhurst. 2013. Carboxyhaemoglobin levels, health and lifestyle perceptions in smokers converting from tobacco cigarettes to electronic cigarettes. *South African Medical Journal. Suid-Afrikaanse Tydskrif Vir Geneeskunde* 103(11):865–868.

Vansickel, A. R., C. O. Cobb, M. F. Weaver, and T. E. Eissenberg. 2010. A clinical laboratory model for evaluating the acute effects of electronic "cigarettes": Nicotine delivery profile and cardiovascular and subjective effects. *Cancer Epidemiology, Biomarkers & Prevention* 19(8):1945–1953.

Wadia, R., V. Booth, H. F. Yap, and D. L. Moyes. 2016. A pilot study of the gingival response when smokers switch from smoking to vaping. *British Dental Journal* 221(11):722–726.

WHO (World Health Organization). 2003. *WHO framework convention on tobacco control*. Geneva, Switzerland: World Health Organization.

Williams, M., A. Villarreal, K. Bozhilov, S. Lin, and P. Talbot. 2013. Metal and silicate particles including nanoparticles are present in electronic cigarette cartomizer fluid and aerosol. *PLoS ONE* 8(3):e57987. https://doi.org/10.1371/journal.pone.0057987 (accessed February 7, 2018).

Yan, X. S., and C. D'Ruiz. 2015. Effects of using electronic cigarettes on nicotine delivery and cardiovascular function in comparison with regular cigarettes. *Regulatory Toxicology and Pharmacology* 71(1):24–34.

Zeller, M., D. Hatsukami, and Strategic Dialogue on Tobacco Harm Reduction Group. 2009. The strategic dialogue on tobacco harm reduction: A vision and blueprint for action in the US. *Tobacco Control* 18(4):324–332.

19

Modeling of E-Cigarette Use

In Section III, the committee presented a conceptual framework of smoking transitions. The framework captures multiple hypothesized pathways by which e-cigarette use could affect combustible tobacco cigarette use. The hypothesized pathways can be used to understand both individual tobacco use trajectories and population-level effects, and include

- Youth and young adults could begin using e-cigarettes and subsequently start using combustible tobacco cigarettes, either completely switching or using both products concurrently (increasing combustible tobacco cigarette initiation).
- Youth and young adults who otherwise would have begun combustible tobacco cigarette smoking could begin using e-cigarettes instead (reducing or delaying combustible tobacco cigarette initiation).
- Adults who smoke combustible tobacco cigarettes could switch to using e-cigarettes alone or quit both products (cessation).
- Adult combustible tobacco cigarette smokers could start using e-cigarettes in addition to combustible tobacco cigarettes (dual use). Some portion of these adult smokers may subsequently transition to e-cigarette use alone (cessation).
- Former smokers could start using e-cigarettes and subsequently transition to combustible tobacco cigarettes (relapse) either alone or concurrently with e-cigarettes (dual use).

Some of these pathways will result in harms while others may confer benefits. In any population, each of these pathways may occur among both individuals and subpopulations. Thus, e-cigarette use could produce harms for some individuals while conferring benefits to others. These benefits and harms can offset each other, making it difficult to draw inferences about the net effect of e-cigarettes at the population level. Thus, to facilitate an assessment of the overall population health effect of e-cigarettes in the U.S. population as a whole, this chapter uses modeling to apply a common metric (years of life lost or gained as a measure of mortality) to these pathways as they occur simultaneously among different subgroups.

Models of population dynamics have been used in tobacco control for more than two decades. The 2014 Surgeon General's report, *The Health Consequences of Tobacco—50 Years of Progress,* presents a summary of those models (HHS, 2014). More recently, several modeling studies have addressed the potential future impact of e-cigarettes under various assumptions, reaching different conclusions (Cherng et al., 2016; Hill and Camacho, 2017; Kalkhoran and Glantz, 2015; Levy et al., 2017; Vugrin et al., 2015). To inform their view of the likely effects of e-cigarette use at a population level, the committee employed a dynamic model of combustible tobacco cigarette smoking prevalence and health effects to examine the potential impact of e-cigarettes on mortality in the U.S. population over the next few decades under various assumptions. Specifically, the committee used a well-established dynamic model of tobacco control (Mendez and Warner, 2004; Mendez et al., 1998) to estimate the cumulative number of life-years lost (or gained) due to e-cigarettes during 2015–2050 and 2015–2070 under different assumptions regarding the harm of e-cigarettes compared with combustible tobacco cigarettes, and their potential effects on the initiation and cessation rates of combustible tobacco cigarettes. The results of the model are not precise forecasts, but rather simulation outputs that inform a qualitative assessment about the potential population health impacts of e-cigarettes.

MODEL

The Mendez-Warner model (Mendez and Warner, 2004; Mendez et al., 1998) tracks individuals in the population from age 0 to a maximum age of 110, additionally differentiated by gender and smoking status. The number of people of age a in year t is computed by multiplying the number of people of age $a - 1$ in year $t - 1$ by the appropriate survival rate (1 – death rate). Birth cohort sizes are supplied exogenously to the model. Death rates are differentiated by year, gender, age, and smoking status. The model tracks the adult population smoking status. At age 18, individuals are characterized as current, former, or never smokers. The definition of an adult current smoker is consistent with that of the National Health Interview Survey (NHIS)—those who have smoked at least 100 cigarettes in their lifetime and are smoking now every day or some days. In this model, adult initiation is measured by the proportion of the population who are current smokers at age 18. Youth smoking history before age 18 is subsumed in the adult initiation measure. Subsequently, current smokers in any given year are estimated as the number of current smokers in the previous year who survived to the current year and did not quit smoking. Former smokers are those who were former smokers the previous year and did not die, plus those who were current smokers the previous year and did not die, but quit. The model differentiates former smokers up to 30 years abstinent, and years-since-quitting–specific death rates are applied accordingly to those individuals.

Smoking prevalence for any specific age group in a specific year is computed by taking the ratio of current smokers to the total number of people within the group that year. Baseline cessation rates were estimated within the model using the NHIS and the National Survey on Drug Use and Health data for the period 1990–2014. The model uses permanent quit rates, that is, quitting net of relapse, so that these rates are smaller than those used in models that include quits that eventually result in relapse. The model is calibrated periodically, and is tracking with excellent accuracy the overall adult smoking prevalence in the United States. At the model baseline (2014), e-cigarette use among working adults was 3.8 percent (Syamlal et al., 2016). However, the model considers that e-cigarette use may increase combustible tobacco cigarette initiation among non-smokers and may also promote cessation among dual users. Thus, the effects of increased e-cigarette prevalence are subsumed in the assumptions of increases in both cessation and initiation of combustible tobacco cigarettes. The model does consider gender differences (e.g., relative risks and death rates), although the committee applied the same values to men and women for some parameters (e.g., background cessation rates). The model uses age, gender, and smoking-status–specific death rates, derived from data from the Cancer Prevention Study II. The model assumes that no smoking-related deaths occur before age 35.

MODELING ASSUMPTIONS

In the model, the committee assumes that the introduction of e-cigarettes has the potential to increase smoking initiation among young adults, and smoking cessation among adults. The committee also assumes that e-cigarettes are not harmless, and that e-cigarette use increases the risk of mortality over that of a non-vaper, non-smoker individual. At the same time, the risk of mortality among e-cigarette users is lower than that among combustible tobacco cigarette smokers. Dual users are treated as current smokers in terms of risk but also as having a different cessation rate than non-vaper smokers. To be conservative, dual users who quit are assumed to continue using e-cigarettes for the rest of their lives and are given a reduction of risk consistent with the direct harm effect assumed for e-cigarettes. For example, if we assume that e-cigarettes are 10 percent as harmful as cigarettes, a dual user who quits smoking will be given 90 percent of the reduction in risk that a non-vaper quitter would attain as a former smoker.

The committee's assumptions about possible effects on smoking initiation among young adults, smoking cessation among adults, and the harm of e-cigarettes in relation to combustible tobacco cigarettes are informed by the committee's review of the literature presented in the preceding chapters. Some of the parameters were also chosen to provide an extreme upper limit for the harmful effects of e-cigarettes and to illustrate the level of such negative effects necessary to counterbalance the potential benefits of e-cigarettes at the population level. In particular, the simulations contain scenarios where e-cigarettes are 50 percent as harmful as cigarettes and/or increase initiation by 50 percent. The committee considers those scenarios to be extreme and highly unlikely.

The committee considered the following specific effect levels:

- E-cigarettes increase the smoking initiation rate by 0 percent, 5 percent, 10 percent, 25 percent, or 50 percent;
- E-cigarettes increase the net smoking cessation rate by –5 percent, 0 percent, 5 percent, 10 percent, or 15 percent; and
- E-cigarettes are 0 percent, 10 percent, 25 percent, or 50 percent as harmful as combustible tobacco cigarettes.

The range of parameter values were selected according to the criteria described in the following sections: e-cigarette effect on initiation, e-cigarette effect on cessation, and e-cigarette harm.

E-Cigarette Effect on Initiation

As concluded in Chapter 16, e-cigarette use likely increases the risk of ever using combustible tobacco cigarettes among youth. However, it is unclear whether this increase in ever use results in an increased adult initiation rate. The committee decided to examine a wide range of effect levels, from no impact on initiation to a 50 percent increase in initiation. The upper limit of 50 percent implies that e-cigarettes will not only stop the currently observed downward trend in the adult initiation rate, but that they will increase initiation from its 2015 value of 13 percent (Jamal et al., 2016) to 19.5 percent, a level not observed since 2011 (CDC, 2012). The committee considers this level extreme and very unlikely, as discussed above.

E-Cigarette Effect on Cessation

Recent meta-analyses including randomized controlled trials and cohort studies report an adjusted odds ratio for cessation around 0.7 (with versus without e-cigarettes); on the other hand, a recent population study (Zhu et al., 2017) reports an adjusted odds ratio of 1.65 (1.40–1.93). Taking the 2014 prevalence of dual users as 16.2 percent (Syamlal et al., 2016), a 0.7 odds ratio translates into 16.2 percent × (0.70 – 1) = –4.86 percent increase (or 4.86 percent decrease) in the overall cessation rate, while 1.65 odds ratio implies a 16.2 percent × (1.65 – 1) = 10.53 percent increase in cessation, with an upper bound of 16.2 percent × (1.93 – 1) = 15 percent. Based on these values, the committee chose to model values between –5 percent and 15 percent for the effect of e-cigarettes on the overall population cessation rate.

An important note is that, as described above, the model uses permanent quit rates (i.e., quitting net of relapse). Thus, cessation in the modeling refers to *net* cessation rates. In other words, a positive value indicates that more people in a population have quit smoking than nonsmokers who have started/relapsed, and a negative value indicates the opposite. This net cessation statistic is not a common measure in the literature, which generally reports only a cessation rate based on the percentage of smokers who successfully quit smoking, without regard to non-active smokers at baseline who started or relapsed within a specified time period. For clarity, the committee uses the term "net cessation" when discussing the modeling.

E-Cigarette Harm

As concluded in previous chapters, e-cigarettes are likely to be less harmful than combustible tobacco cigarettes. Estimates of how harmful they are relative to combustible tobacco cigarettes range from 5 percent estimated by the UK Royal College of Physicians (TAG, 2008) to 30–50 percent estimated by Glantz (2016), with most agreement concentrated around the lower figure. The committee examined a wide range of values for the relative harm of e-cigarettes compared with combustible tobacco cigarettes, from 0 to 50 percent as harmful as combustible tobacco cigarettes. The upper limit of 50 percent was selected as an extreme and improbable value, used to set an upper limit to the potential harm of e-cigarettes. The likelihood that e-cigarettes have none of the harm of combustible tobacco cigarettes is equally extreme and improbable.

SIMULATION SCENARIOS

The model runs were designed as follows: First, to establish a base case, the model was used to estimate the number of life-years lost due to smoking over the periods 2015–2050 and 2015–2070, under the assumption that the annual initiation and net cessation rates observed in 2015 (13 percent among young adults age 18–24 and 4.35 percent among adult smokers, respectively [Jamal et al., 2016; Mendez et al., 2017]) would remain constant in the future. Then, starting in 2015, the committee increased the base initiation and net cessation rates by different percentages that reflect the impact of e-cigarettes on those rates and again calculated the cumulative life-years lost or gained over the same periods as in the base-case scenario. As described in the model assumptions, the committee also assumed that individuals who quit smoking because of e-cigarettes will continue to use e-cigarettes for the remainder of their lives, and so they only achieve a fraction of the health benefits due to quitting combustible tobacco smoking. Finally, the committee compared the different scenarios with the base case to calculate the extra number of life-years gained or lost due to the effects of e-cigarettes.

Overall, the committee considered 85 different simulation scenarios. They reflect a range of likely real-world scenarios as well as scenarios that the committee views as extreme and unlikely, for heuristic purposes. The committee only considered five cases in which e-cigarette use reduces net cessation because it chose not to increase the relative risk of death for anyone beyond that of a current smoker. That is, the differential effect of reducing the net cessation rate would be to increase the number of smokers, who would then be subject to the mortality risk of a current smoker, regardless of the harm associated with e-cigarettes.

The entirety of the simulation runs is summarized in Table 19-1.

RESULTS

All scenarios show a decrease in combustible tobacco cigarette smoking prevalence, which reflect effects from past tobacco policies. Table 19-2 presents the model-estimated life-years lost during 2015–2050 due to e-cigarettes, under the assumption that e-cigarettes cause no harm directly, but their health consequences stem from their effects on initiation and net cessation of combustible tobacco cigarettes. The first section of the table (upper part) shows the life-years lost due to combustible tobacco cigarettes and e-cigarettes combined; the second section shows

TABLE 19-1 Summary of Simulation Runs Considered by the Committee

Case	Percent Initiation Increases	Percent Net Cessation Increases	Percent E-Cigarette Harm
1	0	0	0
2	5	0	0
3	10	0	0
4	25	0	0
5	50	0	0
6	0	5	0
7	5	5	0
8	10	5	0
9	25	5	0
10	50	5	0
11	0	10	0
12	5	10	0
13	10	10	0
14	25	10	0
15	50	10	0
16	0	15	0
17	5	15	0
18	10	15	0
19	25	15	0
20	50	15	0
21	0	0	10
22	5	0	10
23	10	0	10
24	25	0	10
25	50	0	10
26	0	5	10
27	5	5	10
28	10	5	10
29	25	5	10
30	50	5	10
31	0	10	10
32	5	10	10

continued

TABLE 19-1 Continued

Case	Percent Initiation Increases	Percent Net Cessation Increases	Percent E-Cigarette Harm
33	10	10	10
34	25	10	10
35	50	10	10
36	0	15	10
37	5	15	10
38	10	15	10
39	25	15	10
40	50	15	10
41	0	0	25
42	5	0	25
43	10	0	25
44	25	0	25
45	50	0	25
46	0	5	25
47	5	5	25
48	10	5	25
49	25	5	25
50	50	5	25
51	0	10	25
52	5	10	25
53	10	10	25
54	25	10	25
55	50	10	25
56	0	15	25
57	5	15	25
58	10	15	25
59	25	15	25
60	50	15	25
61	0	0	50
62	5	0	50
63	10	0	50
64	25	0	50

TABLE 19-1 Continued

Case	Percent Initiation Increases	Percent Net Cessation Increases	Percent E-Cigarette Harm
65	50	0	50
66	0	5	50
67	5	5	50
68	10	5	50
69	25	5	50
70	50	5	50
71	0	10	50
72	5	10	50
73	10	10	50
74	25	10	50
75	50	10	50
76	0	15	50
77	5	15	50
78	10	15	50
79	25	15	50
80	50	15	50
81	0	–5	0
82	5	–5	0
83	10	–5	0
84	25	–5	0
85	50	–5	0

the life-years lost attributable to e-cigarettes; and the third section shows the same figure as in the second section, as a fraction of the total toll of combustible cigarettes over 2015–2050. In this table, as in all subsequent tables, results shown in red text in parentheses indicate life-years saved compared with a baseline scenario of no effect of e-cigarettes on initiation or net cessation of combustibles.

For example, under the scenario that e-cigarette use causes a decrease of 5 percent (from 4.35 percent to 4.13 percent) on the net cessation rate, and an increase of 5 percent on the initiation rate (from 13 percent to 13.65 percent), the estimated total life-years lost due to smoking (counting the extra smokers because of e-cigarettes) would be 296,067,599. Given

TABLE 19-2 Model-Estimated Life-Years Lost During 2015–2050 Due to E-Cigarettes[a]

Percent Initiation Increases	Percent Net Cessation Increases				
	–5%	0%	5%	10%	15%
	Life-Years Lost Due to Smoking and E-Cigarettes				
0%	296,001,655	294,605,788	293,312,834	292,068,581	290,870,879
5%	296,067,599	294,670,840	293,377,037	292,131,976	290,933,506
10%	296,133,543	294,735,891	293,441,240	292,195,371	290,996,133
25%	296,331,375	294,931,046	293,633,848	292,385,557	291,184,015
50%	296,661,095	295,256,304	293,954,861	292,702,533	291,497,151
	Life-Years Lost Due to E-Cigarettes				
0%	1,395,867	0	(1,292,954)	(2,537,207)	(3,734,909)
5%	1,461,811	65,052	(1,228,751)	(2,473,812)	(3,672,282)
10%	1,527,755	130,103	(1,164,549)	(2,410,417)	(3,609,655)
25%	1,725,587	325,258	(971,940)	(2,220,231)	(3,421,773)
50%	2,055,307	650,516	(650,927)	(1,903,255)	(3,108,638)
	Percentage of Life-Years Lost Due to E-Cigarettes				
0%	0.5%	0.0%	–0.4%	–0.9%	–1.3%
5%	0.5%	0.0%	–0.4%	–0.8%	–1.3%
10%	0.5%	0.0%	–0.4%	–0.8%	–1.2%
25%	0.6%	0.1%	–0.3%	–0.8%	–1.2%
50%	0.7%	0.2%	–0.2%	–0.7%	–1.1%

[a] Under the assumptions that e-cigarettes cause no harm directly and a range of assumptions about smoking initiation and net cessation. E-cigarettes = 0% × risk of combustibles.

NOTE: Results shown in red text in parentheses indicate life-years saved compared with a baseline scenario of no effect of e-cigarettes on initiation or net cessation of combustible tobacco cigarettes.

that approximately 50 percent of life-long smokers die prematurely of smoking-related causes, losing an average of 20 years of life, this figure translates into 14,803,380 total premature deaths over a span of 35 years, or an average of 422,954 premature deaths per year. Out of this figure, the extra toll imposed by e-cigarettes is 1,461,811 life-years lost (or 2,088 premature deaths per year), representing 0.5 percent of the total toll of smoking over the 35-year span.

If, on the other hand, e-cigarettes increased net smoking cessation rates by 5 percent (4.57 percent) while still increasing initiation by 5 percent, 1,228,751 life-years would be saved in 2015–2050, representing approximately 1,755 premature deaths averted per year. Under the scenario of a 5 percent increase in the net smoking cessation rate due to e-cigarettes, even assuming that e-cigarettes increase the initiation rate by 50 percent (to 19.5 percent), there would still be 650,927 life-years saved by 2050.

Scenarios extending outcomes through 2070 under the same assumptions indicate worse outcomes in all scenarios compared with those through 2050. This is because, under any scenario that increases adult initiation, the benefits of increased net cessation are felt much sooner than the negative effects of increased initiation. Of note, the committee chose to keep the background rates on smoking initiation and cessation constant, to avoid forecasting future values of those parameters. In reality, current trends indicate that the adult smoking initiation rate is decreasing while the cessation rate is increasing. If those trends continue into the future, the negative effects of e-cigarettes on smoking initiation will be smaller while the positive effects on cessation will be larger.

Table 19-3 illustrates this fact. It shows cumulative life-years lost (or saved) over 2015–2070. For example, assuming that e-cigarettes increase the initiation rate by one-quarter (to 16.3 percent), and the net cessation rate by 5 percent (to 4.57 percent) in 2015, around 577,000 life-years would be lost by 2070 due to e-cigarettes. However, under the same conditions, there would be 971,940 extra life-years by 2050; by 2070, this gain would be offset by the excess mortality brought by the increased initiation.

The rest of the scenarios show the same results as Tables 19-2 and 19-3, considering different levels of harm associated with e-cigarettes.

Tables 19-4 and 19-5 show the life-years lost by 2050 and 2070, respectively, under the assumption that e-cigarettes cause 10 percent of the harm of (i.e., are 90 percent less harmful than) combustible tobacco cigarettes. These tables show that, if net smoking cessation increases by 5 percent, by 2050, there would be life-years gained. The gains would range from 467,228 life-years if smoking initiation increases by 50 percent to 1,110,728 life-years if there is no increase in smoking initiation. By 2070, if net smoking cessation increases by 5 percent, there would be life-years gained

TABLE 19-3 Model-Estimated Life-Years Lost During 2015–2070 Due to E-Cigarettes[a]

Percent Initiation Increases	Percent Net Cessation Increases				
	–5%	0%	5%	10%	15%
	Life-Years Lost Due to Smoking and E-Cigarettes				
0%	451,006,794	448,561,255	445,791,244	443,165,422	440,674,738
5%	451,693,674	449,239,108	446,460,647	443,826,916	441,328,825
10%	452,380,554	449,916,960	447,130,050	444,488,409	441,982,911
25%	454,441,193	451,950,517	449,138,260	446,472,889	443,945,172
50%	457,875,591	455,339,779	452,485,276	449,780,357	447,215,606
	Life-Years Lost Due to E-Cigarettes				
0%	2,445,539	0	(2,770,011)	(5,395,833)	(7,886,518)
5%	3,132,418	677,852	(2,100,608)	(4,734,340)	(7,232,431)
10%	3,819,298	1,355,705	(1,431,205)	(4,072,846)	(6,578,344)
25%	5,879,937	3,389,262	577,005	(2,088,366)	(4,616,083)
50%	9,314,336	6,778,523	3,924,021	1,219,101	(1,345,649)
	Percentage of Life-Years Lost Due to E-Cigarettes				
0%	0.5%	0.0%	–0.6%	–1.2%	–1.8%
5%	0.7%	0.2%	–0.5%	–1.1%	–1.6%
10%	0.8%	0.3%	–0.3%	–0.9%	–1.5%
25%	1.3%	0.7%	0.1%	–0.5%	–1.0%
50%	2.0%	1.5%	0.9%	0.3%	–0.3%

[a] Under the assumptions that e-cigarettes cause no harm directly and a range of assumptions about smoking initiation and net cessation. E-cigarettes = 0% × risk of combustibles.

NOTE: Results shown in red text in parentheses indicate life-years saved compared with a baseline scenario of no effect of e-cigarettes on initiation or net cessation of combustible tobacco cigarettes.

TABLE 19-4 Model-Estimated Life-Years Lost During 2015–2050 Due to E-Cigarettes[a]

Percent Initiation Increases	Percent Net Cessation Increases				
	–5%	0%	5%	10%	15%
	Life-Years Lost Due to Smoking and E-Cigarettes				
0%	296,001,655	294,605,788	293,495,061	292,426,926	291,399,483
5%	296,067,599	294,670,840	293,559,410	292,490,610	291,462,534
10%	296,133,543	294,735,891	293,623,760	292,554,294	291,525,585
25%	296,331,375	294,931,046	293,816,810	292,745,345	291,714,738
50%	296,661,095	295,256,304	294,138,560	293,063,763	292,029,994
	Life-Years Lost Due to E-Cigarettes				
0%	1,395,867	0	(1,110,728)	(2,178,862)	(3,206,305)
5%	1,461,811	65,052	(1,046,378)	(2,115,178)	(3,143,254)
10%	1,527,755	130,103	(982,028)	(2,051,494)	(3,080,203)
25%	1,725,587	325,258	(788,978)	(1,860,443)	(2,891,050)
50%	2,055,307	650,516	(467,228)	(1,542,025)	(2,575,794)
	Percentage of Life-Years Lost Due to E-Cigarettes				
0%	0.5%	0.0%	–0.4%	–0.7%	–1.1%
5%	0.5%	0.0%	–0.4%	–0.7%	–1.1%
10%	0.5%	0.0%	–0.3%	–0.7%	–1.1%
25%	0.6%	0.1%	–0.3%	–0.6%	–1.0%
50%	0.7%	0.2%	–0.2%	–0.5%	–0.9%

[a] Under the assumptions that e-cigarettes are 90 percent less harmful than combustible tobacco cigarettes and a range of assumptions about smoking initiation and net cessation. E-cigarettes = 10% × risk of combustibles.

NOTE: Results shown in red text in parentheses indicate life-years saved compared with a baseline scenario of no effect of e-cigarettes on initiation or net cessation of combustible tobacco cigarettes.

TABLE 19-5 Model-Estimated Life-Years Lost During 2015–2070 Due to E-Cigarettes[a]

Percent Initiation Increases	Percent Net Cessation Increases				
	–5%	0%	5%	10%	15%
	Life-Years Lost Due to Smoking and E-Cigarettes				
0%	451,006,794	448,561,255	446,234,477	444,031,875	441,945,525
5%	451,693,674	449,239,108	446,905,736	444,696,985	442,604,900
10%	452,380,554	449,916,960	447,576,995	445,362,095	443,264,275
25%	454,441,193	451,950,517	449,590,773	447,357,426	445,242,400
50%	457,875,591	455,339,779	452,947,068	450,682,976	448,539,275
	Life-Years Lost Due to E-Cigarettes				
0%	2,445,539	0	(2,326,778)	(4,529,380)	(6,615,731)
5%	3,132,418	677,852	(1,655,519)	(3,864,270)	(5,956,356)
10%	3,819,298	1,355,705	(984,260)	(3,199,160)	(5,296,981)
25%	5,879,937	3,389,262	1,029,517	(1,203,830)	(3,318,856)
50%	9,314,336	6,778,523	4,385,812	2,121,721	(21,981)
	Percentage of Life-Years Lost Due to E-Cigarettes				
0%	0.5%	0.0%	–0.5%	–1.0%	–1.5%
5%	0.7%	0.2%	–0.4%	–0.9%	–1.3%
10%	0.8%	0.3%	–0.2%	–0.7%	–1.2%
25%	1.3%	0.7%	0.2%	–0.3%	–0.7%
50%	2.0%	1.5%	1.0%	0.5%	0.0%

[a] Under the assumptions that e-cigarettes are 90 percent less harmful than combustible tobacco cigarettes and a range of assumptions about smoking initiation and net cessation. E-cigarettes = 10% × risk of combustibles.

NOTE: Results shown in red text in parentheses indicate life-years saved compared with a baseline scenario of no effect of e-cigarettes on initiation or net cessation of combustible tobacco cigarettes.

TABLE 19-6 Model-Estimated Life-Years Lost During 2015–2050 Due to E-Cigarettes[a]

Percent Initiation Increases	Percent Net Cessation Increases				
	–5%	0%	5%	10%	15%
	Life-Years Lost Due to Smoking and E-Cigarettes				
0%	296,001,655	294,605,788	293,762,024	292,951,883	292,173,826
5%	296,067,599	294,670,840	293,826,594	293,015,998	292,237,512
10%	296,133,543	294,735,891	293,891,164	293,080,114	292,301,197
25%	296,331,375	294,931,046	294,084,875	293,272,460	292,492,255
50%	296,661,095	295,256,304	294,407,727	293,593,038	292,810,683
	Life-Years Lost Due to E-Cigarettes				
0%	1,395,867	0	(843,764)	(1,653,905)	(2,431,962)
5%	1,461,811	65,052	(779,194)	(1,589,790)	(2,368,277)
10%	1,527,755	130,103	(714,624)	(1,525,674)	(2,304,591)
25%	1,725,587	325,258	(520,913)	(1,333,328)	(2,113,534)
50%	2,055,307	650,516	(198,061)	(1,012,750)	(1,795,105)
	Percentage of Life-Years Lost Due to E-Cigarettes				
0%	0.5%	0.0%	–0.3%	–0.6%	–0.8%
5%	0.5%	0.0%	–0.3%	–0.5%	–0.8%
10%	0.5%	0.0%	–0.2%	–0.5%	–0.8%
25%	0.6%	0.1%	–0.2%	–0.5%	–0.7%
50%	0.7%	0.2%	–0.1%	–0.3%	–0.6%

[a] Under the assumptions that e-cigarettes are 75 percent less harmful than combustible tobacco cigarettes and a range of assumptions about smoking initiation and net cessation. E-cigarettes = 25% × risk of combustibles.

NOTE: Results shown in red text in parentheses indicate life-years saved compared with a baseline scenario of no effect of e-cigarettes on initiation or net cessation of combustible tobacco cigarettes.

TABLE 19-7 Model-Estimated Life-Years Lost During 2015–2070 Due to E-Cigarettes[a]

Percent Initiation	Percent Net Cessation Increases				
Increases	–5%	0%	5%	10%	15%
	Life-Years Lost Due to Smoking and E-Cigarettes				
0%	451,006,794	448,561,255	446,878,122	445,290,048	443,790,754
5%	451,693,674	449,239,108	447,552,145	445,960,546	444,458,007
10%	452,380,554	449,916,960	448,226,169	446,631,044	445,125,260
25%	454,441,193	451,950,517	450,248,241	448,642,538	447,127,019
50%	457,875,591	455,339,779	453,618,360	451,995,029	450,463,284
	Life-Years Lost Due to E-Cigarettes				
0%	2,445,539	0	(1,683,134)	(3,271,207)	(4,770,501)
5%	3,132,418	677,852	(1,009,110)	(2,600,709)	(4,103,248)
10%	3,819,298	1,355,705	(335,086)	(1,930,211)	(3,435,995)
25%	5,879,937	3,389,262	1,686,985	81,283	(1,434,236)
50%	9,314,336	6,778,523	5,057,105	3,433,774	1,902,029
	Percentage of Life-Years Lost Due to E-Cigarettes				
0%	0.5%	0.0%	–0.4%	–0.7%	–1.1%
5%	0.7%	0.2%	–0.2%	–0.6%	–0.9%
10%	0.8%	0.3%	–0.1%	–0.4%	–0.8%
25%	1.3%	0.7%	0.4%	0.0%	–0.3%
50%	2.0%	1.5%	1.1%	0.8%	0.4%

[a] Under the assumptions that e-cigarettes are 75 percent less harmful than combustible tobacco cigarettes and a range of assumptions about smoking initiation and net cessation. E-cigarettes = 25% × risk of combustibles.

NOTE: Results shown in red text in parentheses indicate life-years saved compared with a baseline scenario of no effect of e-cigarettes on initiation or net cessation of combustible tobacco cigarettes.

TABLE 19-8 Model-Estimated Life-Years Lost During 2015–2050 Due to E-Cigarettes[a]

Initiation Increases	Percent Net Cessation Increases				
Percent	–5%	0%	5%	10%	15%
	Life-Years Lost Due to Smoking and E-Cigarettes				
0%	296,001,655	294,605,788	294,190,793	293,794,957	293,417,330
5%	296,067,599	294,670,840	294,255,730	293,859,791	293,482,070
10%	296,133,543	294,735,891	294,320,666	293,924,624	293,546,811
25%	296,331,375	294,931,046	294,515,476	294,119,124	293,741,033
50%	296,661,095	295,256,304	294,840,160	294,443,290	294,064,736
	Life-Years Lost Due to E-Cigarettes				
0%	1,395,867	0	(414,995)	(810,831)	(1,188,458)
5%	1,461,811	65,052	(350,059)	(745,998)	(1,123,718)
10%	1,527,755	130,103	(285,122)	(681,164)	(1,058,977)
25%	1,725,587	325,258	(90,312)	(486,664)	(864,755)
50%	2,055,307	650,516	234,371	(162,498)	(541,052)
	Percentage of Life-Years Lost Due to E-Cigarettes				
0%	0.5%	0.0%	–0.1%	–0.3%	–0.4%
5%	0.5%	0.0%	–0.1%	–0.3%	–0.4%
10%	0.5%	0.0%	–0.1%	–0.2%	–0.4%
25%	0.6%	0.1%	0.0%	–0.2%	–0.3%
50%	0.7%	0.2%	0.1%	–0.1%	–0.2%

[a] Under the assumptions that e-cigarettes are half as harmful as combustible tobacco cigarettes and a range of assumptions about smoking initiation and net cessation. E-cigarettes = 50% × risk of combustibles.

NOTE: Results shown in red text in parentheses indicate life-years saved compared with a baseline scenario of no effect of e-cigarettes on initiation or net cessation of combustible tobacco cigarettes.

TABLE 19-9 Model-Estimated Life-Years Lost During 2015–2070 Due to E-Cigarettes[a]

Percent Initiation Increases	Percent Net Cessation Increases: –5%	0%	5%	10%	15%
	Life-Years Lost Due to Smoking and E-Cigarettes				
0%	451,006,794	448,561,255	447,897,792	447,283,134	446,713,620
5%	451,693,674	449,239,108	448,576,373	447,962,514	447,393,860
10%	452,380,554	449,916,960	449,254,955	448,641,895	448,074,101
25%	454,441,193	451,950,517	451,290,700	450,680,036	450,114,822
50%	457,875,591	455,339,779	454,683,609	454,076,939	453,516,024
	Life-Years Lost Due to E-Cigarettes				
0%	2,445,539	0	(663,464)	(1,278,122)	(1,847,636)
5%	3,132,418	677,852	15,118	(598,741)	(1,167,395)
10%	3,819,298	1,355,705	693,700	80,639	(487,155)
25%	5,879,937	3,389,262	2,729,445	2,118,781	1,553,567
50%	9,314,336	6,778,523	6,122,353	5,515,683	4,954,769
	Percentage of Life-Years Lost Due to E-Cigarettes				
0%	0.5%	0.0%	–0.1%	–0.3%	–0.4%
5%	0.7%	0.2%	0.0%	–0.1%	–0.3%
10%	0.8%	0.3%	0.2%	0.0%	–0.1%
25%	1.3%	0.7%	0.6%	0.5%	0.3%
50%	2.0%	1.5%	1.3%	1.2%	1.1%

[a] Under the assumptions that e-cigarettes are half as harmful as combustible tobacco cigarettes and a range of assumptions about smoking initiation and net cessation. E-cigarettes = 50% × risk of combustibles.

NOTE: Results shown in red text in parentheses indicate life-years saved compared with a baseline scenario of no effect of e-cigarettes on initiation or net cessation of combustible tobacco cigarettes.

under scenarios with 0 percent, 5 percent, and 10 percent increases in smoking initiation, and life-years lost if smoking increased by 25 or 50 percent.

Tables 19-6 and 19-7 show the life-years lost by 2050 and 2070, respectively, under the assumption that e-cigarettes cause 25 percent of the mortality harm of combustible tobacco cigarettes. If e-cigarettes increase the net cessation rate by 5 percent, by 2050 there would be life-year gains, ranging from 198,061 if e-cigarettes increase the initiation rate by 50 percent to 843,764 if e-cigarettes have no impact on the initiation rate. Extending the same scenarios to 2070, the results show that, with an increase of 5 percent in net cessation, there would be cumulative life-year gains under the 0, 5, and 10 percent increase in initiation scenarios, but life-year losses below 25 percent and 50 percent increase in initiation assumptions.

Tables 19-8 and 19-9 show the life-years lost by 2050 and 2070, respectively, under the assumption that e-cigarettes are half as harmful as combustible tobacco cigarettes. If e-cigarettes increase the net cessation rate by 5 percent, by 2050 there would be life-year gains if net smoking initiation increases by 0, 5, 10, or 25 percent, but life-year losses if initiation increases by 50 percent. By 2070, if e-cigarettes increase the net cessation rate by 5 percent, there are life-year gains only if there are no increases in smoking initiation.

SUMMARY

The specific time frame and magnitude of population health effects of e-cigarettes will depend on their impact on the rates of initiation and net cessation of combustible tobacco cigarettes and their intrinsic harm. Any population health effect includes the possibility of some groups incurring harm (e.g., youth who initiate combustible tobacco cigarettes), while others benefit (e.g., adult combustible tobacco cigarette users who completely quit or reduce smoking). As with other models of population health effects of tobacco use, the effects of changing net cessation rates are seen earlier than effects of changing initiation rates, due to the lag in time for serious chronic health effects of combustible tobacco cigarettes to manifest.

Under the assumption that the use of e-cigarettes increases the net cessation rate of combustible tobacco cigarette smoking among adults (i.e., the increase in permanent quitting offsets the potential relapsing of former smokers because of e-cigarettes), the modeling projects that use of these products will generate a net public health benefit, at least in the short run. The harms from increased initiation by youth will take time to manifest, occurring decades after the benefits of increased cessation are seen. However, for long-range projections (e.g., 50 years out), the net public health benefit is substantially less, and is negative under some scenarios. With the range of assumptions used, the model projects that there would be net public health harm in the short and long term if the products do not increase net combustible tobacco cessation in adults.

Factors that would maximize potential health benefits associated with these products include determining with more precision whether and under which conditions e-cigarettes could serve as an effective smoking cessation aid; discouraging their use among youth through standard tobacco control strategies, such as education and access restrictions; and increasing their safety through data-driven engineering and design.

REFERENCES

CDC (Centers for Disease Control and Prevention). 2012. Current cigarette smoking among adults—United States, 2011. *Morbidity and Mortality Weekly Report* 61(44):889–894.

Cherng, S. T., J. Tam, P. J. Christine, and R. Meza. 2016. Modeling the effects of e-cigarettes on smoking behavior: Implications for future adult smoking prevalence. *Epidemiology* 27(6):819–826.

Glantz, S. 2016. *Accumulating evidence suggests e-cigs 1/3 to 1/2 as bad as cigs (maybe higher).* https://tobacco.ucsf.edu/accumulating-evidence-suggests-e-cigs-13-12-bad-cigs-maybe-higher (accessed November 30, 2017).

HHS (U.S. Department of Health and Human Services). 2014. *The health consequences of smoking—50 years of progress: A report of the Surgeon General.* Atlanta, GA: U.S. Department of Health and Human Services, Centers for Disease Control and Prevention, National Center for Disease Prevention and Health Promotion, Office on Smoking and Health.

Hill, A., and O. M. Camacho. 2017. A system dynamics modelling approach to assess the impact of launching a new nicotine product on population health outcomes. *Regulatory Toxicology and Pharmacology* 86:265–278.

Jamal, A., B. A. King, L. J. Neff, J. Whitmill, S. D. Babb, and C. M. Graffunder. 2016. Current cigarette smoking among adults—United States, 2005–2015. *Morbidity and Mortality Weekly Report* 65(44):1205–1211.

Kalkhoran, S., and S. A. Glantz. 2015. Modeling the health effects of expanding e-cigarette sales in the United States and United Kingdom: A Monte Carlo analysis. *JAMA Internal Medicine* 175(10):1671–1680.

Levy, D. T., Z. Yuan, Y. Luo, and D. B. Abrams. 2017. The relationship of e-cigarette use to cigarette quit attempts and cessation: Insights from a large, nationally representative U.S. survey. *Nicotine & Tobacco Research*. https://doi.org/10.1093/ntr/ntx166 (accessed February 8, 2018).

Mendez, D., and K. E. Warner. 2004. Adult cigarette smoking prevalence: Declining as expected (not as desired). *American Journal of Public Health* 94(2):251–252.

Mendez, D., K. E. Warner, and P. N. Courant. 1998. Has smoking cessation ceased? Expected trends in the prevalence of smoking in the United States. *American Journal of Epidemiology* 148(3):249–258.

Mendez, D., J. Tam, G. A. Giovino, A. Tsodikov, and K. E. Warner. 2017. Has smoking cessation increased? An examination of the U.S. adult smoking cessation rate 1990–2014. *Nicotine & Tobacco Research* 19(12):1418–1424.

Syamlal, G., A. Jamal, B. A. King, and J. M. Mazurek. 2016. Electronic cigarette use among working adults—United States, 2014. *Morbidity and Mortality Weekly Report* 65(22): 557–561.

TAG (Tobacco Advisory Group of the Royal College of Physicians). 2008. *Ending tobacco smoking in Britain: Radical strategies for prevention and harm reduction in nicotine addiction.* https://cdn.shopify.com/s/files/1/0924/4392/files/ending-tobacco-smoking.pdf?2801907981964551469 (accessed October 11, 2017).

Vugrin, E. D., B. L. Rostron, S. J. Verzi, N. S. Brodsky, T. J. Brown, C. J. Choiniere, B. N. Coleman, A. Paredes, and B. J. Apelberg. 2015. Modeling the potential effects of new tobacco products and policies: A dynamic population model for multiple product use and harm. *PLoS ONE* 10(3):e0121008. https://doi.org/10.1371/journal.pone.0121008 (accessed February 8, 2018).

Zhu, S. H., Y. L. Zhuang, S. Wong, S. E. Cummins, and G. J. Tedeschi. 2017. E-cigarette use and associated changes in population smoking cessation: Evidence from U.S. current population surveys. *BMJ* 358:j3262. https://doi.org/10.1136/bmj.j3262 (accessed February 8, 2018).

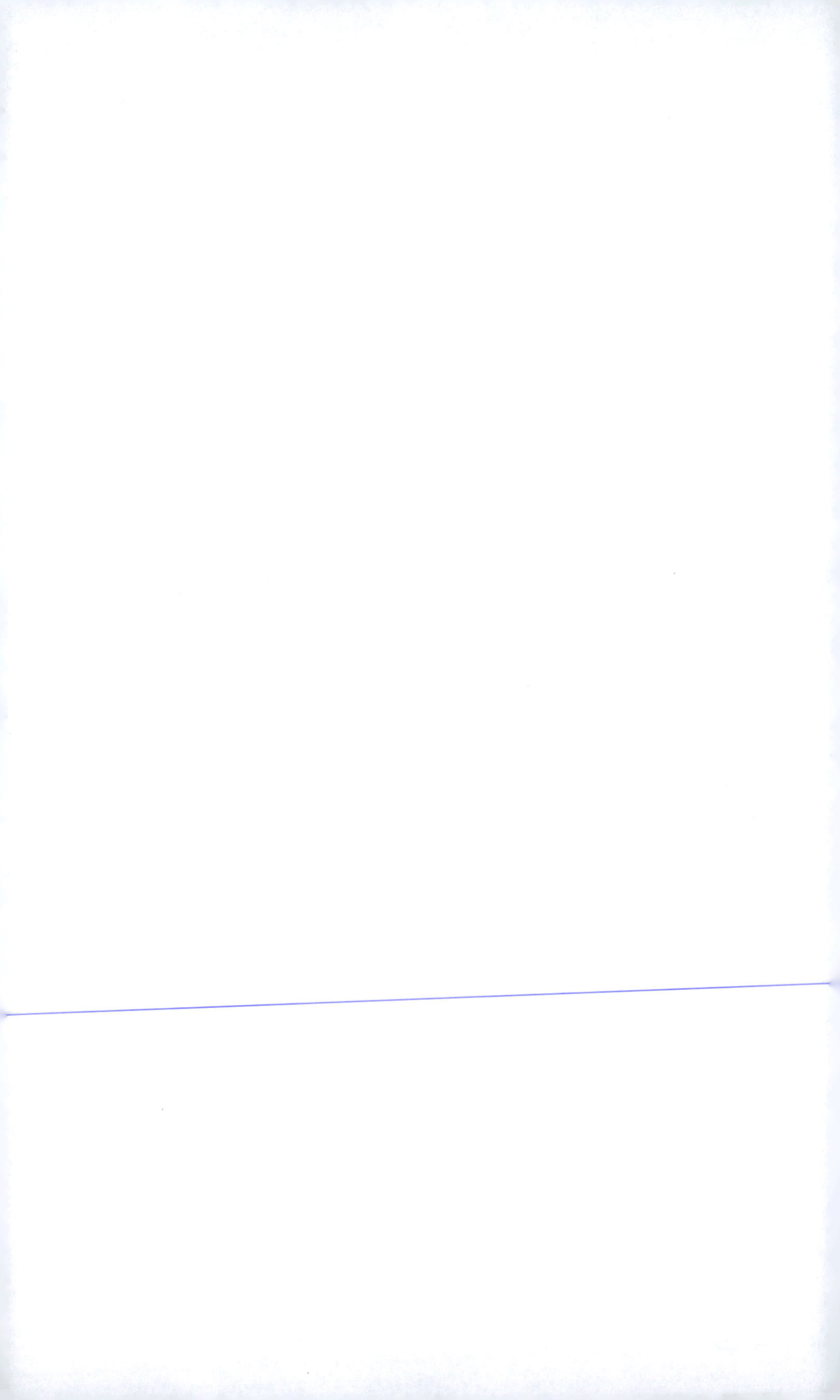

20

Research Needs: Public Health Implications of E-Cigarettes

The committee was tasked to provide a list of research needs to inform Food and Drug Administration (FDA) and e-cigarette regulation that will be prioritized with respect to

- Research to gather information of most importance for the regulation of electronic cigarettes to protect the population health
- Research that should be a priority for federal funding

The committee identified many gaps in the literature during its review and identified dozens of important specific research needs for understanding the harm reduction potential and public health implications of e-cigarettes, as other research groups have documented (Walton et al., 2015). As described in Chapters 6 and 15, the committee identified two overarching research needs: addressing gaps in substantive knowledge and improving research methods and quality. Specific items for consideration identified by the committee are noted for each of these and appear in approximately the order in which the underlying research need emerged within Section III.

ADDRESSING GAPS IN SUBSTANTIVE KNOWLEDGE

Recommendation 20-1: The committee recommends that the Food and Drug Administration and other federal research sponsors and/or device manufacturers prioritize e-cigarette research

that addresses key gaps regarding harm reduction and the public health implications of e-cigarettes. This might include rapid response funding opportunities. Specific items for consideration follow.

- **Potential of e-cigarettes to influence the ever use of combustible tobacco cigarettes:**
    - Research that addresses potential dose–response associations between e-cigarette use and combustible tobacco cigarette smoking in adolescents and young adults, including detailed assessment of the use frequency and intensity, and dependence symptoms, for both products.
    - Studies that follow an entire population of youth beginning at an age in which risk of use of any product is negligible (e.g., 10 years old) and investigate time-varying associations between e-cigarette use and later combustible tobacco cigarette use at multiple developmental stages throughout the entire period of risk (e.g., up until age 29), while using multiple methods to establish temporal precedence of e-cigarette use relative to smoking.
    - Whether use of e-cigarettes with specified product characteristics is associated with different risk of ever smoking and progression to inform product standard.
- **Potential of e-cigarettes to promote smoking cessation and/or harm reduction:**
    - Carefully designed studies, especially adequately powered randomized controlled trials, of the effectiveness of e-cigarettes as cessation aids, using standards that have been used to evaluate smoking cessation pharmacotherapies:
        - Trials that compare e-cigarettes to FDA-approved smoking cessation pharmacotherapies and other evidence-based cessation treatments are most informative.
        - Trials could also compare the effectiveness of e-cigarettes as used in combination with existing FDA-approved cessation aids.
        - Trials should be conducted not only in general populations of smokers, but also among subgroups of smokers with higher smoking rates, among smokers less likely to use or respond to existing cessation treatments, and among individuals for whom tobacco smoking is especially harmful.
        - Trials should assess adverse events in a detailed and standardized manner to permit assessment of the harms of these devices compared with other smoking cessation aids.

    - Analyses should be conducted of the frequency and intensity of use, the reach and appeal, and the affordability and accessibility of e-cigarettes compared with other cessation treatments, and the specific product characteristics that are most closely associated with use and appeal.
    - Trials should be conducted to compare effects of e-cigarettes with different product characteristics on cessation outcomes to inform product standards.
    - To the extent possible, clinical outcomes should be collected in these trials, in addition to the primary outcome, tobacco cessation.
  - Research to develop effective communication strategies about the relative risk of e-cigarettes compared with combustible tobacco cigarettes.
  - Research on potential harm reduction to bystanders exposed involuntarily to tobacco smoke after secondhand or thirdhand exposure to combustible tobacco smoke is replaced by secondhand or thirdhand exposure to emissions of e-cigarettes.
  - Research to evaluate the trade-offs between effects of different product characteristics, product regulation, and policy changes on different populations, for example, increases in youth ever use versus adult cessation.
  - Research on the mechanisms through which e-cigarette use affects combustible tobacco cigarette smoking (both ever use among youth and quitting among current tobacco cigarette smokers).

IMPROVING RESEARCH METHODS AND QUALITY

Recommendation 20-2: The committee recommends that the Food and Drug Administration and other federal research sponsors and/or device manufacturers prioritize research on the public health implications of e-cigarettes that improves the quality of e-cigarette research. This includes protocol and methods validation and development and use of appropriate study designs, including the use of appropriate control groups.

- Prospective observational studies to assess the association of e-cigarettes with smoking cessation that include careful, detailed assessment of factors that existing research suggests may be important to moderate the effect of e-cigarettes on cessation, including frequency and duration of use as well as nicotine dependence, reason for use, and intention to quit.

- Studies that build on existing nationally representative population surveys of adults to monitor patterns of e-cigarette use in detail on an ongoing basis to include characterization of patterns of e-cigarette use such as the frequency and duration of use, type of device used, and reason for use.

REFERENCE

Walton, K. M., D. B. Abrams, W. C. Bailey, D. Clark, G. N. Connolly, M. V. Djordjevic, T. E. Eissenberg, M. C. Fiore, M. L. Goniewicz, L. Haverkos, S. S. Hecht, J. E. Henningfield, J. R. Hughes, C. A. Oncken, L. Postow, J. E. Rose, K. L. Wanke, L. Yang, and D. K. Hatsukami. 2015. NIH electronic cigarette workshop: Developing a research agenda. *Nicotine & Tobacco Research* 17(2):259–269.

21

Concluding Observations

Based on the findings of this report, e-cigarettes cannot be simply categorized as either beneficial or harmful to health. The net public health outcome depends on the balance between adverse outcomes (increased youth initiation of combustible tobacco cigarettes, low or even decreased cessation rates in adults, and a high-risk profile) and positive outcomes (very low youth initiation, high cessation rates in adults, and a low-risk profile). In some circumstances, adverse effects of e-cigarettes clearly warrant concern, such as the use of e-cigarettes among non-smoking adolescents and young adults, devices that are prone to explosion, and the presence of constituents in e-cigarette liquids that are of major health concern (e.g., diacetyl and some other flavorings). In other circumstances, namely regular combustible tobacco cigarette smokers who use e-cigarettes to successfully quit smoking, e-cigarettes may represent an opportunity to reduce smoking-related illness. For these reasons, e-cigarette regulation that merely considers whether to be restrictive or permissive to the marketing, manufacture, and sales of all e-cigarettes for all populations is unlikely to maximize benefits and minimize the risks.

A number of federal regulatory tools exist to maximize the benefits and minimize the harms of e-cigarettes. One of those is the adoption of product standards, which require that product characteristics related to e-cigarette devices (e.g., electrical power, heating element, customizability), e-liquid constituents (e.g., nicotine concentration, flavoring additives, solvents such as propylene glycol and glycerol), and packaging meet certain criteria to ensure maximal benefit to the population as a whole. The

Food and Drug Administration (FDA) has recently announced its intention to "explore clear and meaningful measures to make tobacco products less toxic, appealing and addictive. For example, the FDA intends to develop product standards to protect against known public health risks such as electronic nicotine delivery systems (ENDS) battery issues and concerns about children's exposure to liquid nicotine" (CTP, 2017). More research that is optimally designed to compare and isolate the health effects of certain product characteristics from one another is needed. Overall, studies typically show that product characteristic variation and patterns of use can meaningfully alter the effects of e-cigarette use on important outcomes.

To provide data to inform regulatory strategies that maximize benefits and minimize the risks of e-cigarettes, research is needed to identify product characteristics with an unfavorable health profile across key outcomes. Evidence is needed that isolates the effects of certain product characteristics on (1) toxicity and long-term health risks; (2) appeal and uptake of e-cigarettes among youth and young adult non-smokers as well as the risk of transition to smoking; (3) appeal, uptake, and efficacy as a smoking cessation aid among regular combustible tobacco cigarette smokers; and (4) appeal, uptake, and effects on maintaining abstinence or precipitating relapse among former combustible tobacco cigarette smokers. Some product characteristics may pose much greater health risks with little potential benefit and be viable candidates for restrictive product standards. For example, if evidence were to identify certain flavor additives that increased toxicity and appeal to youth, but did not enhance appeal or efficacy as a smoking cessation aid, the development of product standards to prohibit the use of such additives would likely have net improvement on the health of the population. As demonstrated in Chapter 19, the effects of e-cigarette use on smoking cessation may carry considerable influence on the overall population health burden over the next 30 years. Consequently, data examining the influence of product-characteristic variation on combustible tobacco cigarette cessation are of particular value.

Other nascent issues that intersect with e-cigarettes are likely to have a major impact on population health and warrant attention, but have yet to receive significant scientific study. E-cigarettes can be placed within a broader class of "non-combustible" tobacco products that, like e-cigarettes, generate inhalable aerosols and may lack certain toxicants found in tobacco smoke (HHS, 2014; TAG, 2008). For example, heat-not-burn tobacco products (e.g., devices that aerosolize tobacco leaf mixtures without combustion) share many similarities to e-cigarettes, including the use of propylene glycol and an electric heating element. Phillip Morris's heat-not-burn product iQOS, which electronically aerosolizes tobacco leaves soaked in the same solvents present in e-liquid, has sold more than 3 million units and is currently available in more than 20 markets, but not in the United States (Reuters, 2017). In May 2017, Phillip Morris submitted modified-risk tobacco product (MRTP) applications to FDA for iQOS products and, if approved, would permit marketing with claims of reduced health risk.[1] It is important for regulatory science to translate the same methodologies and research questions directed toward e-cigarettes addressed in this report to heat-not-burn products. Furthermore, patterns of poly-tobacco product use and transitions in use among e-cigarettes, heat-not-burn tobacco products, and combustible tobacco products will also necessitate study.

The use of e-cigarettes and other e-cigarette devices to aerosolize cannabis plants, oils, and waxes is another emergent issue. Estimates of ever using an e-cigarette device to use cannabis products in youth and young adult samples across North America range from 8 percent to 29 percent (Johnston et al., 2017; Leventhal, 2016; Morean et al., 2015). With increasing legalization of cannabis in the United States, the e-cigarette and cannabis commercial industries and customer bases are likely to become increasingly enmeshed. The retail market is flooded with devices and e-liquids devised for aerosolizing liquid cannabis preparations, including products that include both nicotine and cannabis (i.e., e-liquid infused with both tetrahydrocannabinol and nicotine). Knowledge and methodologies about e-cigarette products addressed in this report can be adapted to address the health impact of cannabis use in e-cigarette devices. Furthermore, use of aerosolized cannabis and cannabis products may become an increasingly common precursor to or outcome of e-cigarette use.

The above-mentioned issues reflect the nuanced and balanced consideration that should be taken with regard to scientific priorities for and policy implications from evidence on the health effects of e-cigarettes. Given how rapidly the e-cigarette product marketplace and user population are changing, there will undoubtedly be many new issues that are currently unknown and will require careful surveillance and scientific scrutiny. The approaches taken by the committee to evaluate the health effects of e-cigarettes in this report are anticipated to provide a generalizable template for future evaluations of the evidence.

REFERENCES

CTP (Center for Tobacco Products). 2017. *FDA announces comprehensive regulatory plan to shift trajectory of tobacco-related disease, death.* https://www.fda.gov/NewsEvents/Newsroom/PressAnnouncements/ucm568923.htm (accessed September 18, 2017).

[1] Swedish Match submitted an MRTP application for a non-combustible tobacco product, Snus, on August 27, 2014.

HHS (U.S. Department of Health and Human Services). 2014. *The health consequences of smoking—50 years of progress: A report of the Surgeon General*. Atlanta, GA: U.S. Department of Health and Human Services, Centers for Disease Control and Prevention, National Center for Disease Prevention and Health Promotion, Office on Smoking and Health.

Johnston, L. D., P. M. O'Malley, R. Miech, J. G. Bachman, and J. E. Schulenberg. 2017. *Monitoring the Future national survey results on drug use, 1975–2016: Overview, key findings on adolescent drug use*. Ann Arbor: Institute for Social Research, University of Michigan.

Leventhal, A. 2016. *Adolescent use of alternative cannabis products: Epidemiology, correlates, and consequences*. Paper presented at the College on Problems of Drug Dependence Annual Meeting, Palm Springs, CA.

Morean, M. E., G. Kong, D. R. Camenga, D. A. Cavallo, and S. Krishnan-Sarin. 2015. High school students' use of electronic cigarettes to vaporize cannabis. *Pediatrics* 136(4): 611–616.

Reuters. 2017. *Philip Morris says it has doubled supply of iQOS tobacco device in Japan*. https://www.reuters.com/article/us-japan-ecigarettes/philip-morris-says-it-has-doubled-supply-of-iqos-tobacco-device-in-japan-idUSKBN1690DX (accessed October 11, 2017).

TAG (Tobacco Advisory Group of the Royal College of Physicians). 2008. *Ending tobacco smoking in Britain: Radical strategies for prevention and harm reduction in nicotine addition*. https://cdn.shopify.com/s/files/1/0924/4392/files/ending-tobacco-smoking.pdf?2801907981964551469 (accessed October 11, 2017).

A

Questions from the Center for Tobacco Products of the Food and Drug Administration Submitted for the Committee's Consideration

SPECIFIC QUESTIONS TO BE CONSIDERED

Health Effects in Users

1. What are the known short- and long-term health effects of electronic cigarettes in users who have not used tobacco products, users of other tobacco products and electronic cigarettes, and users who switch completely from smoking combustible tobacco cigarettes or other combustible tobacco products to using electronic cigarettes?
   a. What unique issues should be considered in the evaluation of the short- and long-term health effects in users of electronic cigarettes in combination with combustible tobacco cigarettes, other combustible products, smokeless tobacco, and other tobacco products?
2. What are the potential short- and long-term health effects of inhaling humectants (e.g., propylene glycol, glycerin), flavorings, and other e-liquid additives or constituents? What are the specific impacts of these constituents on the following systems:
   a. Cardiovascular
   b. Immune
   c. Oropharyngeal (e.g., the oral microbiome)
   d. Pulmonary
   e. Other

3. What biomarkers and clinical endpoints should be used to assess the impact of electronic cigarettes on user health?
4. What other risks are associated with electronic cigarette exposures in users (e.g., overheating or explosion resulting in burn injuries)?

Effects of Electronic Cigarettes on Smoking Cessation

5. Do electronic cigarettes help combustible tobacco cigarette smokers quit smoking?
6. Do cigarette smokers who quit smoking using electronic cigarettes continue using electronic cigarettes, and if so, for how long? Is there evidence that there is relapse of smoking after smokers quit cigarettes and use electronic cigarettes for some time?
7. Do electronic cigarettes promote current smokers to completely switch to electronic cigarette products or is dual or poly-tobacco use common?
8. Does the type of electronic cigarette product used or e-liquid flavor impact any of the above questions in 1A?

Health Effects in Vulnerable Populations

9. What populations of users may be at lower or higher risk of adverse effects related to electronic cigarette use?
10. What unique health effects may be of concern for users with underlying disease (e.g., chronic obstructive pulmonary disease, cardiovascular disease, diabetes mellitus, cancers, mental health disorders)?
11. What factors should be considered in the evaluation of risk in vulnerable populations?

Health Effects in Youth

12. What unique health effects may be of concern in youth e-cigarette users?
13. How should the short- and long-term health risks associated with youth initiation and ongoing use be evaluated?

Health Effects of Use During Pregnancy

14. What are the short- and long-term health effects of e-cigarette use during pregnancy? What is the impact of e-cigarette use during pregnancy on the pregnant woman and on the fetus?

15. How should the short- and long-term effects of e-cigarette use during pregnancy be evaluated?

Health Effects in Non-Users

16. What chemicals/toxicants are delivered to non-users who are exposed to electronic cigarette aerosols?
17. What are the impacts of electronic cigarette use on the levels of particulate matter and chemicals/toxicants from the e-cigarette in enclosed spaces such as cars, homes, office settings, and public buildings?
18. What are the short- and long-term health risks, including cancer and non-cancer–related illnesses, of secondary exposure to electronic cigarette aerosols?
19. What are the short- and long-term health risks, including cancer and non-cancer–related illnesses, of tertiary exposure to electronic cigarette aerosols?
20. What populations of non-users are at higher risk of adverse health effects related to electronic cigarette exposures?
21. What other risks are associated with electronic cigarette exposures in non-users (e.g., overheating or explosion resulting in burn injuries)?
22. What are the hazards associated with inadvertent exposure to electronic cigarettes by young children (e.g., accidental dermal exposure or oral ingestion of liquid nicotine, choking on e-cigarette components, e-cigarette inhalation)?

Research Needs

23. What research should be conducted to evaluate the short- and long-term health effects of electronic cigarettes in users and non-users to better address the questions above?
24. What research on short- and long-term health effects is the highest priority to inform Food and Drug Administration regulation of electronic cigarettes?

B

Search Strategy and Quality Assessment

The Statement of Task charges the committee with conducting a "comprehensive and systematic assessment and review of the literature" on the health effects of e-cigarettes. The committee's approach was informed by published guidelines for conducting systematic reviews as well as the approaches taken by prior National Academies committees (CRD, 2009; Higgins and Green, 2011; IOM, 2008, p. 45, 2011a, pp. 10–24, 2011b, 2016, pp. 8–10; NASEM, 2017; NRC, 2014; OHAT, 2015; Sena et al., 2014; Whiting et al., 2016). For its assessment on the health effects of e-cigarettes, the committee conducted structured reviews of the literature on the effects of e-cigarette exposure on any biological outcome (whether human, animal, or in vitro). Because assessment of the overall public health impact of e-cigarettes requires understanding the relationship between e-cigarettes and combustible tobacco cigarettes, the committee also undertook comprehensive literature reviews of the effects of e-cigarette use on combustible tobacco cigarette smoking initiation and cessation. The committee did not systematically review the health effects of known constituents and contaminants of e-cigarette devices or their refill solutions (e.g., nicotine, certain metals). Because many of these constituents have been widely studied in other settings, the committee draws on existing bodies of evidence to describe potential health effects of these constituent parts. This appendix describes the committee's strategy for identifying and reviewing literature in detail.

LITERATURE SEARCH

The committee conducted a series of searches in six databases—PubMed, Scopus, Web of Science, PsycINFO (ProQuest), MEDLINE (Ovid), and Embase (Ovid)—between February 1, 2017, and August 31, 2017, to identify all literature on e-cigarettes. Due to e-pub ahead of print and online first articles, 2018 citations were captured. In addition, a few 2016 and 2017 studies may not have been captured due to lags and discrepancies in database indexing. The committee applied no limits on date, language, or country to any of its searches. The following sections describe the committee's search strategies to identify literature on the health effects of e-cigarettes and on the e-cigarettes and smoking transitions.

Health Effects of E-Cigarettes

Because the committee is interested primarily in the effects of e-cigarettes as a whole product, rather than the effects of their individual constituent parts, the committee conducted a search to identify literature on human, animal, and in vitro exposure to e-cigarettes. Human epidemiological evidence provides the strongest evidence, but due to the lack of available human studies, the committee also chose to review animal and in vitro exposure to e-cigarettes from which they could draw informed inferences. The committee's initial search included all literature pertaining to e-cigarette exposures and was conducted as a series of six searches between February 1, 2017, and February 6, 2017. The search was conducted in five databases—PubMed, Scopus, Web of Science, PsycINFO (ProQuest), and MEDLINE (Ovid). All literature on e-cigarettes used the following key words and phrases: e-cigarette, e-cigarettes, "electronic cigarette," "electronic cigarettes," "electronic nicotine delivery," "electronic nicotine device," vape, vaping, and e-liquid. (The committee excluded the term "e-liquid" from searches in Scopus and Web of Science, which are multidisciplinary databases, where the term "e-liquid" produced results related to geothermal energy.) Searches in PubMed and MEDLINE also used the Medical Subject Headings (MeSH) term "electronic cigarettes." This initial series of searches identified 3,494 unique results. The complete search syntax can be found in Boxes B-1A through B-1F. Titles and abstracts for all references were reviewed using inclusion criteria developed through a preliminary title and abstract review process. The final inclusion criteria for human, animal, and in vitro studies are listed in Box B-2.

The committee conducted a special search to identify literature on e-cigarette use and dependence. The search was conducted between July 14, 2017, and August 31, 2017, in the same five databases as the initial search. In addition to the e-cigarette terms described above, the committee added the following terms: dependence, withdrawal, craving, appeal, addition, "abuse liability," "subjective effects, "smoking urge," "urge to smoke," "smoking desire," and "desire to smoke." In PubMed and MEDLINE, they also used the MeSH terms "tobacco use disorder," "substance withdrawal syndrome," and "craving." The complete search syntax can be found in Box B-3. This initial search identified 957 unique results. Titles and abstracts were reviewed for all literature that included an assessment of dependence using a validated instrument.

E-Cigarettes and Transitions to and from Combustible Tobacco Cigarette Smoking

To identify literature on the effects of e-cigarette use on smoking transitions (initiation and cessation), the committee conducted a series of subsearches within its initial search to identify epidemiological and experimental data on these smoking transitions. To do so, the committee added terms to the original search to restrict results to smoking transition outcomes of interest. Additionally, because there are many recent, systematic reviews on the effects of e-cigarettes on smoking initiation and cessation but few original studies, the committee chose to assess first these review articles rather than duplicating these efforts. The committee then complemented the evidence identified through these reviews with new studies published after the search dates of the most recent literature reviews, and also met the most rigorous inclusion/exclusion criteria used in the existing, prior systematic reviews.

To identify literature on smoking initiation, the key terms "smoking initiation" and "initiation" were added to the e-cigarette terms described in the section above. This search included all literature published through May 4, 2017, in six databases—PubMed, Scopus, Web of Science, PsycINFO (ProQuest), MEDLINE (Ovid), and Embase (Ovid). The complete search syntax can be found in Box B-4. The committee applied no limits on date, language, or country, and the search yielded 138 unique studies.

The committee conducted two searches on smoking cessation, one limited to reviews, and one limited to original, peer-reviewed research. The search of systematic reviews published through March 1, 2017, was conducted in seven databases—PubMed, Scopus, Web of Science, PsycINFO (ProQuest), MEDLINE (Ovid), Embase (Ovid), and Cochrane (Ovid). The key terms "smoking cessation" and "cessation," and the MeSH term "smoking cessation" were added to the e-cigarette terms described above. The committee applied no limits on date, language, or country. This search produced 209 unique results. The search of primary literature published through May 3, 2017, was conducted in six databases—PubMed, Scopus, Web of Science, PsycINFO, MEDLINE (Ovid),

BOX B-1A
Search Strategy for E-Cigarettes in Human Populations

PubMed:
"e-cigarette" OR "e-cigarettes" OR "electronic cigarette" OR "electronic cigarettes" OR "electronic nicotine delivery" OR "electronic nicotine device" OR "vape" OR "vaping" OR "e-liquid" OR "Electronic Cigarettes" [MeSH]
Limit: Humans
Limit: Peer-Reviewed Journal Article
Results: 1,060

Scopus:
TITLE-ABS-KEY ("e-cigarette" OR "e-cigarettes" OR "electronic cigarette" OR "electronic cigarettes" OR "electronic nicotine delivery" OR "electronic nicotine device" OR "vape" OR "vaping") AND NOT TITLE-ABS-KEY (animal OR animals OR mice OR mouse OR rat OR rats)
Source Type: Journal
Document Type: Article, Review, Article in Press, Erratum
Note: Scopus is a multidisciplinary database. The term "e-liquid" produced results related to geothermal energy.
Results: 1,724

Web of Science:
TS=("e-cigarette" OR "e-cigarettes" OR "electronic cigarette" OR "electronic cigarettes" OR "electronic nicotine delivery" OR "electronic nicotine device" OR "vape" OR "vaping") NOT TS=(animal OR animals OR mice OR mouse OR rat OR rats)
Document Type: Article
Note: Web of Science is a multidisciplinary database. The term "e-liquid" produced results related to geothermal energy.
Results: 1,036

PsycINFO (ProQuest):
"e-cigarette" OR "e-cigarettes" OR "electronic cigarette" OR "electronic cigarettes" OR "electronic nicotine delivery" OR "electronic nicotine device" OR "vape" OR "vaping" OR "e-liquid" OR SU.EXACT ("Electronic Cigarettes")
Population: Human
Source Type: Scholarly Journals; Peer-Reviewed
Record Type:
Include: Journal, Peer-Reviewed Journal, Journal Article
Exclude: Comment/Reply, Editorial, Letter, Column/Opinion, Review-Book
Results: 617

MEDLINE (Ovid):

Search No.	Search Syntax
1	(e-cigarette or e-cigarettes or electronic cigarette or electronic cigarettes or electronic nicotine delivery or electronic nicotine device or vape or vaping or e-liquid).ti,ab.
2	Electronic Cigarettes/
3	1 or 2
4	3
5	limit 4 to humans
6	limit 5 to (case reports or clinical study or clinical trial, all or clinical trial, phase i or clinical trial, phase ii or clinical trial, phase iii or clinical trial, phase iv or clinical trial or comparative study or controlled clinical trial or "corrected and republished article" or evaluation studies or historical article or introductory journal article or journal article or meta-analysis or multicenter study or observational study or pragmatic clinical trial or published erratum or randomized controlled trial or "review" or "scientific integrity review" or systematic reviews or technical report or twin study or validation studies)

Results: 1,058

Totals:
Citations Downloaded: 5,495
After Removing Duplicates: 2,094

BOX B-1B
Search Strategy for E-Cigarettes in In Vivo Animal Populations

PubMed:
"e-cigarette" OR "e-cigarettes" OR "electronic cigarette" OR "electronic cigarettes" OR "electronic nicotine delivery" OR "electronic nicotine device" OR "vape" OR "vaping" OR "e-liquid" OR "Electronic Cigarettes" [MeSH]
Limit: Other Animals
Limit: Peer-Reviewed Journal Article
Results: 68

Scopus:
TITLE-ABS-KEY ("e-cigarette" OR "e-cigarettes" OR "electronic cigarette" OR "electronic cigarettes" OR "electronic nicotine delivery" OR "electronic nicotine device" OR "vape" OR "vaping") AND TITLE-ABS-KEY (animal OR animals OR mice OR mouse OR rat OR rats)
Note: Scopus is a multidisciplinary database. The term "e-liquid" produced results related to geothermal energy.
Source Type: Journal
Document Type: Article, Review, Article in Press, Erratum
Results: 88

Web of Science:
TS=("e-cigarette" OR "e-cigarettes" OR "electronic cigarette" OR "electronic cigarettes" OR "electronic nicotine delivery" OR "electronic nicotine device" OR "vape" OR "vaping") AND TS=(animal OR animals OR mice OR mouse OR rat OR rats)
Note: Web of Science is a multidisciplinary database. The term "e-liquid" produced results related to geothermal energy
Document Type: Article
Results: 62

PsycINFO (ProQuest):
"e-cigarette" OR "e-cigarettes" OR "electronic cigarette" OR "electronic cigarettes" OR "electronic nicotine delivery" OR "electronic nicotine device" OR "vape" OR "vaping" OR "e-liquid" OR SU.EXACT ("Electronic Cigarettes")
Population: Animal
Source Type: Scholarly Journals; Peer-Reviewed
Record Type:
Include: Journal, Peer-Reviewed Journal, Journal Article
Exclude: Comment/Reply, Editorial, Letter, Column/Opinion, Review-Book
Results: 21

MEDLINE (Ovid):

Search No.	Search Syntax
1	(e-cigarette or e-cigarettes or electronic cigarette or electronic cigarettes or electronic nicotine delivery or electronic nicotine device or vape or vaping or e-liquid).ti,ab.
2	Electronic Cigarettes/
3	1 or 2
4	3
5	limit 4 to (animals and (case reports or clinical study or clinical trial, all or clinical trial, phase i or clinical trial, phase ii or clinical trial, phase iii or clinical trial, phase iv or clinical trial or comparative study or controlled clinical trial or "corrected and republished article" or duplicate publication or evaluation studies or historical article or introductory journal article or journal article or meta-analysis or multicenter study or observational study or pragmatic clinical trial or published erratum or randomized controlled trial or "review" or "scientific integrity review" or systematic reviews or technical report or twin study or validation studies))

Results: 56

Totals:
Citations Downloaded: 295
After Removing Duplicates: 133

BOX B-1C
Search Strategy for E-Cigarettes in In Vitro Populations

PubMed:
("e-cigarette" OR "e-cigarettes" OR "electronic cigarette" OR "electronic cigarettes" OR "electronic nicotine delivery" OR "electronic nicotine device" OR "vape" OR "vaping" OR "e-liquid" OR "Electronic Cigarettes" [MeSH]) AND ("In Vitro Techniques" [MeSH] OR "in vitro")
Limit: Other Animals
Limit: Peer-Reviewed Journal Article
Results: 46

Scopus:
TITLE-ABS-KEY ("e-cigarette" OR "e-cigarettes" OR "electronic cigarette" OR "electronic cigarettes" OR "electronic nicotine delivery" OR "electronic nicotine device" OR "vape" OR "vaping") AND TITLE-ABS-KEY ("in vitro")
Note: Scopus is a multidisciplinary database. The term "e-liquid" produced results related to geothermal energy.
Source Type: Journal
Document Type: Article, Review, Article in Press, Erratum
Results: 40

Web of Science:
TS=("e-cigarette" OR "e-cigarettes" OR "electronic cigarette" OR "electronic cigarettes" OR "electronic nicotine delivery" OR "electronic nicotine device" OR "vape" OR "vaping") AND TS=("in vitro")
Note: Web of Science is a multidisciplinary database. The term "e-liquid" produced results related to geothermal energy.
Document Type: Article
Results: 42

PsycINFO (ProQuest):
("e-cigarette" OR "e-cigarettes" OR "electronic cigarette" OR "electronic cigarettes" OR "electronic nicotine delivery" OR "electronic nicotine device" OR "vape" OR "vaping" OR "e-liquid" OR SU.EXACT ("Electronic Cigarettes")) and ("in vitro")
Source Type: Scholarly Journals; Peer-Reviewed
Record Type:
Include: Journal, Peer-Reviewed Journal, Journal Article
Exclude: Comment/Reply, Editorial, Letter, Column/Opinion, Review-Book
Results: 6

MEDLINE (Ovid):

Search No.	Search Syntax
1	(e-cigarette or e-cigarettes or electronic cigarette or electronic cigarettes or electronic nicotine delivery or electronic nicotine device or vape or vaping or e-liquid).ti,ab.
2	Electronic Cigarettes/
3	1 or 2
4	In Vitro Techniques/
5	in vitro.ti,ab.
6	or/4–5
7	3 and 6
8	limit 7 to (case reports or classical article or clinical study or clinical trial, all or clinical trial, phase i or clinical trial, phase ii or clinical trial, phase iii or clinical trial, phase iv or clinical trial or comparative study or controlled clinical trial or "corrected and republished article" or duplicate publication or evaluation studies or historical article or introductory journal article or journal article or meta-analysis or multicenter study or observational study or pragmatic clinical trial or published erratum or randomized controlled trial or "review" or "scientific integrity review" or systematic reviews or technical report or twin study or validation studies)

Results: 17

Totals:
Citations Downloaded: 151
After Removing Duplicates: 73

BOX B1-D
Search Syntax for E-Cigarettes with No Population Limits, Excluding Results from Earlier Searches (Boxes B-1A, B-1B, B-1C)

PubMed:
No Population Limit:
("e-cigarette" OR "e-cigarettes" OR "electronic cigarette" OR "electronic cigarettes" OR "electronic nicotine delivery" OR "electronic nicotine device" OR "vape" OR "vaping" OR "e-liquid" OR "Electronic Cigarettes" [MeSH])
Limit: Peer-Reviewed Journal Article
Results: 1,910

Humans:
"e-cigarette" OR "e-cigarettes" OR "electronic cigarette" OR "electronic cigarettes" OR "electronic nicotine delivery" OR "electronic nicotine device" OR "vape" OR "vaping" OR "e-liquid" OR "Electronic Cigarettes" [MeSH]
Limit: Humans
Limit: Peer-Reviewed Journal Article
Results: 1,060

Animals:
"e-cigarette" OR "e-cigarettes" OR "electronic cigarette" OR "electronic cigarettes" OR "electronic nicotine delivery" OR "electronic nicotine device" OR "vape" OR "vaping" OR "e-liquid" OR "Electronic Cigarettes" [MeSH]
Limit: Other Animals
Limit: Peer-Reviewed Journal Article
Results: 68

In Vitro:
("e-cigarette" OR "e-cigarettes" OR "electronic cigarette" OR "electronic cigarettes" OR "electronic nicotine delivery" OR "electronic nicotine device" OR "vape" OR "vaping" OR "e-liquid" OR "Electronic Cigarettes" [MeSH]) AND ("In Vitro Techniques" [MeSH] OR "in vitro")
Limit: Peer-Reviewed Journal Article
Results: 46

Animals + Humans + In Vitro = 1,174
No Population – (Animals + Humans + In Vitro) = 736

Scopus:
No Population Limit:
TITLE-ABS-KEY ("e-cigarette" OR "e-cigarettes" OR "electronic cigarette" OR "electronic cigarettes" OR "electronic nicotine delivery" OR "electronic nicotine device" OR "vape" OR "vaping")
Source Type: Journal
Document Type: Article, Review, Article in Press, Erratum
Results: 1,814

Humans:
TITLE-ABS-KEY ("e-cigarette" OR "e-cigarettes" OR "electronic cigarette" OR "electronic cigarettes" OR "electronic nicotine delivery" OR "electronic nicotine device" OR "vape" OR "vaping") AND NOT TITLE-ABS-KEY (animal OR animals OR mice OR mouse OR rat OR rats)
Source Type: Journal
Document Type: Article, Review, Article in Press, Erratum
Results: 1,727

Animals:
TITLE-ABS-KEY ("e-cigarette" OR "e-cigarettes" OR "electronic cigarette" OR "electronic cigarettes" OR "electronic nicotine delivery" OR "electronic nicotine device" OR "vape" OR "vaping") AND TITLE-ABS-KEY (animal OR animals OR mice OR mouse OR rat OR rats)
Source Type: Journal
Document Type: Article, Review, Article in Press, Erratum
Results: 87

In Vitro:
TITLE-ABS-KEY ("e-cigarette" OR "e-cigarettes" OR "electronic cigarette" OR "electronic cigarettes" OR "electronic nicotine delivery" OR "electronic nicotine device" OR "vape" OR "vaping") AND TITLE-ABS-KEY ("in vitro")
Source Type: Journal
Document Type: Article, Review, Article in Press, Erratum
Results: 40

Animals + Humans + In Vitro = 1,854
No Population – (Animals + Humans + In Vitro) = no additional results

Web of Science:
No Population:
TS=("e-cigarette" OR "e-cigarettes" OR "electronic cigarette" OR "electronic cigarettes" OR "electronic nicotine delivery" OR "electronic nicotine device" OR "vape" OR "vaping")
Document Type: Article
Results: 1,101

Animals:
TS=("e-cigarette" OR "e-cigarettes" OR "electronic cigarette" OR "electronic cigarettes" OR "electronic nicotine delivery" OR "electronic nicotine device" OR "vape" OR "vaping") AND TS=(animal OR animals OR mice OR mouse OR rat OR rats)
Document Type: Article
Results: 62

Humans:
TS=("e-cigarette" OR "e-cigarettes" OR "electronic cigarette" OR "electronic cigarettes" OR "electronic nicotine delivery" OR "electronic nicotine device" OR "vape" OR "vaping") NOT TS=(animal OR animals OR mice OR mouse OR rat OR rats)
Document Type: Article
Results: 1,039

continued

BOX B1-D Continued

In Vitro:
TS=("e-cigarette" OR "e-cigarettes" OR "electronic cigarette" OR "electronic cigarettes" OR "electronic nicotine delivery" OR "electronic nicotine device" OR "vape" OR "vaping") AND TS=("in vitro")
Document Type: Article
Results: 42

Animals + Humans + In Vitro = 1,140
No Population – (Animals + Humans + In Vitro) = no additional results

PsycINFO (ProQuest):
No Population:
"e-cigarette" OR "e-cigarettes" OR "electronic cigarette" OR "electronic cigarettes" OR "electronic nicotine delivery" OR "electronic nicotine device" OR "vape" OR "vaping" OR "e-liquid" OR SU.EXACT ("Electronic Cigarettes")
Source Type: Scholarly Journals; Peer-Reviewed
Results: 779

Animals:
"e-cigarette" OR "e-cigarettes" OR "electronic cigarette" OR "electronic cigarettes" OR "electronic nicotine delivery" OR "electronic nicotine device" OR "vape" OR "vaping" OR "e-liquid" OR SU.EXACT ("Electronic Cigarettes")
Population: Animal
Results: 21

Humans:
"e-cigarette" OR "e-cigarettes" OR "electronic cigarette" OR "electronic cigarettes" OR "electronic nicotine delivery" OR "electronic nicotine device" OR "vape" OR "vaping" OR "e-liquid" OR SU.EXACT ("Electronic Cigarettes")
Population: Human
Source Type: Scholarly Journals; Peer-Reviewed
Results: 721

In Vitro:
("e-cigarette" OR "e-cigarettes" OR "electronic cigarette" OR "electronic cigarettes" OR "electronic nicotine delivery" OR "electronic nicotine device" OR "vape" OR "vaping" OR "e-liquid" OR SU.EXACT ("Electronic Cigarettes")) and ("in vitro")
Source Type: Scholarly Journals; Peer-Reviewed
Results: 6

Animals + Humans + In Vitro = 748
No Population – (Animals + Humans + In Vitro) = 31

MEDLINE (Ovid):
No Population:

Search No.	Search Syntax
1	(e-cigarette or e-cigarettes or electronic cigarette or electronic cigarettes or electronic nicotine delivery or electronic nicotine device or vape or vaping or e-liquid).ti,ab.
2	Electronic Cigarettes/
3	1 or 2
4	3
5	limit 4 to (case reports or clinical study or clinical trial, all or clinical trial, phase i or clinical trial, phase ii or clinical trial, phase iii or clinical trial, phase iv or clinical trial or comparative study or controlled clinical trial or “corrected and republished article” or evaluation studies or historical article or introductory journal article or journal article or meta-analysis or multicenter study or observational study or pragmatic clinical trial or published erratum or randomized controlled trial or “review” or “scientific integrity review” or systematic reviews or technical report or twin study or validation studies)

Results: 1,144

Animals:

Search No.	Search Syntax
1	(e-cigarette or e-cigarettes or electronic cigarette or electronic cigarettes or electronic nicotine delivery or electronic nicotine device or vape or vaping or e-liquid).ti,ab.
2	Electronic Cigarettes/
3	1 or 2
4	3
5	limit 4 to (animals and (case reports or clinical study or clinical trial, all or clinical trial, phase i or clinical trial, phase ii or clinical trial, phase iii or clinical trial, phase iv or clinical trial or comparative study or controlled clinical trial or “corrected and republished article” or duplicate publication or evaluation studies or historical article or introductory journal article or journal article or meta-analysis or multicenter study or observational study or pragmatic clinical trial or published erratum or randomized controlled trial or “review” or “scientific integrity review” or systematic reviews or technical report or twin study or validation studies))

Results: 56

continued

BOX B1-D Continued

Humans:

Search No.	Search Syntax
1	(e-cigarette or e-cigarettes or electronic cigarette or electronic cigarettes or electronic nicotine delivery or electronic nicotine device or vape or vaping or e-liquid).ti,ab.
2	Electronic Cigarettes/
3	1 or 2
4	3
5	limit 4 to humans
6	limit 5 to (case reports or clinical study or clinical trial, all or clinical trial, phase I or clinical trial, phase ii or clinical trial, phase iii or clinical trial, phase iv or clinical trial or comparative study or controlled clinical trial or "corrected and republished article" or evaluation studies or historical article or introductory journal article or journal article or meta-analysis or multicenter study or observational study or pragmatic clinical trial or published erratum or randomized controlled trial or "review" or "scientific integrity review" or systematic reviews or technical report or twin study or validation studies)

Results: 1,058

In Vitro:

Search No.	Search Syntax
1	(e-cigarette or e-cigarettes or electronic cigarette or electronic cigarettes or electronic nicotine delivery or electronic nicotine device or vape or vaping or e-liquid).ti,ab.
2	Electronic Cigarettes/

3	1 or 2
4	In Vitro Techniques/
5	in vitro.ti,ab.
6	or/4–5
7	3 and 6
8	limit 7 to (case reports or classical article or clinical study or clinical trial, all or clinical trial, phase i or clinical trial, phase ii or clinical trial, phase iii or clinical trial, phase iv or clinical trial or comparative study or controlled clinical trial or "corrected and republished article" or duplicate publication or evaluation studies or historical article or introductory journal article or journal article or meta-analysis or multicenter study or observational study or pragmatic clinical trial or published erratum or randomized controlled trial or "review" or "scientific integrity review" or systematic reviews or technical report or twin study or validation studies)

Results: 17

Animals + Humans + In Vitro = 1,131
No Population – (Animals + Humans + In Vitro) = 13

EndNote Totals:
Animals Exposure: 133
Humans Exposure: 2,094
In Vitro: 73
No Population Limit: 780
After removing duplicates and comparing No Population to Animals, Humans + In Vitro: 265

BOX B-1E
Search Syntax for E-Cigarettes and Dermal and Ingestion Exposure

PubMed:
("e-cigarette" OR "e-cigarettes" OR "electronic cigarette" OR "electronic cigarettes" OR "electronic nicotine delivery" OR "electronic nicotine device" OR "vape" OR "vaping" OR "e-liquid" OR "Electronic Cigarettes" [MeSH]) AND ("Poisoning" [MeSH] OR dermal OR ingestion OR poison OR poisoning or ingest)
Results: 78

Scopus:
TITLE-ABS-KEY ("e-cigarette" OR "e-cigarettes" OR "electronic cigarette" OR "electronic cigarettes" OR "electronic nicotine delivery" OR "electronic nicotine device" OR "vape" OR "vaping") AND TITLE-ABS-KEY (poisoning OR poison OR dermal OR ingestion OR ingest)
Results: 63

Web of Science:
TS=("e-cigarette" OR "e-cigarettes" OR "electronic cigarette" OR "electronic cigarettes" OR "electronic nicotine delivery" OR "electronic nicotine device" OR "vape" OR "vaping") AND TS=(poisoning OR poison OR dermal OR ingestion OR ingest)
Results: 58

PsycINFO (ProQuest):
"e-cigarette" OR "e-cigarettes" OR "electronic cigarette" OR "electronic cigarettes" OR "electronic nicotine delivery" OR "electronic nicotine device" OR "vape" OR "vaping" OR "e-liquid" OR SU.EXACT ("Electronic Cigarettes") AND (poisoning OR poison OR dermal OR ingestion OR ingest)
Results: 21

MEDLINE (Ovid):

Search No.	Search Syntax
1	(e-cigarette or e-cigarettes or electronic cigarette or electronic cigarettes or electronic nicotine delivery or electronic nicotine device or vape or vaping or e-liquid).ti,ab.
2	Electronic Cigarettes/
3	1 or 2
4	3
5	Poisoning/
6	(dermal or ingestion or poison or poisoning or ingest).ti,ab.
7	or/5–6
8	4 and 7

Results: 29

Totals:
Citations Downloaded: 249
After Removing Duplicates: 124

BOX B-1F
Search Syntax for E-Cigarettes with No Limit on Population or Publication, Excluding Results from Prior Searches (see Boxes B-1A, B-1B, B-1C, B-1D, B-1E)

PubMed
("e-cigarette" OR "e-cigarettes" OR "electronic cigarette" OR "electronic cigarettes" OR "electronic nicotine delivery" OR "electronic nicotine device" OR "vape" OR "vaping" OR "e-liquid" OR "Electronic Cigarettes" [MeSH])
Results: 2,304

Scopus:
TITLE-ABS-KEY ("e-cigarette" OR "e-cigarettes" OR "electronic cigarette" OR "electronic cigarettes" OR "electronic nicotine delivery" OR "electronic nicotine device" OR "vape" OR "vaping")
Results: 2,597

Web of Science:
TS=("e-cigarette" OR "e-cigarettes" OR "electronic cigarette" OR "electronic cigarettes" OR "electronic nicotine delivery" OR "electronic nicotine device" OR "vape" OR "vaping")
Results: 2,013

PsycINFO (ProQuest):
"e-cigarette" OR "e-cigarettes" OR "electronic cigarette" OR "electronic cigarettes" OR "electronic nicotine delivery" OR "electronic nicotine device" OR "vape" OR "vaping" OR "e-liquid" OR SU.EXACT ("Electronic Cigarettes")
Results: 804

MEDLINE (Ovid):

Search No.	Search Syntax
1	(e-cigarette or e-cigarettes or electronic cigarette or electronic cigarettes or electronic nicotine delivery or electronic nicotine device or vape or vaping or e-liquid).ti,ab.
2	Electronic Cigarettes/
3	1 or 2
4	3

Results: 1,493

Totals:
Total Citations Downloaded: 9,211
After Removing Duplicates Compared to All Populations, Peer-Reviewed Literature: 805

BOX B-2
Inclusion Criteria for the Literature Review on the Health Effects of E-Cigarettes

Human Studies:

- Human subjects
- Exposure: e-cigarettes or e-cigarette product/s (e.g., e-liquid, aerosol)—primary, secondary, tertiary
- Outcome: Any physiological response or biological effect—such as biomarkers of exposure, biomarkers of risk, adverse events (including self-reported symptoms, injury), disease endpoints (including mental health)
- Peer-reviewed, original research

Animal Studies:

- (Other) animal subjects
- Exposure: e-cigarettes or e-cigarette product/s (e.g., e-liquid, aerosol)—primary, secondary, tertiary
- Outcome: Any physiological response or biological effect—including biomarkers of exposure, biomarkers of risk, adverse events (including self-reported symptoms, injury), disease endpoints (including behavioral changes)
- Peer-reviewed, original research

In Vitro Studies:

- Human or animal cells
- Exposure: e-cigarettes or e-cigarette product/s (e.g., e-liquid, aerosol)—primary, secondary, tertiary
- Outcome: Any physiological response or biological effect—cytotoxicity, etc.
- Peer-reviewed, original research

BOX B-3
Search Syntax for E-Cigarettes and Dependence

Search Syntax:
MEDLINE (Ovid):

Search No.	Syntax	Results
1	(e-cigarette or e-cigarettes or electronic cigarette or electronic cigarettes or electronic nicotine delivery or electronic nicotine device or vape or vaping or e-liquid).ti,ab.	1,668
2	Electronic Cigarettes/	1,306
3	1 or 2	1,787
4	"Tobacco Use Disorder"/	10,292
5	Substance Withdrawal Syndrome/	20,572
6	Craving/	676
7	(dependence or withdrawal or craving or appeal or addiction).ti,ab.	257,569
8	(smok* adj3 urge).ti,ab.	283
9	(smok* adj3 desire).ti,ab.	317
10	"abuse liability".ti,ab.	970
11	"subjective effects".ti,ab.	1,686
12	or/4–11	269,923
13	3 and 12	370
14	limit 13 to (comment or editorial or letter)	37
15	13 not 14	333

Embase (Ovid):

Search No.	Syntax	Results
1	(e-cigarette or e-cigarettes or electronic cigarette or electronic cigarettes or electronic nicotine delivery or electronic nicotine device or vape or vaping or e-liquid).ti,ab.	2,749
2	electronic cigarette/	2,754
3	withdrawal syndrome/ or tobacco dependence/	43,252
4	addiction/	49,320
5	(dependence or withdrawal or appeal or addiction).ti,ab.	352,865
6	crav*.ti,ab.	10,313
7	(smok* adj3 urge).ti,ab.	354
8	(smok* adj3 desire).ti,ab.	418
9	"abuse liability".ti,ab.	1,389
10	"subjective effects".ti,ab.	2,256
11	1 or 2	3,159
12	or/3–10	406,827
13	11 and 12	722
14	limit 13 to (editorial or letter or note)	136
15	13 not 14	586

continued

BOX B-3 Continued

PubMed:
Note: PubMed does not perform adjacency searching
("e-cigarette" OR "e-cigarettes" OR "electronic cigarette" OR "electronic cigarettes" OR "electronic nicotine delivery" OR "electronic nicotine device" OR "vape" OR "vaping" OR "e-liquid" OR "Electronic Cigarettes" [MeSH]) AND ("Tobacco Use Disorder" [MeSH] OR "Substance Withdrawal Syndrome" [MeSH] OR "Craving" [MeSH] OR dependence or withdrawal or craving or appeal or addiction OR "abuse liability" OR "subjective effects" OR "smoking urge" OR "urge to smoke" OR "smoking desire" OR "desire to smoke")
Results: 565

Scopus:
TITLE-ABS-KEY ("e-cigarette" OR "e-cigarettes" OR "electronic cigarette" OR "electronic cigarettes" OR "electronic nicotine delivery" OR "electronic nicotine device" OR "vape" OR "vaping") AND TITLE-ABS-KEY (dependence OR withdrawal OR craving OR appeal OR addiction OR "abuse liability" OR "subjective effects" OR (smok* w/3 urge) OR (smok* w/3 desire))
Results: 489

Web of Science:
TS=("e-cigarette" OR "e-cigarettes" OR "electronic cigarette" OR "electronic cigarettes" OR "electronic nicotine delivery" OR "electronic nicotine device" OR "vape" OR "vaping") AND TS=(dependence OR withdrawal OR craving OR appeal OR addiction OR "abuse liability" OR "subjective effects" OR (smok* NEAR/3 urge) OR (smok* NEAR/3 desire))
Results: 341

PsycINFO (ProQuest):
("e-cigarette" OR "e-cigarettes" OR "electronic cigarette" OR "electronic cigarettes" OR "electronic nicotine delivery" OR "electronic nicotine device" OR "vape" OR "vaping" OR "e-liquid" OR SU.EXACT ("Electronic Cigarettes")) AND (ti(dependence OR withdrawal OR craving OR appeal OR addiction OR "abuse liability" OR "subjective effects" OR (smok* NEAR/3 urge) OR (smok* NEAR/3 desire)) OR ab(dependence OR withdrawal OR craving OR appeal OR addiction OR "abuse liability" OR "subjective effects" OR (smok* NEAR/3 urge) OR (smok* NEAR/3 desire)))
Results: 246

Total:
Results After Removing Duplicates: 957

BOX B-4
Search Syntax for E-Cigarettes and Combustible Tobacco Cigarette Smoking Initiation

Search Strategy:

Scopus:

TITLE-ABS-KEY ("e-cigarette" OR "e-cigarettes" OR "electronic cigarette" OR "electronic cigarettes" OR "electronic nicotine delivery" OR "electronic nicotine device" OR "vape" OR "vaping") AND TITLE-ABS-KEY ("smoking initiation" OR initiation)

Results: 81

Web of Science:

TS=("e-cigarette" OR "e-cigarettes" OR "electronic cigarette" OR "electronic cigarettes" OR "electronic nicotine delivery" OR "electronic nicotine device" OR "vape" OR "vaping") AND TS=("smoking initiation" OR initiation)

Results: 86

PsycINFO (ProQuest):

("e-cigarette" OR "e-cigarettes" OR "electronic cigarette" OR "electronic cigarettes" OR "electronic nicotine delivery" OR "electronic nicotine device" OR "vape" OR "vaping" OR "e-liquid" OR SU.EXACT ("Electronic Cigarettes")) AND (ti("smoking initiation" OR initiation) OR ab("smoking initiation" OR initiation))

Results: 46

MEDLINE (Ovid):

Search No.	Search Syntax	Results
1	(e-cigarette or e-cigarettes or electronic cigarette or electronic cigarettes or electronic nicotine delivery or electronic nicotine device or vape or vaping or e-liquid).ti,ab.	1,548
2	Electronic Cigarettes/	1,193
3	1 or 2	1,657
4	3	1,657
5	(smoking adj initiation).ti,ab.	1,179
6	initiation.ti,ab.	175,727
7	or/5–6	175,727
8	4 and 7	42
9	limit 8 to (meta-analysis or "review" or systematic reviews)	12
10	limit 8 to (comment or editorial or letter)	0
11	8 not (9 or 10)	30

Results: 42

continued

BOX B-4 Continued

Embase (Ovid):

Search No.	Search Syntax	Results
1	(e-cigarette or e-cigarettes or electronic cigarette or electronic cigarettes or electronic nicotine delivery or electronic nicotine device or vape or vaping or e-liquid).ti,ab.	2,389
2	Electronic Cigarettes/	1,900
3	1 or 2	2,659
4	3	2,659
5	(smoking adj initiation).ti,ab.	1,410
6	initiation.ti,ab.	247,094
7	or/5–6	247,094
8	4 and 7	77
9	limit 8 to (meta-analysis or "systematic review")	3
10	limit 8 to (editorial or erratum or letter or note)	1
11	8 not (9 or 10)	73

Results: 77

PubMed:

("e-cigarette" OR "e-cigarettes" OR "electronic cigarette" OR "electronic cigarettes" OR "electronic nicotine delivery" OR "electronic nicotine device" OR "vape" OR "vaping" OR "e-liquid" OR "Electronic Cigarettes" [MeSH]) AND ("smoking initiation" OR initiation)

Results: 75

Totals:

Total Citations Downloaded: 407

After Removing Duplicates: 138

and Embase (Ovid). The key terms "smoking cessation," "cessation," "quit," and "abstinence" and the MeSH term "smoking cessation" were added to the e-cigarette terms from the original search, and the committee applied no limits on date, language, or country. The complete search syntax can be found in Boxes B-5 and B-6. This search yielded 1,759 unique results.

Finally, the committee conducted a search of literature on e-cigarette exposure and smoking reduction. For this search, the key terms "smoking reduction" and "harm reduction" were added to the e-cigarette terms described in the section above. This search included all literature published through May 4, 2017, in six databases—PubMed, Scopus, Web of Science, PsycINFO (ProQuest), MEDLINE (Ovid), and Embase (Ovid).

BOX B-5
Search Syntax for Systematic Reviews and Meta-Analyses on E-Cigarettes and Combustible Tobacco Cigarette Smoking Cessation

PubMed:
("e-cigarette" OR "e-cigarettes" OR "electronic cigarette" OR "electronic cigarettes" OR "electronic nicotine delivery" OR "electronic nicotine device" OR "vape" OR "vaping" OR "e-liquid" OR "Electronic Cigarettes" [MeSH]) AND ("Smoking Cessation" [MeSH] OR "smoking cessation" OR cessation)
Limit: Meta-Analysis, Systematic Reviews
Results: 53

Scopus:
TITLE-ABS-KEY ("e-cigarette" OR "e-cigarettes" OR "electronic cigarette" OR "electronic cigarettes" OR "electronic nicotine delivery" OR "electronic nicotine device" OR "vape" OR "vaping") AND TITLE-ABS-KEY ("smoking cessation" OR cessation)
Source Type: Journal
Document Type: Review
Results: 143

Web of Science:
TS=("e-cigarette" OR "e-cigarettes" OR "electronic cigarette" OR "electronic cigarettes" OR "electronic nicotine delivery" OR "electronic nicotine device" OR "vape" OR "vaping") AND TS=("smoking cessation" OR cessation)
Document Type: Review
Results: 57

PsycINFO (ProQuest):
("e-cigarette" OR "e-cigarettes" OR "electronic cigarette" OR "electronic cigarettes" OR "electronic nicotine delivery" OR "electronic nicotine device" OR "vape" OR "vaping" OR "e-liquid" OR SU.EXACT ("Electronic Cigarettes")) AND (SU.EXACT ("Smoking Cessation") OR "smoking cessation" OR cessation)
Source Type: Scholarly Journals; Peer-Reviewed
Methodology: Literature Review, Meta-Analysis, Meta-Synthesis, Systematic Review
Results: 22

continued

BOX B-5 Continued

MEDLINE, Embase, Cochrane (Ovid):

Search No.	Search Syntax
1	electronic cigarette/
2	(e-cigarette or e-cigarettes or electronic cigarette or electronic cigarettes or electronic nicotine delivery or electronic nicotine device or vape or vaping or e-liquid).ti,ab.
3	or/1–2
4	smoking cessation/
5	"smoking cessation".ti,ab.
6	cessation.ti,ab.
7	or/4–6
8	3 and 7
9	limit 8 to (meta-analysis or systematic reviews)

MEDLINE Results: 31
Embase Results: 44
Cochrane Results: 1

Totals:
Citations Downloaded: 351
After Removing Duplicates: 209

The complete search syntax can be found in Box B-7. The committee applied no limits on date, language, or country. This search yielded 455 unique results.

Literature Updates

After the initial searches, the committee continued to collect literature through the end date of August 31, 2017. A total of 641 unique results were identified.

QUALITY ASSESSMENT

Each relevant study was reviewed and assessed by committee members. The committee began by identifying what questions the literature addresses and then assessed the extent to which each study was able to answer each question of interest. In their assessment, the committee considered study design, elements of study design, study results, and other potential sources of conflict of interest or bias. Where committee members co-authored studies to be assessed, committee members who

BOX B-6
Search Syntax for Original Studies on E-Cigarettes and Smoking Cessation

Search Strategy:
PubMed:
((“e-cigarette” OR “e-cigarettes” OR “electronic cigarette” OR “electronic cigarettes” OR “electronic nicotine delivery” OR “electronic nicotine device” OR “vape” OR “vaping” OR “e-liquid” OR “Electronic Cigarettes” [MeSH]) AND (“Smoking Cessation” [MeSH] OR “smoking cessation” OR cessation or quit or abstinence))
Document Type: Editorial, Comment, Letter Results: 148
Document Type: Case Reports, Classical Article, Clinical Study, Clinical Trial, Comparative Study, Controlled Clinical Trial, Evaluation Studies, Government Publications, Historical Article, Introductory Journal Article, Multicenter Study, Randomized Controlled Trial, Twin Study, Validation Studies, Journal Article Results: 864
Results: 1,012

Scopus:
TITLE-ABS-KEY (“e-cigarette” OR “e-cigarettes” OR “electronic cigarette” OR “electronic cigarettes” OR “electronic nicotine delivery” OR “electronic nicotine device” OR “vape” OR “vaping”) AND TITLE-ABS-KEY (“smoking cessation” OR cessation or quit or abstinence)
Source Type: Journal
Document Type: Note, Letter, Editorial, Erratum: 345
Document Type: Article, Article in Press: 694
Results: 1,039

Web of Science:
TS=(“e-cigarette” OR “e-cigarettes” OR “electronic cigarette” OR “electronic cigarettes” OR “electronic nicotine delivery” OR “electronic nicotine device” OR “vape” OR “vaping”) AND TS=(“smoking cessation” OR cessation or quit or abstinence)
Document Type: Article: 540
Document Type: Editorial Material, Letter, Note: 78
Results: 618

PsycINFO (ProQuest):
(“e-cigarette” OR “e-cigarettes” OR “electronic cigarette” OR “electronic cigarettes” OR “electronic nicotine delivery” OR “electronic nicotine device” OR “vape” OR “vaping” OR “e-liquid” OR SU.EXACT (“Electronic Cigarettes”)) AND (SU.EXACT (“Smoking Cessation”) OR “smoking cessation” OR cessation or quit or abstinence)
Source Type: Journal, Journal Article, Peer-Reviewed Journal: 490
Document Type: Comment/reply, Editorial, Letter: 73
Results: 563

continued

BOX B-6 Continued

MEDLINE (OVID):

Search No.	Search Syntax	Results
1	electronic cigarette/	1,169
2	(e-cigarette or e-cigarettes or electronic cigarette or electronic cigarettes or electronic nicotine delivery or electronic nicotine device or vape or vaping or e-liquid).ti,ab.	1,522
3	or/1–2	1,630
4	smoking cessation/	24,810
5	"smoking cessation".ti,ab.	18,167
6	cessation.ti,ab.	57,497
7	quit.ti,ab.	11,598
8	abstinence.ti,ab.	17,729
9	or/4–8	83,943
10	3 and 9	741
11	limit 10 to (comment or editorial or letter)	123
12	limit 10 to (meta-analysis or "review" or systematic reviews)	118
13	10 not (11 or 12)	503

Results: 626

Embase (Ovid):

Search No.	Search Syntax	Results
1	electronic cigarette/	2,366
2	(e-cigarette or e-cigarettes or electronic cigarette or electronic cigarettes or electronic nicotine delivery or electronic nicotine device or vape or vaping or e-liquid).ti,ab.	2,379
3	or/1–2	2,735
4	smoking cessation/	47,313
5	"smoking cessation".ti,ab.	25,202
6	cessation.ti,ab.	78,749
7	quit.ti,ab.	15,339
8	abstinence.ti,ab.	23,856
9	or/4–8	123,500
10	3 and 9	1,263
11	limit 10 to (editorial or letter or note)	322
12	limit 10 to (meta-analysis or "systematic review")	37
13	10 not (11 or 12)	906

Results: 1,228

Totals:

Total Results: 5,086

After Removing Duplicates: 1,759

BOX B-7
Search Syntax for E-Cigarettes and Combustible Tobacco Cigarette Smoking Reduction

Search Strategy:
Scopus:
TITLE-ABS-KEY ("e-cigarette" OR "e-cigarettes" OR "electronic cigarette" OR "electronic cigarettes" OR "electronic nicotine delivery" OR "electronic nicotine device" OR "vape" OR "vaping") AND TITLE-ABS-KEY ("smoking reduction" OR "harm reduction")
Results: 327

Web of Science:
TS=("e-cigarette" OR "e-cigarettes" OR "electronic cigarette" OR "electronic cigarettes" OR "electronic nicotine delivery" OR "electronic nicotine device" OR "vape" OR "vaping") AND TS=("smoking reduction" OR "harm reduction")
Results: 221

PsycINFO (ProQuest):
("e-cigarette" OR "e-cigarettes" OR "electronic cigarette" OR "electronic cigarettes" OR "electronic nicotine delivery" OR "electronic nicotine device" OR "vape" OR "vaping" OR "e-liquid" OR SU.EXACT ("Electronic Cigarettes")) AND (ti("smoking reduction" OR "harm reduction") OR ab("smoking reduction" OR "harm reduction"))
Results: 75

MEDLINE (Ovid):

Search No.	Search Syntax	Results
1	(e-cigarette or e-cigarettes or electronic cigarette or electronic cigarettes or electronic nicotine delivery or electronic nicotine device or vape or vaping or e-liquid).ti,ab.	1,548
2	Electronic Cigarettes/	1,193
3	1 or 2	1,657
4	3	1,657
5	(smoking adj reduction).ti,ab.	486
6	Harm Reduction/	2,157
7	(harm adj reduction).ti,ab.	2,488
8	or/5–7	4,119
9	4 and 8	156
10	limit 9 to (meta-analysis or "review" or systematic reviews)	26
11	limit 9 to (comment or letter or editorial)	20
12	9 not (10 or 11)	110

Results: 156

continued

BOX B-7 Continued

Embase (Ovid):

Search No.	Search Syntax	Results
1	(e-cigarette or e-cigarettes or electronic cigarette or electronic cigarettes or electronic nicotine delivery or electronic nicotine device or vape or vaping or e-liquid).ti,ab.	2,389
2	Electronic Cigarettes/	1,900
3	1 or 2	2,659
4	3	2,659
5	(smoking adj reduction).ti,ab.	555
6	Harm Reduction/	4,026
7	(harm adj reduction).ti,ab.	3,715
8	or/5–7	6,315
9	4 and 8	280
10	limit 9 to (meta analysis or "systematic review")	9
11	limit 9 to (editorial or erratum or letter or note)	74
12	9 not (10 or 11)	198

Results: 280

PubMed:
("e-cigarette" OR "e-cigarettes" OR "electronic cigarette" OR "electronic cigarettes" OR "electronic nicotine delivery" OR "electronic nicotine device" OR "vape" OR "vaping" OR "e-liquid" OR "Electronic Cigarettes" [MeSH]) AND ("smoking reduction" OR "harm reduction")
Results: 253

Totals:
Total Downloaded: 1,312
Total After Removing Duplicates: 455

did not participate in the study independently reviewed the work, with particular attention to the study design, results, and the interpretation of the results (i.e., conclusions). This section briefly describes these study characteristics; strengths and weaknesses of individual studies are best understood in the context in which they are being used. Thus, considerations for optimal study design and special considerations for different outcomes are discussed in each relevant section in the report text.

Study Design

In general, randomized controlled trials (RCTs) are the gold standard for assessing the effectiveness of an intervention compared with nothing or other interventions. For areas where experimental studies are feasible, but RCTs are not available, the committee considered next-best designs—controlled studies (without randomization). In some cases, RCTs are not feasible because they would be unethical, in which case longitudinal observational designs offer the next strongest evidence. These include prospective cohort studies and crossover trials. For all studies, the committee considered multiple elements pertinent for assessing the studies' internal and external validity. These elements include the study sample, such as sampling methods, basic demographic information (age, gender, and race/ethnicity), as well as study setting. The committee also considered analytical methods, such as statistical tests used, and their appropriateness. Finally, the committee considered the study results (including adjusted and unadjusted results where available), including the outcomes assessed and how these outcomes were operationalized.

Special Considerations for Interventions

As described in Chapter 3, the e-cigarette product and how it is used shape e-cigarette aerosol composition, exposure, and thus health effects. Therefore, when assessing experimental studies, the committee considered the device and e-liquid used, the nicotine concentration, the device settings (e.g., power, temperature, resistance), as well as the puffing protocols used. The committee also considered the comparison or control conditions.

Special Considerations for Observational Studies

Confounding is a challenge inherent in observational studies. Confounders are a third variable related to both an exposure and an outcome and not in the causal pathway. If confounders are distributed unequally across groups (e.g., e-cigarette users and non-users), they can statistically bias the association between the exposure and outcome (i.e., observed effect or study results). Thus, the committee considered confounders and other covariates controlled for in observational studies.

For longitudinal (or cohort) studies, the committee considered follow-up periods and time points assessed. Additionally, loss to follow-up is a challenge in these studies. Because those lost could be systematically different from those who remain in the study, this systematic difference could bias study results. This may be important for the generalizability of findings. Methods exist to account for loss to follow-up. The committee therefore considered the treatment of the study sample lost to follow-up in longitudinal studies.

External Influences

Potential bias in the studies based on sponsorship, particularly by industry, is a concern in the health effects literature on e-cigarettes given the tobacco industry's history of manipulating evidence to support their interests. The committee recognizes that there is a range of non-scientific influences that affect the ways in which investigators design, conduct, analyze, and interpret their data, including but not limited to research sponsorship and source of employment. The committee focused its assessment of the evidence on the quality of the research and the results that were reported, but recognized that financial interests raise concerns to varying degrees with the credibility of the findings. For completeness, the committee documents, in a table available as an online supplement the source of research sponsorship or other external involvement, noting whether each study was funded by industry, government, other (university, foundation), or not stated. The committee also notes other industry involvement, such as if industry is a source of employment. The table can be downloaded at https://www.nap.edu/catalog/24952.

REFERENCES

CRD (Centre for Reviews and Dissemination). 2009. *Systematic reviews: CRD's guidance for undertaking reviews in health care.* https://www.york.ac.uk/crd/SysRev/!SSL!/WebHelp/SysRev3.htm (accessed November 27, 2017).

Higgins, J. P. T., and S. Green, eds. 2011. *Cochrane handbook for systematic reviews of interven¬tions version 5.1.0.* The Cochrane Collaboration. http://www.handbook.-5-1-cochrane.org (accessed November 27, 2017).

IOM (Institute of Medicine). 2008. *Treatment of posttraumatic stress disorder: An assessment of the evidence.* Washington, DC: The National Academies Press.

IOM. 2011a. *Adverse effects of vaccines: Evidence and causality.* Washington, DC: The National Academies Press.

IOM. 2011b. *Finding what works in health care: Standards for systematic reviews.* Washington, DC: The National Academies Press.

IOM. 2016. *Veterans and Agent Orange: Update 2014.* Washington, DC: The National Academies Press.

NASEM (National Academies of Sciences, Engineering, and Medicine). 2017. *The health effects of cannabis and cannabinoids: The current state of evidence and recommendations for research.* Washington, DC: The National Academies Press.

NRC (National Research Council). 2014. *Review of EPA's Integrated Risk Information System (IRIS) process.* Washington, DC: The National Academies Press.

OHAT (National Toxicology Program Office of Health Assessment and Translation). 2015. *Handbook for conducting a literature-based health assessment using OHAT approach for systematic review and evidence integration.* https://ntp.niehs.nih.gov/ntp/ohat/pubs/handbookjan2015_508.pdf (accessed November 27, 2017).

Sena, E. S., G. L. Currie, S. K. McCann, M. R. Macleod, and D. W. Howells. 2014. Systematic reviews and meta-analysis of preclinical studies: Why perform them and how to appraise them critically. *Journal of Cerebral Blood Flow & Metabolism* 34(5):737–742.

Whiting, P., J. Savovic, J. P. Higgins, D. M. Caldwell, B. C. Reeves, B. Shea, P. Davies, J. Kleijnen, R. Churchill, and ROBIS Group. 2016. ROBIS: A new tool to assess risk of bias in systematic reviews was developed. *Journal of Clinical Epidemiology* 69:225–234.

C

Glossary of Terms Related to E-Cigarettes

Term	Definition
advanced personal vaporizer (APV)	Generally used to refer to second- or third-generation e-cigarette devices with regulated variable voltage or variable wattage, APV can also be called a mod.
analog (slang)	Combustible tobacco cigarette.
atomizer	The atomizer is the component in an electronic cigarette that is responsible for heating the e-liquid to the point of aerosolization. The atomizer contains the heating coil and wick. It is most often contained within the metal, glass, or plastic housing called a cartomizer, tank, or clearomizer, which is screwed into the battery.
base liquid	This is the liquid to which nicotine and flavoring are added to create e-juice. The two most common base liquids are glycerol and propylene glycol.

Term	Definition
battery	The battery is used to power an electronic cigarette's atomizer, and is usually a rechargeable lithium ion battery available in a variety of sizes/capacities expressed in mAh, commonly in 600, 900, and 1,100 mAh.
cartomizer	A combined atomizer and cartridge, the cartomizer combines a heating element and a juice delivery system into a single unit. Cartomizers can be made of plastic, metal, or a combination of both. They are disposable and not considered to be refillable, although some users manage to do so. Cartomizers can come in single-coil, dual-coil, or multiple-coil configurations. Having more than one coil produces twice as much aerosol or the same amount twice as fast from the standard. There are top-coil and bottom-coil configurations.
cartridge	The mouthpiece that contains the absorbent filler material soaked with e-liquid. This is a plastic or metal covered part of an e-cigarette, primarily of first-generation devices. A single cartridge contains about 1 ml of e-liquid.
cigalike	An electronic cigarette having a form factor similar to a combustible tobacco cigarette. It is generally considered to be the first generation of e-cigarette products.
clearomizer	A cartomizer that is made of a clear material (usually plastic, Pyrex, or glass) so that the user can see the quantity of e-juice remaining in the unit. Many have milliliter graduations for the capacity of e-liquid left. The common capacity of clearomizers varies from 3 to 6 ml.

Term	Definition
coil/heating coil	A coil is generally a piece of nichrome or kanthal wire that has been wrapped around a wick. Current flows through the coil; the coil gets hot and aerosolizes e-liquid. Cartomizers can come in single-coil, dual-coil, or multiple-coil configurations. Having more than one coil in an atomizer results in increased production of aerosol as compared to single coil.
disposable e-cigarette	The disposable e-cigarette is designed to be used once and usually comes with no charger. It is a single-piece e-cigarette device.
do it yourself (DIY)	Commonly used to refer to preparing and customizing your own e-juice or refillable solution.
dripping	Putting e-juice directly on the atomizer.
dry puff	This refers to the unpleasant taste reported by an e-cigarette user when not enough e-liquid is supplied to an atomizer or cartomizer, resulting in poor aerosol and flavor.
e-cigar	E-cigarette device designed to resembles a traditional tobacco cigar in shape.
e-juice, e-liquid	The liquid that produces the aerosol in an electronic cigarette. E-liquid is aerosolized by the heating element, and generated aerosol is inhaled by the e-cigarette user. Typically contains glycerol, propylene glycol, nicotine, and flavorings.
e-pipe	E-cigarette device designed to resemble a tobacco pipe.
flavoring	The flavorings used in e-liquids, which are usually the same flavorings used in food and drinks. Certain ingredients (particularly sugars and sweeteners) are avoided, however, because of the damage they can do to atomizers.

Term	Definition
mod	Short for modification. This originally referred to modifying a flashlight or a battery to be used in vaping, but is now commonly used to refer to any vaping device of second or third generation that is not a cigalike.
pen style	A style of first-generation e-cigarette device that resembles a pen.
personal vaporizer	The entire e-cigarette device; usually refers to second- and third-generation products.
starter kit	A kit that includes basic e-cigarette equipment, typically a battery, cartomizer, charger, and instruction manual for the user.
sub-ohming	Sub-ohming involves vaping using an atomizer coil with a resistance of $<1\ \Omega$. This increases the overall power output (wattage) of the device allowing more energy to reach the coil which, in turn, heats up faster and reaches a higher temperature so more aerosol is produced.
tank	The part of second- or third-generation e-cigarette that holds the refillable solution. Tank is a common name for a refillable clearomizer and it usually holds more e-liquid than cartridges and it is usually manually refilled with e-liquid by the user.
throat hit	The sensation on the back of the throat that e-cigarette users commonly report after taking a puff on an e-cigarette.
vape/vaping	The act of using an electronic cigarette. The equivalent of "smoking" for combustible tobacco cigarettes.
vaper	Someone who uses an electronic cigarette (a person who vapes).

Term	Definition
vaper's tongue	Used by experienced e-cigarette users to describe the sensation of not being able to taste the flavor in e-liquid when inhaled.
vaporizer	Used by experienced e-cigarette users to refer to their e-cigarette device.
variable voltage/ variable wattage	E-cigarette with variable voltage or variable wattage allows users to control battery output voltage or power of the e-cigarette. Increasing the voltage/ wattage leads to increased coil temperature and, as a result, increased production of aerosol.
wick	Deliver e-liquid to the coil in electronic cigarettes. Most commonly made from silica cord, the wick can also be made from rolled-up steel mesh, ceramic, fiberglass, cotton, or a host of other materials.
wire	Generally refers to resistance wire used in building coils for atomizers.

D

Cytotoxicity Tables

This appendix contains summary tables (Tables D-1, D-2, and D-3) of in vitro studies in which cytotoxicity is assessed.

TABLE D-1 Summary of Exposure, Comparison, and Control Conditions and Cell or Tissue Type Used in In Vitro Studies of E-Cigarettes Assessing Cytotoxicity

Reference	Exposure: Aerosol (A), Extracts (X), E-liquid (L)	Humectant Only as an Exposure	Nicotine Only as an Exposure	Combustible Tobacco Cigarette Smoke as a Control	Compares Flavors	Cell or Tissue Type Used and Comments
Aufderheide and Emura, 2017	A			✓		• Immortalized primary NHBE cell line (CL-1548) • Study used 3D constructs of cells.
Bahl et al., 2012	L	✓	✓		✓	• hESC • mNSC • hPF • Although all are primary cells, consideration must be given to the low capacity of some embryonic cells to metabolize chemicals via Phase I and II enzymes and efflux processes.
Barber et al., 2016	X		✓	✓		• HUVEC
Behar et al., 2014	L	✓	✓		✓	• hPF • hESC • Primary cells (embryonic and adult) tested for aerosol effect using cinnamon Ceylon.

Behar et al., 2016	L and A	✓			✓	• hPF • Human lung epithelial carcinoma cells (A549) • hESC • Combination of primary cell line and embryonic cells to test cinnamonaldehyde cytotoxicity by exposure to aerosols made from refill fluids.
Bharadwaja et al., 2017	L and A					• Stress-specific recombinant bacterial cells: *E. coli*-RecA, *E. coli*-SodA, *E. coli*-CopA, and *E. coli*-DMO1 (as biosensors) • Not a primary or mammalian-derived cell. These bioluminescent *E. coli* strains are engineered to serve as biosensors of DNA strand breaks (*E. coli*-RecA), reactive oxygen species generation (*E. coli*-SodA), presence of heavy metals such as copper (*E. coli*-CopA), and cell membrane damage (*E. coli*-DMO1).
Cervellati et al., 2014	A	✓		✓		• Immortalized human keratinocytes (HaCaT) • Human lung epithelial carcinoma cells (A549)

continued

TABLE D-1 Continued

Reference	Exposure: Aerosol (A), Extracts (X), E-liquid (L)	Humectant Only as an Exposure	Nicotine Only as an Exposure	Combustible Tobacco Cigarette Smoke as a Control	Compares Flavors	Cell or Tissue Type Used and Comments
Farsalinos et al., 2013	A	✓	✓	✓	✓	• Monolayer-cultured cardiomyoblast cells (H9c2) • Reason provided for cell selection is the better culture stability and reproducibility than human cardiomyocytes.
Husari et al., 2016	X			✓		• Human lung epithelial carcinoma cells (A549)
Leigh et al., 2016	A	✓	✓	✓	✓	• Human lung mucoepidermoid cells (NCI-H292 cell line)
Lerner et al., 2015	A	✓	✓	✓	✓	• Human bronchial airway epithelial cells (H292) • HFL1
Lerner et al., 2016	A					• HFL1
Misra et al., 2014	X		✓	✓		• Human lung epithelial carcinoma cells (A549)
Neilson et al., 2015	A			✓		• EpiAirway™: a human 3D airway tissue model • Fully differentiated in vitro reconstructs of primary human tracheobronchial epithelium. Cultures express mucus-producing

					goblet cells, ciliated cells with actively beating cilia, basal cells, and club cells (Clara). However, cells were obtained from a single donor and therefore may not be representative of responses from a heterogeneous population (e.g., polymorphisms, ethnicities, sex-related factors).
Romagna et al., 2013	L		✓	✓	• Mouse BALB/3T3 fibroblasts
Sancilio et al., 2016	L	✓			• HGF • Cells were obtained from healthy gingival tissue taken from adult subjects during surgical dental extractions. However, fibroblasts are considered to be mesenchymal stem cells because of their self-renewing and multipotent character.
Sancilio et al., 2017	L	✓			• HGF
Scheffler et al., 2015a	A	✓	✓		• Primary NHBE cells • Human lung epithelial carcinoma cells (A549) • Immortalized primary NHBE cell line (CL-1548)

continued

TABLE D-1 Continued

Reference	Exposure: Aerosol (A), Extracts (X), E-liquid (L)	Humectant Only as an Exposure	Nicotine Only as an Exposure	Combustible Tobacco Cigarette Smoke as a Control	Compares Flavors	Cell or Tissue Type Used and Comments
Scheffler et al., 2015b	A	✓	✓	✓		• Primary NHBE cells • Primary cells came from two donors (cells named NHBE48 and NHBE33). Responses and endpoints vary depending on the origin (donor) of the cells. In some instances, changes and differences are quite significant.
Welz et al., 2016	L				✓	• Spheroidal cultures of oropharyngeal mucosa • Freshly isolated specimens were cut 1 mm^3 mucosal cubes. Cultures became spheroidal in shape and recoated with interacting endogenous epithelium. In vitro system used in this study is much closer to actual in vivo situation than other in vitro systems tested for e-liquid toxicity.
Willershausen et al., 2014	L	✓	✓		✓	• Clonetics® HPdLF • Fibroblasts are considered to be mesenchymal stem cells because of their self-renewing and multipotent character.

Wu et al., 2014	L	✓		• Normal hTBE cells from young, healthy, non-smoking organ donors
Yu et al., 2016	X	✓		• Spontaneously transformed immortal keratinocyte (HaCaT) • HNSCC cell lines: HN30 and UMSCC10B • The HN30 and UMSCC10B cell lines were originally derived from the oropharynx; HN30 was derived from primary laryngeal tumor and UMSCC10B was derived from metastatic lymph node.

NOTE: hESC = human embryonic stem cell; HFL1 = human fetal lung fibroblast; HGF = human gingival fibroblast; HNSCC = head and neck squamous cell carcinoma; HPdLF = human periodontal ligament fibroblast; hPF = human pulmonary fibroblast; hTBE = human tracheobronchial epithelial; HUVEC = human umbilical vein endothelial cell; mNSC = mouse neural stem cell; NHBE = normal human bronchial epithelial.

TABLE D-2 Summary of Test Agents, Cell or Tissue Type Used, and Assays Employed in In Vitro Studies of E-Cigarettes Assessing Cytotoxicity

Reference	Test Agent(s)	Cell or Tissue Type Used	Dose and Time Course	Assay Employed
Aufderheide and Emura, 2017	• Mainstream combustible tobacco cigarette smoke from reference 3R4F cigarettes (University of Kentucky) • E-liquid aerosol (Tennessee cured flavor, no nicotine, Johnsons Creek, Hartland, WI)	• Immortalized primary NHBE cell line CL-1548	• Samples taken after 0, 4, 6, and 8 smoke/aerosol exposure repetitions and analyzed microscopically after histopathological preparation of the cultures.	• Histopathology
Bahl et al., 2012	• 35 different flavors	• hESC • mNSC • hPF	• 6 concentrations: 0.001%, 0.01%, 0.03%, 0.1%, 0.3%, and 1% • Incubation at 37°C, 5% CO_2, and 95% relative humidity for 48 hours	• MTT assay
Barber et al., 2016	• Combustible tobacco cigarette smoke extracts from Marlboro 100 cigarettes (16 mg tar, 1.2 mg/ml nicotine, Philip Morris)	• HUVECs	• 48-hour exposure to the extracts	• Endothelial cell viability, density and metabolic activity after exposure to mainstream and sidestream tobacco smoke extracts, e-aerosol extracts, and pure nicotine

	• E-cigarette aerosol extract from NJoy OneJoy device, traditional flavor with 1.2% (12 mg/ml) or 1.8% (18 mg/ml) nicotine and eGo (OKC Vapes), desert sands flavor with 0, 12, or 18 mg/ml nicotine			• Activation/deposition of complement proteins onto endothelial cells was quantified as a means to monitor the progression of innate immune responses
Behar et al., 2014	• 10 cinnamon-flavored e-cigarette refill liquids from online vendors; various concentrations of nicotine, cinnamon flavoring, and percentages of PG and/or glycerol • Cinnamaldehyde and 2-MOCA	• hPF • hESC	• 48 hours	• MTT assay

continued

TABLE D-2 Continued

Reference	Test Agent(s)	Cell or Tissue Type Used	Dose and Time Course	Assay Employed
Behar et al., 2016	• 39 e-cigarette refill fluids purchased from online vendors • Laboratory-made refill fluids • Aerosols produced from the refill fluids (produced with unused cartomizer or tank using smoking machine) • Cinnamon Ceylon aerosol produced from cartomizer-style e-cigarette	• hPF • Human lung epithelial carcinoma cells (A549) • hESC	• The Vea cartomizer device and unfilled cartomizers (Johnson Creek, Hartland, Wisconsin) operated at 2.9 V, 2.1 Ω, and 4 W. An Innokin iTaste MVP 3.0 battery with variable voltage and wattage and Innokin iClear 16D bottom dual-coil clearomizers (tanks) were operated at 3 V, 2.1 Ω, and 4.2 W or at 5 V, 2.1 Ω, and 11.9 W. 2 ml of fluid for each sample. Puff duration was 4.3 seconds. • Time course varied by assay and cell type.	• GC/MS • MTT assay • Nuclei stained with DAPI • Live cell imaging assay • Alkaline comet assay
Bharadwaja et al., 2017	• E-cigarette liquid (NJOY brand containing glycerol, PG, 10 mg/ml nicotine, flavoring chemicals)	• Stress-specific recombinant bacterial cells: *E. coli*-RecA, *E. coli*-SodA, *E. coli*-CopA, and *E. coli*-DMO1 (as biosensors)	• Cells were exposed to various concentrations of e-liquid and soluble e-liquid aerosol.	• UV-Vis spectroscopy • Bioluminescence assay • DNA fragmentation assay

	• Soluble e-liquid aerosol produced from the e-cigarette liquid			
Cervellati et al., 2014	• E-cigarette aerosol (e-cigarette Mini Touch T-Fumo T-TEX with e-liquid in balsamic flavors with or without nicotine, Cloudsmoke, Terna Trade) • E-cigarette aerosol with humectants only (no additives such as flavors or nicotine). • Combustible tobacco cigarette smoke (United Kingdom research cigarette, 12 mg tar, 1.1 mg nicotine)	• Immortalized human keratinocytes (HaCaT) • Human lung epithelial carcinoma cells (A549)	• HaCaT cells were exposed to fresh combustible tobacco cigarette smoke in an exposure system that generated smoke by burning one UK research cigarette, and to e-cigarette mixtures using a vacuum pump to draw air through the cigarette and leading the smoke stream over the cell cultures for 50 minutes.	• Ultrastructural morphology • Trypan Blue exclusion test • LDH assay • Pro-inflammatory cytokines were measured in culture medium by the Bio-Plex cytokine assay kit

continued

TABLE D-2 Continued

Reference	Test Agent(s)	Cell or Tissue Type Used	Dose and Time Course	Assay Employed
Farsalinos et al., 2013	• Combustible tobacco cigarette with 0.8 mg nicotine, 10 mg tar, and 10 mg carbon monoxide yields (Marlboro, Philip Morris Italia S.r.l., Rome, Italy) • 20 commercially available e-liquids (17 tobacco flavored, 3 sweet or fruit flavored), with 6–24 mg/ml nicotine, manufactured or distributed by 5 different companies	• Monolayer-cultured cardiomyoblast cells (H9c2)	• Two sets of experiments were performed; one using regular voltage and a second using higher voltage, for e-cigarette aerosol production. • The medium was aspirated and replaced by medium containing the combustible tobacco smoke and e-cigarette liquid extracts in one undiluted (100%) and 4 diluted samples (50%, 25%, 12.5%, and 6.25%). For the e-cigarette extract, 100% e-cigarette extract is equal to an aerosol extract concentration of 1%.	• MTT assay

Husari et al., 2016	• E-cigarette aerosol was generated using pre-filled V4L CoolCart cartomizer cartridges (strawberry flavor, 3.5 Ω, 18 mg/ml labeled nicotine) and 4.2-V battery (Vapor Titan Soft Touch) • Reference 3R4F combustible tobacco cigarettes (University of Kentucky, 9.4 mg tar, 0.726 mg nicotine per cigarette)	• Human lung epithelial carcinoma cells (A549)	• Exposure to e-cigarette aerosol or combustible tobacco cigarette smoke extract was initiated 24 hours post-seeding by diluting smoke extract in complete media to the desired final concentration (e.g., 0.5, 1, 2, 4, 8 mg/ml). Images were taken 24 hours post-treatment.	• Trypan blue exclusion assay

continued

TABLE D-2 Continued

Reference	Test Agent(s)	Cell or Tissue Type Used	Dose and Time Course	Assay Employed
Leigh et al., 2016	• 6 types of commercially available e-cigarettes (purchased from gas stations, convenience stores, online retailers, and local vape shops in Buffalo, New York, Daly City, California, and online) • eGo tank system (Vision Spinner) e-cigarette device with battery output voltage fixed at 3.3 V and refill solutions in tobacco, piña colada, menthol, coffee, and strawberry flavors (purchased from a local vape shop in Buffalo, New York) • Reference 3R4F combustible tobacco cigarettes (University of Kentucky)	• Human lung mucoepidermoid cells (NCI-H292 cell line)	• Air–liquid interface (ALI) exposure • Health Canada Intense method, using the following conditions: 3-second puff duration, every 30 seconds, with a 55-ml puff volume, implemented continuously for 30 minutes, and resulting in a total of 55 puffs. • Air exposures (control) generated using smoking machines were run during each experiment. • Reference 3R4F combustible tobacco cigarettes (comparison) were smoked using the same method as for the e-cigarette products.	• Neutral red uptake assay • Trypan blue assay • Cytokine release was measured as an indicator of cell inflammatory response

- 5 nicotine concentrations were examined: 0, 6, 12, 18, and 24 mg/ml.
- To study effects of humectants, H292 cells were exposed at the ALI to aerosols generated from the e-GO device filled with unflavored liquids containing the same nicotine concentration of 24 mg/ml in (1) PG-only; (2) glycerol-only; or (3) a 50/50 mixture of PG/glycerol.
- Three battery output voltage settings were tested: 3.3, 4.0, and 4.8 V.

continued

TABLE D-2 Continued

Reference	Test Agent(s)	Cell or Tissue Type Used	Dose and Time Course	Assay Employed
Lerner et al., 2015	• Refillable pen-style e-cigarette device (eGo Vision Spinner, China) and compatible clearomizer chamber (Anyvape, China) with 2.2-Ω heating element • blu e-cigarettes (classic tobacco flavor containing 16 mg nicotine) • CSE from a research-grade combustible tobacco cigarette	• Human bronchial airway epithelial cells (H292) • HFL1	• H292: blu e-cigarette aerosol using a CSM-SSM machine (CH-Technologies Inc.) was drawn into the chamber every 30 seconds with a 4-second pulse for different time durations of 5, 10, and 15 minutes. • HFL1 was treated with the following e-liquids: PG, glycerol, Vape Dudes (classic tobacco with or without nicotine), Vape Dudes (cinnamon roll without nicotine), Vape Dudes (grape vape without nicotine), Ecto (American tobacco with or without nicotine) and other e-liquids for 24 hours and then examined for morphological changes by phase-contrast microscopy.	• HFL1: Violet B 405-nm laser and 440/40 bandpass filter to detect increases in cellular fluorescence • FlowJo V.10 for data compilation

Lerner et al., 2016	• blu classic tobacco e-cigarette with 16 mg nicotine (Lorillard, Greensboro, NC)	• HFL1	• E-cigarette puffs were regulated with 4-second puffs every 30 seconds for various sessions (5, 10, 15, or 20 minutes).	• Mitochondria superoxide staining • Mitochondria membrane potential staining • DNA fragmentation assay • IL-8 and IL-6 cytokine secretion
Misra et al., 2014	• blu e-cigarettes containing glycerol-based e-liquids, with and without nicotine and two market flavors (classic tobacco and magnificent menthol) • Reference 3R4F, 1R5F, and Marlboro gold combustible tobacco cigarettes	• Human lung epithelial carcinoma cells (A549)	• 0–20 mg/ml	• Neutral red uptake • IL-8 release

continued

TABLE D-2 Continued

Reference	Test Agent(s)	Cell or Tissue Type Used	Dose and Time Course	Assay Employed
Neilson et al., 2015	• NJOY bold (4.5% labeled nicotine) and NJOY menthol (3.0% labeled nicotine) • Reference 3R4F combustible tobacco cigarettes	• EpiAirway™: a human 3D airway tissue model	• A VITROCELL VC 01 Smoking Robot (VC1/110613) and a 12/6 CF stainless-steel exposure module (VITROCELL Systems GmbH) • Reference 3R4F cigarettes were smoked to the ISO smoking regime: 8 puffs/cigarette. E-cigarettes were puffed for 30 minutes, equating to 60 puffs at an independent intense puffing regime, defined as an 80-ml puff drawn over 3 seconds with 30-second intervals.	• MTT assay • Integrity of the airway epithelium tight junctions was measured by TEER8 conducted according to the MatTek Corporation's standard protocol.
Romagna et al., 2013	• Combustible tobacco cigarette smoke extract • 21 different e-cigarette liquids. Composition of e-liquids was (w/w) 46.17% PG USP,	• Mouse BALB/3T3 fibroblasts	• E-cigarette aerosol and combustible tobacco cigarette smoke extracts simulating e-cigarette use added to culture medium. 100%, 50%, 25%, 12.5%, 6.25%,	• MTT assay

	glycerol USP, 8.11% water, 0.8% nicotine USP, and < 0.5% flavorings		3.12% for 24 hours at 37°C	
Sancilio et al., 2016	• Two different cartridge solutions (nicotine content [w/v] 0 and 24 mg/ml) from Halo Company (Pompton Plains, NJ, USA) containing PG, glycerol, and natural and artificial flavorings (concentrations not provided by the manufacturer), diluted from 4.8 to 48 times	• HGF	• HGFs treated with pre-warmed fluids with or without nicotine. Cell medium was replaced every 24 hours. In the vaped samples, 1.5 ml of the cartridge solution was put in the cartomizer, warmed for 1 minute before the dilution and then harvested with a syringe from the cartomizer to a vial.	• MTT assay • Apoptosis • Increase in green fluorescence for reactive oxygen species production • Bax expression (pro-apoptotic protein)

continued

TABLE D-2 Continued

Reference	Test Agent(s)	Cell or Tissue Type Used	Dose and Time Course	Assay Employed
Sancilio et al., 2017	• Two different cartridge solutions (nicotine content [w/v] 0 and 24 mg/ml) containing PG, glycerol, and natural and artificial flavorings (concentrations not provided by the manufacturer), diluted 24 times with DMEM	• HGF	• HGFs treated with 1 mg/ml nicotine (obtained by diluting 24 times the 24 mg/ml nicotine-containing fluid), warmed and not warmed before administration • HGFs treated with the fluid without nicotine diluted 24 times, warmed and not warmed before administration • HGFs also left untreated	• TEM • LDH assay • Lysosome compartment analysis • Human collagen type I concentration in supernatants was assayed using an ELISA • Western blot for LC3 expression in HGF
Scheffler et al., 2015a	• Reevo Mini-S e-cigarette (In-Smoke, Winnenden, Germany) with a 3.3-V/900-mAh battery and 2.2-Ω resistance with e-liquids purchased from Johnsons Creek (Hartland, WI, USA) in Tennessee cured flavor (75% PG USP, 25%	• Primary NHBE cells • Human lung epithelial carcinoma cells (A549) • Immortalized primary NHBE cell line (CL-1548)	• The e-cigarette was connected to the piston pump of a smoking robot and 200 puffs were taken with a puff volume of 35 ml, puff duration of 2 seconds, blow-out time of 7 seconds, and an interpuff interval of 10 seconds.	• ROS-Glo™ H_2O_2 Assay (Promega, Madison, WI, USA) for oxidative stress • CellTiter-Blue® Assay (Promega, Madison, WI, USA) for cell viability

glycerol USP, 0.0% and 2.4% nicotine USP). Other ingredients listed on the bottle include deionized water, natural flavors, artificial flavor, and USP-grade citric acid (as a preservative).
- Reference 3R4F combustible tobacco cigarettes (Kentucky) with a standard cellulose acetate filter tip

- For combustible tobacco cigarette smoke exposure, 10 K3R4F cigarettes were each puffed by the smoking robot using the same parameters as described for the e-cigarette.

continued

TABLE D-2 Continued

Reference	Test Agent(s)	Cell or Tissue Type Used	Dose and Time Course	Assay Employed
Scheffler et al., 2015b	• Aerosols from two e-cigarette liquids purchased from Johnsons Creek (Hartland, WI, USA) in Tennessee cured flavor (0% and 2.4% nicotine). Liquids contained USP-grade PG, USP-grade glycerol, deionized water, natural and artificial flavors, USP-grade nicotine, and USP-grade citric acid. • Aerosols from humectants (glycerol and PG) obtained from Alfa Aesar (Karlsruhe, Germany), with a purity of 99.5%. • Combustible tobacco cigarette smoke from 10 reference K3R4F combustible tobacco cigarettes (Lexington, Kentucky) with a standard cellulose acetate filter tip.	• Primary NHBE cells	• The e-cigarette was connected to the piston pump of a smoking robot and 200 puffs were taken with a puff volume of 35 ml, puff duration of 2 seconds, blow-out time of 7 seconds. • For combustible tobacco cigarette smoke exposure, 10 K3R4F cigarettes were smoked by the smoking robot using the same parameters as described for the e-cigarette. Each cigarette was puffed 6 times. • Cultures were analyzed 24 hours after exposure.	• ROS-Glo™ H_2O_2 Assay (Promega, Madison, WI, USA) for oxidative stress • CellTiter-Blue® Assay (Promega, Madison, WI, USA) for cell viability

Welz et al., 2016	• E-liquids in three flavors (apple, cherry, and tobacco) with a base mixture of 80% PG, 10% glycerol, and 10% water and 12 mg/ml nicotine	• Spheroidal cultures of oropharyngeal mucosa	• 24-hour one-time incubation • 2.5-hour incubation on 5 sequential days	• MTT assay
Willershausen et al., 2014	• E-liquids (eSmokerShop, GmbH, Hannover, Germany) in hazelnut, lime, and menthol flavors with 20–22 mg/ml nicotine in a PG-base	• Clonetics® HPdLF	• Up to 96-hour incubation depending on assay	• PrestoBlue Cell Viability Assay • ATP detection • Cell visualization • Migration assay
Wu et al., 2014	• Tobacco-flavored e-liquid at various concentrations (0, 0.01, 0.1, 0.3% v/v) without nicotine or with 18 mg/ml of nicotine (InnoVapor LLC., Boise, ID)	• Normal hTBE cells from young, healthy, non-smoking organ donors	• 24- and 48-hour exposures. The final nicotine concentrations were within the serum nicotine range of e-cigarette users.	• Pro-inflammatory cytokines • HRV-16 infection in e-liquid-–exposed normal hTBE cells • LDH • IL-6 levels by ELISA • Taqman quantitative real-time RT-PCR to detect HRV RNA and human SPLUNC1 mRNA

continued

TABLE D-2 Continued

Reference	Test Agent(s)	Cell or Tissue Type Used	Dose and Time Course	Assay Employed
Yu et al., 2016	• V2 (red American tobacco flavor) and VaporFi (classic tobacco flavor) e-cigarette brands in a 70% PG/30% glycerol base with 0.0% and 1.2% nicotine	• Spontaneously transformed immortal keratinocyte (HaCaT) • HNSCC cell lines: HN30 and UMSCC10B	• HaCaT cells were treated for 8 weeks with 1% v/v extract • UMSCC10B and HN30 were each treated for 1 week with 1% v/v extract. • HaCaT cells were treated for 10 days at 0.5%, 1.0%, and 2.0% v/v aerosolized e-cigarette liquid. • HaCaT cells were treated for 10 days, and UMSCC10B and HN30 for 12 days prior to colony counting.	• Neutral comet assay • γ-H2AX immunostaining • Cell cycle changes by flow cytometry • Trypan Blue staining • Clonogenic survival • Annexin V apoptotic assay

NOTE: 2-MOCA = 2-methoxycinnamaldehyde; CSE = cigarette smoke extract; DAPI = 4′,6-diamidino-2-phenylindole; GC/MS = gas chromatography/mass spectrometry; hESC = human embryonic stem cell; HFL1 = human fetal lung fibroblast; HGF = human gingival fibroblast; HNSCC = head and neck squamous cell carcinoma; HPdLF = human periodontal ligament fibroblast; hPF = human pulmonary fibroblast; HRV = human rhinovirus; hTBE = human tracheobronchial epithelial; HUVEC = human umbilical vein endothelial cell; LDH = lactate dehydrogenase; mNSC = mouse neural stem cell; MTT = 3-(4,5-dimethylthiazol-2-yl)-2,5-diphenyltetrazolium bromide; NHBE = normal human bronchial epithelial; PG = propylene glycol; TEM = transmission electron microscopy.

TABLE D-3 Summary of Results from In Vitro Studies of E-Cigarettes Assessing Cytotoxicity

Reference	Results and Observations
Aufderheide and Emura, 2017	Cultures exposed to both mainstream combustible tobacco cigarette smoke and e-liquid aerosol showed a clear reduction in mucus production and cilia bearing, but the effect was weaker for the aerosol than for the smoke.
Bahl et al., 2012	The MTT assay showed effects of refill solutions on cell survival that ranged from no evidence of cytotoxicity to high levels of toxicity. Cinnamon Ceylon had the strongest effects and was the only sample that was cytotoxic for all three cell types. Fifteen refill samples were moderately cytotoxic to hESC, and in general, mNSC responded similarly to these samples. In general, hESC were more sensitive than hPF, but Freedom Smoke menthol arctic and Global Smoke caramel produced stronger cytotoxic effects on hPF than on the other two cells. The humectants (PG and glycerol) were non-cytotoxic for all cell types. Five butterscotch- or caramel-flavored samples were also non-cytotoxic at the highest dose tested. The relevance of exposure to refill liquid (as compared with aerosols) in cytotoxicity studies is a concern.
Barber et al., 2016	Most of the exposure conditions resulted in significant effects on cell density. There was also a slight reduction in viability, independent of nicotine concentration or the exact formulation of the extract. Authors observed a significant decrease in metabolic activity for cells that were exposed to combustible tobacco cigarette smoke or e-cigarette aerosol extracts, independent of the formulation of the extract. Exposure to pure nicotine did not alter endothelial cell metabolic activity. Results showed significant increase in the deposition of C1q and C5b-9, and in C3b to a lesser extent. There were no changes in C4d.
Behar et al., 2014	The study established NOAELs of 0.03% for hESC and 0.01% for hPF; hESC was more sensitive than hPF. Of 4 chemical additives tested, CAD and 2-MOCA were the most cytotoxic, producing similar IC_{50} for both hESC and hPF cells. By contrast, dipropylene glycol and vanillin were the least cytotoxic, and their IC_{50} were higher than a user would likely experience.

continued

TABLE D-3 Continued

Reference	Results and Observations
Behar et al., 2016	In the 48-hour MTT assay, hESC (embryonic stem cells) were more sensitive to cinnamon Ceylon and cinnamaldehyde aerosols than hPF and A549 (respiratory) cells. By contrast, hESC tolerated short-term exposure to cinnamaldehyde for a longer time (8 hours) than hPF (2 hours). Cytoskeletal structure disruption (e.g., depolymerization of actin microfilaments and microtubules) was observed for both hESC and hPF exposed to cinnamaldehyde at MTT NOAEL and IC_{50} concentrations.
Bharadwaja et al., 2017	Following exposure to e-liquids and e-cigarette aerosol at various concentrations, bioluminescent recombinant bacterial cells (as biosensors) showed dose-dependent and stress-specific responses. Interestingly, cells exposed to e-liquid showed greater inhibition of bioluminescence at high concentrations, which declined dose-dependently with dilutions, whereas cells exposed to e-cigarette aerosols showed the opposite effect, with bioluminescence increasing in a dose-dependent manner with exposure to decreasing concentrations of e-cigarette aerosol. These changes in bioluminescence expression indicate potential cellular damage, such as DNA damage, oxidative stress, ion homeostasis, and membrane damage. Both e-liquid and aerosol exposure resulted in cellular damage, but e-cigarette aerosol exposure showed damage without significant growth inhibition. Results of the DNA fragmentation assay showed considerable DNA breaks at high doses of e-liquid exposure, compared with lower doses (which showed partial DNA fragmentation) and controls.

TABLE D-3 Continued

Reference	Results and Observations
Cervellati et al., 2014	Exposure to e-cigarette aerosol with humectants only (no flavorings or nicotine) resulted in no change in either cell viability or LDH release over 24 hours. Exposure to e-cigarette aerosol with flavoring caused significant progressive loss of viability and increased LDH release in both cell types. E-cigarette aerosol with both flavoring and nicotine caused rapid (50 minutes) and marked loss in viability and enhanced LDH release. This is similar to effects of combustible tobacco cigarette smoke exposure, which caused an early (6 hours) and progressive decrease in cell viability and increased LDH release. The authors observed a similar trend during the different time points in both cell lines, but keratinocytes appeared more susceptible to combustible tobacco cigarette smoke–induced toxicity after 24 hours. The morphology of the cells exposed to combustible tobacco cigarette smoke shows clear signs of cellular damage and presence of vacuoles. By contrast, cells treated with e-cigarette aerosol with humectants only (no flavors or nicotine), remained intact with the same ultrastructural aspect of control cells, even 24 hours after treatment. In cells exposed to e-cigarette with flavors, an increase in vacuolization and alteration of cytoplasmic membrane was observed. The degeneration of intracellular organelles was more pronounced after exposure to e-cigarette aerosols with flavors and nicotine, especially in HaCaT cells, which showed a marked vacuolization consequent to the expansion of the mitochondria and the endoplasmic reticulum. Results suggest that e-liquid and/or aerosol components contain some pro-inflammatory stimuli leading to a change in the secretome pattern depending on the cells lines employed. Fluctuations in cytokine release after other e-cigarette and combustible tobacco cigarette smoke exposures were also observed, but interpreting these effects was possible due to subsequent cell death.

continued

TABLE D-3 Continued

Reference	Results and Observations
Farsalinos et al., 2013	Of 20 samples tested, 4 samples exhibited a cytotoxic effect in the 3.7-V experiments: Cinnamon cookies flavor was slightly cytotoxic at the highest extract concentration, while both samples of El Toro cigarillos and El Toro puros were cytotoxic at both 100% and 50% extract concentrations. The range of myocardial cell survival for all e-cigarette samples at 3.7 V was 89.7%–112.1% at 6.25%, 90.6%–115.3% at 12.5%, 81.0%–106.6% at 25%, 7.4%–106.8% at 50%, and 2.2%–110.8% at 100% extract concentration. The "base" sample was not cytotoxic at any extract concentration. Combustible tobacco cigarette smoke extract was significantly cytotoxic at concentrations above 6.25%, with viability rates being 76.9 ± 2.0% at 6.25%, 38.2 ± 0.6% at 12.5%, 3.082 ± 0.2% at 25%, 5.2 ± 0.8% at 50%, and 3.9 ± 0.2% at 100% extract concentration. The absolute mean difference in viability between 3.7-V and 4.5-V experiments was 7.1 ± 4.1% at 6.25%, 5.0 ± 5.3% at 12.5%, 4.2 ± 4.8% at 25%, 5.0 ± 3.8% at 50%, and 17.0 ± 12.2% at 100% extract concentration. Only the difference at 6.25% extract concentration was statistically significant ($p = 0.039$). None of the 4 samples was considered cytotoxic. IC_{50} could be determined only for combustible tobacco cigarette smoke extract and for El Toro cigarrillos and El Toro puros, since for every other e-cigarette sample, viability was higher than 50% at all extract concentrations. The lowest NOAEL and IC_{50} were observed in combustible tobacco cigarette smoke extract.
Husari et al., 2016	Combustible tobacco cigarette smoke total particulate matter extract at concentrations of 2 mg/ml and higher attenuated cellular growth and triggered cell death. Similar effects only occurred from exposure to e-cigarette total particulate matter extract at concentrations of 64 mg/ml.

TABLE D-3 Continued

Reference	Results and Observations
Leigh et al., 2016	Effects of e-cigarette aerosols on toxicity to bronchial epithelial cells differed significantly. Flavors have a significant and differential effect on toxicity: e-cigarette aerosols with menthol, coffee, and strawberry flavors significantly reduced cell viability and metabolic activity compared to air controls. E-cigarette aerosols with coffee and strawberry flavors also significantly increased cytokine levels compared to both air controls and reference combustible tobacco cigarettes.
	No significant differences ($p < 0.05$) in metabolic activity and cell viability were observed between the e-cigarette aerosols with various nicotine concentrations and the air control, or among the varying nicotine concentrations when compared against each other. However, significant differences ($p < 0.05$) were found between the various nicotine concentrations and combustible tobacco cigarette smoke. Of note, metabolic activity of exposed cells was measured by neutral red uptake assay, but the definition of this endpoint is not clear because neutral red assay is a quantitative estimation of the number of viable cells in culture.
	With respect to cytokine release, compared with air controls, exposure to aerosol with 18 mg/ml nicotine resulted in significant decreases in IL-1β, CXCL1, and CXCL2, while exposure to aerosol with 24 mg/ml nicotine resulted in significantly increased IL-6. IL-1β and CXCL2 levels were also significantly decreased between 18 mg/ml nicotine aerosol and the reference combustible tobacco cigarette. Significant differences were observed among aerosols with variable nicotine concentrations for IL-1β, IL-6, CXCL1, and CXCL2.
	Exposure of H292 cells to e-cigarette humectant-only aerosols significantly decreased cell viability ($p < 0.05$) compared to air controls, but toxic effects were significantly less than from exposure to combustible tobacco cigarette smoke. Effects of humectant aerosols on cell metabolic activity differed significantly, decreasing significantly in cells exposed to PG/glycerol and glycerol-only aerosols, but not to PG-only compared with air controls. With respect to cytokine release, all tested cytokines increased significantly except CXCL1 and CXCL10 in cells exposed to PG-only compared with air controls.
	Aerosol from the 4.0-V and 4.8-V devices significantly decreased ($p < 0.05$) metabolic activity and cell viability compared with the air control. Aerosol generated with the 3.3-V device was not different than air and significantly less toxic than combustible tobacco cigarette smoke ($p < 0.05$). Aerosol generated with the device at the highest (4.8-V) setting significantly increased all tested cytokines compared with air controls.

continued

TABLE D-3 Continued

Reference	Results and Observations
Lerner et al., 2015	Fibroblasts cultured with e-liquid or combustible tobacco CSE exhibited a reduction in the number of cells per count area. Many of the treated cells were enlarged and vacuolarized, and this effect was greater in CSE-treated cells and cells treated with 5% e-liquids. Compared to control cells, e-liquid and CSE-treated cells showed morphological changes—enlarged cells and spindle formation. Morphological changes were similar in cells exposed to e-liquid without nicotine added to cells at 1% concentration and 1% PG. In contrast, fibroblasts cultured in 1% e-liquid with nicotine resulted in morphological changes that resemble cells treated with 1% CSE. Lung fibroblast viability following treatments with 2.5% PG, glycerol, or commercial e-liquids was not significantly different than control after 24 hours (% viability in means ± SD; control: 90.53 ± 5.34, PG: 88.40 ± 2.99, glycerol: 91.97 ± 6.23, Ecto American tobacco flavor 0 mg nicotine: 92.7 ± 2.55, Ecto American tobacco flavor 24 mg nicotine: 78.57 ± 6.67, $p > 0.05$). Exposure to humectants only (PG, glycerol) elicited no significant increase in release of IL-8 compared with the control group (15.9 ± 12.02 pg/ml) after 24-hour treatment. Of the four commercially available e-liquids, only cinnamon roll-flavored e-liquid stimulated a significant increase in IL-8 secretion (458.14 ± 26.20 pg/ml). IL-8 and IL-6 secretion at 16 hours post-exposure was significantly higher for cells exposed to e-cigarette aerosols than air controls for each exposure time period. The release of IL-6 into culture media was dose dependent. IL-6 secretion was significantly higher after 10-minute exposure than 5-minute exposure. The IL-8 levels were all significantly increased in cells exposed to e-cigarette aerosol compared with the air controls. In cells exposed to e-cigarette aerosols, small but significant increases in fluorescence were observed.

TABLE D-3 Continued

Reference	Results and Observations
Lerner et al., 2016	Results showed a small but significant reduction in the amount of mtROS present after 20 minutes of aerosol exposure compared to 10- or 15-minute exposures.
	The level of ARE-inducible Nqo1 expression increased for the 10- and 20-minute exposure sessions. Similarly, 10 minutes of exposure of HFL-1 to e-cigarette aerosol increased average Nqo1 levels when total cellular proteins were collected 18 hours following the exposures.
	After 24 hours, the level of mtROS in cells treated with the copper metal nanoparticles increased significantly.
	E-cigarette aerosol-exposed cells exhibited Complex IV sensitivity as observed by decreased levels of COX-2 (MTCO2) subunit in cell lysates collected 18 hours after aerosol exposure. A reduced level of Complex I NDUFB8 subunit in addition to reduced COX-2 was observed in cell lysates harvested 90 minutes after exposure.
	5-minute aerosol exposure did not produce any difference in DNA fragmentation, whereas, 10- and 15-minute exposures resulted in significant increases in DNA fragmentation compared to air control groups. However, as the exposure duration increased, the likelihood for DNA damage increased in the air control group as well.
	10-minute aerosol exposure resulted in increased IL-6 secretion (45.70 pg/ml) at 18 hours post-e-cigarette exposure, compared with IL-6 levels (7.34 pg/ml) from the air control group. IL-8 levels (28.02 pg/ml) also increased compared with the air control group (16.42 pg/ml).
Misra et al., 2014	No cytotoxicity was observed for any of the e-liquids tested up to their respective highest sample doses.
	E-liquid exposure resulted in greater IL-8 release at high doses (6.9–13.8 mg/ml). Any IL-8 release from blu MM e-liquid treatments that were significant when compared with IL-8 release from exposure to combustible tobacco cigarettes occurred at doses approximately 42-fold higher than the combustible tobacco cigarettes.

continued

TABLE D-3 Continued

Reference	Results and Observations
Neilson et al., 2015	Tissue cell viability following combustible tobacco cigarette smoke exposure was reduced in a time- and dose-dependent manner from 100% to 12% viability after 6 hours of exposure, relative to untreated controls. Exposure of EpiAirway™ tissue to either variety of e-cigarette did not reduce tissue viability relative to untreated control tissues. Thus, an ET50 for e-cigarette aerosol could not be calculated. No statistical difference in viability was seen between NJOY bold or NJOY menthol and diluting air controls. A dose-dependent decrease in cell viability was seen following incremental hourly exposures to cigarette smoke for up to 6 hours, resulting in reductions of around 90% at the highest dose. By contrast, the two e-cigarettes did not cause cytotoxic effects under any of the test conditions, despite a much larger puff volume and exposure frequency in the e-cigarette machine smoking regime.
Romagna et al., 2013	From the 21 samples examined, only the coffee-flavored e-liquid exhibited a cytotoxic effect, and this only at the highest extract concentration. For this sample, the viability rate was 114.5 ± 2.0% at 3.125%, 112.2 ± 3.6% at 6.25%, 101.5 ± 3.1% at 12.5%, 92.0 ± 8.9% at 25%, 85.9 ± 11.8% at 50%, and 51.0 ± 2.6% at 100% extract concentration. Combustible tobacco cigarette smoke extract exhibited significant cytotoxicity at extract concentrations greater than 12.5%. For the majority of e-liquids (13 of 21), viability was not statistically different between extract concentrations. Thus, NOAEL for these samples was defined as 100% concentration. None of the 12 tobacco-flavored e-cigarette liquids tested were associated with a statistically significant difference in fibroblast viability.

TABLE D-3 Continued

Reference	Results and Observations
Sancilio et al., 2016	E-liquid exposure resulted in reduced metabolic activity in a time- and dose-dependent manner in HGFs. For e-liquids both with and without nicotine at 5 mg/ml and 2 mg/ml concentrations, the metabolic activity was reduced up to 20% of the control. There were no significant changes in apoptosis in the treated HGFs compared with untreated cells. After 48 hours, cell viability decreased in all the experimental conditions (about 60% versus about 85% in the controls), with a higher range in the 1-N sample (35.85% of viable cells). The reactive oxygen species production showed a peak after 24 hours of treatment compared with untreated controls (771.6 [nicotine], 798.6 [warmed nicotine], 458.9 [no nicotine], and 687.6 [warmed, no nicotine] versus 200 [untreated]). In the nicotine-free fluid-treated HGFs, the ROS production was lower than in the other experimental conditions. However, effects were seen after 48 hours (540.7 nicotine-free versus 271.1 untreated), whereas the other samples showed no significant changes compared with the control after 48 hours. Bax protein expression did not appear to be affected after 6 hours of exposure, but after 24 hours, it was higher in the e-liquid–exposed conditions than in the control sample (1.485-fold increase [nicotine], 1.605-fold increase [warmed nicotine], 1.490-fold increase [no nicotine], and 1.405-fold increase [warmed no nicotine] on the untreated samples). After 48 hours, Bax expression in the nicotine, warmed nicotine, and nicotine-free conditions remained higher than in the untreated HGFs (1.735-, 1.695-, and 1.385-fold increase on the untreated samples, respectively) while in the warmed e-liquid without nicotine, the increase was close to onefold.
Sancilio et al., 2017	E-liquids with nicotine exerted cytotoxicity as demonstrated by the increased levels of LDH, in parallel to the presence of numerous vacuoles in the cytoplasm, as well as a decrease in collagen I production and an augmented LC3 II expression. Autophagic vesicles and an increased number of pro-collagen I molecules were present in the cytoplasm of fibroblasts exposed to nicotine-free fluids. In the same samples, the time-dependent activation of the lysosomal compartment with no changes in LC3 expression was detected.

continued

TABLE D-3 Continued

Reference	Results and Observations
Scheffler et al., 2015a	Primary NHBE48 cells were the most sensitive, responding to e-liquid aerosol exposure with a decrease in viability up to 60% and 52% compared to clean air-exposed cells. In comparison, combustible tobacco cigarette mainstream smoke–exposed cells showed only 7% viability of clean air–exposed cells. Immortalized CL-1548 cells are less sensitive to e-liquid aerosol (75% and 70% viability) and combustible tobacco cigarette smoke exposure (10% viability) compared to primary NHBE48 cells, but are still significantly more sensitive than A549 cells (88% viability for e-liquid aerosol, 21% for mainstream smoke exposure). In all cell types, no significant differences were seen after exposure to nicotine-containing and nicotine-free aerosol. The oxidative stress level is elevated in CL-1548 cells compared to A549 cells, but lower than those of primary NHBE48 cells.
Scheffler et al., 2015b	The authors found toxicological effects of e-cigarette aerosol and the humectant-only substances, whereas the nicotine concentration did not have an effect on cell viability. The viability of combustible tobacco cigarette mainstream smoke–exposed cells was 4.5–8 times lower and the oxidative stress levels 4.5–5 times higher than those of e-cigarette aerosol–exposed cells, depending on the donor.
Welz et al., 2016	Both fruit- and tobacco-flavored extracts were cytotoxic to oropharyngeal tissue, but fruit-flavored liquids showed a higher toxicity than tobacco-flavored ones. Additionally, incubation of mucosal tissue cultures with fruit-flavored extracts showed DNA fragmentation, but no serious DNA damage was seen in tissue cultures incubated in tobacco-flavored extracts.

TABLE D-3 Continued

Reference	Results and Observations
Willershausen et al., 2014	Starting at 24 hours, the highest reduction in the proliferation was observed for the treatment with menthol-flavored liquids, which was the only statistically significant reduction as compared to control cells. After an incubation time of 48 hours with the menthol-flavored liquid, the difference in comparison both to the control cells and the nicotine-treated cells was highly statistically significant ($p < 0.001$). Hazelnut flavor or lime flavor only caused a slight not statistically significant reduction of the proliferation rates at 48 hours. After 96 hours of incubation this strong growth-reducing effect of the menthol-flavored liquids persisted and was still statistically significant. In comparison to the untreated cells, incubation with hazelnut-flavored ($p < 0.024$), lime-flavored ($p < 0.009$), or menthol-flavored liquids ($p < 0.001$) led to a statistically significant reduction of ATP detection. The untreated human periodontal ligament fibroblasts and those incubated for 24 hours with PG showed good proliferation. Those incubated with nicotine-, hazelnut-, or lime-flavored liquids showed a slight growth reduction, while incubation with the menthol-flavored liquid produced a strong growth inhibition. The inhibitory effect of menthol flavor exposure on the fibroblast cells was especially noticeable in the migration assay. Only the menthol-flavored liquid caused a highly statistically significant reduction ($p < 0.001$) of cell migration after 72 hours in comparison to the control cells as well as to the cells treated with nicotine.
Wu et al., 2014	Within the physiological nicotine range, e-liquid exposure did not cause noticeable cytotoxicity at either 24 or 48 hours. Exposure to e-liquid without nicotine increased IL-6 protein levels in a dose-dependent manner at both 24 and 48 hours. Addition of nicotine to e-liquid only marginally enhanced the IL-6 levels. Cells exposed to tobacco-flavored e-liquid (without or with nicotine) had higher levels of HRV load than unexposed cells at both 6 and 24 hours. Compared with e-liquid without nicotine, the addition of nicotine into e-liquid either did not alter (at 6 hours) or slightly increased (at 24 hours, $p = 0.05$) HRV load. HRV infection significantly increased IL-6 production at both 6 and 24 hours in cells that were pre-exposed to the control (medium alone) or e-liquid with and without nicotine.

TABLE D-3 Continued

Reference	Results and Observations
Yu et al., 2016	E-cigarette exposure without nicotine induced a 10-fold increase in cell death, while e-cigarette exposure with nicotine induced a 10-fold increase compared with controls.
	UMSCC10B showed a statistically significant increased accumulation of arrest in G1, and HN30 showed an increase in G2, both independently of e-cigarette nicotine content.
	A stepwise decrease in colony count and decreased survival was observed with increasing e-cigarette doses in both brands, independently of nicotine content. After exposure to 0.5% v/v nicotine-free e-cigarette aerosol, greater than a twofold decrease in survival was seen in all cell lines.

NOTE: 2-MOCA = 2-methoxycinnamaldehyde; CSE = cigarette smoke extract; hESC = human embryonic stem cell; HFL1 = human fetal lung fibroblast; HGF = human gingival fibroblast; HNSCC = head and neck squamous cell carcinoma; HPdLF = human periodontal ligament fibroblast; hPF = human pulmonary fibroblast; HRV = human rhinovirus; hTBE = human tracheobronchial epithelial; HUVEC = human umbilical vein endothelial cell; LDH = lactate dehydrogenase; mNSC = mouse neural stem cell; MTT = 3-(4,5-dimethylthiazol-2-yl)-2,5-diphenyltetrazolium bromide; NHBE = normal human bronchial epithelial; NOAEL = no observed adverse effect level; PG = propylene glycol.

REFERENCES

Aufderheide, M., and M. Emura. 2017. Phenotypical changes in a differentiating immortalized bronchial epithelial cell line after exposure to mainstream cigarette smoke and e-cigarette vapor. *Experimental and Toxicologic Pathology* 69(6):393–401.

Bahl, V., S. Lin, N. Xu, B. Davis, Y. H. Wang, and P. Talbot. 2012. Comparison of electronic cigarette refill fluid cytotoxicity using embryonic and adult models. *Reproductive Toxicology* 34(4):529–537.

Barber, K. E., B. Ghebrehiwet, W. Yin, and D. A. Rubenstein. 2016. Endothelial cell inflammatory reactions are altered in the presence of e-cigarette extracts of variable nicotine. *Cellular and Molecular Bioengineering* 10(1):124–133.

Behar, R. Z., B. Davis, Y. Wang, V. Bahl, S. Lin, and P. Talbot. 2014. Identification of toxicants in cinnamon-flavored electronic cigarette refill fluids. *Toxicology in Vitro* 28(2):198–208.

Behar, R. Z., W. T. Luo, S. C. Lin, Y. H. Wang, J. Valle, J. F. Pankow, and P. Talbot. 2016. Distribution, quantification and toxicity of cinnamaldehyde in electronic cigarette refill fluids and aerosols. *Tobacco Control* 25(Supplement 2):ii94–ii102. http://tobaccocontrol.bmj.com/content/25/Suppl_2/ii94 (accessed February 5, 2018).

Bharadwaj, S., R. J. Mitchell, A. Qureshi, and J. H. Niazi. 2017. Toxicity evaluation of e-juice and its soluble aerosols generated by electronic cigarettes using recombinant bioluminescent bacteria responsive to specific cellular damages. *Biosensors and Bioelectronics* 90:53–60.

Cervellati, F., X. M. Muresan, C. Sticozzi, R. Gambari, G. Montagner, H. J. Forman, C. Torricelli, E. Maioli, and G. Valacchi. 2014. Comparative effects between electronic and cigarette smoke in human keratinocytes and epithelial lung cells. *Toxicology in Vitro* 28(5):999–1005.

Farsalinos, K. E., G. Romagna, E. Allifranchini, E. Ripamonti, E. Bocchietto, S. Todeschi, D. Tsiapras, S. Kyrzopoulos, and V. Voudris. 2013. Comparison of the cytotoxic potential of cigarette smoke and electronic cigarette vapour extract on cultured myocardial cells. *International Journal of Environmental Research and Public Health* 10(10):5146–5162.

Husari, A., A. Shihadeh, S. Talih, Y. Hashem, M. El Sabban, and G. Zaatari. 2016. Acute exposure to electronic and combustible cigarette aerosols: Effects in an animal model and in human alveolar cells. *Nicotine & Tobacco Research* 18(5):613–619.

Leigh, N. J., R. I. Lawton, P. A. Hershberger, and M. L. Goniewicz. 2016. Flavourings significantly affect inhalation toxicity of aerosol generated from electronic nicotine delivery systems (ENDS). *Tobacco Control* 25(Supplement 2):ii81–ii87. http://tobaccocontrol.bmj.com/content/25/Suppl_2/ii81 (accessed February 5, 2018).

Lerner, C. A., I. K. Sundar, H. Yao, J. Gerloff, D. J. Ossip, S. McIntosh, R. Robinson, and I. Rahman. 2015. Vapors produced by electronic cigarettes and e-juices with flavorings induce toxicity, oxidative stress, and inflammatory response in lung epithelial cells and in mouse lung. *PLoS ONE* 10(2):e0116732. https://doi.org/10.1371/journal.pone.0116732 (accessed February 5, 2018).

Lerner, C. A., P. Rutagarama, T. Ahmad, I. K. Sundar, A. Elder, and I. Rahman. 2016. Electronic cigarette aerosols and copper nanoparticles induce mitochondrial stress and promote DNA fragmentation in lung fibroblasts. *Biochemical and Biophysical Research Communications* 477(4):620–625.

Misra, M., R. D. Leverette, B. T. Cooper, M. B. Bennett, and S. E. Brown. 2014. Comparative in vitro toxicity profile of electronic and tobacco cigarettes, smokeless tobacco and nicotine replacement therapy products: E-liquids, extracts and collected aerosols. *International Journal of Environmental Research & Public Health* 11(11):11325–11347.

Neilson, L., C. Mankus, D. Thorne, G. Jackson, J. DeBay, and C. Meredith. 2015. Development of an in vitro cytotoxicity model for aerosol exposure using 3D reconstructed human airway tissue; application for assessment of e-cigarette aerosol. *Toxicology in Vitro* 29(7):1952–1962.

Romagna, G., E. Allifranchini, E. Bocchietto, S. Todeschi, M. Esposito, and K. E. Farsalinos. 2013. Cytotoxicity evaluation of electronic cigarette vapor extract on cultured mammalian fibroblasts (ClearStream–LIFE): Comparison with tobacco cigarette smoke extract. *Inhalation Toxicology* 25(6):354–361.

Sancilio, S., M. Gallorini, A. Cataldi, and V. di Giacomo. 2016. Cytotoxicity and apoptosis induction by e-cigarette fluids in human gingival fibroblasts. *Clinical Oral Investigations* 20(3):477–483.

Sancilio, S., M. Gallorini, A. Cataldi, L. Sancillo, R. A. Rana, and V. di Giacomo. 2017. Modifications in human oral fibroblast ultrastructure, collagen production and lysosomal compartment in response to e-cigarette fluids. *Journal of Periodontology* 88(7):673–680.

Scheffler, S., H. Dieken, O. Krischenowski, and M. Aufderheide. 2015a. Cytotoxic evaluation of e-liquid aerosol using different lung-derived cell models. *International Journal of Environmental Research and Public Health* 12(10):12466–12474.

Scheffler, S., H. Dieken, O. Krischenowski, C. Forster, D. Branscheid, and M. Aufderheide. 2015b. Evaluation of e-cigarette liquid vapor and mainstream cigarette smoke after direct exposure of primary human bronchial epithelial cells. *International Journal of Environmental Research and Public Health* 12(4):3915–3925.

Welz, C., M. Canis, S. Schwenk-Zieger, S. Becker, V. Stucke, F. Ihler, and P. Baumeister. 2016. Cytotoxic and genotoxic effects of electronic cigarette liquids on human mucosal tissue cultures of the oropharynx. *Journal of Environmental Pathology, Toxicology and Oncology* 35(4):343–354.

Willershausen, I., T. Wolf, V. Weyer, R. Sader, S. Ghanaati, and B. Willershausen. 2014. Influence of e-smoking liquids on human periodontal ligament fibroblasts. *Head & Face Medicine* 10:39. https://doi.org/10.1186/1746-160X-10-39 (accessed February 5, 2018).

Wu, Q., D. Jiang, M. Minor, and H. W. Chu. 2014. Electronic cigarette liquid increases inflammation and virus infection in primary human airway epithelial cells. *PLoS ONE* 9(9):e108342. https://doi.org/10.1371/journal.pone.0108342 (accessed February 5, 2018).

Yu, V., M. Rahimy, A. Korrapati, Y. Xuan, A. E. Zou, A. R. Krishnan, T. Tsui, J. A. Aguilera, S. Advani, L. E. Crotty Alexander, K. T. Brumund, J. Wang-Rodriguez, and W. M. Ongkeko. 2016. Electronic cigarettes induce DNA strand breaks and cell death independently of nicotine in cell lines. *Oral Oncology* 52:58–65.

E

Public Meeting Agenda

Committee on the Review of the Health Effects
of Electronic Nicotine Delivery Systems

An Information-Gathering Workshop
National Academy of Sciences Building
Room 120
2101 Constitution Avenue, NW
Washington, DC 20418

AGENDA

Tuesday, February 21, 2017

8:45 AM Welcome and Opening Remarks
David Eaton, Committee Chair

Understanding Vaping: Who, What, and Why

9:00 User and Retailer Perspective
Spike Babaian, VapeNY

9:20 Insights from Qualitative Research
Jennifer Alexander, RTI

9:40 Patterns of Use and Disparities
Daniel Giovenco, Mailman School of Public Health, Columbia University

10:00 Role of Flavorings in Sensory Perceptions of ENDS
Paul Wise, Monell Center

10:20 Panel Discussion and Q&A

10:45 Break

Systematic Reviews: Methodology and Lessons Learned

11:00 Integrating In Vitro and In Vivo Data
Jon Samet, University of Southern California (via WebEx)

11:20 Human Health Effects
Allison Glasser and Ray Niaura, Truth Initiative

11:40 Discussion and Q&A

12:00 PM Lunch Available in Cafeteria (lower level)

Preclinical and Clinical Testing of ENDS

1:00 AEMSA Standards
Lou Ritter, American E-Liquid Manufacturing Standards Association

1:15 Key Variables Important in Assessing ENDS Devices
John Bellinger, Evolv Inc.

1:35 Key Variables Important in Assessing E-Liquids
Kurt Kistler, The Pennsylvania State University, Brandywine

1:55 Clinical Studies in ENDS Users
James Murphy, British American Tobacco

2:15 Particle Deposition
Kirsten Koehler, Johns Hopkins Bloomberg School of Public Health

2:35 In Vitro Models Available for Testing of ENDS
Holger Behrsing, Institute for In Vitro Sciences, Inc.

2:55 Results from In Vitro Assays
Marianna Gaça, British American Tobacco

3:15 Panel Discussion and Q&A

3:45 Break

Use of Population Dynamic Models to Understand the Population Health Effects of ENDS: Data Gaps and Uncertainties

4:00 Population Dynamic Modeling
Eric Vugrin, Sandia National Labs

4:20 Panel Discussion
Annette Bachand, Environ
Rafael Meza, University of Michigan
David Levy, Georgetown University

5:00 Public Comment

5:15 Adjourn

Wednesday, February 22, 2017

Human Studies of ENDS Exposure

9:30 AM Virtual Session: Functional Changes in Airway Resistance and Inflammatory Cytokine Profiles After Human ENDS Exposures
Pam Dalton, Monell Center (via WebEx)

10:00 Closed Session Resumes

F

Committee Biosketches

David L. Eaton, Ph.D. (*Chair*), is the dean and vice provost of the Graduate School at the University of Washington and professor of environmental and occupational health sciences and of public health genetics. Dr. Eaton's research has focused on the metabolism of drugs and environmental carcinogens. He is interested in determining how useful animal toxicity testing data are to predicting human response, as well as understanding how individuals may differ in their susceptibility to cancer-causing chemicals. He served as president of the Society of Toxicology, as vice president of the Toxicology Education Foundation, and on the Board of Trustees of the Academy of Toxicological Sciences, of which he is an Elected Fellow. He previously served on seven committees convened by the National Academies of Sciences, Engineering, and Medicine on a variety of environmental health topics. Dr. Eaton received his Ph.D. in pharmacology from the University of Kansas Medical Center. He is an elected member of the National Academy of Medicine.

Anthony J. Alberg, Ph.D., M.P.H., is a professor and the chair of the Department of Epidemiology and Biostatistics, Arnold School of Public Health, University of South Carolina. He was previously the Blatt Ness Endowed Chair in Oncology, professor of Public Health Sciences, and the associate director of Population Sciences of the Hollings Cancer Center at the Medical University of South Carolina. Dr. Alberg is an epidemiologist whose research focuses on non-melanoma skin cancer, cigarette smoking, health effects of secondhand smoke, etiology of tobacco-associated malignancies, and tobacco prevention and control. He currently serves on the Cancer Screening and Prevention Editorial Board of the National Cancer Institute's Physician Data Query, as the chair-elect of the Cancer Prevention Committee of the American Society of Clinical Oncology and has served as editor for the Epidemiology Section of the American College of Chest Physician's Lung Cancer Guidelines II and III, associate editor of the *American Journal of Epidemiology*, and has been a contributing author to two Surgeon General's reports on the health consequences of smoking. In South Carolina, he is a member of the state's Cancer Control Advisory Committee (CCAC) and is chair of the CCAC's Cancer Surveillance Committee. He has previously served on the National Academies committee addressing the health implications of raising the minimum age for purchasing tobacco products. Dr. Alberg received his M.P.H. from the Yale University School of Medicine and his Ph.D. from the Johns Hopkins Bloomberg School of Public Health.

Maciej Goniewicz, Ph.D., is an associate professor of oncology at the Department of Health Behavior, Roswell Park Comprehensive Cancer Center in Buffalo, New York. Dr. Goniewicz's primary research area is in nicotine pharmacology, with a focus on nicotine dependence and smoking cessation. He has research experience in smoking cessation behavioral treatment, pharmacotherapy, and pharmacokinetics in both clinical and community-based settings. His current research is focused on new nicotine-containing products and alternative forms of tobacco. These studies include the laboratory evaluation of the products, pharmacological and toxicological assessment, surveys among their users, and their potential application in harm reduction and smoking cessation. Dr. Goniewicz received his Pharm.D. and Ph.D. in toxicology and pharmacology from the Medical University of Silesia, Poland.

Adam Leventhal, Ph.D., is a professor of preventive medicine and psychology at the University of Southern California. Dr. Leventhal is a clinical psychologist who conducts longitudinal cohort research, laboratory studies, and clinical trials. Major foci of his work include adolescent and young adult substance use, comorbidity between psychiatric disorders and addiction, e-cigarette use and tobacco regulatory science, addiction psychopharmacology and genetics, and addiction among populations subject to health disparities (e.g., African Americans, women). He directs the University of Southern California Health, Emotion, & Addiction Laboratory, a multidisciplinary team of scholars, staff, and students that supports scientific and educational activities in the health promotion and disease prevention field. Dr. Leventhal received his M.A. in psychology and Ph.D. in clinical psychology from the University of Houston.

José E. Manautou, Ph.D., is a professor of pharmacology and toxicology and interim chair of the Department of Pharmaceutical Sciences at the University of Connecticut School of Pharmacy. Dr. Manautou's research interests include target organ toxicity, hepatic detoxification and disposition mechanisms, and hepatotoxicants and interference affecting susceptibility to chemical injury. He is a former councilor of the Society of Toxicology and of the society's Mechanisms Specialty Section. He previously served on a committee of the National Academies addressing health risks of trichloroethylene. Dr. Manautou received his Ph.D. in pharmacology and toxicology from the Purdue University School of Pharmacy.

Sharon McGrath-Morrow, M.D., M.B.A., is a professor in the Department of Pediatrics at the Johns Hopkins University School of Medicine with a joint appointment in the Department of Environmental Health Sciences at the Bloomberg School of Public Health. Dr. McGrath-Morrow is also the Johns Hopkins Pediatric Pulmonary Fellowship Director, a fellow of the American Academy of Pediatrics, and a member of the American Academy of Pediatric Tobacco Consortium. She is a pediatric pulmonologist and clinician scientist who runs a translational laboratory modeling neonatal lung injury. Her research interests include understanding the neonatal immune response to acute lung injury, respiratory outcomes in preterm infants with chronic lung disease, and the impact of secondhand and thirdhand smoke on postnatal lung growth and adult lung function. Dr. McGrath-Morrow received her M.D. from the University of Virginia.

David Mendez, Ph.D., is an associate professor in the Department of Health Management and Policy at the University of Michigan School of Public Health. His research focuses on the application of mathematical/computational models for public health policy, particularly in the field of tobacco control. He has conducted research on the impact of tobacco control policies on smoking prevalence and health outcomes. He has also been involved in research to evaluate policies regarding residential radon and the uptake of the human papillomavirus vaccine. He is currently engaged in a study to evaluate the impact of peer pressure on smoking uptake among teenagers using systems dynamics and agent-based models. He served on a prior committee of the National Academies assessing agent-based modeling in tobacco control. Dr. Mendez received his M.S. in applied statistics, M.S. in operations research/systems science, and Ph.D. in management science from Michigan State University.

Richard Miech, Ph.D., is a research professor at the Survey Research Center, Institute for Social Research, University of Michigan. Previously, Dr. Miech had been a professor and department chair in the Department of Health and Behavioral Sciences at the University of Colorado Denver. His work focuses on trends in substance use, with an emphasis on disentangling how these trends vary by age, historical period, and birth cohort membership. His research interests also include the causes and consequences of substance use over the life course. Dr. Miech received his M.A. and Ph.D. in sociology from the University of North Carolina at Chapel Hill and an M.P.H. from Johns Hopkins University.

Ana Navas-Acien, M.D., is a professor of environmental health sciences at Columbia University Mailman School of Public Health. Dr. Navas-Acien's research investigates the long-term health effects of widespread environmental exposures (arsenic and other metals, tobacco smoke, air pollution), their interactions with genetic and epigenetic variants, and effective interventions for reducing involuntary environmental exposures. For more than 10 years, she has been working on environment-related research in population-based cohort studies such as the Strong Heart Study, a study of cardiovascular disease and its risk factors in American Indian communities, and the Multi-Ethnic Study of Atherosclerosis, a study of cardiovascular, metabolic, and lung disease in urban settings across the United States. She has served on National Academies committees addressing inorganic arsenic and the scientific capabilities of the Environmental Protection Agency. Dr. Navas-Acien received her M.D. from the University of Granada, M.P.H. from the National School of Health, Madrid, Spain, and Ph.D. from Johns Hopkins University.

Kent E. Pinkerton, Ph.D., is a professor in the Department of Pediatrics in the School of Medicine and the Department of Anatomy, Physiology, and Cell Biology in the School of Veterinary Medicine at the University of California, Davis. Dr. Pinkerton also serves as director of the university's Center for Health and the Environment. Dr. Pinkerton's research interests focus on the health effects of environmental air pollutants on lung structure and function, the interaction of gases and airborne particles within specific sites and cell populations of the lungs in acute and chronic lung injury, and the effects of environmental tobacco smoke on lung growth and development. Prior to 2008, he received research support from Phillip Morris and has collaborated with other researchers who received research support from Phillip Morris. He previously served on committees of the National Academies related to estimating mortality risk reduction from decreasing tropospheric ozone exposure, formaldehyde risk assessment, and particulate matter surveillance. Dr. Pinkerton received his Ph.D. in pathology from Duke University.

Nancy A. Rigotti, M.D., is a professor of medicine at Harvard Medical School and associate chief of the Division of General Internal Medicine at Massachusetts General Hospital. Dr. Rigotti has pioneered research on interventions to reduce smoking prevalence and the burden of tobacco-related morbidity and mortality. A general internist, her clinical research focuses on developing and disseminating interventions for smoking cessation within primary care practices and inpatient settings. She founded and directs the Massachusetts General Hospital Tobacco Research and Treatment Center. She is a past president of the Society of General Internal Medicine and a past president of the Society for Research in Nicotine and Tobacco. She was a scientific editor of the 1989 Surgeon General's report on tobacco, a comprehensive review that provided scientific support for policy making and she was a deputy editor of *Nicotine & Tobacco Research*. Dr. Rigotti received her M.D. from Harvard Medical School.

David A. Savitz, Ph.D., is a professor of epidemiology in the Brown University School of Public Health, with a joint appointment in obstetrics and gynecology and pediatrics in the Alpert Medical School. His epidemiological research has addressed a wide range of many important public health issues including environmental hazards in the workplace and community, reproductive health outcomes, and environmental influences on cancer. He has done extensive work on health effects of nonionizing radiation, pesticides, drinking water treatment by-products, and perfluorinated compounds. He was the president of the Society for Epidemiologic Research and the Society for Pediatric and Perinatal Epidemiologic Research and North American Regional Councilor for the International Epidemiological Association. He was compensated by Best Practice Management Inc. through an unrestricted grant from Star Scientific to chair a panel discussion and author a 2006 summary paper on the public health implications of smokeless tobacco use as a harm reduction strategy. Dr. Savitz received his master's degree in preventive medicine from The Ohio State University and Ph.D. in epidemiology from the University of Pittsburgh Graduate School of Public Health. He is an elected member of the National Academy of Medicine.

Gideon St.Helen, Ph.D., is an assistant professor of medicine, Division of Clinical Pharmacology, Department of Medicine, at the University of California, San Francisco. The focus of his research program is the utility and evaluation of biological markers of tobacco use and exposure for epidemiology, risk assessment, product regulation, and identification of susceptibility factors for tobacco-related diseases. His ongoing research on the clinical pharmacology of e-cigarettes includes studies on nicotine pharmacokinetics, cardiovascular and subjective effects of e-cigarette use, patterns of use, and influence of e-cigarette device characteristics such as flavors on the clinical pharmacology and safety of e-cigarettes. Dr. St.Helen received his Ph.D. in toxicology from the University of Georgia.